MAYO CLINIC
DIET MANUAL

Sixth Edition

A Handbook of Dietary Practices

MAYO CLINIC
DIET
MANUAL

Sixth Edition

A Handbook of Dietary Practices

Cecilia M. Pemberton, R.D.
Karen E. Moxness, M.S., R.D.
Mary J. German, M.S., R.D.
Jennifer K. Nelson, M.S., R.D.
Clifford F. Gastineau, M.D., Ph.D.

By the Dietetic Staffs of
Mayo Clinic, Rochester Methodist Hospital and Saint Marys Hospital

1988
B.C. Decker Inc • Toronto • Philadelphia

Publisher

B.C. Decker Inc
3228 South Service Road
Burlington, Ontario   L7N 3H8

B.C. Decker Inc
320 Walnut Street
Suite 400
Philadelphia, Pennsylvania   19106

Sales and Distribution

United States and Possessions	**The C.V. Mosby Company** 11830 Westline Industrial Drive Saint Louis, Missouri 63146
Canada	**The C.V. Mosby Company, Ltd.** 5240 Finch Avenue East, Unit No. 1 Scarborough, Ontario M1S 4P2
United Kingdom, Europe and the Middle East	**Blackwell Scientific Publications, Ltd.** Osney Mead, Oxford OX2 OEL, England
Australia	**Harcourt Brace Jovanovich** 30–52 Smidmore Street Marrickville, N.S.W. 2204 Australia
Japan	**Igaku-Shoin Ltd.** Tokyo International P.O. Box 5063 1-28-36 Hongo, Bunkyo-ku, Tokyo 113, Japan
Asia	**Info-med Ltd.** 802-3 Ruttonjee House 11 Duddell Street Central Hong Kong
South Africa	**Libriger Book Distributors** Warehouse Number 8 "Die Ou Looiery" Tannery Road Hamilton, Bloemfontein 9300
South America (non-stock list representative only)	**Inter-Book Marketing Services** Rua das Palmeriras, 32 Apto. 701 222-70 Rio de Janeiro RJ, Brazil

Mayo Clinic Diet Manual

ISBN 1-55664-032-3

Library of Congress catalog card number: 87–72382

10 9 8 7 6 5 4 3 2 1

CONTRIBUTORS

Mary Ames, R.D.

Myocardial Infarction
Urolithiasis–Calcium, Oxalate, and
Purine Restriction
Acid-Ash and Alkaline-Ash Diets

Constance Bayne, M.S., R.D.

Chronic Renal Failure (Adult)
Hemodialysis (Adult)
Continuous Ambulatory Peritoneal
Dialysis (Adult)
Continuous Cyclic Peritoneal
Dialysis (Adult)
Chronic Renal Failure (Pediatric)
Hemodialysis (Pediatric)
Continuous Ambulatory Peritoneal
Dialysis (Pediatric)
Food Exchange List for Protein,
Sodium, and Potassium Control
Common Foods High in Phosphorous
Potassium Control

Sandra A. Bjerkness, R.D.

Diet and Cancer Protection
Food Allergy and Intolerance
Penicillin and Mold-Controlled Diet
Low Salicylate and Tartrazine-Free Diet
Yeast-Controlled Diet
Nickel Restriction
Sulfite Restriction
Monosodium Glutamate Intolerance

Jenny Buccicone, M.S., R.D.

Hypertension
Approximate Sodium Content of
Selected Foods

Ann Cronin, R.D.

Cancer

Sara R. DiCecco, M.S., R.D.

Esophageal Reflux
High Fiber Diet
Restricted Fiber Diet
Low Residue Diet
Liver Transplant
Low Bacteria Diet

Janet C. Finkelson, M.S., R.D.

Congestive Heart Failure
Myocardial Infarction
Hyperlipidemia

Molly Freeman, R.D.

General Hospital Diet
Clear Liquid Diet
Full Liquid Diet
Pureed Diet
Mechanical Soft Diet
Soft Diet
Transitional Feeding Progression
Preoperative Diet
Postoperative Diet

Joan Gartner, R.D.

Gluten Sensitivity: Celiac Sprue
and Dermatitis Herpetiformis
Lactose Intolerance

Clifford F. Gastineau, M.D., Ph.D.

Hypoglycemia

Mary Jane German, M.S., R.D.

Nutritional Assessment
Geriatric Nutrition
Jewish Dietary Practices

Beth Gillio, M.S., R.D.

Hepatic Encephalopathy

Jeanne Grant, R.D., C.D.E.

Nutritional Assessment
Diabetes Mellitus (Adult)
Food Exchange List for Diabetes

Kelley Green, R.D.

Nutritional Assessment

Karen Harelson-Meyer, M.S., R.D.

Nutritional Assessment

Diane M. Huse, M.S., R.D.

Anorexia Nervosa and Bulimia
Allergy (Pediatric)
Gluten Sensitive Enteropathy: Celiac
    Disease (Pediatric)
Constipation and Encopresis
Cystic Fibrosis
Diabetes Mellitus (Pediatric)
Hyperlipidemia and Hypertension
    (Pediatric)
Inflammatory Bowel Disease (Pediatric)
Ketogenic Diet
Weight Control (Pediatric)
Fat Absorption Test Diet (Pediatric)

Virginia Hiatt, R.Ph.

Parenteral Nutrition Support of Adults

Michael Jensen, M.D.

Obesity

Rita Jones, R.D., C.D.E.

Diabetes Mellitus (Adult)
Food Exchange List for Diabetes

Janet M. Kaehler, R.D.

Geriatric Nutrition

Ann Klause, R.D.

Osteoporosis
Pregnancy and Lactation

Marty Kochevar, R.Ph.

Parenteral Nutrition Support of
    Adults

Mary Kopriva, R.D.

Diarrhea

A. R. Lucas, M.D.

Anorexia Nervosa and Bulimia

Kathy Mack, R.D.

Acute Renal Failure

Deb Marcella, R.D.

Diabetes Mellitus (Adult)
Food Exchange List for Diabetes

Dennis McCallum, Pharm.D.

Parenteral Nutrition Support of Adults

Peggy A. Menzel, R.D.

Congestive Heart Failure
Hyperlipidemia
Vegetarian Diet

Zachary J. Meyer, R.D.

Diabetes Mellitus (Adult)
Food Exchange List for Diabetes

Karen L. Montgomery, R.D.

Peptic Ulcer Disease
Renal Transplant (Adult)
Nephrotic Syndrome (Adult)
Food Exchange List for Protein, Sodium,
    and Potassium Control
Common Foods High in Phosphorous
Potassium Control

Jean Mortensen, R.D., C.D.E.

Diabetes Mellitus (Adult)
Food Exchange List for Diabetes

Karen E. Moxness, M.S., R.D.

Dysphagia
Constipation and Encopresis
Enteral Nutrition Support (Pediatrics)
Nutritional Assessment

Jennifer K. Nelson, M.S., R.D.

Fat Malabsorption
Medium Chain Triglycerides
Inflammatory Bowel Disease (Adult)
Nutritional Assessment
Enteral Nutrition Support of Adults
Appendix 13, Enteral Nutrition Formulas
Breath Hydrogen Concentration
Appendices (Adult)

Lavonne Oenning, R.D.

Copper Metabolism
Copper Content of Foods

Diane Olson, R.D., C.D.E.

Burn
Cancer (Pediatric)
Inborn Errors of Metabolism
Glycogen Storage Diseases
Maple Syrup Urine Disease
Nutritional Therapy for
Phenylketonuria

F. Karen Olson, R.D.

Geriatric Nutrition

Cecilia M. Pemberton, R.D.

Principles of Nutritional Care
Obesity
Gastroplasty
Fat Absorption Test Diet
Carbohydrate Metabolism
5-HIAA

Karen Rooney, M.S., R.D.

Pregnancy and Lactation
Pediatric Nutritional Assessment
Sick Infants, Children,
and Adolescents
Low Birth Weight Infant
Failure to Thrive
Developmental Disability
Parenteral Nutrition Support (Pediatric)
Pediatric Appendices

Jacalyn A. See, M.S., R.D.

Nutritional Assessment
Abdominal Gas and Flatulence
Delayed Gastric Emptying
Postgastrectomy Dumping Syndrome
Cancer

Nicole Spelhaug, M.S., R.D.

Nutritional Needs for Physical
Performance

Joan Vruwink, R.D.

Bone Marrow Transplant

Elizabeth J. Weiners, R.D.

Liver Transplant
Normal Nutrition–Healthy Infants,
Children, and Adolescents
Vegetarian Diet
Pediatric Nutritional Assessment

Denise J. Weisenbeck, R.D.

Pregnancy and Lactation
Young Athletes

Linda Wenig, R.D.

General Hospital Diet
Clear Liquid Diet
Full Liquid Diet
Pureed Diet
Mechanical Soft Diet
Soft Diet
Transitional Feeding Progression
Preoperative Diet
Postoperative Diet
Intermaxillary Fixation
Diabetes Mellitus (Adult)
Food Exchange List for Diabetes

Rosemary White, R.D.

Cardiac Surgery
Tyramine Controlled Diet

Carol L. Willett, R.D., C.D.E.

Diabetes Mellitus (Adult)
Food Exchange List for Diabetes

J. Denise Wilson, R.D.

Basic Four Food Guide
Dietary Guidelines for Americans
American Heart Association Dietary
Recommendations
Recommended Dietary Allowances
Food Labeling

Georgia Ziegler, R.D., C.D.E.

Diabetes Mellitus (Adult)
Food Exchange List for Diabetes

FOREWORD

The sixth edition of the *Mayo Clinic Diet Manual* represents a continuing commitment to excellence in clinical nutrition by the Mayo Clinic and its affiliated hospitals, Rochester Methodist and Saint Marys. This manual is provided as a comprehensive and expanded resource for healthful nutrition from infancy through adulthood and for the evaluation and management of problems in clinical nutrition. The Mayo Clinic has had a longstanding tradition in nutrition in clinical practice, in education, and in research dating back to the early 1920s. The Section of Dietetics has been in existence for over 60 years. The Mayo Clinic has long recognized the important role of the dietitian in the health care team. The manual was developed as a resource for dietitians and for practicing physicians.

At first, the manual primarily provided information regarding diets for appropriate clinical disorders. As information regarding nutritional management increased, the manual continued to meet the challenge of an expanding body of knowledge. The fifth edition of the work provided guidelines for healthy nutrition and introduced the scientific basis for various dietary modifications with appropriate references. The present edition of the manual demonstrates further evolution with expansion, reorganization, and revamping of clinically relevant nutritional information in a more readable and logical fashion. There is more general information regarding the principles of nutritional care, nutritional assessment of adults, and normal nutritional consideration for infants, children, adolescents, and adults. There is an expanded section in pediatric nutrition for both the ambulatory patient and the hospitalized patient. There are sections addressing the nutritional needs of young athletes, the young cancer patient, the young person with hypertension, diabetes mellitus, obesity, renal disease, or inborn errors of metabolism.

There is a new section on guides for meal planning and promotion of wellness that incorporates the latest information and recommendations for healthful nutrition. This section should be particularly helpful for the practicing clinician and the dietitian in assisting individuals with developing healthy nutritional practices in their lifestyles.

To meet the ever-continuing challenge of nutritional problems, the manual contains information regarding the needs of patients who have undergone gastroplasty for morbid obesity, the nutritional assessment and needs of patients undergoing bone marrow or liver transplantation, the role of nutrition in the management of osteoporosis, and the management of bulimia.

The section on nutritional support for hospitalized patients, both adults and children, has been expanded. The appendices contain important, pertinent reference information with ease of access.

The sixth edition of the *Mayo Clinic Diet Manual* is not a cookbook or a dictionary; it is a textbook of healthful nutrition and of the nutritional management of clinical problems, thereby providing a resource for the practicing clinician and the dietitian, as well as for the research scientist. This manual has something for everyone; use it well!

P. J. Palumbo, M.D.
Director of Clinical Nutrition
Mayo Clinic

PREFACE

The *Mayo Clinic Diet Manual* is intended as a reference tool for dietitians, medical and nursing staff, and students of nutrition and diet therapy. The manual is intended for use in providing nutritional care for both hospitalized and ambulatory patients. The manual can serve as a guide for nutritional assessment and intervention; however, it is not to be regarded as a collection of diets to be used without further thought or modification.

The manual is not intended for lay public use or as an educational tool for patient counseling. When written materials are needed for education and counseling, we recommend that materials designed specifically for that purpose be used. The Mayo Clinic has developed a wide array of educational materials with varying levels of difficulty and scope. Many of these materials are available for purchase by writing directly to, Dietetics, Mayo Clinic, Rochester, Minnesota 55905.

The *Mayo Clinic Diet Manual* provides guidelines for nutritional care practices in the Mayo Medical Center. It is recognized that other health care organizations who use this manual may need to adapt it to patient populations and protocols specific to that organization. The manual is published in both bound and loose-leaf form to facilitate its adaptation to individual institutional practices.

Owing to the nature of some diets, brand names of certain products must be stated in the manual. This is not intended as an endorsement of a specific product when an equivalent product exists.

CONTENTS

CHAPTER 1

PRINCIPLES OF NUTRITIONAL CARE

Nutritional care includes (1) an assessment of the patient's needs that are relative to his or her health status; (2) the development of a nutrition care plan; (3) the implementation of that plan, which includes provision of nutrients via oral, enteral, or parenteral routes; (4) the education of the patient; and (5) the evaluation of the effectiveness of the intervention. This manual is designed to assist the health care provider in all aspects of nutritional care.

This is a manual of therapeutic nutrition. Nutritional recommendations for a particular disease or disorder are often complex and multifaceted. In order to address the often numerous considerations, many of the chapters in the manual are organized by disease, by disorder, or by health state rather than by dietary constituents. Reference to other sections is made throughout the text because of the overlap of nutritional practices among disorders. Normal nutrition serves as the foundation for therapeutic diet modifications. Essential references for normal nutrition are included in addition to a more detailed discussion of the needs at life cycle stages within sections on *Pregnancy and Lactation,* on *Normal Nutritional Requirements of Infants, Children, and Adolescents,* and on *Geriatrics.*

A nutritional assessment is a necessary antecedent to intervention. Therefore, the chapters on nutritional assessment precede both the adult and the pediatric sections and are referred to in the subsequent sections.

Many of the chapters are organized to include a general description of a diet and discussion of the nutritional inadequacies, indications and rationale, of the goals of dietary management, of the dietary recommendations, and of the guidelines for ordering diets.

The *General Description* is intended to be a brief summary of the key aspects of nutritional intervention or of dietary modifications.

The section titled *Nutritional Inadequacy* points out those diet plans that, if adhered to for a long period of time, have the potential for nutrient deficiencies. The Recommended Dietary Allowances (RDA) are used as the reference standard. The National Research Council states that the RDA were not intended to cover the needs of those who are ill.[1] However, for lack of more suitable guidelines, the RDA were used in evaluating the therapeutic diets that are presented in this manual.

The *Indications and Rationale* for dietary modifications is provided so that

1

nutritional practices can be carried out with the choice of type and the degree of control of dietary components that are appropriate to the individual situation. We have stated when diet regimens are based on traditional practices rather than on documented scientific evidence.

The section on *Goals of Dietary Management* is intended as a brief summary of the key objective or the purpose of nutritional intervention.

The *Dietary Recommendations* section includes a discussion of the aspects of assessment, which are unique to a particular disease or disorder, and the specific guidelines for diet modification and for development of a nutritional care plan. This section expands on the practices and on the philosophy in the Mayo Medical Center. Tables that summarize food composition are included in many sections. As compared to previous editions of the Mayo Clinic Diet Manual, the sixth edition provides fewer standard meal patterns or sample menus. The science of nutrition is rarely so exacting or so accurate that a single, ideal plan is advised for all persons.

A section titled *Physicians: How to Order Diet* indicates the preferred terms for the request of nutritional assessment and intervention. The diet order should convey the treatment modality or the goal of dietary treatment. The diet order may be general or specific.

Various terms are used throughout this text to indicate the degree of restriction or the quantity of a dietary constituent. The term "minimum" indicates that the diet provides as small an amount of the substance as possible without making the diet distinctly inconvenient or unpalatable. "Low," "limited," and "restricted" are used to indicate an intermediate reduction in the amount of the substance in the diet. The term "high" indicates an increase of the substance in the diet that can be achieved with reasonable convenience. When practical, a range for the quantity, which is implied by these general terms, is specified with the diet.

The physician should discuss the diet with the patient as one component of the treatment plan. The patient is more likely to accept the recommended changes if he or she is aware of the importance with which the physician regards the dietary modification. Altering food habits is often a difficult task. Adequate time for education is essential. Requests for education and counseling should be made as early in the patient's stay as possible.

REFERENCE

1. Food and Nutrition Board, National Research Council. Recommended Dietary Allowances. 9th Ed. Washington, D.C.; National Research Council, 1980.

CHAPTER 2

NUTRITIONAL ASSESSMENT

Introduction

Nearly every visit of a dietitian with a patient, whether in the hospital or in an outpatient setting, involves a nutritional assessment to some degree. This assessment may be a structured process that consists of a series of questions to be answered by the patient or by the medical record, of certain anthropometric procedures, and of laboratory tests; or it may be a less structured procedure that consists of asking key diet-related questions, noting the general appearance of the patient, reviewing the medical record, and considering a plan of therapy.

The assessment of the nutritional state involves both the initial visit and a continuation of observations during the following days and weeks to determine whether changes in the nutritional status have occurred. Whether the assessment is formalized or less structured, certain elements are involved, such as a review of the medical history, a patient interview, an examination of the patient, anthropometric measurements, an analysis of laboratory data, an estimation of nutritional requirements, nutritional intervention, and an evaluation of the outcome of the intervention. In 1986 the American Society for Parenteral and Enteral Nutrition published Standards of Practice for the Nutritional Support Dietitian. These standards of practice may also be used in conjunction with established protocols for nutritional assessment and support and appear in Appendix I.

There is information available on nutritional assessment techniques and on criteria for diagnosing nutritional risks.[1-4] Such methods, however, are open to criticism,[5] and one should understand their limitations when interpreting findings.

There are several important questions that need to be considered when an evaluation of nutritional status is performed.

1. Which nutritional assessment techniques can be utilized?
2. What are the limitations of the data thus gathered?
3. How are the results of the assessment utilized?
4. Does nutritional intervention favorably influence the outcome of the care?

With these issues in mind, it has been our usual practice to approach nutritional assessment globally rather than by utilizing specific protocols per se.[6,7] Data that are routinely available are used by the clinician in identifying a nutritional diagnosis rather than utilizing a standard nutritional assessment battery. The following information is a description of this approach to nutritional assessment.

Review of Medical History

The initial step in the screening of patients for nutritional problems should be a review of the medical history for high risk conditions that may accompany malnutrition or that may predispose a patient to malnutrition. This permits early intervention in both the treatment of established malnutrition and its prevention in individuals at high risk.

Malnutrition usually results from one or more of the following pathophysiological mechanisms (Table 2–1): alterations in nutrient intake, digestion, absorption, metabolism, excretion, and/or requirements. Knowledge of medical conditions and of their pathophysiology is helpful in identifying patients who are at risk for malnutrition owing to hypermetabolic states, nutrient losses, chronic illness, etc.

TABLE 2–1 Pathophysiological Mechanisms of Malnutrition

Mechanism	Disorder
Intake	Impairment or inability to regulate ingestion of nutrients. Found in, but not limited to, such diseases or disorders as: Anorexia nervosa Inability to chew and swallow Bulimia GI motility disorders Altered level of consciousness Hyperemesis GI tract obstruction
Digestion	Impairment or inability to break down nutrients into absorbable entities. Found in, but not limited to, such diseases or disorders as: Disaccharidase deficiency Cystic fibrosis Gastrectomy Pancreatitis and biliary insufficiency
Absorption	Impairment or inability to assimilate nutrients. Found in, but not limited to, such diseases or disorders as: Inflammatory bowel (Crohn's) disease Short bowel syndrome Fistula Radiation enteritis
Excretion	Impairment or inability to rid the body of waste products of metabolized nutrients or increased losses of nutrients. Found in, but not limited to, such diseases or disorders as: Chronic renal disease Dialysis Draining abscesses or wounds Blood loss
Metabolism	Impairment or inability to utilize assimilated nutrients. Found in, but not limited to, such diseases or disorders as: Inborn errors of metabolism Chronic obstructive pulmonary Liver disease disease Drug-nutrient interactions Chronic renal disease
Requirements	Alteration in quantity of nutrients needed to obtain or maintain health that is beyond the ability of the individual to consume. Found in, but not limited to, such conditions as: Trauma Burns Sepsis Hypermetabolic states

Patient Interview

After becoming acquainted with the course of the patient's medical history, the dietitian interviews the patient and, if necessary, the family members. A knowledge of various disease states (see Table 2–1), their impact on nutritional status, and rationales for different diets aid in knowing which questions to ask.

In general, questions should be directed to (1) the nature and the duration of the illness and their effect on eating patterns and on the integrity of the digestive process; (2) weight loss or gain over a period of time; (3) usual eating habits and food preferences; (4) intake of medications, nutrition supplements, and alcohol.

The method that is selected to obtain the diet history is determined by the time and the personnel available, by the setting (e.g., hospital, outpatient clinic), and by the degree of accuracy that is needed. After the dietary intake data have been collected and summarized, they may be compared to one of several established nutrient intake guidelines and/or standards to determine nutritional adequacy in meeting the individual's needs.

The dietitian should review medications recently and currently used by the patient, noting those medications that have known drug-nutrient interactions (*Appendix* 2).[8] The amounts and types of vitamin and/or of mineral preparations that are ingested by the patient should be determined and evaluated for potential toxicities. If nutritional supplements have been ingested, their nutrient and caloric contribution should be included as a part of the dietary analysis. Alcohol intake should be noted for its potential effect on nutrient utilization as well as its caloric contribution to the diet. (See *Appendix* 3.)

Clinical Assessment

A physical examination of the patient can provide valuable assistance in identifying patients who are malnourished or who are at high risk of becoming malnourished. Many of these variable signs can be detected by observation during the interview.

Anthropometrics

Anthropometrics may be defined as the measurement of size, weight, and proportions of the body. Methods most frequently utilized include height, weight, triceps skinfold thickness, and midarm muscle circumference measurements. Anthropometric indices assist in establishing a basis for determining protein and caloric malnutrition. The selection of the most appropriate method depends on whether the intent is for general nutritional screening or for more indepth nutritional assessment.

Body Height and Weight. An accurate measurement of the patient's height and weight on admission and the weight at regular intervals is important, as these provide crude measures of body fat stores and muscle mass and, therefore, metabolic fuels. Height and weight are the measurements most frequently used in nutritional assessments.

Such measurements may be utilized in comparison to height and weight norms (*Appendix* 4). Such norms, however, are often mistaken as an ideal weight for height for an individual. These standards do not account for variations in patient age, heredity, degree of athletic training, or possible effect of illness. Therefore, it is preferred practice to utilize a more physiologic norm for weight comparisons. An individual's pre-illness weight or the usual weight during health can serve as a more realistic norm for determining the effect of illness on body weight. The clinician must be aware of factors that affect weight status (such as edema, dehydration, amputation).

When there is a loss of body parts, the estimation of weight loss or gain becomes more difficult. Table 2–2 shows the approximate percentage of body weight that is contributed by various body parts. These percentages can be used to adjust body weight norms.

TABLE 2–2 Percentage Total Body Weight Contributed by Individual Body Parts[9]

Body Part	Percent
Trunk without limbs	42.7
Hand	0.8
Forearm with hand	3.1
Entire arm with hand	6.5
Foot	1.8
Lower leg with foot	7.1
Entire leg	18.6

With permission and adapted from: Grant A, DeHoog S. Anthropometrics. In: Grant A, DeHoog S, eds. Nutritional assessment and support. 3rd ed. Seattle: Grant A, DeHoog S, 1985:12.

Weight Change.   A history of a very rapid weight loss suggests a catabolic state with a substantial loss of protein tissue, dehydration, or both. Protein tissue with muscle as its prototype represents only about 400 Kcal per pound, whereas adipose tissue represents a storage of about 3,500 Kcal per pound. Hence, a negative caloric balance from the destruction of protein tissue can be expected to cause a weight loss eight to ten times greater than would be the case if the weight loss from the same negative caloric balance were only in the form of adipose tissue.

The most significant usage of body weight as an index for determining nutritional status is the percent of recent weight change. The following equations are helpful in calculating the degree of weight change:

$$\text{Percent of Usual Body Weight} = \frac{\text{Current Body Weight}}{\text{Usual Body Weight}} \times 100$$

$$\text{Percent of Recent Weight Change} = \frac{\text{Usual Body Weight} - \text{Current Body Weight}}{\text{Usual Body Weight}} \times 100$$

It is difficult to know how much weight loss is significant, since one does not know that the stated level of weight loss is body tissue rather than fluid loss. Approximately 50 to 60 percent of a healthy adult is fluid. A weight loss of 10 percent in a six-month period probably is important to consider. However, if the patient is or has been edematous, such a weight change may not be of nutritional importance.

Skin Fold Measurements.   More detailed estimates of body fat reserves can be made by skin fold measurements. The determination of body fat reserves may permit an estimate of the duration and the severity of pre-existing malnutrition. It also may provide an indication of a patient's nonprotein caloric reserves. Considerable practice is needed for reliable and accurate measurements and, ideally, one should learn this technique from a competent instructor.[10–13]

Biochemical Assessment

A number of laboratory procedures that can serve as indicators of nutritional status are available in most clinics and hospitals. Serum proteins provide an estimation of long and short term changes in nutritional status and correlate with patient morbidity and mortality. However, to detect changes that have occurred rapidly in response to an acute problem, prealbumin may be needed in addition to albumin and transferrin (which reflect longer term malnutrition). The interpretation of a single measurement must be done with caution, as over or under hydration can alter concentrations.

Other tests that are useful in assessing nutritional status include glucose, alkaline phosphatase, hematocrit, hemoglobin, mean corpuscular volume, lymphocytes, and urine analysis studies. (See *Appendix* 5 for normal ranges for these tests.)

In summary, for most clinical purposes adequate assessment may be achieved by routine blood and urine studies, especially when these studies are combined with careful history and physical examinations and supported by a systematic analysis of the data so obtained.

Estimation of Nutrient Requirements

In arriving at an estimate of nutrient needs, the following must be considered: (1) the requirements for a normal individual; (2) the nature of the disease or injury; (3) the known capacity of the body to store certain nutrients; (4) the known losses through skin, urine, or intestinal tract; (5) the interactions of drugs and nutrients; and (6) the interrelationships of various nutrients.

Estimating Energy Needs

Several methods exist for estimating resting energy requirements. The most widely used formulas are those of Harris and Benedict.[14]

For Males, $BEE = 66.4 + 13.7(W) + 6(H) - 6.8(A)$

For Females, $BEE = 655 + 9.6(W) + 1.8(H) - 4.7(A)$

BEE is basal energy expenditure, A is age in years, W is actual weight in kilograms, and H is height in centimeters. The Mayo Clinic Nomogram is also used (see *Appendix* 6). Adjustments to the calculated BEE for various forms of stress, fever, surgery, sepsis, or burns often overestimate the actual BEE when measured by indirect calorimetry.[15] Therefore, for patients who are suspected of having greatly increased energy requirements, a measurement of the oxygen consumption is recommended.

The energy expenditure is indirectly determined by measuring the oxygen consumption. By also determining carbon dioxide production, the substrate(s) being oxidized can be assessed and the respiratory quotient calculated. A caloric equivalent for a liter of oxygen is assigned based on this respiratory quotient, which results in a more accurate measure of energy requirement than is accomplished by using oxygen consumption alone. The respiratory service of the hospital should be able to measure the oxygen consumption and, if necessary, the carbon dioxide that is expired and to express the result as Kilocalories expended. To evaluate the adequacy of nutritional support, energy expenditure can be calculated and can be compared with the amount of energy that is provided to the patient.[15]

For unstressed patients, measured energy expenditures range between 20 and 25 Kcal per kilogram. Thus, caloric intakes between 25 and 35 Kcal per kilogram of actual body weight should be adequate for nearly all hospitalized patients. There appears to be no advantage to regimens that provide less than 20 Kcal per kilogram, even in obese patients.

Estimating Protein Needs

The recommended dietary allowance (RDA) of protein for normal healthy adults is 0.8 g per kilogram of body weight. The minimum requirement for the maintenance of nitrogen balance in healthy adults is between 0.4 and 0.5 g per kilogram. Fever, sepsis, surgery, trauma, and burns increase the protein catabolism, and therefore greater amounts of amino acids and/or of protein must be supplied in order to achieve nitrogen balance. The most direct way for assessing protein requirements in acutely ill patients is to measure 24-hour urinary nitrogen. This can be determined by multiplying the grams of urinary nitrogen per 24 hours (plus an allowance of 1 to 2 g for fecal and for other nitrogen losses) times 6.25 or daily protein = (24 hour urinary nitrogen + 2 g) × 6.25. The calculation of the allowance for fecal and for other nitrogen losses is adequate unless these losses are large, as seen in diarrheal stool or in fistula fluids.

Most hospitalized patients can be adequately maintained on protein intakes between 1.0 and 1.5 g per kilogram per day of actual body weight. Intakes greater than 2 g per kilogram per day should not be considered in the absence of documentation of the rate of protein catabolism by 24-hour urinary nitrogen. In some rare instances (e.g., graft-versus-host reactions), it may be necessary to give as much as 3 to 4 g per kilogram per day of protein in order to meet nitrogen requirements. Such patients require close monitoring to assure that they do not receive excess nitrogen loads.

Vitamins

Vitamin allowances for healthy persons are well standardized, but the altered needs that are associated with specific disease states remain poorly defined. Supplemental vitamins should be provided to ensure the RDA when the quantity or the quality of the intake does not provide adequate vitamins.

Minerals and Trace Elements

As with vitamins, mineral requirements have been established for healthy adults, but less is known about the needs during the stress of disease and of trauma. An adequate supply of minerals is essential for anabolism. Potassium and phosphorus, the major intracellular ions, are deposited in new cells during nutritional repletion, and serum levels may fall if potassium and phosphorus are not supplied in sufficient amounts. It is also important to note that pseudohypocalcemia may result from reduced serum albumin, as approximately one-half of serum calcium is loosely bound to serum albumin. The "routine chemistry and hematology group" usually indicates in some degree the mineral status. As with vitamins, the mineral intake should assure 100 percent of the RDA, and supplements should be provided to correct for increased requirements or losses or for inadequate intake.

After the goals of nutritional therapy are determined, the nutritional care plan can guide the selection of appropriate nutritional support. A nutritional care plan should consist of a completed nutritional assessment, the identification of any nutritional problems, and a statement of nutritional objectives that must be realistic and quantifiable. Therapeutic measures to provide estimated nutrient needs may include oral feeding, enteral tube feeding, and/or parenteral nutrition. The reader is referred to the remaining sections of this manual to aid in the establishment of nutritional support practices and of patient education efforts according to the needs in health and in specific diseases. Finally, monitoring or reassessment of the nutritional status should be performed at appropriate intervals to evaluate the effectiveness of the nutritional intervention.

REFERENCES

1. Mullen JL, Gertner MH, Buzby GP, Goodhart SL, Rosato EF. Implications of malnutrition in surgical patients. Arch Surg 1979;114:121–125.
2. Bistrian BR, Blackburn GL, Vitale B, Cochran D, Naylor B. Prevalance of malnutrition in general medical patients. JAMA 1976;230:1567–1570.
3. Bistrian BR, Blackburn GL, Hallowell E, Heddle R. Protein status of general surgical patients. JAMA 1974;230:858–860.
4. Dreblow DM, Anderson CF, Moxness KE. Nutritional assessment of orthopedic patients. Mayo Clin Proc 1981;56:51–54.
5. Grant JP. Nutritional assessment in clinical practice. Nutr Clin Pract 1986;1:3–11.
6. Baker JP, Detsky AS, Wesson DE, Walman SL, Stewart S, Whitewell J, Langer B, Jeejeebhoy KN. Nutritional assessment: A comparison of clinical judgment and objective measurements. N Engl J Med 1982;306:969–972.
7. Collins JA. Editorial: Clinical judgment versus the laboratory. N Engl J Med 1982;306:987.
8. Smith CH, Bidlade WR. Dietary concerns associated with the use of medications. J Am Diet Assoc 1984;84:901–914.
9. Grant A, DeHoog S. Anthropometrics. In: Grant A, DeHoog S, eds. Nutritional assessment and support. 3rd ed. Seattle: Grant A, DeHoog S, 1985:12.
10. Durnin JVGA, Womersley J. Body fat assessed from total body density and its estimation from skin fold thickness: Measurement on 81 men and women aged from 16 to 72 years. Br J Nutr 1974;32:77–97.
11. Gray GE, Gray LK. Anthropometric measurements and their interpretation: principles, practices, and problems. J Am Diet Assoc 1980;77:534–539.
12. Jackson AS, Pollock ML, Ward A. Generalized equations for predicting body density of women. Med Sci Sports Exer 1980;12:175–182.
13. Jackson AS, Pollock ML. Generalized equations for predicting body density of men. Br J Nutr 1978;40:497–504.
14. Harris JA, Benedict FG. A biometric study of basal metabolism in man. Washington, D.C.: Carnegie Institution, 1919 (Carnegie Institution of Washington, Publication No. 279).
15. Anderson CF, Loosbrock LM, Moxness KE. Nutrient intake in critically ill patients: Too many or too few calories? Mayo Clin Proc 1986;61:853–858.

CHAPTER 3

NORMAL NUTRITION

PREGNANCY AND LACTATION

General Description

Many studies have shown that nutrition during pregnancy affects the pregnancy's course and outcome. Nutritional status before pregnancy is also a major factor that affects the health of a pregnant woman and of her infant. The best diet for any pregnancy is one that begins before conception.

"Optimum development of an infant is necessarily a function of parental diet—an ongoing, long-term, as well as immediate relationship. The mother's preconception diet and possibly that of her mother is important."[1]

Women who have been on oral contraceptives, especially long-term users with poor dietary habits, are at a nutritional risk for probable folic acid and vitamin B_6 deficiency[2] and may be best advised to wait several months before attempting pregnancy.

The following situations presented in Table 3–1 during or prior to pregnancy also increase nutritional risk. Pregnant women in these situations should have a more extensive evaluation of their nutritional status and of the adequacy of their dietary intake.

Nutritional considerations for normal pregnancy and the three common situations of adolescence, obesity, and diabetes, which are associated with increased nutritional risk, are discussed. Table 3–2 summarizes dietary recommendations for pregnancy and lactation.

TABLE 3–1 Nutritional Risk and Pregnancy

Adolescence
Diabetes
High Parity
Frequent Conceptions
Low Pre-Pregnancy Weight
Insufficient Weight Gain During Pregnancy
Obesity
Previous Obstetrical Complications
Low Income
Smoking, Alcoholism, Drug Addiction
Dietary Faddism and Pica

TABLE 3–2 The Suggested Daily Dietary Intake During Pregnancy and Lactation

Food Group	Normal Pregnancy Servings	Pregnant Adolescent* Servings	Lactation Servings
Dairy Group (one cup or calcium equivalent)	4	5	4
Meat Group (2–3 oz or protein equivalent)	3	3	3
Fruit and Vegetable Group (about 1/2 cup edible portion) 1 rich source of vitamin A 2 rich sources of vitamin C	4	4 or more	5
Starch Group (1 slice bread or 1/2 cup enriched or whole grain)	4	5 or more	4 or more
Other Foods	To meet caloric needs	To meet caloric needs	To meet caloric needs

*The dietary pattern meets the Recommended Dietary Allowance for pregnant adolescents except for iron and folic acid.

Normal Pregnancy

Weight Gain. The goal of weight management during pregnancy is to promote optimum nutrition for the mother and for the child. An inadequate maternal weight gain may result in a low birth weight of the fetus and in an increase in perinatal mortality. The American College of Obstetrics and Gynecology recommends a pregnancy weight gain of 10 to 12.3 kg (22 to 27 lb) for normal weight women.[3] For underweight women, the best outcomes occur when a gain of about 13.6 kg (30 lb) is achieved.[4]

Rosso[5] has developed a weight gain grid that monitors the weight gain during pregnancy. Although it is not yet known if this grid is suitable for all populations, it may serve as a guide for evaluating the rate and the amount of weight gain. It may be especially useful to determine an appropriate weight gain for the woman who is overweight or who is underweight at the beginning of her pregnancy. A nomogram is used first to calculate values of the percentage of the "standard weight" at various gestational ages for pregnant women (Fig. 3–1). This maternal body weight, as a percentage of the standard, is then plotted according to the appropriate weeks of gestation (Fig. 3–2). The chart establishes a desirable weight-near term, which is equivalent to 120 percent of the "standard weight" for women with a pre-pregnancy weight equal to or lower than 100 percent of the "standard weight." For women with a pre-pregnancy weight that is above 100 percent of the "standard weight," the desirable weight-near term varies according to the initial weight, but includes a minimal weight gain of 7 kg (15.4 lb) for women with a pre-pregnancy weight over 120 percent of the standard.

Caloric Intake. In order to achieve an optimal weight gain, the Food and Nutrition Board has recommended an intake of 300 Kcal per day in excess of the number of kilocalories that are required to maintain an ideal weight in the nonpregnant state.[6] This results in a total of approximately 2,200 to 2,400 Kcal per day for the average-sized pregnant woman, which is about a 15 percent increase over her usual intake. The increased kilocalories and nutrients needed

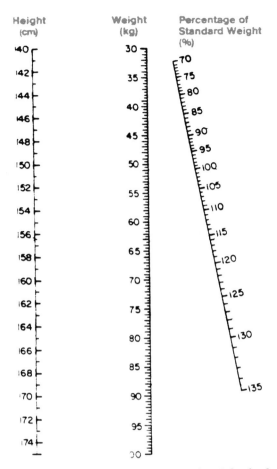

Figure 3–1 Nomogram to determine the adequacy of weight for height. (Connect the height and the pre-pregnancy weight using a straight edge. Read the percentage of the standard weight at the point the straight edge crosses that line.) Reprinted with permission.[5]

during pregnancy can be met by consuming a nutritionally balanced diet from the basic food groups (see Table 3–2). Additional food may be added according to individual energy and nutrient needs.

Protein. Current recommendations by the National Research Council for protein intake during pregnancy are for an increase of 30 g per day over the amount (45 to 50 g) needed by a nonpregnant adult woman.[6] This makes an increased need of about 60 percent more protein, or a total of about 75 to 80 g. Some high risk or active women may need even more, perhaps nearer 100 g.[6]

Iron. An increase in the body stores of iron of about 670 mg is needed for the expansion of the maternal red blood cell volume and for the synthesis of fetal and of placental tissues.[4] This level cannot be met by the recommended diet without adding too many kilocalories; therefore, the National Research Council recommends that pregnant women receive an oral iron supplement of 30 to 60 mg of elemental iron per day. This amount should maintain hemoglobin levels in normal pregnant women, but those who are anemic when they enter the pregnancy need a larger dose. Simple ferrous salts should be used.

Folic Acid. The question of oral supplementation of folic acid during pregnancy is still a debatable issue. Folic acid is not stored in the body, but it can

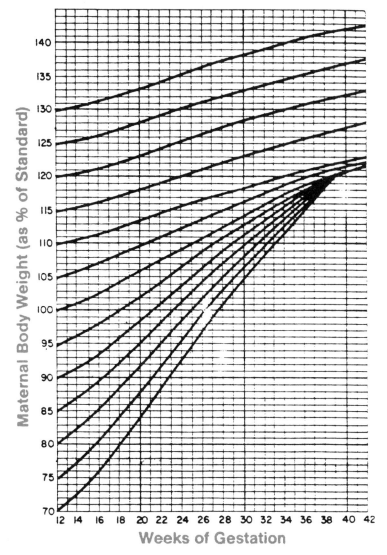

Figure 3–2 A chart to monitor the weight gain during pregnancy, considering the pre-pregnancy weight and height. This grid should be used only as a guide. Reprinted with permission.[5]

be supplied by an appropriate diet that contains raw fruits and vegetables. Although megaloblastic anemia attributable to folate deficiency is infrequent, routine supplementation appears desirable. In order to protect the fetus and to maintain maternal stores, the National Research Council recommends that a pregnant woman take an oral supplement of 400 μg per day of folic acid in the last half of her pregnancy.[6]

Other Supplemental Vitamins. With the exception of iron and of folic acid, routine dietary supplementation with vitamin and mineral preparations is of doubtful value. Vitamin and mineral preparations should not be regarded as corrective measures for inadequate dietary habits.

Sodium. During pregnancy, there is a cumulative retention of about 950 mEq of sodium that is distributed between the products of conception, which include the fetus (290 mEq), the placenta (57 mEq), and the amniotic fluid (100 mEq), and the maternal extracellular volume, which includes the uterus (80 mEq), the breasts (35 mEq), the plasma (140 mEq), and the edema fluid (240 mEq). The pregnant woman's volume receptors sense these gains as normal. When salt restriction or diuretic therapy limits this physiologic hypervolemia, the maternal response is similar to the response observed in salt-depleted, nonpregnant subjects. Thus, there is evidence that sodium restriction can be harmful in normotensive pregnancies and also in hypertensive pregnancies.[7]

Smoking. Factors that are adversely affected by smoking, which include altered respiration, health of lung tissue, and oxygen-carrying capacity of the blood, may contribute to an increased incidence of low birth weight, of prematurity, of stillbirth, and of late fetal and infant mortality.[4] These effects are dose-dependent in that the more the mother smokes, the more significant the potential adverse outcome.

Alcohol. Fetal alcohol syndrome, which consists of congenital malformations, of growth failure, and of central nervous system effects, may result from the excessive consumption of alcohol during pregnancy.[8-10]

The exact mechanism of cause and of effect is not yet known. It is uncertain whether the damage is a direct toxic effect from alcohol or from its metabolites. The defects and the growth deficiency may be the result of a reduced number of fetal cells. The effect upon the fetus may be dose related. A high blood alcohol level during a critical time in the fetal development may be as devastating as a continually high intake of alcohol throughout the pregnancy. This presents the possibility that fetal damage may occur shortly after conception before the woman even knows that she is pregnant.

Since no one knows for sure if there is a safe level of alcohol that can be used during pregnancy, it is prudent to recommend the total abstinence of alcohol for the pregnant woman.[10]

Caffeine. Caffeine, a stimulant drug found in coffee, tea, cocoa, colas and some other soft drinks, chocolate, some over the counter pain medications, cold remedies, stimulants, and weight control aids, can cross the placenta. Caffeine acts mainly on the brain, the central nervous system, the heart, the kidneys, the lungs, and the arteries that supply blood to the heart and the brain.[11]

The effects of caffeine on the reproduction in animals include fetal deaths, low birth weights, small litters, delayed bone development, and limb abnormalities.[12] Few studies have examined the effects of caffeine on the reproductive outcomes in humans. Some retrospective studies have found an association between a high caffeine intake of greater than 600 mg per day and fetal death, stillbirth, premature birth, and birth defects.[12]

As a precautionary measure, the Food and Drug Administration and the American Dietetic Association have advised pregnant women to avoid or to limit their consumption of foods and of drugs that contain caffeine,[2,13] although conclusions about the teratogenicity of caffeine in humans cannot be made at this time.

ADOLESCENT PREGNANCY

The adolescent age group has started to represent a statistically greater percentage of total pregnancies in the United States,[13] although the number of pregnant teenage girls who give birth has declined slightly in the decade from 1970 to 1980. Also, the incidence of perinatal problems, such as toxemia, anemia, premature births, infants with low birth weight,* and increased maternal and neonatal mortality, has remained significantly higher among teenagers than for adult women. The average birth weight of infants rises as the maternal age increases, and the percent of infants with low birth weight decreases as the maternal age rises from less than 15 years to 19 years of age.[14,15] Numerous studies that investigate the causes of the increased perinatal risks suggest that the etiologies are related more to factors such as delayed prenatal care, low socioeconomic status, poor health habits, race, greater incidence of prematurity, and lower pre-pregnancy weight than to maternal biologic immaturity.[16–19] Thus factors that are amenable to intervention, such as nutrition, early prenatal care, and improved health habits, gain more importance in assuring a better outcome among pregnant teenagers.[20]

The average age of menarche today is 12 to 13 years. Growth usually continues for 4 years postmenarche although at a much slower rate than during prepuberty. Teenage girls who become pregnant within 4 years of menarche are generally considered biologically immature. The girls' nutritional needs for pregnancy must be estimated in addition to their needs for growth. After growth is complete (more than 4 years postmenarche or at about 17 years of age), the adolescent's nutritional requirements are similar to the adult pregnant woman's requirements. The dietary intake of nutrients must meet not only the pregnancy requirements, but also the individual needs of the patient at the different stages of growth. Thus, the nutritional requirements for the immature teenager can be estimated by summing the Recommended Dietary Allowances for the specific age and the additional recommendations for pregnant adults.[6,21]

The total estimated average energy requirement for adolescents is 2,500 to 2,700 Kcal per day.[21] However, since energy expenditure is variable, the best assurance of an adequate intake is a satisfactory weight gain. This should be accomplished by individual counseling on the basis of estimates of body size, of growth rate, of age, and of activity level. Many young girls in today's society limit their food intake severely to be fashionably slim. This is an additional nutritional risk for pregnant teenagers both in terms of having a low pre-pregnancy weight, which is associated with higher perinatal risks, and in terms of their ability to meet their nutritional needs for growth.[22]

Protein. Protein needs in the pregnant teenager are understandably high. Jacobson delineates the protein recommendations for girls 15 to 18 years of age at 1.5 g of protein per kilogram of pregnant body weight and at 1.7 g of protein per kilogram of pregnant body weight for girls who are less than 15 years of age.[21] Adequate caloric intake is essential in order for protein to be used for nitrogen retention and for growth.[23,24]

Special attention is required to meet the calcium and the iron needs of pregnant teenagers because of their historically poor intake of these two nutrients. The National Research Council recommends an intake of 1,600 mg of calcium for a growing pregnant adolescent.[6] This level is believed necessary to provide sufficient calcium for normal fetal development without depleting maternal stores. The long-term consequences of maternal depletion of calcium stores remains unknown.[21] The iron needs of the growing adolescent are high because of their enlarging muscle mass and blood volume. Nevertheless, the National Research Council recommendation of a daily supplement of 30 to 60 mg of elemental iron

---

*Infant with low birth weight: less than 2,500 g

during pregnancy should be adequate for the pregnant adolescent as well as for the adult woman.[6]

Nutritional assessment and education for the pregnant teenager require on-going individual counseling. Assessment should include the growth history, the present height and weight, the gynecologic age (the chronologic age minus the age at menarche),[18] and the dietary intake history. Attention should be given to the adequacy of the dietary intake prior to the pregnancy, to bizarre dietary patterns, to the amount of snacking, to meals being skipped, to a low intake of nutrient-dense foods, and to caloric restriction. United States' teenagers have been found to have low intakes of calcium, of iron, of vitamins A, D, and C, of folic acid, and of kilocalories.[22] Pregnant teenagers tend to eat what their non-pregnant peers do.[22] Dietary counseling must be realistic in setting goals with the pregnant adolescent for dietary changes. Vitamins and/or minerals or other nutritional supplements should be used when the diet is likely to be inadequate.

PREGNANCY AND OBESITY

Obesity in pregnancy is associated with an increased risk for gestational diabetes, for hypertension, for pre-eclampsia, for cesearean section, for perinatal mortality, for induced labor, and for decreased milk production.

Lower weight gains are acceptable for overweight women because the fetus can receive part of its needed kilocalories from the maternal energy stores. Three to 5 kg (6.6 to 11 lb) of the expected gestational weight gain involves the ex-panding maternal fat stores that the overweight mother does not need. One study has shown that mothers who were grossly overweight had the best outcomes when they gained approximately 7 kg (15.4 lb) during the pregnancy.[25] A gain of 7 to 9 kg (15.4 to 19.8 lb) is recommended in order to avoid the risk of in-creased perinatal mortality.

Weight management in the overweight pregnant woman should be flexible and personalized. An evaluation of the weight status at conception as well as the dietary and the activity patterns are necessary in determining the appro-priate weight gain for each woman.

To achieve the desired intake, it is essential to counsel each patient in the selection of foods that meet the nutritional requirements of normal pregnancy and that are also appealing and conducive to a weight gain that is within the optimum range.

PREGNANCY AND DIABETES

Women with previously diagnosed diabetes mellitus account for 0.1 to 0.5 percent of all pregnancies, plus an additional 2.5 percent of pregnant women develop gestational diabetes.[26] It has been recommended that all pregnant women be screened between 24 to 28 weeks gestation with a 50 g glucose challenge test. An oral glucose tolerance test is indicated if the plasma glucose is greater than 150 mg per deciliter one hour after the test. The criteria for the diagnosis of gestational diabetes include two or more of the following plasma glucose con-centrations that are met or exceeded following a 100 g glucose load. (1) A fasting plasma glucose—105 mg per deciliter; (2) at 1 hr—190 mg per deciliter; (3) at 2 hr—165 mg per deciliter; and (4) at 3 hr—145 mg per deciliter. If the fasting plasma glucose levels of the gestational diabetic cannot be kept below 105 mg per deciliter by diet alone, insulin therapy should be started. Sulfonylureas are contraindicated during pregnancy.

Good control of the blood glucose levels during pregnancy is critical both to the health of the mother and to the fetus. Studies have shown that perinatal mortality rates have dropped to within normal ranges for those patients who demonstrate good glycemic control (i.e., 80 to 120 mg per deciliter while fasting and before meals) during their pregnancy. Increased blood glucose levels during the first 6 to 8 weeks of conception increase the chances of fetal malformations, and increased blood glucose levels later in the pregnancy are associated with macrosomia, fetal hypoglycemia, and respiratory distress syndrome. On the other hand, the fetus does not seem to be adversely affected by transient maternal hypoglycemia.

Dietary recommendations follow the basic principles of the standard diabetic diet (see section on Diabetes).

The caloric level of the diet is based on the number of kilocalories that are required to maintain the patient's pre-pregnancy weight with an increase of approximately 300 Kcal per day or on the number of kilocalories that are sufficient to achieve a weight gain of 7 to 13.6 kg (15.4 to 30 lb). The rate of weight gain can be monitored using the grid presented in Figure 3–2. A weight loss during the pregnancy is to be avoided because of the need for adequate fetal nutrition and because of an increased incidence of maternal ketonurea associated with very low kilocalorie diets.[26] The conceptus can be linked to a "glucose sink," which constantly removes glucose from the maternal circulation and renders the woman vulnerable to hypoglycemia before meals as well as to ketosis, especially early in the pregnancy. Between meal feedings minimize fluctuations in the plasma glucose and reduce the risk of ketosis. Therefore, the caloric allotment should be divided into three meals and three snacks (a midmorning, a midafternoon, and a bedtime snack). The regularity of meals and of exercise is stressed to prevent wide fluctuations in the blood glucose levels. The use of complex carbohydrates should be emphasized. The use of artificial sweeteners is not recommended.

The diet should be reviewed frequently and adjusted to reflect maternal weight gain, changes in activity, and food tolerances and preferences. Two important goals are an adequate weight gain and an absence of urinary ketones.

LACTATION

The maternal nutritional status and the diet can influence the quantity and the quality of human milk, although lactational performance can be maintained over a wide range of maternal states. A moderate to a severe caloric restriction or actual starvation reduces the milk supply more so than the nutrient composition, although the latter is reduced as well.[27] An adequate weight gain during pregnancy and a normal infant birth weight are indirect indicators of good maternal nutritional status, which can improve the likelihood of successful lactation.

Kilocalories. The caloric requirement for the lactating woman is related to the amount of milk that is produced and to the amount of caloric reserve found in the form of the mother's body fat. The National Research Council recommends an extra 500 Kcal a day over the pre-pregnancy needs for the first 3 months and more according to maternal needs after that (see Table 4–1). Breast milk has a caloric content of 70 Kcal per 100 milliliters but, because of a 90 percent efficiency in energy conversion, approximately 40 Kcal are required for the production of 100 ml of milk. The average amount of milk produced per day is 850 ml, which necessitates an additional 800 Kcal per day. Normally during pregnancy about 3 kg of body fat is stored, which can be mobilized to provide 200 to 300 Kcal per day for 3 months. Therefore, the average nonpregnant diet should be increased by 500 Kcal per day for the first 3 months, then 800 Kcal per day after that. A gradual weight reduction in the mother is compatible with successful lactation. Additional energy recommendations should be adjusted to meet the individual woman's needs. More recently, however, it has been found that women could maintain adequate milk production on fewer kilocalories than that recommended by the National Research Council, and that the energy expenditure for lactation was only about 350 Kcal per day.[28] Women who have a low pregnancy weight gain, who have decreased weight for height in lactation, who nurse longer than 3 months, and who nurse more than one infant most likely need additional kilocalories. Severe caloric restriction to achieve rapid weight reduction should be discouraged.

Protein. Protein requirements are also related to the amount of milk produced. An extra 20 g of protein is recommended based on an average of 10 g of protein secreted per day. Since the efficiency of the conversion of dietary protein to milk protein is about 70 percent, and individual variations must be accounted for, the recommended allowance for lactation is an additional 20 g of protein[6] per day.

Other Nutrients. The requirements for other nutrients are all increased and reflect the need for milk production and the need to replenish maternal stores.[29] The human milk levels generally reflect the maternal intake and the stores for all vitamins and for all types of fat. The mineral content of human milk remains relatively constant with various maternal intakes. Deficits in the intake are made up for by the maternal stores. The Recommended Dietary Allowance for calcium and for vitamin D involves an additional 400 mg and 5 μg per day, respectively, to prevent maternal demineralization.[6]

The lactating woman should be counseled to add an extra serving from the meat group, to add 2 cups of milk or the equivalent, to add an extra serving of a vitamin C-rich food, and to include raw fruits and vegetables in her diet to provide adequate folic acid to her adequate pre-pregnancy diet. An iron supplement of 30 to 60 mg of elemental iron per day should be continued for the first 2 to 3 months of lactation to replete maternal iron stores.[5] Vitamin supplementation is not necessary unless a deficiency in water-soluble vitamins is detected.[30] Breast milk concentrations of iron, of fluoride, and of vitamin D can be low and are not affected by dietary supplementation; therefore, supplementation to the infant is advisable.

Fluids. An increase of fluid intake does not increase the milk volume; however, additional fluid is needed to maintain a normal maternal fluid balance. Mothers should be encouraged to drink when they are thirsty.[26]

Special attention should be given, when assessing the adequacy of the diet of the vegetarian woman who is lactating, to include adequate kilocalories, iron, protein, calcium, vitamin D, and zinc. (Zinc may be poorly absorbed from a vegetarian diet.) A vitamin B_{12} supplement of up to 4 μg per day is also recommended.[27]

Caffeine, Alcohol, and Drugs. Most chemicals ingested by the lactating woman cross into her milk. Therefore, the mother should seek the advice of her physician before taking any dietary supplement, any medication, or any drugs.

Caffeine and alcohol also pass into the milk. Excess caffeine may make the infant irritable and wakeful. Ethanol appears in the human milk in a similar concentration to that in the maternal blood, although acetaldehyde, which is the major toxic breakdown product of ethanol, does not appear in the milk. Nevertheless, an excessive maternal intake of alcohol should be avoided.

REFERENCES

1. Gibbs CE, Seitchik J. Nutrition in pregnancy. In: Goodhart RS, Shils ME, eds. Modern nutrition in health and disease. 6th ed. Philadelphia: Lea & Febiger, 1980:743–752.
2. Tyrer LB. Nutrition and the pill. J Reprod Med 1984;29(Suppl 7):547–550.
3. Sutter C, Ott D. Maternal and infant nutrition recommendations: a review. J Am Diet Assoc 1984;84:572–573.
4. Williams SR. Nutritional therapy in special conditions of pregnancy. In: Worthington-Roberts BS, Vermeersch J, Williams SR, eds. Nutrition in pregnancy and lactation. St. Louis: CV Mosby, 1981:105–134.
5. Rosso P. A new chart to monitor weight gain during pregnancy. Am J Clin Nutr 1985;41:644–652.
6. National Research Council, National Academy of Sciences, Committee on Dietary Allowances, Food and Nutrition Board. Recommended Dietary Allowances. 9th ed. Washington, D.C., 1980.
7. Lindheimer M. Current concepts of sodium metabolism and use of diuretics in pregnancy. Contemp Ob Gyn 1980;15:207.
8. Suter C, Ott D. Maternal and infant nutrition recommendations: a review. J Am Diet Assoc 1984;84:572.
9. Rosett HL, Weiner L. Alcohol and pregnancy. Annu Rev Med 1985;36:73–80.
10. Council on Scientific Affairs, American Medical Association. Fetal effects of maternal alcohol use. JAMA 1983;249:2517–2521.
11. Friedman F. Caffeine and pregnancy: answers to common questions. J Pract Nurs 1981;31:31–37.
12. Brooten D, Jordan CH. Caffeine and pregnancy. JOGN Nurs May/June 1983;12:190–195.
13. Food and Drug Administration: alcohol, caffeine and pregnancy. FDA consumer update. 1982;April:16(2):25–26.
14. National Center for Health Statistics. Trends in teenage childbearing, United States 1970–1981. Hyattsville, MD: National Center for Health statistics, September 1984. (Vital and health statistics. Series 21, no. 41) (DHHS publication no. (PHS) 84–1919).
15. U.S. Department of Health and Human Services, Hyattsville, MD: 1982:1–61. (Vital statistics of the United States, 1978 Volume 1 Natality) (DHHS publication no. (PHS) 81–1100).
16. Zuckerman B, Alpert JJ, Dooling E, Hingson R, Kayne H, Morelock S, Oppenheimer E. Neonatal outcome: is adolescent pregnancy a risk factor? Pediatrics 1983;71:489–493.
17. Elster AB. The effect of maternal age, parity, and prenatal care on perinatal outcome in adolescent mothers. Am J Obstet Gynecol 1984;149:845–847.
18. Horon IL, Strobino DM, MacDonald HM. Birth weights among infants born to adolescent and young adult women. Am J Obstet Gynecol 1983;146:444–449.
19. Hollingsworth DR, Katchen JM. Gynecologic age and its relation to neonatal outcome. Birth Defects Original Article Series 1981;17:91–105.
20. Committee on adolescence, American Academy of Pediatrics. Statement on teenage pregnancy. Pediatrics 1979;63:795–797.
21. Worthington-Roberts BS. Nutritional needs of the pregnant adolescent. In: Worthington-Roberts BS, Vermeersch J, Williams SR, eds. Nutrition in pregnancy and lactation. St. Louis: CV Mosby, 1981:135–154.

22. Jacobson HN. Nutritional risk of pregnancy during adolescence. Birth Defects Original Article Series 1981;17:69–83.
23. King JC, Calloway DH, Margen S. Nitrogen retention, total body 40^K and weight gain in teenage pregnant girls. J Nutr 1973;103:772–785.
24. Calloway DH. Recommended dietary allowances for protein and energy. J Am Diet Assoc 1974;64:157–162.
25. Naeye RL. Weight gain and the outcome of pregnancy. Am J Obstet Gynecol 1979;135:3.
26. Nelson RL. Diabetes and pregnancy. Primary Care 1983;10:225–240.
27. Lawrence RA. Diet and dietary supplements for the mother and infant. In: Lawrence RA, ed. Breast feeding: a guide for the medical profession. St. Louis: CV Mosby, 1980:135.
28. Butte NF, Garza C, Stuff JE, Smith E, Nichols BL. Effect of maternal diet and body composition on lactational performance. Am J Clin Nutr 1984;39:296–306.
29. Committee on Nutrition, American Academy of Pediatrics. Nutrition and lactation. Pediatrics 1981;68:435–443.
30. Worthington-Roberts BS. Lactation and human milk: nutritional considerations. In: Worthington-Roberts BS, Vermeersch J, Williams SR, eds. Nutrition in pregnancy and lactation. St. Louis: CV Mosby, 1981:155.

NUTRITIONAL NEEDS FOR PHYSICAL PERFORMANCE

General Description

There is no specific diet that provides optimum athletic performance. In general, physical activity does not increase the needs for specific nutrients. Whether an individual is professionally competitive, recreationally active, or sedentary, a variety of normal foods can satisfy both the energy and the nutrient needs.

Kilocalories

As with the nonathletic, healthy individual, the energy intake should consist of about 55 to 60 percent carbohydrate, preferably complex carbohydrates, 15 percent protein, and 25 to 30 percent fat. Specific caloric needs depend on a number of variables, such as the body size, the age, the sex (determinents of basal metabolic rate), and the level of activity. Experience is often the best measure. Methods of estimating kilocalories are included in the *Nutritional Assessment* section of this manual (see page 3).

Often, athletes who are involved in intensely active training programs have to consciously eat more to match their energy output. Meals should be frequent and based on a variety of foods.

In some athletic activities, the individual wants to increase muscle strength and embarks on a weight gaining program. The aim should be to increase the lean body mass at 0.5 lb per week.[1] This can be done by a gradual increase in food intake with a concomitant increase in physical activity.

Casual exercisers, who do not attain high levels of physical training, do not usually expend a noticeably greater number of kilocalories.[2] To lose weight, they have to eat fewer kilocalories. Athletes who are involved in sports with weight categories should be advised against fasting and very low caloric diets before competition.

Carbohydrate

Carbohydrate is the preferred fuel for working muscles. The diet should obtain at least 55 to 60 percent of its kilocalories from predominantly complex carbohydrates. Carbohydrate loading or "glycogen packing" of the muscles may be beneficial for endurance athletes who exercise at an intensity between 65 and 85 percent of VO_2 max for longer than about 80 minutes.[3] However, the classic two-phase procedure of carbohydrate loading, which consists of glycogen depletion followed by loading, has been abandoned for a modified approach that is safer, yet effective. It is now recommended that athletes follow a high carbohydrate diet throughout training and begin a tapered rest about 7 days before an endurance event, with complete rest the day of the event.[3,4] Athletes should try to achieve a diet that provides 60 to 65 percent of the total kilocalories as complex carbohydrates (or 550 g of carbohydrates, whichever is greater) during the 72 hours before competition.[4] This should maximize muscle glycogen stores.

Exercise that lasts less than 1 hour requires only normal muscle glycogen levels.[3] A diet that provides 55 to 60 percent of its kilocalories as carbohydrates should be sufficient. Meals that are rich in carbohydrates can restore muscle glycogen to pre-exercise levels within 24 hours.[3]

Protein

The Recommended Dietary Allowance (RDA) for protein intake is 0.8 g of protein per kilogram of body weight. Needs might be higher (1 to 1.5 g per kilogram of body weight for periods of intense training [greater than 70 percent VO_2 max]), but there is little evidence that indicates a need for larger increases.[5] When kilocalories from protein exceed the amount that is needed for the maintenance of body tissue, the kilocalories are used as energy or may be converted to fat and stored in adipose tissue. In addition, high protein diets often deliver an increased percentage of kilocalories from fat.

Fat

Kilocalories from fat should not exceed 25 to 30 percent of the total energy. Since fatty foods are slow to leave the stomach, they sometimes cause nausea and indigestion if eaten shortly before competition. High fat, low carbohydrate diets can also deplete muscle and liver glycogen stores and compromise endurance and muscle strength. Active persons should be advised on how to identify and how to avoid high carbohydrate foods that also contain large amounts of hidden fat.

Fluid and Electrolyte Replacement

The most serious consequence of heavy sweating, which may accompany exercise, is the loss of body water. A replacement of fluids during exercise of at least 50 percent of the predicted weight loss is adequate to prevent heat illnesses on performance decrements. To prevent dehydration, Table 3–3 offers guidelines for fluid replacement before, during, and after exercise.

Thirst is not considered a reliable indicator of the water needs.[1,6,7,8] Therefore, it is suggested that athletes weigh themselves before and after an event, then drink 1 pint of fluid for every pound lost. After recreational activity, it

TABLE 3–3 Suggested Times and Intervals for Fluid Ingestion Before, During, and After Exercise[4]

Time or Interval of Ingestion for Competition or Workout	Amount to Ingest
2 hr prior to competition or workout	16 to 20 oz fluid
10–20 min prior to competition or workout	16 to 20 oz fluid
At 10- to 15-min intervals during competition or workout	4 to 6 oz fluid
After competition or workout	Replace each pound of weight lost with 16 oz of fluid

may be more practical to drink a greater amount of water than might be necessary to satisfy the thirst.

Plain, cold fluids cool and hydrate the body best because they leave the stomach faster than warm liquids.[6,7] Fluids that contain sugar in the form of glucose, fructose, or sucrose at concentrations greater than 2.5 percent slow gastric emptying and should not be encouraged. Many popular drinks contain 5 percent glucose solutions and are contraindicated for this reason.

On the other hand, trained athletes who exercise for at least 2 hours may benefit from glucose polymer drinks. These solutions have a lower osmolality than sports drinks that contain high concentrations of simple sugars. Therefore, they do not induce gastrointestinal distress and are absorbed almost as rapidly as plain water.[9] Glucose polymers aid endurance athletes by maintaining adequate blood sugar while preventing dehydration because they provide an easily absorbed carbohydrate.

Sweat is hypotonic and contains sodium at approximately 40 mEq per per liter and potassium at approximately 3 mEq per per liter.[2,10] In most situations, both sodium and potassium losses can be easily replaced by eating a variety of foods after competition. Salt tablets should not be recommended because they can irritate the gastric mucosa and cause nausea and vomiting. High concentrations of sodium can draw water into the stomach, further inducing dehydration.[7] Commercial electrolyte replacements are therefore not necessary. In extreme situations where fluid losses exceed 3 L per day, sodium and other electrolytes should be individually assessed and replaced.[5]

Vitamins and Minerals

There is little evidence to suggest that vitamin supplementation, in the absence of a specific vitamin deficiency, is necessary for active individuals.[11,12] Athletes as well as nonathletes should avoid taking large doses of vitamins and concentrate on eating nutritionally balanced meals. Women who exercise regularly may have greater requirements for riboflavin.[13] However, supplementation does not appear to enhance performance by improving maximum oxygen consumption.[14] Further research is needed in this area.[4]

An iron deficiency can impair physical performance, and manifests itself most often in distance runners or in endurance athletes.[15] Strenuous physical exercise may create a state of hemodilution and a low hemoglobin concentration as a normal physiologic response.[15] This low hemoglobin level should be carefully distinguished from a true anemia. Rigorous running regimens may cause small intestinal losses of blood that may, over time, result in iron depletion. Therefore, some experts suggest endurance athletes double their RDA for iron.[1] Other athletes who are at high risk for iron deficiency include menstruating females, children, vegetarians, and other individuals who do not meet their iron needs through diet.[11] Consequently, iron supplementation as ferrous sulfate may be advisable. However, the need for iron supplementation should be determined by a physician after an evaluation of the hematology status and of the diet history.

The calcium needs of the athlete are no greater than the needs of the non-athlete.[11] However, since calcium intake is frequently inadequate for many people, the athlete should also be advised regarding sufficient dietary calcium to promote proper bone growth and to maintain adequate bone density. Counseling should determine individual calcium requirements after assessing the factors that influence calcium retention or absorption.

Drugs and Special Dietary Supplements

During endurance activities, the availability of muscle glycogen is a critical factor. Caffeine mobilizes free fatty acids, thereby exerting a glycogen sparing effect.[4,8,16] However, because caffeine may also trigger adverse physiologic responses, controversy exists regarding the use of this drug in exercise. The American College of Sports Medicine and the American Orthopedic Society for Sports Medicine do not advocate caffeine tablets or caffeine-containing stimulants to enhance performance. Caffeine is also banned as an illegal drug for international competition.[17]

Although illegal, anabolic steroids are popular among many athletes who desire a large muscle mass. There is little scientific evidence that anabolic steroids enhance aerobic work capacity.[18,19] In addition, such steroids may lead to liver damage, liver cancer, cardiovascular disease, mood changes, masculinizing effects in women, and testicular atrophy with temporary sterility in men.[20]

There is no evidence that "ergogenic" foods such as amino acids, wheat germ, wheat germ oil, lecithin, bee pollen, gelatin, honey, kelp, brewer's yeast, pangamic acid, ginseng, or sunflower seeds improve physical performance.[4]

The Pre-Competition Meal

What an athlete eats before competition is both physically and psychologically important. It is not a time to experiment with new foods or eating styles. The purpose of the meal is to prevent hunger during the competition in a way that is both pleasant and satisfying. The meal should be eaten 3 1/2 to 4 hours before the event to ensure gastric emptying and to avoid discomfort or cramping.[4] The meal may range from 300 to 1,000 Kcal and should consist primarily of complex carbohydrates.[4]

REFERENCES

1. Manjarrez C, Birrer R. Nutrition and athletic performance. Am Fam Phys 1983;28:105–115.
2. Nelson R. Nutrition and physical performance. Presentation for the 22nd AMA National Conference on the medical aspects of sports. January 24, 1981.
3. Sherman WM. Carbohydrate, muscle glycogen, and improved performance. Phys Sports Med 1987;15:157–164.
4. Nutrition for physical fitness and athletic performance for adults: Technical support paper. J Am Diet Assoc 1987;87:934–939.
5. Sports and cardiovascular nutritionists dietetic practice group. Sports nutrition. Marcus JB, ed. Chicago: American Dietetic Association, 1986.

6. Costill DL, Grisolfi C, Murphy RJ, Westerman RL. Balancing heat stress, fluids, and electrolytes. Phys Sports Med 1975;43:43–52.

7. Food power: a coach's guide to improving performance. Nat Dairy Council, 1984.

8. O'Neil FT, Hynak-Hankinson MT, Gorman J. Research and application of current topics in sports nutrition. J Am Diet Assoc 1986;86:1007–1015.

9. Seiple R, Vivian V. Gastric-emptying characteristics of two glucose polymer-electrolyte solutions. Med Sci Sports Exerc 1983;15:366–369.

10. Costill DL, Miller J. Nutrition for endurance sport: carbohydrate and fluid balance. Int J Sports Med 1980;1:2–14.

11. A statement by the American Dietetic Association. Nutrition and physical fitness. J Am Diet Assoc 1980;76:437–443.

12. Grandjean AC. Vitamins, diet, and the athlete. Clin Sports Med 1983;2:105–115.

13. Belko AZ, Obarzanek E, Roach M, Rotter R, Urban G, Weinberg S, Roe DA. Effects of aerobic exercise and weight loss on riboflavin requirements of moderately obese, marginally deficient young women. Am J Clin Nutr 1984;40:553–561.

14. Belko M, Kalward HJ, Obarzanek E, Weinberg S, Roach R, McKeon G, Roe DA. Effects of exercise on riboflavin requirements: Biological validation in weight-reducing women. Am J Clin Nutr 1985;41:270–277.

15. Selby GB, Eichner ER. Endurances swimming, intravascular hemolysis, anemia, and iron depletion. New perspective on athletes anemia. Am J Med 1986;81:791–794.

16. Wilmore JH, Freund BJ. Nutritional enhancement of athletic performance. Nutr Abstr and Rev Clin Nutr 1984;54:1–16.

17. Sherman WM, Costill DL. The marathon: dietary manipulation to optimize performance. Am J Sports Med 1984;12:44–50.

18. Lamb DR. Anabolic steroids in athletics: how well do they work and how dangerous are they? Am J Sports Med 1984;12:31–36.

19. Haupt HA, Rovere GD. Anabolic steroids: a review of the literature. Am J Sports Med 1984;12:469–483.

20. Martikainen H, Alen M, Rahkila P, Vihko R. Testicular response to human chorionic gonadotrophin during transient hypogonadotrophic hypogonadism induced by androgenic/anabolic steroids in power athletes. J Steroid Biochem 1986;25:109–112.

GERIATRIC NUTRITION

General Description

The aging process is a continuum throughout adult life marked by the steady deterioration in bodily functions and by the accumulation of chronic disabilities and of diseases. The rate of the aging process is influenced by genetic and by environmental forces and differs among individuals from physiologic, psychological, and social viewpoints. Thus, chronologic age by itself becomes less reliable as an index of the physiologic or the psychological condition when nutritional needs of the geriatric population are determined.[1]

Factors Affecting Nutritional Status Of The Elderly. There is a general agreement that metabolic, physiologic, and biochemical processes change with increasing age, and these changes tend to have an adverse effect on the nutritional status of the elderly (Table 3–4). A decrease in the acuity of taste, of smell, and of vision may interfere with the act of eating and with the enjoyment of food. The loss of teeth and poorly fitting dentures further interfere with eating. The digestion and the absorption of nutrients are affected by a decrease in the secretion of stomach acid, a delay in gastric emptying, a diminished secretion of enzymes in the small intestine, and a decrease in peristalsis. The cardiac output declines along with the capacity of the cardiovascular system to respond to stress. The kidney size and the number of functioning nephrons decrease with age, which causes a diminished capacity to eliminate metabolic waste products. Liver size decreases, and there is a progressive loss in the liver's functional capacity. Changes in body composition also occur with age. Lean body mass decreases, and adipose tissue increases. A lower metabolic rate and a decline in carbohydrate tolerance render the older person vulnerable to obesity and diabetes.

TABLE 3–4 Physiologic Changes with Aging

Physiologic Changes	Potential Impact on Nutritional Status
Decreased salivary secretion; atrophic taste buds	Decreased taste sensation, anorexia, dry mouth → decreased food intake
Decreased sense of smell	Decreased taste sensation, foods lose appeal → decreased food intake
Missing teeth, periodontitis	Poorly fitting dentures cause difficulty chewing → restricted variety of or decreased food intake. Dentures interfere with sense of taste → food loses appeal → decreased food intake
Impaired vision and hearing	Interferes with socialization at mealtimes, difficulty in food preparation → diminished enjoyment of food → decreased intake
Decreased secretion of acid in stomach, enzymes in small intestine, and decreased peristalsis	Diminished digestion and absorption of nutrients
Decreased capacity of kidney to concentrate urine	Dehydration
Decreased lean body mass, increased adipose tissue, lower metabolic rate	Vulnerable to obesity
Decline in glucose tolerance	Vulnerable to development of diabetes → restricted dietary selections → decreased food intake

Other factors that may alter the food intake and, consequently, the nutritional status are socioeconomic in nature. Social isolation, limited financial resources, lack of education regarding nutrition, minority status, lack of family support, and decreased mobility that results from physical disabilities or from neighborhood safety concerns can lessen the availability of a selection of foods. Frequently, the elderly are dependent on others for care, and this dependency may result in the potential for abuse, such as the withholding of food or the providing of inadequate or unacceptable food. Food items in large packages and information labels that are difficult to read and to interpret can contribute to inappropriate food purchasing. The elderly are also susceptible to the misleading claims of advertisers and may unnecessarily use nutritional supplements and over the counter drugs.

The presence of chronic diseases, such as diabetes, hypertension, or arthritis, and associated diet or drug therapy contribute further to the potential for inadequate nutrition in the elderly. Many commonly used drugs may interfere with digestion, with absorption, or with the utilization or the excretion of essential nutrients. Drugs also have an effect on appetite, on taste, and on smell acuity (see *Appendix* 2). Alcohol abuse may be a further contributor to malnutrition in the elderly by way of its effect on the nutrient absorption and by its displacement of nutrient dense foods in the diet.

Special Dietary Considerations. Physician-prescribed and self-imposed diets in the elderly population are common because of the frequency of chronic diseases. However, each therapeutic dietary modification limits the selection of foods available to the individual. The psychological effects of having favorite foods restricted, the loss of flavor by the elimination of customary seasonings, and the alterations in meal preparation methods may have an adverse effect on the desire to eat. In an institutional setting, the elderly person's loss of control of any food selection may be disruptive enough that he or she no longer enjoys eating. The resulting decreased food consumption can be detrimental to the maintenance of a sound nutritional state.

Dietary modifications should be imposed only when such an intervention can be expected to result in a significant health improvement.[2,3] The benefits of aggressive therapeutic dietary measures must be balanced with the elderly person's willingness and ability to comply with dietary changes. Dietary modifications, such as the avoidance of saturated fats and cholesterol, are generally less beneficial when initiated late in life. However, one should consider the reassuring effect of continuing previously established dietary restrictions that are directed toward a progressive disease.

Nutritional Needs Of The Elderly. The information that is available to determine the specific requirements of essential nutrients for the elderly is inconclusive.[2,4–7] Based on the data available, the nutrient requirements of the aging population do not seem to be significantly different than the RDAs for the younger adult. However, there is some evidence that an increased need for protein in the elderly exists above the current RDA level of 0.8 g per kilogram per day.[8]

There are diminished energy needs with aging because of (1) the decreases in lean body mass, (2) the lower metabolic rate, and (3) the decrease of physical activity. However, a concern for the very old is that the amounts of food that are consumed are not enough to meet even these decreased energy requirements. The lower energy requirement, coupled with the same RDAs as for younger adults, has been used as an argument for a more nutrient dense diet, but if the convention were to express RDA per 1,000 kilocalories expended by the individual, the apparent need for a greater nutrient density would disappear.

Although vitamin and mineral deficiencies are presumed to be more common in the elderly, there are few experimental data on which to estimate the exact dietary requirements of the micronutrients. An increased need, with age, for vitamins and for minerals may result from less efficient absorption, from more frequent illness, and perhaps from the use of certain medications. The administration of specific vitamin or mineral supplements should be based on need and defined by clinical and by biochemical assessment of the nutritional status.

Constipation is one of the most frequent gastrointestinal complaints of the elderly owing to diminished muscle tone and to decreased peristalsis. Dietary fiber should be increased in addition to the consumption of six to eight glasses of water daily. Mineral oil should be avoided since it may contribute to vitamin A and D losses.

The heterogeneity of the older population must not be overlooked. Nutritional assessment of the elderly and recommendations for nutritional care should consider individual abilities, capabilities, and levels of function. The presence

Continuum of Nutrition Care for Older Americans	
Community-Based Long-Term Care	
Obstacle to Adequate Intake	Nutrition Service
Lack of socialization, motivation, income, or physical strength to prepare meals	—Congregate nutrition program (1 hot lunch 5–7 days)
	—Nutrition education: importance of nutrition; motivational activities; easy, inexpensive, and nutritious meals; special requirements (e.g., low sodium, ethnic)
Limited income	—Congregate meals + Food Stamps or other income supplement
	—Congregate meals + nutrition education: increasing food purchasing power, low-cost, and nutritious meals
Limited access to food stores, inability to carry groceries	—Congregate meals + transportation (with assistance) to food store
Physical inability to food shop	—Congregate meals + food shopping services
	—Congregate meals + delivery of basic food supplies every two weeks
Inability to participate in congregate nutrition program, limited ability to prepare foods; can reheat foods	—Home delivery of prepared frozen or shelf-stable foods every two weeks or once a month
	—Nutrition education: maintaining intake at home
	—Home health aide for meal preparation
	—Home delivery of chilled prepared foods every 2–3 days
Limited socialization	—Telephone assurance, friendly visitors, or equivalent program
Inability to safely prepare foods	—Home-delivered nutrition services: hot, daily delivery of 1 meal; provision of ready-to-eat food for remainder of meals or home health aide/neighbor/ family assistance
	—Nutrition education for family/caregivers
	—Adult day care programs with nutrition services
Severe physical or mental debilitation	—Home health aide assistance with feeding
	—Nutrition education for family/caregivers
	—Hospice care including dietary counseling
Institutionalization	

Figure 3–3 Continuum of nutrition care for older Americans; community-based long-term care.[9] Copyright The American Dietetic Association. Reprinted with permission from ADA takes proactive stance, testifies on Older Americans Act Reauthorization. J Am Diet Assoc 1984;84:822–835.

or the absence of chronic diseases, the general health, and the amount of physical activity may affect dietary requirements of the older person. Whether the individual is living independently or in an institution, such as a nursing home, should also be considered in planning the dietary requirements for elderly persons.[9,10] The American Dietetic Association has proposed a continuum of nutrition care for older adults based on their level of independence (Fig. 3–3).

REFERENCES

1. Morley JE. Nutritional status of the elderly. Am J Med 1986;81:679–698.
2. Gastineau CF. Nutrition and aging. In: Spitell JA, ed. Clinical medicine. Philadelphia: Harper and Row, 1984:1.
3. Luros E. A rational approach to geriatric nutrition. Ross Dietetic Currents 1983; 6:1–4.
4. Munro HN. Nutrition and the elderly: a general overview. J Am Coll Nutr 1984;3:341–350.
5. Schneider EL, Vining EM, Hadley EC, Farnham SA. Recommended dietary allowances and the health of the elderly. N Engl J Med 1986;314:157–160.
6. Young EA. Nutrition, aging and the aged. Symposium on clinical geriatric medicine. Med Clin North Am 1983;67:295–313.
7. Watkin DM. Nutrition for the aging and aged. In: Goodhart RS, Shils ME, eds. Modern nutrition in health and disease. 6th ed. Philadelphia: Lea & Febiger, 1980:781.
8. Gersovitz M, Motil K, Munro HN, Scrimshaw NS, Young VR. Human protein requirements: assessment of the adequacy of the current RDA for dietary protein in elderly men and women. Am J Clin Nutr 1982;35:6–14.
9. ADA takes proactive stance, testifies on Older Americans Act Reauthorization. J Am Diet Assoc 1984;84:822–835.
10. Lecos C. Diet and the elderly. FDA Consumer 1984; September:22–25.

VEGETARIAN DIET

General Description

Vegetarianism is interesting an increasing number of people for reasons of health, of economy, of religion, of ecology, or of philosophy. This term embraces a variety of dietary practices. Vegetarian diets are most frequently classified (Table 3–5) according to the extent by which animal foods are excluded.

TABLE 3–5 Classification of Vegetarian Diets[1]

Total vegetarians or "vegan" eat only foods of plant origin
Fruitarians consume only raw or dried fruits and nuts, honey and/or olive oil
Lactovegetarians eat plant foods plus milk and other dairy products
Lacto-ovovegetarians consume plant foods, milk and dairy products, and eggs
Semivegetarians or partial vegetarians* consume some groups of animal foods but not all

*Meat is usually excluded; either poultry or fish and seafood may be excluded. This category includes persons who are nonred meat eaters and/or may exclude some animal food groups completely; because of this, semivegetarians often consider themselves vegetarians.

The reader is referred to section on *Vegetarian Diet*, page 311 for a discussion on vegetarian diets for infants, for children, and for adolescents.

Nutritional Inadequacy

The American Dietetic Association recognizes that well-planned vegetarian diets can be consistent with a good nutritional intake.[1] The extent to which food selection and feeding patterns meet the dietary recommendations for an individual is dependent upon the type of vegetarian diet chosen and upon the degree of careful food selection and meal planning. Nutrients that may be limited or lacking in vegetarian diets are high quality protein, vitamin B_{12}, vitamin D, riboflavin, calcium, zinc, and iron. An individual's intake should be assessed for nutritional adequacy and supplemented accordingly.

In addition, there are times when individuals may be physiologically stressed and at nutritional risk if vegetarian diets are not carefully planned. Such periods of physiologic stress include pregnancy and lactation, growth (see section on *Vegetarian Diet*, page 311), and when health problems or disease limit the intake or increase the nutrient requirements beyond normal.

Goals of Dietary Management

The nutritional goal in vegetarianism is to achieve an intake that meets all known nutrient needs. A well-planned diet that consists of a variety of largely unrefined plant foods supplemented with some milk and eggs (lacto-ovovegetarian diet) meets all known nutrient needs. A total dietary intake of plant foods can be made adequate by careful planning. Give proper attention to specific nutrients that may be in a less available form or in a lower concentration or absent in plant foods.[1]

Dietary Recommendations

Lacto-ovovegetarian and lactovegetarian diets are nutritionally sound, but a conscious effort must be made to select the proper foods in sufficient amounts to maintain optimal weight and health. If selected appropriately, these diets are also adequate in meeting the needs induced by the stress of growth, of pregnancy, and of lactation.

Care must be taken in planning the "pure" vegetarian diet, since this diet lacks concentrated sources of a single protein with desirable proportions of essential amino acids and also is limited in calcium, iron, zinc, riboflavin, vitamin B_{12}, and vitamin D.

Protein. Plant proteins have a lower biologic value than do proteins of animal origin. The biologic value of a protein is defined as its ability to support growth and to maintain body structure, and this ability depends on the number, the proportion, and the type of amino acids the protein contains. The proteins of legumes, of whole grains, of nuts, and of vegetables contain all the essential amino acids, but yield certain ones at lower levels than do proteins of animal origin. The lower biologic value of plant proteins is the result of low levels of one or more of the essential amino acids. However, when plant proteins from a variety of sources are consumed, supplementation occurs and results in a mixture of all essential amino acids in proportions similar to those found in proteins of animal origin. Vegetable mixtures that supply the essential amino acids in appropriate proportions are as efficient as proteins of animal origin in meeting the protein needs at minimal levels of intake.[2] In fact when different proteins are combined in appropriate ways, vegetable proteins cannot be distinguished nutritionally from those of animal origin. Therefore, the amino acid profile that is derived from the mixture of proteins and not the origin or "value" of a single protein should be considered as the criterion whether the protein needs are being met in vegetarian diets.

The sources of protein must be combined in such a way that the amount and the proportion of amino acids that result support normal growth and maintenance. To supply enough derived protein of high biologic value that contains all the essential amino acids in desirable proportions, meals should consist of a combination of grains and legumes, of grains and nuts or seeds, or of grains and vegetables.

Vitamin B₁₂. The lacto-ovovegetarian and the lactovegetarian categories, in general, have an adequate intake of vitamin B_{12}. Vitamin B_{12} is not present in plant foods in large enough amounts to be considered a significant dietary source. However, some persons eating "pure" vegetarian or vegan diets appear to remain in good health for many years, or nearly a lifetime, without developing symptoms of deficiency. Others are forced to use supplementary vitamin B_{12} or to adopt a lactovegetarian or lacto-ovovegetarian diet after a few months or a few years. The reason for this variation is not clear, and the results of nutritional studies are not uniform. Supplementary vitamin B_{12} for the "pure" vegetarian can be obtained from soybean milk (fortified with vitamin B_{12}) or commercial meat analogues (fortified with vitamin B_{12}).

Riboflavin, Calcium, Vitamin D, Iron, and Zinc. The lacto-ovovegetarians are able to meet their needs for calcium and for riboflavin from dairy products, while the pure vegetarian's intake of these elements may only be marginal. Sources of calcium for the vegetarian include dark green leafy vegetables (avoid those high in oxalic acid, such as spinach, chard, and beet greens), some nuts and seeds, and fortified soybean milk. Those individuals who may not consume milk or soybean milk in adequate quantities may need supplemental calcium (see the section on *Osteoporosis*). Vitamin D may be obtained by the exposure of the skin to sunlight or by supplementation.

The absorptional availability of iron and of zinc can be influenced by a number of dietary maneuvers. One can increase the use of fortified grains and cereals, but limit those high in bran and in phytates since phytic acid tends to reduce iron and zinc absorption. The proportion of the iron that is available for absorption can be increased by including a source of ascorbic acid at the same meal. Finally, it is important to recommend good food sources of iron (enriched cereals and grains, legumes, dates, prunes and raisins, greens) and of zinc (leavened breads, legumes and nuts, spinach) and to emphasize their inclusion in each meal (see also *Vegetarian Diet,* Table 8–10 on page 313).

Planning and Evaluating Vegetarian Diets

Table 3–6 presents a scheme for planning a nutritionally adequate vegetarian diet.[3] It can also be utilized to evaluate the adequacy of vegetarian dietary practices.

Whole grains and their products ("A" box) should be used in generous amounts in any vegetarian diet. They are sources of protein, of iron, and of riboflavin in addition to being the complementary protein to the legumes ("B" box), the nuts and the seeds ("C" box), and the vegetables ("D" box). In order to yield a balance of amino acids, a meal pattern should include food from the "A" box and a supplementing protein from the "B", the "C", or the "D" box. If a particular meal in a day's pattern does not include a selection of food from the "A" box, the resulting amino acid mixture is not in balance, and the diet should be supplemented either by eggs or by dairy products or by food from the appropriate protein box.

Table 3–7 is a modification to the basic four food guide that may be useful in planning vegetarian diets for pregnancy and for lactation.[4]

TABLE 3–6 AD-BAC Protein Complement Guide[3]

	D Vegetables	
B Legumes	A Whole Grains & Cereals	C Nuts & Seeds

"A" Box—Whole Grains and Cereals	Limiting Amino Acids[4]
Wheat	Lysine, threonine
Rye	(sometimes tryptophan)
Barley	
Corn	
Millet	
Oats	
Rice	
Buckwheat	
Triticale	
Bulgur	
"B" Box—Legumes	
Peanuts	Methionine, tryptophan
Peas	
Mung beans	
Broad beans	
Black-eyed peas	
Lentils	
Lima beans	
Soybeans	
Black beans	
Kidney beans	
Garbanzos (chick peas)	
Navy beans	
"C" Box—Nuts and Seeds	
Cashews	Lysine
Pistachios	
Walnuts	
Brazil nuts	
Almonds	
Pecans	
Pumpkin seeds	
Squash seeds	
Sunflower seeds	
Sesame seeds	
Filberts	
Pine nuts	
"D" Box—Vegetables	
Potato	Methionine
Dark green vegetables	
Other vegetables	

Physicians: How to Order Diet

The diet order should indicate *vegetarian diet*. The dietitian determines food preferences and establishes a nutritionally adequate diet.

TABLE 3–7 Modified Basic Four Food Guide for Vegetarian Diets[5]

Food Group	Number of Servings	
	Adult	Pregnancy or Lactation
Milk and milk products, and fortified soybean milk	4	4+
Protein foods		
Legumes	2	2
Nuts	1	1+
Whole grain products and enriched cereals	6	6
Vegetables and fruits		
Rich in vitamin C	3	3
Dark green	$1\frac{1}{2}$	$1\frac{1}{2}$
Other	3	3

REFERENCES

1. ADA Reports. Position paper on the vegetarian approach to eating. J Am Diet Assoc 1980;77:61–69.
2. Bressani R, Behar M. The use of plant protein foods in preventing malnutrition. In: Edinburgh E, Livingstone S, eds. Proceedings of the 6th International Congress of Nutrition. 1964:182.
3. Pemberton CM, Gastineau CF. Vegetarian diets. In: Pemberton CM, Gastineau CF, eds. Mayo Clinic Diet Manual. 5th ed. Philadelphia: W B Saunders, 1981:16.
4. Hui YH. Principles and issues in nutrition. Monterey, CA: Wadsworth Division, 1985:143.
5. King JC, Cohenour SH, Corruccini CG, Schneeman P. Evaluation and modification of the basic four food guide. J Nutr Ed 1978;10:27–29.

JEWISH DIETARY PRACTICES

The following discussion of Jewish dietary habits is presented to promote better understanding and to facilitate service to the patient who follows kosher practices. The Mayo Clinic and its associated hospitals do not have a kosher food service. Commercially prepared kosher dinners (regular and salt-free) are available.

"Kosher" means "fit." The term refers to foods that can be eaten in accordance with Jewish dietary laws, which include specific foods and food combinations that are allowed or prohibited. The stringency with which these practices are followed varies among communities and among individuals.

1. Meat and poultry must be slaughtered and processed in a specified manner to be kosher. Proper kosher procedure involves soaking the meat in water for at least 30 minutes and then salting the meat with kosher salt; an alternative method is to broil the meat until it is well done. Kosher meat may come only from cloven-hooved animals (such as cows, sheep, and goats) that graze and chew their cud. Pork is not allowed.

2. Only fish with fins and scales are permitted; shellfish and eels are not allowed.

3. Dairy and meat products may not be eaten at the same meal. Dairy products may be eaten just before a meal that contains meat; there should be

an interval of 3 to 6 hours after a meal that contains meat before dairy products may be consumed again.

4. Separate facilities for food preparation and separate dishes and utensils for food service should be used for meat and for dairy foods. In a nonkosher food service, disposable dishes and utensils may be used for serving the food; disposable foil containers may be used for heating foods.

5. Leavened bread products are not allowed for 8 days during Passover. Foods leavened with eggs or with steam may be used. During Passover, bread products are unleavened and are made from specially approved flour.

6. Most fruits, vegetables, fish, eggs, grains, coffees, and teas are "pareve," meaning "inherently kosher." They may be eaten in any combination with other foods. Therefore, nondairy creamers, margarine, and soy products may be included in meals that contain either meat or milk products. (Grape juice and any jams or jellies that contain grapes are kosher only if the preparation is supervised.)

7. Symbols are used on processed foods to certify that the food is kosher. These include the emblem Ⓤ, copyrighted by the Union of Orthodox Jewish Congregations; the letter K, indicating rabbinical supervision by the individual company (not always approved by Orthodox rabbis; each item should be cleared with a local rabbi for suitability); the emblem Ⓚ, copyrighted by the Organized Kasrus Laboratories; ⓋⒽ, the emblem used by Vaad-Harobonim of Massachusetts; ⓂⓀ, the emblem used by Montreal Vaad-Hair; Ⓒ.Ⓞ.Ⓡ., copyrighted emblem of the Council of Orthodox Rabbis of Toronto; and △C.R.C., emblem of the Chicago Rabbinical Council.

8. Some therapeutic food products and some dietary supplements are permissible for those who follow kosher practices. For information on the acceptability of a particular product, ask a rabbi or the Union of Orthodox Jewish Congregations of America, 84 Fifth Avenue, New York, New York.

9. Nonkosher food products may be used if they are considered to be essential to the treatment of an extremely ill person. A rabbi should be consulted on this or on any similar matter.

10. There is a toll-free Kosher hotline where questions on Jewish dietary practices can be answered:

> 1 (800) 843-8825 (outside New York)
> 1 (914) 667-1001 (inside New York)
> through
> Union for Traditional Conservative Judaism
> 145 North Fifth Avenue
> Mount Vernon, NY 10550

CHAPTER 4

GUIDES FOR MEAL PLANNING AND PROMOTION OF WELLNESS

BASIC FOUR FOOD GUIDE

The Basic Four Food Guide or the Four Food Groups were developed by the United States Department of Agriculture (USDA) in the mid 1950s.[1] These food groups were designed to aid individuals in their selection of appropriate types and amounts of foods that would form the foundation of an adequate diet. A subsequent revision took place in 1979 when the USDA added a fifth food group that allowed for increased energy needs that are essential for growth, for activity, and for the maintenance of a desirable weight. There continues to be some debate as to whether or not this food guide, if followed, provides the essential amounts of all nutrients, and whether the guide functions as an effective communication tool in nutrition education programs today.

The Four Food Groups were never intended to be a complete diet, but to serve as a foundation for meal planning. Nearly 80 percent of the protein, the vitamin, and the mineral (except iron) needs are met by this plan, and the caloric levels are approximately sufficient to meet basal energy requirements. Portion sizes should be modified for preschool, for school children, and for teenagers. To fully meet the energy needs, more servings from the Four Food Groups or from others may be selected.

REFERENCES

1. Essentials of Adequate Diet, USDA, Home Economics Report No. 3, Agricultural Research Service, United States Department of Agriculture, 1957.
2. Science and Education Administration. Food, Home and Garden Bulletin No. 228. United States Department Agriculture. Superintendent of Documents. U.S. Government Printing Office, Washington, D.C., 1980.
3. Anon. How to eat for good health. Rosemont, IL: National Dairy Council, 1986.

Daily Food Guide[2,3]

Milk Group	*Minimum Number of Servings*	*Serving Size—Food Selections*
Children < 9	2–3	1 cup milk
Children 9–12	3	1 cup yogurt (plain)
Teenagers	4	$1\frac{1}{2}$ oz cheese
Adults	2	2 cups cottage cheese
Pregnant Women	3	$1\frac{3}{4}$ cup ice cream or ice milk
Nursing Mothers	4	4 Tbsp cheese spread or Parmesan cheese

Meat Group	*Minimum Number of Servings*	*Serving Size—Food Selections*
Children	2	2–3 oz cooked lean meat, poultry or fish.
Teenagers	2	2 eggs
Adults	2	$1–1\frac{1}{2}$ cup dried peas or beans
Pregnant Women	3	1/2–1 cup nuts and seeds
Nursing Mothers	2	4 Tbsp of peanut butter

Fruit and Vegetable Group	*Minimum Number of Servings*	*Serving Size—Food Selections*
Children	4	1/2 cup juice
Teenagers	4	1/2 cup fruit or vegetable (canned, cooked)
Adults	4	1 cup fruit or vegetable (raw)
Pregnant Women	4	Medium size fresh fruit
Nursing Mothers	4	1/2 grapefruit or cantaloupe

Grain Group	*Minimum Number of Servings*	*Serving Size—Food Selections*
Children	4	1 slice bread
Teenagers	4	1 cup ready-to-eat cereal
Adults	4	1/2 cup cooked cereal or grits
Pregnant Women	4	1/2 cup rice
Nursing Mothers	4	1/2 cup pasta

Fats–Sweets– Alcohol	*Minimum Number of Servings*	*Serving Size—Food Selections*
	Select if additional calories are needed, after eating the recommended number of servings from the above groups.	1 tsp margarine or butter
		1 tsp sugar
		1 Tbsp mayonnaise, salad dressing
		1 Tbsp jelly
		1 cup soft drink
		$3\frac{1}{2}$ oz wine
		1/6 of 9-in pie
		1/16 of 9-in pie

DIETARY GUIDELINES FOR AMERICANS

The United States Senate Select Committee on Nutrition and Human Needs issued the Dietary Goals for the United States in 1977 with the intent of encouraging healthy eating habits. In 1980 the United States Department of Agriculture and the United States Department of Health and Human Services is-sued *Nutrition and Your Health: Dietary Guidelines for Americans* to provide practical dietary advice based on current research. In addition, the United States Senate Appropriations Committee requested that a Dietary Guidelines Advisory Committee be established to periodically review comments that are received and to incorporate new pertinent scientific data, thereby maintaining key references from which to derive the guidelines. The latest revision of the Dietary Guide-lines for Americans occurred in 1985 and appears below.[1]

1. Eat a variety of foods.
2. Maintain an ideal weight.
3. Avoid too much fat, too much saturated fat, and too much cholesterol.
4. Eat foods with adequate starch and fiber.
5. Avoid too much sugar.
6. Avoid too much sodium.
7. If you drink alcohol, do so in moderation.

These guidelines are for healthy people, not for people who need special diets because of diseases and conditions that interfere with normal nutrition.

REFERENCE

1. USDA and USDHHS. Nutrition and your health: Dietary guidelines for Americans, 2nd ed., Rev. August 1985. Home and Garden Bulletin No. 232, Washington, D.C.: USDA/USDHHS. August 1985.

AMERICAN HEART ASSOCIATION DIETARY RECOMMENDATIONS

Since 1957, there has been a deep interest on the part of the American Heart Association (AHA) to provide dietary guidelines that would prevent or reduce the incidence of coronary heart disease and of other atherosclerotic dis-eases. The first dietary recommendations were authorized by the AHA in 1961. Periodic reviews of the research data that describe the relationship of diet to coronary heart disease and the subsequent recommendations have been the re-sponsibility of the American Heart Association Nutrition Committee. State-ments from the AHA that regard diet and heart disease generally appear every 3 to 5 years. The 1986 AHA Dietary Guidelines for Healthy American Adults appear below.[1]

1. The saturated fat intake should be less than 10 percent of the total kilocalories.

2. The total fat intake should be less than 30 percent of the total kilo-calories.

3. The cholesterol intake should be less than 100 mg per 1,000 kilocalories and should not exceed 300 mg each day.

4. The protein intake should be approximately 15 percent of the total kilocalories.

5. The carbohydrate intake should constitute 50 to 55 percent or more of the total kilocalories with the emphasis on an increase of the complex carbohydrates.

6. The sodium intake should be reduced to approximately 1 g per 1,000 kilocalories and not exceed 3 g daily.

7. If alcoholic beverages are consumed, the caloric intake from this source should be limited to 15 percent of the total kilocalories, but should not exceed 50 ml of ethanol per day.

8. The total kilocalories should be of a sufficient amount to maintain the individual's best body weight.

9. A wide variety of foods should be consumed.

REFERENCE

1. American Heart Association. Dietary guidelines for healthy American adults. A statement for physicians and health professionals by the Nutrition Committee, American Heart Association, Dallas, TX, 1986.

DIET AND CANCER PROTECTION

The role of the diet and its effect on cancer risk has been one of great interest to the public.[1,2] In 1984 the National Cancer Institute and the American Cancer Society recommended the following dietary guidelines.[3,4] It is important to note that the Institutes' dietary recommendations are consistent with the United States Department of Agriculture, Department of Health and Human Services' dietary guidelines for Americans.

1. Achieve and keep a normal body weight. An excessive caloric intake and obesity have been linked to increased death rates for some cancers in humans, particularly those of the prostate, the pancreas, the breast, the ovary, the colon, the gallbladder, and the uterus.

2. Avoid too much fat, both saturated and unsaturated fats. Evidence from epidemiologic studies have shown a direct correlation between dietary fat levels and the occurrence of several cancers, especially prostate and colorectal cancer. Exact underlying mechanisms are far from clear. Recent reports suggest that dietary fat intake may, however, be unrelated to the incidence of breast cancer.[5] No level for the fat intake has been established, but it is believed the lower the fat intake, the more decreased the risk of cancer. A prudent guideline for the fat intake may be 30 percent of the total caloric intake.

3. Eat foods that are rich in fiber. The National Cancer Institute recommends a fiber intake of 25 to 35 g each day.[2] Dietary fiber appears to protect the body against some forms of cancer, particularly colorectal. Which specific types of fiber and how they may work are not clear at this point; therefore, fiber from all dietary sources, such as fresh fruits, vegetables, and whole grain products, are recommended on a daily basis.

4. Include foods rich in vitamins A and C daily. The carotenoids (plant precurser of vitamin A) and vitamin A have been found to decrease the incidence of a number of cancers, which includes those cancers of the oral cavity, the pharynx, the larynx, and the lung.

Animal studies show that ascorbic acid (vitamin C) can inhibit the formation of carcinogenic N-nitroso compounds from ingested nitrates, a well-known carcinogen.[6]

It is important to note that an adequate consumption of vitamin A or the carotenoids and vitamin C is important; no suggestion is made to consume levels higher than the U.S. RDA's.

5. Include cruciferous vegetables in your diet. Vegetables in this family include cabbage, broccoli, Brussels sprouts, kohlrabi, kale, cauliflower, mustard greens, and Swiss chard. Research has revealed that these foods appear to offer protection from the development of colorectal, of stomach, and of lung cancers.

6. Eat only moderate amounts of salt-cured, of smoked, and of nitrate-cured foods. The incidence of cancers of the esophagus and of the stomach are higher in those populations where large quantities of the aforementioned foods are consumed. Some cooking methods such as barbecuing, grilling, or smoking can also produce possible cancer-causing substances.

7. Keep alcohol consumption moderate if you drink. The consumption of large amounts of alcohol increases the risk of liver cancer. Alcohol intake that is accompanied by smoking or by chewing tobacco increases the risk of cancer of the mouth, of the larynx, of the throat, and of the esophagus. A limit of two or fewer drinks a day is recommended.

Further research is being conducted on the topic of nutrition and of cancer protection at this point. This research may provide more conclusive recommendations at a future date.

REFERENCES

1. Pariza M. Analyzing current recommendations on diet, nutrition and cancer. Food Nutr Jan/Feb 1986;58.
2. Heatley RV. Do dietary factors cause cancer in man? Clin Nutr 1985;4:1–6.
3. National Cancer Institute/Office of Cancer Communication. Statement—diet and cancer. May 1986.
4. American Cancer Society. Nutrition, common sense and cancer. 84-(2.5MM)-Rev. July 1985-No. 2096-LE. 1984.
5. Willett WC, Stampfer MJ, Colditz GA, Rosner BA, Hennekens CH, Sneizer FE. Dietary fat and the risk of breast cancer. N Engl J Med 1987;316:22–28.
6. Mettlin C. Dietary factors for cancer of specific sites. Surg Clin North Am (Nutr and Cancer I) 66:920–923.

RECOMMENDED DIETARY ALLOWANCES

The Recommended Dietary Allowances (RDA) were first established in 1941 by the National Research Council of the National Academy of Sciences as a "guide for planning and procuring food supplies for national defense" and to "provide standards serving as a goal for good nutrition." The Food and Nutrition Board of the National Research Council defines the recommended daily dietary allowances as the "suggested nutrient intake levels of various essential dietary components necessary for meeting the needs of most healthy persons." An attempt is made to publish the RDA every 5 years in order to allow for possible updating as new scientific data becomes available.

The function of the RDA has evolved with each revision. Some applications of the guide include its use in planning and in evaluating group and individual diets as well as feeding programs, in evaluating dietary survey data and other scientific research that establishes the U.S. RDAs used in food labeling, and in teaching about food and nutrition. The 1980 RDAs are presented in Table 4–1.[1] The 10th edition of the RDA is not yet available.

TABLE 4–1 FOOD AND NUTRITION BOARD, NATIONAL ACADEMY OF SCIENCES-NATIONAL RESEARCH COUNCIL RECOMMENDED DAILY DIETARY ALLOWANCES,[a] Revised 1980

Designed for the maintenance of good nutrition of practically all healthy people in the U.S.A.

	Age (yr)	Weight (kg)	Weight (lb)	Height (cm)	Height (in)	Protein (g)	Fat-Soluble Vitamins Vita-min A (µg RE)[b]	Vita-min D (µg)[c]	Vita-min E (mg α-TE)[d]	Water-Soluble Vitamins Vita-min C (mg)	Thia-min (mg)	Ribo-flavin (mg)	Niacin (mg NE)[e]	Vita-min B6 (mg)	Fola-cin (µg)[f]	Vitamin B12 (µg)	Minerals Cal-cium (mg)	Phos-phorus (mg)	Mag-nesium (mg)	Iron (mg)	Zinc (mg)	Iodine (µg)
Infants	0.0–0.5	6	13	60	24	kg × 2.2	420	10	3	35	0.3	0.4	6	0.3	30	0.5[g]	360	240	50	10	3	40
	0.5–1.0	9	20	71	28	kg × 2.0	400	10	4	35	0.5	0.6	8	0.6	45	1.5	540	360	70	15	5	50
Children	1–3	13	29	90	35	23	400	10	5	45	0.7	0.8	9	0.9	100	2.0	800	800	150	15	10	70
	4–6	20	44	112	44	30	500	10	6	45	0.9	1.0	11	1.3	200	2.5	800	800	200	10	10	90
	7–10	28	62	132	52	34	700	10	7	45	1.2	1.4	16	1.6	300	3.0	800	800	250	10	10	120
Males	11–14	45	99	157	62	45	1,000	10	8	50	1.4	1.6	18	1.8	400	3.0	1,200	1,200	350	18	15	150
	15–18	66	145	176	69	56	1,000	10	10	60	1.4	1.7	18	2.0	400	3.0	1,200	1,200	400	18	15	150
	19–22	70	154	177	70	56	1,000	7.5	10	60	1.5	1.7	19	2.2	400	3.0	800	800	350	10	15	150
	23–50	70	154	178	70	56	1,000	5	10	60	1.4	1.6	18	2.2	400	3.0	800	800	350	10	15	150
	51+	70	154	178	70	56	1,000	5	10	60	1.2	1.4	16	2.2	400	3.0	800	800	350	10	15	150
Females	11–14	46	101	157	62	46	800	10	8	50	1.1	1.3	15	1.8	400	3.0	1,200	1,200	300	18	15	150
	15–18	55	120	163	64	46	800	10	8	60	1.1	1.3	14	2.0	400	3.0	1,200	1,200	300	18	15	150
	19–22	55	120	163	64	44	800	7.5	8	60	1.1	1.3	14	2.0	400	3.0	800	800	300	18	15	150
	23–50	55	120	163	64	44	800	5	8	60	1.0	1.2	13	2.0	400	3.0	800	800	300	18	15	150
	51+	55	120	163	64	44	800	5	8	60	1.0	1.2	13	2.0	400	3.0	800	800	300	10	15	150
Pregnant						+30	+200	+5	+2	+20	+0.4	+0.3	+2	+0.6	+400	+1.0	+400	+400	+150	h	+5	+25
Lactating						+20	+400	+5	+3	+40	+0.5	+0.5	+5	+0.5	+100	+1.0	+400	+400	+150	h	+10	+50

[a] The allowances are intended to provide for individual variations among most normal persons as they live in the United States under usual environmental stresses. Diets should be based on a variety of common foods in order to provide other nutrients for which human requirements have been less well defined.

[b] Retinol equivalents. 1 retinol equivalent = 1 µg retinol or 6 µg β carotene. See text for calculation of vitamin A activity of diets as retinol equivalents.

[c] As cholecalciferol. 10 µg cholecalciferol = 400 IU of vitamin D.

[d] α-tocopherol equivalents. 1 mg d-α tocopherol = 1 α-TE. See text for variation in allowances and calculation of vitamin E activity of the diet as α-tocopherol equivalents.

[e] 1 NE (niacin equivalent) is equal to 1 mg of niacin or 60 mg of dietary tryptophan.

[f] The folacin allowances refer to dietary sources as determined by *Lactobacillus casei* assay after treatment with enzymes (conjugases) to make polyglutamyl forms of the vitamin available to the test organism.

[g] The recommended dietary allowance for vitamin B_{12} in infants is based on average concentration of the vitamin in human milk. The allowances after weaning are based on energy intake (as recommended by the American Academy of Pediatrics) and consideration of other factors, such as intestinal absorption; see text.

[h] The increased requirement during pregnancy cannot be met by the iron content of habitual American diets nor by the existing iron stores of many women; therefore the use of 30–60 mg of supplemental iron is recommended. Iron needs during lactation are not substantially different from those of nonpregnant women, but continued supplementation of the mother for 2–3 months after parturition is advisable in order to replenish stores depleted by pregnancy.

REFERENCE

1. Recommended Dietary Allowances, 9th ed. Committee on Dietary Allowances, Food and Nutrition Board, National Research Council, Washington, D.C., 1980.

FOOD LABELING

In 1973, the Food and Drug Administration developed standards to be used in the labeling of foods for which manufacturers make a nutritional claim or for any food to which a nutrient has been added.[1] The United States Recommended Dietary Allowance (U.S. RDA) was derived from the 1968 Recommended Dietary Allowances (RDA). The U.S. RDA expresses the highest allowance for nutrients for adults and for children over 4 years of age.* (Other sets of U.S. RDAs for children under 4 years, for infants, and for pregnant and lactating women are used for foods and for supplements marketed specifically for these individuals.)

A food label contains (1) the serving size; (2) the caloric, protein, carbohydrate, and fat content; (3) the percentage of the U.S. RDA for protein, for five vitamins (Vitamin A, Vitamin C, thiamin, riboflavin, and niacin), and for two minerals (calcium and iron); and (4) the ingredients in descending order by weight. A manufacturer may also decide to list 12 more vitamins and minerals for which the U.S. RDA has been established. Labels can be used as a tool for nutrition education at the point of purchase. (See also the sections on *Hypertension* and *Dietetic Food Labeling* for examples of labels.)

REFERENCE

1. Anon. Food Labeling. Fed Reg 1973;38:2124–2164.

---

*The U.S. RDA for biotin, pantothenic acid, copper, and zinc were specified even though these nutrients were not included in the 1968 RDAs. The U.S. RDA for calcium and phosphorous were set at 1 g rather than the highest allowance.

CHAPTER 5

GENERAL HOSPITAL DIET AND CONSISTENCY MODIFICATION

GENERAL HOSPITAL DIET

General Description

The general diet utilizes the *Basic Four Food Guide*,[1] the *Dietary Guidelines for Americans*,[2] the *American Dietetic Association* and the *Diabetes Association Exchange Lists*,[3] or other guides for meal planning (see pages 114–123) to provide a nutritionally adequate diet. Menus are either selected by or planned for the patient according to food preferences.

Nutritional Inadequacy

The general diet is planned to be consistent with the Recommended Dietary Allowances. Nutritional adequacy depends on the patient's selection of food as well as the patient's intake of food. In the hospital setting, the dietitian evaluates the selection of foods to ensure adequate nutritional intake. Patients who consistently select less than adequate food choices, who eat less than adequate food portions, or whose hospital stay is of 10 days duration or longer are monitored by the dietitian.

Indications and Rationale

The general diet is intended for the hospitalized patient whose medical condition does not warrant a therapeutic modification.

There are two general philosophies on the composition of a general hospital diet. One focuses on educating the patient in the principles of nutrition by example, and the other focuses on providing food the patient is willing and is able to eat. Usually, a compromise is reached between these philosophies, with the emphasis adjusted to meet the needs of a particular patient.

Some consider the implementation of a diet based on the control of the sodium, of the cholesterol, and of the fat intake to foster advantageous health practices. If the patient is able to eat adequately, hospitalization may provide an opportune time to teach these principles to the patient. Either the *Dietary Guidelines for Americans* or the *American Heart Association Dietary Recommendations* (see pages 36 and 37) may be used as a guide. If such modifications are considered desirable, the physician should notify the dietitian, who will discuss the modifications with the patient.

In many instances, hospitalization is not an appropriate time to impose undue dietary restrictions, especially if the modifications keep the patient from consuming enough protein and calories to meet the nutritional needs of convalescence from illness, injury, or surgery. The importance of an adequate and of an appropriate food intake during these situations may warrant compromise in traditional meal planning practices.

Meal Plan

The following meal plan (Table 5–1) uses portion sizes that are approximately equal to those of the American Dietetic Association and the Diabetes Association Exchange List with additional groupings for desserts and for sweets. It represents a typical or a usual content of the general hospital diet on a daily basis.

TABLE 5–1   The General Hospital Meal Plan

Meat or Meat Substitute	4–6 oz
Milk or Dairy Products	2–3 servings
Cereals or Starches	6–8 servings
Vegetables	2–3 servings
Fruits	2–3 servings
Fats	4–6 servings
Sweets	0–2 servings
Desserts	0–2 servings

Approximate Composition

The approximate composition (Table 5–2) varies depending on food choices.

TABLE 5–2   Composition of the General Hospital Diet

Calories (Kcal)	Protein (g)	Fat (g)	Carbohydrate (g)
1,600–2,200	60–80	60–80	200–300

Physicians: How to Order Diet

The diet order should indicate *general diet.*

REFERENCES

1. National Dairy Council. How to eat for good health. Rosemont, IL, 1985.
2. U.S. Department of Agriculture. Nutrition and your health—dietary guidelines for Americans. 2nd ed. U.S. Department of Health and Human Services. Home and Garden Bulletin No. 232, 1985.

3. American Diabetes Association and American Dietetic Association. Exchange lists for meal planning. Alexandria, VA and Chicago, IL, 1986.

CLEAR LIQUID DIET

General Description

The diet provides foods that are clear and liquid at room temperature (Table 5–3).

Nutritional Inadequacy

The diet is inadequate in calories and in essential nutrients. It should seldom be used for more than 1 to 3 days. If a residue-free liquid diet is required for longer periods of time, commercially prepared nutritional supplements are advised. See page 264.

Indications and Rationale

The purpose of the diet is to provide an oral source of fluids that is easily absorbed and leaves minimal residue in the gastrointestinal tract. The clear liquid diet minimizes stimulation of the gastrointestinal tract. Some liquids, particularly carbonated beverages and juices, are not tolerated by some surgical patients.

The diet is used as an initial feeding progression between intravenous feeding and a full liquid diet or a solid diet that follows surgery, as a dietary preparation for bowel examination or for surgery, for an acute disturbance of gastrointestinal function, and for a severely debilitated patient as a first step in oral feeding.

Physicians: How to Order Diet

The diet order should indicate *clear liquid diet*. The diet order should also indicate if modifications are desired following a particular surgical procedure or if additional supplements are desired. If it is anticipated that the patient will require therapeutic diet modifications, such as diabetic or sodium restrictions, these modifications should be indicated on the diet order.

FULL LIQUID DIET

General Description

The diet provides foods that are liquid or semiliquid at room temperature (see Table 5–3).

TABLE 5-3 Liquid Diets—Recommended Foods

Food Group	Clear Liquid Diet	Full Liquid Diet
Soup	Clear fat-free broth, bouillon	Broth, bouillon, strained or blenderized cream soup
Beverages	Coffee, tea, decaffeinated coffee and tea, cereal beverages, carbonated beverages,* artificially flavored fruit drinks	Coffee, tea, decaffeinated coffee and tea, cereal beverages, carbonated beverages, artificially flavored fruit drinks
Meat	—	—
Fat	—	Butter, margarine, cream
Milk	—	Milk and milk beverages,† yogurt without seeds, nuts or fruit, cocoa
Starch	—	Cooked refined cereal
Vegetables	—	Juices
Fruit	Fruit juice* (exclude nectars, tomato, and prune juice)	Juices
Dessert	Gelatin, fruit ice, popsicle	Gelatin, sherbet, ice cream, custard, pudding, popsicle, fruit ice
Sweets	Sugar, hard candy, honey, Polycose	Sugar, honey, hard candy, Polycose, flavorings
Miscellaneous	Salt	Salt, pepper, mild seasonings as tolerated
Supplements	Residue-free, e.g., Citrotein, Ross SLD (Surgical Liquid Diet)	All, see page 264

*Carbonated beverages and juices may not be tolerated by some surgical patients
†Some patients postoperatively exhibit a temporary lactose intolerance. The diet may be modified by substituting lactose-hydrolyzed milk or lactose-free products.

Nutritional Inadequacy

The diet is inadequate in all nutrients except protein, calcium, and ascorbic acid. If the full liquid diet is used for more than 2 to 3 days, liquid nutritional supplements (see page 264) or blenderized foods (see *Appendix* 13) should be used to improve nutritional adequacy.

Indications and Rationale

The purpose of the diet is to provide an oral source of fluids for individuals who are incapable of chewing, swallowing, or digesting solid food.

The full liquid diet is used as an intermediate progression to solid foods following surgery, in conjunction with parenteral nutrition, in the presence of chewing or swallowing disorders, following oral or plastic surgery of the face and neck, in the presence of esophageal or gastrointestinal strictures during moderate gastrointestinal inflammations, and for acutely ill patients.

Physicians: How to Order Diet

The diet order should indicate *full liquid diet*. If it is anticipated that the patient will require therapeutic diet modifications, such as a diabetic or a sodium restriction, these modifications should be indicated on the diet order.

Sample Menus

Clear Liquid Diet:	*Breakfast*	*Noon and Evening*
	Juice	Broth
	Beverage	Juice
		Gelatin
		Beverage
	Between-meal feedings:	Available if desired
Full Liquid Diet:	*Breakfast*	*Noon and Evening*
	Juice	Juice
	Cooked cereal	Strained cream soup
	Milk or cream	Ice cream
	Beverage	Milk
	Sugar or honey	Beverage
	Between-meal feedings:	Available if desired

Approximate Composition of Liquid Diets

The composition varies depending on the quantity and the type of liquids that are consumed by the patient. The following values represent a usual intake (Table 5–4).

TABLE 5–4 Composition of Liquid Diets

Diet	Protein, (g)	Fat (g)	Carbohydrate (g)	Sodium* (mEq)	Potassium (mEq)	Calories (Kcal)
Clear liquid diet	5	trace	70–95	65	20	375+
Clear liquid plus three 6 oz servings of Citrotein[†]	30	1	140–165	80	30	750+
Clear liquid plus 9 Tbsp of Polycose[‡]	5	trace	125–150	68	20	580+
Full liquid diet	50	55	205	110	65	1,500+

*Value is for amount of sodium in food
[†]Sandoz Nutrition, Minneapolis, MN
[‡]Ross Laboratories, Columbus, OH

PUREED DIET

General Description

The pureed diet includes strained, pureed, or liquid foods (Tables 5–5 and 5–6).

Nutritional Inadequacy

The diet is not inherently inadequate in nutrients in comparison with the Recommended Dietary Allowance (RDA) providing that the patient is able to consume adequate amounts of food. The dietitian monitors the nutrient intake and modifies the diet with supplements if the intake is insufficient.

Indications and Rationale

The purpose of the diet is to provide foods that don't need mastication and that are easily swallowed (see Table 5–5).

The diet is used for patients with inflammation, ulceration, or structural or motor deficits of the oral cavity and the esophagus, or for patients without teeth. The diet may also be used following esophageal or oral surgery or after radiation of the oral or of the pharyngeal region.

Extreme temperatures are usually not well tolerated. The dietitian evaluates the individual's acceptance and tolerance of the diet and progresses the patient to a mechanical soft diet when indicated. If a syringe is needed to feed the patient, further modifications in texture may be necessary.

Physicians: How to Order Diet

The diet order should indicate *pureed diet.*

MECHANICAL SOFT DIET

General Description

The mechanical soft diet is a general diet that is modified only in texture for ease of mastication. Initially, it includes ground meat and pureed fruits and vegetables. The dietitian modifies the texture to include soft, easy to chew foods in accordance to the patient's tolerance and acceptance (see Tables 5–5 and 5–6).

Nutritional Inadequacy

The diet is not inherently inadequate in nutrients in comparison with the Recommended Dietary Allowance (RDA) providing the patient is able to consume adequate amounts of food. The dietitian monitors the nutrient intake and modifies the diet with nutritional supplements if the nutrient intake is insufficient.

Indications and Rationale

The purpose of the diet is to provide moist foods that are easy to chew and to swallow (see Table 5–5).

The mechanical soft diet may be appropriate for patients with poorly fitting dentures or with no teeth; for severely debilitated patients who are unable to chew; for patients with dysphagia that is secondary to neurologic, esophageal, oral, or laryngeal disorders or surgeries; for patients with strictures of the intestinal tract; for patients after laser or radiation treatment to the oral cavity; and for patients who are progressing from tube feeding or from parenteral nutrition to solid food.

TABLE 5–5 Consistency Modifications—Recommended Foods

Food Group	Pureed Diet	Mechanical Soft Diet	Soft Diet
Soups	Broth; bouillon; strained or blenderized cream soup	Broth; bouillon; strained or blenderized cream soup	Broth; bouillon; cream soup
Beverages	All	All	All
Meat	Strained or pureed meat or poultry; cheese used in cooking	Ground, moist meats, or poultry; flaked fish; eggs; cottage cheese; cheese; creamy peanut butter; soft casseroles	Moist, tender meat, fish, or poultry; eggs, cottage cheese; mild flavored cheese; creamy peanut butter; soft casseroles
Fat	Butter; margarine; cream; oil; gravy	Butter; margarine; cream; oil; gravy; salad dressing	Butter; margarine; cream; oil; gravy; crisp bacon; avocado; salad dressing
Milk	Milk; milk beverages; yogurt without fruit, nuts, or seeds; cocoa	Milk, milk beverages, yogurt without seeds or nuts; cocoa	Milk; milk beverages; yogurt without seeds or nuts; cocoa
Starch	Cooked, refined cereal; mashed potatoes	Cooked or refined ready-to-eat cereal; potatoes; rice; pasta; white, refined wheat, light rye bread or rolls; graham crackers as tolerated	Cooked or ready-to-eat cereal; potatoes; rice; pasta; white, refined wheat, light rye or graham bread, rolls, or crackers
Vegetables	Strained or pureed; juice	Soft, cooked, without hulls or tough skin (e.g., peas and corn); juice	Soft, cooked, vegetables; limit strongly flavored vegetables and whole kernal corn, lettuce and tomatoes
Fruit	Strained or pureed; juice	Cooked or canned fruit without seeds or skins; banana; juice	Cooked or canned fruit; banana; citrus fruit without membrane; melon; juice
Desserts	Gelatin; sherbet; ice cream without nuts or fruit; custard; pudding; fruit ice; popsicle	Gelatin; sherbet; ice cream without nuts or fruit; custard; pudding; fruit ice; popsicle	Gelatin; sherbet; ice cream without nuts; custard; pudding; cake; cookies without nuts or coconut; fruit ice; popsicle
Sweets	Sugar; honey; jelly; candy; flavorings	Sugar; honey; jelly; candy; flavorings	Sugar; honey; jelly; candy; flavorings
Miscellaneous	Seasonings; condiments	Seasonings; condiments	Seasonings; condiments

Extreme temperatures are usually not well tolerated. Bread and bread products are often not well tolerated and, therefore, not served to patients who have difficulty swallowing until the dietitian evaluates the patient's tolerance.

Physicians: How to Order Diet

The diet order should indicate *mechanical soft diet.*

SOFT DIET

General Description

The diet provides soft whole food that is lightly seasoned and moderately low in fiber. Small volume meals are offered until the patient's tolerance of solid food is established (see Tables 5–5 and 5–6).

Nutritional Inadequacy

The diet is not inherently inadequate in nutrients in comparison with the Recommended Dietary Allowance (RDA) providing the patient is able to consume adequate amounts of food. Supplements or between meal feedings may be used, if needed, to increase the intake.

Indications and Rationale

The soft diet is used for a variety of reasons. It provides a transition between a liquid and a general diet (see Table 5–5).

The soft diet may be used for debilitated or other patients who are unable to consume a general diet or for patients with mild gastrointestinal problems.

The soft diet should be individualized according to the type of illness or surgery, the patient's appetite, food tolerances, previous nutritional status, and chewing and swallowing ability.

Some patients who require a soft diet do not tolerate highly seasoned foods or strongly flavored vegetables. Spices and seasonings are usually kept to a minimum, but may be increased in accordance to the patient's tolerance. Strongly flavored vegetables are usually served only in small amounts, but may be increased according to the patient's tolerance.

Physicians: How to Order Diet

The diet order should indicate *soft diet*.

Sample Menus

Pureed Diet:	*Breakfast*	*Noon and Evening Meal*
	Juice or pureed fruit	Broth or strained cream soup
	Cooked cereal	Pureed meat
	Milk	Mashed potatoes
	Beverage	Pureed vegetable
	Cream and sugar	Butter or margarine
		Pureed fruit or juice
		Pudding
		Milk
		Beverage
		Cream and sugar

Mechanical Soft Diet:	*Breakfast*	*Noon and Evening Meal*
	Juice	Broth or strained cream soup
	Cooked cereal	Ground meat
	Egg	Mashed potatoes
	Bread	Soft cooked vegetable
	Butter or margarine	Soft, canned fruit or juice
	Milk	Bread
	Beverage	Butter or margarine
	Cream and sugar	Pudding
	Jelly or honey	Milk
		Beverage
		Cream and sugar

Soft Diet:	*Breakfast*	*Noon and Evening*
	Juice or fruit	Soup
	Cereal	Meat
	Egg	Mashed potatoes
	Toast	Cooked vegetable
	Butter or margarine	Canned fruit or juice
	Milk	Bread
	Beverage	Butter or margarine
	Cream and sugar	Pudding
	Jelly or honey	Milk
		Beverage
		Cream and sugar

Approximate Composition

The composition varies depending on the quantity and the type of food consumed by the patient (see Table 5–6). These values represent a usual intake.

TABLE 5–6 Composition of Pureed, Mechanical Soft, and Soft Diets

	Protein (g)	Fat (g)	Carbohydrate (g)	Sodium* (mEq)	Potassium (mEq)	Calories (Kcal)
Pureed Diet	70	80	190	100	80	1,750
Mechanical Soft Diet	70	75	210	125	80	1,800
Soft Diet	65	75	215	150	90	1,800

*Value is for the amount of sodium in usual foods and does not include salt added in preparation.

TRANSITIONAL FEEDING PROGRESSION

PREOPERATIVE DIET

A general diet may be ordered the night before general surgery. Usually nothing is permitted by mouth after this evening meal.

If it is necessary to limit foods that produce residue in the gastrointestinal tract, a diet that is controlled in residue (see page 146) may be used before the surgery. A clear liquid diet may also be preferred for patients having colon surgery.

POSTOPERATIVE DIET

General Description

Diets that are included in the standard postoperative regimens are clear liquid, full liquid, and soft diets. The rate of progression depends on the type of surgery, the physician's personal philosophy, and the response of the patient.

Indications and Rationale

Oral intake of food should be resumed as soon as possible, although intravenous glucose and electrolyte solutions are sufficient to sustain most patients for short periods of time postsurgically without serious depletion of body protein and of other stored nutrients. Oral intake of a liquid diet can begin when, in the judgment of the surgeon, the gastrointestinal tract is functioning. Commonly, feedings are not begun until peristaltic sounds are heard and there is passage of flatus. In all instances, one should be ready to discontinue feeding or to revert to an earlier stage in the dietary progression if there is abdominal distention, cramping, or other evidence of intolerance.

Alternate methods of feeding, such as tube feedings or peripheral parenteral or central parenteral nutrition, should be considered for patients who are severely debilitated and malnourished or who, for prolonged periods, are unwilling or unable to eat adequately. See page 261 for a discussion of supplements and of tube feedings and page 275, which addresses parenteral nutritional support.

General Postoperative Dietary Progressions

The following diet progressions (Table 5–7) permit the surgeon to designate how rapidly the feeding is to be resumed after surgery. The dietitian and the surgeon evaluate each patient's acceptance and tolerance of the diet and may adjust the rate of progression.

TABLE 5–7 Diet Progression

Start with a clear liquid diet (first meal) and advance to a general diet by the meal indicated for the rate of progression desired.

Progression	Meal
Rapid	Third
Regular	Sixth
Slow	Ninth

Diet Progression Following Tonsillectomy or Adenoidectomy (T & A)

The diet progression is a modification of the full liquid and the mechanical soft diets. Foods that are considered nonirritating following throat surgery are provided. The use of straws is usually prohibited.

Standard Progression

The first meal is a T & A, full liquid diet. The second and the third meals are a mechanical soft diet, and subsequent meals are a general diet as tolerated.

Physicians: How to Order Diet

The diet order may indicate either the rate of progression (rapid, regular, or slow progression) or the specific diet (clear liquid, full liquid, or soft diet) at each stage in the patient's convalescence. Following tonsillectomy or adenoidectomy, the diet order should indicate *T & A diet.*

INTERMAXILLARY FIXATION

General Description

The diet consists of liquids and of foods that are blenderized to a smooth, liquid consistency. Generally, six to eight small meals are recommended.

Nutritional Inadequacy

The diet is not inherently inadequate in nutrients in comparison with the Recommended Dietary Allowance (RDA) providing the patient is able to consume adequate amounts of food. Special consideration may be needed for patients who are not able to consume adequate amounts of food to maintain their weight, for patients who undergo a surgical procedure because of a traumatic accident, or for patients who are in a compromised nutritional state prior to surgery.

Indications or Rationale

Intermaxillary fixation is a surgical procedure used for craniofacial reconstruction. This includes fixation of fractures of the mandible or the maxilla secondary to trauma or to repair of developmental malocclusions. The jaws are wired together with the aid of arch bars or with braces attached to the teeth. The amount of space between the upper and the lower teeth is minimal unless teeth have been pulled to correct the occlusion of the teeth or unless teeth are missing secondary to facial fractures. Fixation of the jaws is usually 4 to 8 weeks in duration.

Dietary Recommendations

Generally, six to eight small meals are recommended to achieve an adequate caloric intake. The tendency of a person with a wired jaw is to decrease the intake dramatically over the duration of jaw wiring because eating causes fatigue, the taste of liquid meals is boring, and the increased liquid intake causes a "full feeling." Patients should be encouraged to consume an adequate caloric intake to maintain their weight. Weekly weighing is recommended to monitor the weight and the adequacy of the caloric intake.

A food processor or a blender is required to blenderize foods to a completely smooth mixture. The blenderized liquid should be strained with a wire mesh strainer if particles remain after processing. The blenderized liquids, when consumed, pass through the space between the teeth. The consistency that is needed is determined by the individual patient's needs and his or her ability to consume liquids.

Suggestions for Blenderizing Foods

1. Meats need to be well cooked and cubed or ground prior to blenderizing. Generally, straining is required to remove chunks.

2. *Foods should be refrigerated or frozen within the hour after preparation since blenderized foods are an excellent culture media for the growth of bacteria.* Extra portions can be frozen in meal size amounts or in ice cube trays.

3. The temperature of liquid foods should be lukewarm to prevent burning the mouth. If a warm liquid is added to foods when blenderizing, additional heating before serving may not be necessary. Extremely cold foods are often not tolerated.

4. The salty or the sweet flavor in foods is magnified when foods are blended. Other strong seasonings may also be enhanced when foods are blended. Extremely sweet foods are usually not tolerated for a long time period.

5. Whole milk should be used rather than a lower fat milk in milk drinks to improve the texture of the liquid and to increase kilocalories.

6. Liquifying foods with sour cream, milk, half and half, cream, juice, broth, cheese sauce, or tomato sauce is recommended instead of water to enhance the flavor and the nutritional value of foods. The liquid should be added gradually, as too much liquid may change or dilute the flavor of foods.

7. To increase kilocalories and protein grate cheese into soups, potatoes, casseroles, and vegetables (processed cheese and cheese spread melt more thoroughly); use whole milk, cream, or half and half instead of water; add powdered milk to casseroles, mashed potatoes, soups, cooked cereals, pudding, or milk drinks at a ratio of 2 Tbsp per cup; add creamy peanut butter to puddings or to milkshakes; add pasteurized eggs to milk drinks, casseroles, and puddings; add extra butter or margarine to foods.

8. Frozen or pasteurized eggs, such as egg substitutes, are recommended to minimize the risk of salmonella poisoning.

9. For ease and for quickness in meal preparation commercial products and supplements may be used. These include canned casseroles, soups, puddings, instant mashed potatoes or cereals, commercial strained baby foods, and supplements, such as instant breakfast mixes, Ensure, Sustacal, or Osmolite (see page 264).

10. If a straw is allowed, plastic straws that have a flexible top are easier to use and are wider in diameter. It may be helpful to cut 1 or 2 inches off the base of the straw, as shorter straws require less suction.

Dietary Progression

Once the wires have been removed, a soft textured diet usually is required for a limited time until the jaw muscles regain strength. The progression to regular food varies with the individual.

Some individuals have a temporary numbness in the lower lip or the chin that is secondary to nerve stretching or to nerve damage. These patients need to be careful in biting and in chewing to prevent injury to the lips.

Physicians: How to Order Diet

The diet order should indicate *diet for wired jaw* or *intermaxillary fixation*.

DYSPHAGIA

General Description

The dietary recommendations for swallowing disorders or for dysphagia include an evaluation of the swallowing disorder and modifications in the consistency of foods for individual abilities and tolerances. The diet may include liquids, pureed foods, or soft foods.

Nutritional Inadequacy

The dietary recommendations are not intended to be inherently inadequate in comparison with the Recommended Dietary Allowance (RDA). However, many patients may not be able to consume an adequate quantity of foods or of liquids. Supplements or enteral nutritional support (see page 261) should be considered if the patient's intake is inadequate.

Indications and Rationale

Dysphagia, a difficulty or a discomfort in swallowing, can occur in any of the three phases of swallowing, which include oral, pharyngeal, and esophageal. Its cause may be mechanical or paralytic. The mechanical type is primarily attributable to surgical resection or to alteration of one or more of the organs of swallowing owing to trauma, to obstruction, or to damaging diseases such as cancer. The paralytic type results from a lesion in the cerebral cortex or from a lesion of the cranial nerves of the brain stem, in particular the medulla oblongata. The most common cause of dysphagia paralytica is a cerebral vascular accident. Head injury, brain tumors, and diseases that involve the neurologic system may also cause dysphagia.

Five cranial nerves function to control swallowing. Dysphagia may be the result of damage to one or more of these nerves. Since each of these nerves has a different role in controlling swallowing, the nature and the severity of dysphagia depends on which nerve or nerves are damaged (Table 5–8).

TABLE 5–8 Nerves That Control Swallowing

Cranial nerve	Stimulates
Trigeminal (5th)	Chewing Sensations of texture and temperature in the mouth Salivation Swallowing
Facial (7th)	Taste (anterior tongue) Facial expression and movement
Glossopharyngeal (9th)	Taste (posterior tongue) Sensations to soft palate, pharynx Sensory component to pharyngeal (gag) reflex Salivation
Vagus (10th)	Movement of soft palate, pharynx, larynx Salivation Gag reflex Peristalsis Speech
Hypoglossal (12th)	Tongue movement Chewing Speaking

Reprinted with permission from Loustau A. Dealing with the dangers of dysphagia. Nursing 1985;15(2):47–50 and the Springhouse Corporation, Springhouse, PA.

Swallowing disorders may be characterized by weak or uncoordinated muscles of the mouth and of the throat, by reduced sensation of the mouth and of the throat, or by deficits of the motor and the sensory nerves that impede chewing and/or swallowing after neurologic damage. Symptoms of dysphagia include drooling, retaining food in the mouth, coughing after swallowing, gurgling voice quality, and a feeling of a "lump in the throat." There is also an increased risk of aspiration and of pneumonia.

The effects of dysphagia on nutritional status include inadequate dietary intake, weight loss, vitamin and mineral deficiencies, and consequently, protein-caloric malnutrition. Factors that contribute to an inadequate dietary intake include swallowing difficulties, a decrease in the olfactory and the gustatory senses, a decrease in the appetite and the saliva, psychological factors such as the fear of choking, and the effects of therapy, such as surgery and medication.

If the patient is to be fed orally, the dietitian coordinates his or her efforts with the speech pathologist or the occupational therapist to evaluate the swallowing deficits and to provide the appropriate food consistency.

It is useful to evaluate the nature of the patient's swallowing disorder prior to the initiation of or a change in oral feedings. The following foods can be used to evaluate various components of swallowing (Table 5–9).

It is imperative that the dietitian, who provides the diet to the patient with dysphagia, considers the individual's particular swallowing deficit. For example, liquids may be the only diet that a dysphagic patient with an obstruction can take with safety, while some neurologically impaired patients may aspirate on

TABLE 5–9 Foods for Evaluation of Swallowing Disorders

To Evaluate	Foods Used
Taste sensation	Honey, salt, cocoa, lemon
Tongue control	Peanut butter, honey
Sucking	Popsicles, pickles
Swallowing	Strained baby foods, cereals, pudding
Chewing	Cheerios, crackers, cheese, marshmallows

liquid and may require a pureed diet. Individualization of diet consistencies is important.

Dietary Recommendations

1. Foods should be mild in taste and served at room temperature.

2. For patients with reduced sensation, small pieces of food should be avoided, as they can become lost in the mouth and can increase the chance of choking.

3. Select foods that form a bolus within the mouth or do not break apart; e.g., bananas, mashed potatoes, souffles, and macaroni and cheese.

4. If the patient has muscle weakness, avoid sticky foods that adhere to the roof of the mouth, as they cause fatigue.

5. If excess mucus formation is a problem, avoid sweet foods, milk products, and citrus juice, as they seem to increase or to thicken the saliva.

6. To compensate for decreased saliva production, moisten foods with small amounts of liquid.

7. Change food items as often as possible to reduce the boredom and the possible reliance on particular foods.

8. Observe patients eating a variety of different foods at mealtime and adjust the diet accordingly.

9. If oral intake and supplements fail to meet the patient's caloric and protein needs, tube feeding (see page 261) should be considered.

Positioning is very important for feeding the patient with dysphagia. Good positioning allows for alignment of the alimentary canal; swallowing is facilitated by flexion. If the patient is seated in a chair, he or she should be sitting upright with the hips flexed at a 90-degree angle, the back straight, and the feet flat on the floor. The patient should be sitting up for 15 to 30 minutes both before and after meals. This decreases the risk of aspiration and of pneumonia. If the patient is in bed, elevate the head of the bed and place pillows behind the patient to achieve the 90-degree hip and neck flexion. This position may be helpful for other patients who are not dysphagic, but who need the assistance of gravity and of proper alignment of the esophagus to aid in swallowing.

Physicians: How to Order Diet

The diet order should indicate *diet as tolerated for dysphagia.*

REFERENCE

1. Loustau A, Lee KA. Dealing with the dangers of dysphagia. Nursing 1985;15:47–50.

CHAPTER 6

NUTRITIONAL MANAGEMENT OF DISEASES AND DISORDERS

ALLERGY

FOOD ALLERGY AND INTOLERANCE

Introduction

A true food allergy is a hypersensitivity reaction that is immunologically mediated in response to a food exposure. Food allergies occur more commonly in children and in infants than in adults. Food allergies may change or disappear altogether and thus need periodic re-evaluation. Food allergies are diagnosed by a history, by a demonstration of allergen-specific antibody (skin testing, or in vitro immuno assay such as RAST or ELISA), and by a double-blind food challenge. Food allergies are treated by the elimination of the offending foods from the diet. The dietitian's expertise can be valuable in assessing the nutritional status of the allergic person and to assure nutritional adequacy during treatment (Table 6–1).

Food intolerances are symptoms that result from the ingestion of specific foods that do not involve immunologic mechanisms. A common example would be a milk intolerance that is caused by lactase deficiency (lactose intolerance). Less common food intolerances may involve various additives, which include butylated hydroxyanisole (BHA), butylated hydroxytoluene (BHT), monosodium glutamate (MSG), sulfites, or tartrazine (FD & C yellow dye No. 5). Toxic substances in food, such as yeast, penicillin, or mold, may also elicit nonimmunologic reactions.

The following sections describe various dietary interventions for food allergies and for intolerances.

TABLE 6–1 Food Allergy Assessment

Examination	Findings
History	Provides detailed description of symptoms, time from ingestion of food to onset of symptoms, most recent reaction, quantity of food necessary to produce a reaction, and suspected foods.*
	Includes family history of allergic disease, enzyme deficiencies, and so forth.*
Physical examination	Includes anthropometric evaluation, assessment of growth and development, and nutritional status.*
	Assesses other chronic disease.
	Evaluates allergic conditions like allergic rhinitis, eczema, and asthma.
Food and symptom diary for 2 weeks	Provides actual record of food, amount and time when eaten, time of appearance of symptoms, and any medication taken.*
	Allows assessment of dietary adequacy.*
Immunological testing (skin tests, RAST, ELISA, other)	Yields list of suspect foods.
	Requires confirmation of positive results by trial elimination diet and food challenge to show clinical sensitivity to food.
Trial elimination diet for 2 to 4 weeks or until symptoms clear	Needs to be nutritionally sound.*
	Requires that patient record all ingested food as the suspect food may be ingested in an alternative form.*
	Begins with a simple elimination diet. Only foods suspected by history, food diary, and/or immunological testing are eliminated.*.
	Progresses to more extensive elimination diet if symptoms do not clear on simple diet. Only one food in each of four food groups or exotic foods never before eaten are allowed.*
	May require use of hypoallergenic diet (i.e., Vivonex,[†] Pregestimil,[‡] Nutramigen[‡]) if symptoms do not clear on an extensive elimination diet.*
Food challenge	Excludes foods known to cause severe reactions such as wheezing, asthma, or anaphylaxis.*
	Returns suspect foods to diet one at a time after symptoms have cleared for 2 to 4 wk.*
	8 to 10 mg (1/2 to 1 tsp) is given for the first dose.
	The amount is increased until it approximates usual intake.
	Is repeated following positive reactions as coincident reactions are common.*
	Is performed as double-blind challenge when uncertainty about reaction persists.*

* Points in the diagnostic process where the dietitian's expertise may be particularly valuable.
† Norwich-Eaton Pharmaceuticals, Norwich, NY.
‡ Mead Johnson Nutritional Division, Evansville, IN.
Butkus SN, Mahan LK. Food allergies: immunologic reactions to food. Copyright The American Dietetic Association. Reprinted by permission from Journal of the American Dietetic Association 1986;86:601.

SUGGESTED FURTHER READING

Bock SA. Food sensitivity. Nutr News 1984; 47:9–11.

Buckley RH, Metcalfe D. Food allergy. JAMA 1982;248:2627–2631.

Butkus SN, Mahan LK. Food allergies: immunological reactions to food. J Am Diet Assoc 1986;86:601–608.

DeShazo RD, Salvaggio JE. Allergy and immunology. JAMA 1985;256:2257–2259.

Mermelstein NH. Food allergies and other food sensitivities. Contemp Nutr 1985;9:9.

Nutrition and the immune response. Dairy Council Digest 1985;56:7–12.

Taylor SI. Food allergies and sensitivities. J Am Diet Assoc 1986;86:599–600.

American Academy of Allergy and Immunology, Committee on Adverse Reactions to Foods and the National Institute of Allergy and Infectious Diseases. Adverse reactions to foods. HHS Publication NIH 84-2442. 1984:117.

LOW SALICYLATE AND TARTRAZINE-FREE DIET

General Description

The diet is designed to minimize the intake of tartrazine or of both salicylates and tartrazine. Salicylates occur naturally in some foods, predominately in the fruit and the vegetable group. Other sources of salicylates are acetylsalicylic acid (in aspirin and in aspirin-containing medications) and methyl salicylate or salicin (wintergreen or mint flavoring that is added to foods, drugs, and cosmetics). It is the intention of this diet to exclude all forms of the salicylate radical.

Tartrazine (FD & C Yellow No. 5) is a certified coloring dye that has been used in foods, drugs, and cosmetics. Since 1980 manufacturers are required to identify tartrazine on food product labels if it is used in the product. Foods listed under the "may contain tartrazine" category are the foods most likely to contain tartrazine. A product is acceptable only if it has been established that it does not contain tartrazine. Patients should check product ingredient labels for the words "FD & C yellow No. 5" or "Yellow #5."

Nutritional Inadequacy

The low salicylate and tartrazine-free diet is likely to be inadequate in nutrients as compared to the RDA because of the limited fruits and vegetables allowed. It should not be used for an extended period without medical supervision. A multiple vitamin supplement (free of salicylate and tartrazine) is recommended daily. The tartrazine-free diet can be planned to meet nutritional needs.

Indications and Rationale

A diet that restricts both salicylates and tartrazine has been used in the treatment of specific types of chronic urticaria. There are no good incidence data regarding what fraction of patients with chronic urticaria actually have a sensitivity to these substances, and many physicians do not use a restricting diet as a form of treatment at all. The mechanisms by which salicylates and tartrazine induce or aggravate urticaria have not been established. It has been hypothesized that the salicylate radical, by acting as an antigen in the development of the allergic reaction or by enhancing the effect of histamine on the skin, promotes urticaria.

In some patients with asthma, particularly those with nasal polyps, the ingestion of aspirin may cause severe asthmatic reactions. In a very small percentage of these patients, asthmatic attacks may also follow the ingestion of tartrazine. Asthmatic patients who are sensitive to aspirin or tartrazine, however, often can ingest choline salicylate without difficulty. There are no well-controlled studies that show that dietary manipulation of salicylate (other than avoidance of the drug aspirin) has important effects on the course of the asthma. In the tartrazine-reactive patient, however, it does seem reasonable to exclude tartrazine from the diet. Food sources of salicylates and of tartrazine are listed separately so the diet can be adjusted to meet the particular need of the patient (Table 6–2).

TABLE 6–2 Food Sources of Tartrazine and Salicylates

Food Groups	May Contain Tartrazine*	Contains Salicylates (>0.4 mg/100 g)	Allowed Foods (low in tartrazine & salicylates [<0.4 mg/100 g])
Beverage	Carbonated beverages, soft drinks and soft drink mixes, orange drinks	Tea, root beer, birch beer	Coffee, decaffeinated coffee, cereal beverage
Meat	Sausage, frankfurters, cheese-flavored foods	Corned beef, meat processed with vinegar	All other meats, fish, and fowl, eggs, cheese
Fat	Nondairy cream	Salad dressing, mayonnaise, avocado, olives, almonds, peanuts, sunflower seeds, cashews, Brazil nuts, Macadamia nuts, pistachio nuts	Butter, margarine, vegetable oil, cream and cream products, other nuts, other fats
Milk	Yogurt, hot chocolate, and cocoa mixes	Fruited yogurt	Milk, cheeses
Starch	Ready-to-eat cereals, variety crackers, noodles, commercial mixes including macaroni and cheese	Yellow corn meal	Bread, spaghetti, macaroni, rice, most commercially prepared breads and rolls, potato, barley, oats, rye and wheat flours
Vegetable		Alfalfa sprouts, asparagus (fresh), bean sprouts, broccoli, cucumbers, green bell peppers, tomatoes (canned), okra, parsnip, pimentos, pumpkin, spinach, squash, sweet potato, zucchini, water-cress, endive, water chestnuts	Asparagus (canned), bamboo shoots, bean sprouts, Brussels sprouts, cabbage, carrots, celery, cauliflower, corn, lentils, lettuce, green peas, split peas, chickpeas, onions, potato (white), spinach (frozen), tomato (fresh), tomato juice, mushrooms (fresh), turnip
Fruit		Apricots, blackberries, boysenberries, cherries, currants, gooseberries, huckleberries, maraschino cherries, grapes, melon, nectarines, peaches, raisins, raspberries, prunes, blueberries, cranberries, dates, grapefruit, loganberries, oranges, pineapple, strawberries	Apple, apple juice, apricot nectar, banana, figs (fresh and canned), light seedless grapes (canned), kiwi, lemon, mango, peach nectar, pear, persimmon, pineapple juice, red plums, pomegranate, rhubarb
Soup	Commercial soups and soup mixes		All made from allowed foods

Dessert	Gelatin, sherbet, ice cream, ice milk, fruit ice, commercially prepared desserts and mixes including cakes, frostings, puddings, and gingerbread		All others made from allowed foods
Sweets	Commercially prepared jam, jelly, and candy; any colored yellow, orange, pink, green, or brown chewing gum	Honey, licorice; any mint, wintergreen or anise flavored	Sugar, syrup, molasses, all others
Miscellaneous	Cocoa and hot chocolate mixes, flavoring extracts	Pickles, catsup, tartar sauce, Tabasco sauce, cider vinegar, wine vinegar, beer, wine, distilled alcoholic beverages (except vodka and gin) curry, paprika, thyme, dill powder, mustard powder, garam masala, oregano, tumeric, other herbs and spices contribute significant amounts of salicylates to the diet if eaten in unusually large quantities	Salt, pepper, distilled white vinegar, cocoa powder, pure chocolate, soy sauce, garlic (fresh), parsley (fresh), coriander (fresh), gin, vodka, whiskey

*These foods are likely to contain tartrazine. If the manufacturer states that a specific brand does not contain tartrazine or FD&C Yellow No. 5, it may be used. This information is available from the product ingredient label.

Physicians: How to Order Diet

The diet order should indicate either *low salicylate and tartrazine-free diet* or *tartrazine-free diet.*

SUGGESTED FURTHER READINGS

Moore-Robinson M, Warin RP. Effect of salicylates in urticaria. Br Med J 1967;4:262–264.
Settipane GA, Chafee FH, Postman IM. Significance of tartrazine sensitivity in chronic urticaria of unknown etiology. J Allergy Clin Immunol 1976;57:541–546.
Swain AR, Dutton SP, Truswell AS. Salicylates in foods. J Am Diet Assoc 1985;85:950–960.

NICKEL RESTRICTION

General Description

Studies have demonstrated that a reduction of the nickel intake in food can be useful in treating one-third to one-half of patients with nickel dermatitis.

However, there is often some discrepancy between the food items known to contain significant amounts of nickel and those mentioned by patients as the cause of exacerbations of their dermatitis.

This diet should not be used over an extended period of time without medical supervision.

Table 6–3 is a list of foods known to contain significant amounts of nickel and should be avoided by those patients with nickel sensitivity.

TABLE 6–3 Food Sources of Nickel

Food Category	Types of Food
Seafood	Oysters, herring and other shellfish, canned fish
Vegetables	Asparagus, beans, mushrooms, onions, corn, tomatoes, spinach, peas, lettuce, carrots, all canned vegetables
Fruit	Cooked or fresh pears, rhubarb, all canned fruits
Cereal Products	Whole-grain flour of all kinds, soy flour, oats
Beverages	Tea, cocoa and chocolate beverages
Miscellaneous	Baking powder, pickles, chocolate, all nuts

Patients should be asked not to cook foods in stainless steel cooking utensils. Instead, use enamel or aluminum utensils.

Foods that are canned in metal containers should be avoided, as they may contain higher concentrations of nickel.

Physicians: How to Order Diet

The diet order should indicate *low-nickel diet.*

SUGGESTED FURTHER READING

Brun R. Nickel in food: the role of stainless-steel utensils. Contact Dermatitis 1979;5:43–45.
Veien N. Dietary treatment of nickel dermatitis. Acta Derm Venereol (Stockh) 1985;65:138–142.

SULFITE RESTRICTION

Sulfites have been implicated in a syndrome with an acute onset of bronchospasm in asthmatics and, in some cases, shock. The prevalence of sulfite intolerance is not clear at this time, but some investigators feel as many as 5 percent of asthmatics could be intolerant. Sulfite sensitivity has been reported in non-asthmatics; however, the incidence appears to be very low.

Sulfiting agents have a number of purposes in food processing. They are used in a number of drug products and in foods as antioxidants (preservatives) Table 6–4.

It is important to remember that only a fraction of the public may be sulfite intolerant, and no studies exist showing a diet that is devoid of sulfites improves asthma.

Recent legislation has banned the use of sulfites on raw fruits and vegetables with the exception of potato products. This regulation is aimed primarily at restaurant salad bars and grocery stores that use sulfites on pre-cut raw produce. This does not necessarily eliminate the preservatives from other foods that are served often in salad bars such as potato or shrimp salads, canned vegetables or fruits, dried fruit, pickled vegetables, and olives.

TABLE 6–4 Common Foods That Contain Sulfites*

Food Category	Types of Food
Alcoholic beverages[†]	Wine, beer, cocktail mixes, wine coolers
Baked goods	Cookies, crackers, mixes with dried fruits or vegetables, pie crust, pizza crust, quiche crust, flour tortillas
Beverage bases	Dried citrus fruit beverage mixes
Condiments and relishes	Horseradish, onion and pickle relishes, pickles, olives, salad dressing mixes, wine vinegar
Confections and frostings	Brown, raw, powdered, or white sugar that is derived from sugar beets
Dairy product analogs	Filled milk (skim milk enriched in fat content by addition of vegetable oils)
Fish and shellfish	Canned clams; fresh, frozen, canned, or dried shrimp; frozen lobster; scallops; dried cod
Pre-cut fresh fruits and vegetables[‡]	Sulfite treatments were banned by FDA regulation (7/9/86) except for fresh pre-cut potatoes
Processed fruits	Canned, bottled, or frozen fruit juices (including lemon, lime, grape, apple); dried fruit; canned, bottled, or frozen dietetic fruit or fruit juices; maraschino cherries; glazed fruit
Processed vegetables	Vegetable juices; canned vegetables (including potatoes); pickled vegetables (including sauerkraut, cauliflower, and peppers); dried vegetables; instant mashed potatoes; frozen potatoes; potato salad
Gelatins, puddings, fillings	Fruit fillings, flavored and unflavored gelatin, pectin, jelling agents
Grain products and pasta	Cornstarch, modified food starch, spinach pasta, gravies, hominy, breadings, batters, noodle or rice mixes
Jams and jellies	Jams and jellies
Nuts and nut products	Shredded coconut
Plant protein products	Soy protein products
Snack foods	Dried fruit snacks, trail mixes, filled crackers
Soups and soup mixes	Canned soups, dried soup mixes
Sweet sauces, toppings, syrups	Corn syrup, maple syrup, fruit toppings, high fructose corn syrup, pancake syrup, molasses
Tea	Instant tea, liquid tea concentrates

* Not all manufacturers of these foods use sulfites. The amounts that are used may vary. Information from this list should be supplemented by reading the labels of packaged foods.
† The use of sulfites in wine and in beer comes under the jurisdiction of the Treasury Department's Bureau of Alcohol, Tobacco and Firearms, which has proposed requiring sulfite labeling for wine, distilled spirits, and malt beverages if sulfite levels are 10 parts per million or more.
‡ Sulfur dioxide is used as a fungicide on grapes, a use regulated by the U.S. Environmental Protection Agency.

Further legislation defines that the presence of sulfites must be declared in a finished food. Any food that contains at least 10 parts per million of sulfites must identify the sulfite in the ingredient list on the label.

Sulfites may be called by any of the following names: sulfur dioxide, potassium bisulfite, potassium metabisulfite, sodium bisulfite, sodium metasulfite, and sodium sulfite or whitening agents. Sulfite intolerant individuals should be instructed to read ingredient labels on all processed foods or to ask restaurant managers if sulfiting agents are present in foods on the menus.

Physicians: How to Order Diet

The diet order should indicate *diet for sulfite-reactive patients.*

SUGGESTED FURTHER READINGS

Hecht W. Sulfites: preservatives that can go wrong. FDA Consumer 1983;17:11.
Lecos CW. Sulfites: FDA limits uses, broadens labeling. FDA Consumer 1986;20:11–13.
Sulfites still here, there, and everywhere. Tufts University Diet and Nutrition Letter. 1986;4:1–3.
Worth Nothing. Nutr News 1985;48(Dec):#4.

MONOSODIUM GLUTAMATE INTOLERANCE

General Description

Some individuals may be intolerant of monosodium glutamate. Symptoms may include a tightness in the chest, a warm and tingling feeling, a stiffness and/or a weakness of the limbs, a headache, light-headedness, facial flush, heartburn, and gastric discomfort. Some investigators have reported severe asthmatic attacks that require ventilatory support. The diagnosis is established by the clinical history and by a specific challenge. This intolerance may not be as common as previously thought.

Monosodium glutamate (MSG) is a flavor enhancer that is widely used in Japanese, Chinese, and Southeastern Asian food preparation. It is also used in various spices and in bouillon cubes.

Patients should be advised to read the ingredient labels of processed foods to determine the presence of monosodium glutamate content prior to purchasing food.

SUGGESTED FURTHER READING

Anderson JA. Food allergy and food intolerance. Contemp Nutr 1984(Sept);9.
Cochran JW, Cochran AH. Monosodium glutamania: the Chinese restaurant syndrome revisited. (letter) JAMA 1984;252:899.
Mermelstein NH. Food allergies and other food sensitivities. Contemp Nutr 1985;10.
Gore KE, Salmon PR. Chinese restaurant syndrome: fact or fiction? (letter) Lancet 1980;1:251–252.
Kenney RA. The Chinese restaurant syndrome: an anecdote revisited. Food Chem Toxicol 1986;24:351–354.
Zautcke JL, Schwartz JA, Mueller EJ. Chinese restaurant syndrome: a review. Ann Emerg Med 1986;15:1210–1213.

PENICILLIN AND MOLD-CONTROLLED DIET

General Description

The diet is intended to eliminate penicillin and molds (Table 6–5). Milk and all dairy products are to be avoided, since they may contain penicillin as a contaminant. Food sources of molds may be categorized as (1) mold foods (such as mushrooms), (2) mold-containing foods, which includes foods to which molds are added to develop a particular flavor (such as cheese, sour cream, buttermilk, bacon, sausage, ham), and (3) mold-acquiring foods, which includes foods that are likely to act as a substrate for mold growth (such as jams, jellies, tea, spices).

TABLE 6–5 Foods to Allow and Foods to Avoid in the Penicillin- and Mold-Controlled Diet

Food Groups	Allow	Avoid
Beverage	Coffee; decaffeinated coffee; cereal beverages; carbonated beverages; soft drink mixes	Tea; cocoa; hot chocolate; beverage mixes that contain milk products
Meat	All except those in the "Avoid" column	Ham; sausage; cottage cheese; cheese; cheese spreads; processed cheese; cold cuts; frankfurters
Fat	Nondairy cream substitutes; all others except those in the "Avoid" column	Bacon or bacon drippings; butter; cream cheese; half and half; cream, sour cream; whipping cream; margarines that contain milk products; salad dressings that contain milk products, cheese, or vinegar; gravy that contains milk
Milk	Soybean milk	All milk and milk products: whole milk, low fat milks, skim milk, buttermilk, evaporated milk, condensed milk, dry powdered milk, yogurt
Starch	Any that do not contain milk products; potatoes; rice; noodles; spaghetti	Any breads, cereals, crackers, or prepared foods that contain milk products
Vegetable	All except those in the "Avoid" column	Any prepared with milk products; mushrooms; truffles; morels
Fruit	All except dried fruit	Dried fruit
Soup	All except those in the "Avoid" column	Cream soups; any made with milk products
Dessert	Fruit ices; gelatin; others made with allowed foods	Ice cream; ice milk; sherbet; puddings; any desserts that contain milk, which includes commercial mixes, bakery products, and homemade foods that contain dried fruit or raisins
Sweets	Sugar, pure sugar candy	Jams; jellies; honey; syrup; molasses; any that contain milk products
Miscellaneous	Salt	Pepper; herbs; spices; seasonings and flavorings that contain milk products; chocolate; cocoa; beer; wine; distilled alcoholic beverages; soy sauce

Nutritional Inadequacy

The diet is low in calcium as compared to the RDA. If the diet is to be followed for an extended period, a calcium supplement should be prescribed.

Indications and Rationale

The diet may be useful in the treatment of some types of chronic urticaria or of other forms of allergic response attributable to penicillin hypersensitivity.

Other than anecdotal case reports, there is little evidence that major dietary manipulations have specific benefit for patients who are allergic to penicillin and have other disorders such as urticaria or asthma.

The contamination of milk occurs when animals with bovine mastitis are treated with penicillin. Although the sale of milk from these animals is legally prohibited for a certain period, small amounts of penicillin may nevertheless be present. Milk processing is not likely to destroy all the penicillin, and it is possible that the degradation products are as sensitizing as penicillin itself, if not more so. Therefore, no dairy products may be used in any form.

Food sources of molds are restricted on the basis that *Penicillium* is one of the most commonly occurring molds. Other molds may produce a reaction that is similar to that of penicillin. The molecular basis for these ideas has not been proven.

An acceptable level of penicillin in the diet has not been determined. The diet is intended to be as free of penicillin and molds as possible.

Food Labeling

The patient should be advised to read product labels carefully and to avoid dairy products (that is, milk and milk products, cheese and cheese products, cream and cream products, milk solids, casein lactalbumin, curds, and whey).

Medications

Antibiotics that are related to penicillin may have the same effect as penicillin itself. Caution should be exercised in the prescription and administration of medications.

Food Storage

Foods should be stored at cool temperatures to inhibit the growth of penicillin and of mold.

The diet should not be followed for a prolonged period without adequate medical supervision and evaluation of symptomatic response.

Physicians: How to Order Diet

The diet order should indicate *penicillin- and mold-controlled diet.*

SUGGESTED FURTHER READING

Bock SA. Food sensitivity. Nutr News 1984;47:9–11.

Kaplan AP. Chronic urticaria. Postgrad Med 1983;74:209–222.

Mold allergy. Washington, D.C.: Asthma and Allergy Foundation of America, 1984;June: 1–7.

Schwartz HJ, Sher TH. Anaphylaxis to penicillin in a frozen dinner. Ann Allergy 1984;52:342–343.

YEAST-CONTROLLED DIET

General Description

It is impossible to eliminate yeast completely, as yeast spores occur naturally in the air and grow rapidly on any source of carbohydrate and of water. This diet, however, attempts to eliminate food sources of yeast and some yeast-like molds.

Patients who are allergic to yeast may "cross-react" and develop symptoms from the ingestion or the inhalation of mold, since both are fungi and may share common allergens.

Sources of yeast are listed in Tables 6–6 and 6–7.

TABLE 6–6 Food Sources of Yeast

Bakers' yeast (used as leavening agent)
Brewers' yeast (used as fermenting agent)
Compressed yeast
Dry yeast
"Natural" vitamins derived from yeast
Enriched flours and fortified cereals that contain vitamins that are derived from yeast
Yeast-forming foods (which include fermented beverages, vinegar, and malt)
Mold foods (such as mushrooms)
Mold-containing foods (such as cheese)

Nutritional Inadequacy

The diet is similar to the general hospital diet and is not inherently inadequate in nutrients as compared to the RDA. It should not be used for an extended period of time without medical supervision. If a vitamin supplement is needed, it should not contain vitamins that are derived from yeast. This information is available from the manufacturer.

Indications and Rationale

The diet may be useful in the treatment of some types of chronic urticaria. The role of yeasts in urticaria is not established. An acceptable level of yeast in the diet has not been established. Therefore, the diet is designed to be as free of yeasts as possible. A modification that allows trace amounts of yeast derivatives may be made later, depending upon individual tolerance.

Physicians: How to Order Diet

The diet order should indicate *yeast-controlled diet.*

Food Labeling

The patient should be advised to read product labels carefully. If the list of ingredients includes "enriched" or "fortified" flour cereal grains, the product

TABLE 6–7 Foods to Allow and Foods to Avoid in the Yeast-Controlled Diet

Food Groups	Allow	Avoid
Beverage	Coffee; decaffeinated coffee; cereal beverages; other carbonated beverages; artificially flavored fruit drink	Black tea; naturally flavored root beer and ginger ale
Meat	Pure meat, fish, fowl, and eggs; peanut butter	Cold cuts; frankfurters; aged and processed cheese; cottage cheese; hamburger (unless pure meat); commercially prepared meat products; meat loaf; breaded meats; meat patties; croquettes; omelets
Fat	Butter; margarine; cream; bacon; vegetable oil; shortening; nuts; gravies and sauces made with allowed thickening agent	Nondairy cream substitutes;* cream cheese; sour cream; commercially prepared gravies and cream sauces; olives; commercially prepared salad dressings
Milk	All except those in the "Avoid" column	Buttermilk; yogurt; malted milk
Starch	Baked products leavened with baking powder or baking soda: biscuits, muffins, quick breads, pancakes, waffles, corn bread	Baked products leavened with yeast: bread, rolls, buns, sourdough, bread products, bread crumbs, crackers, stuffings; commercially prepared baked goods,* mixes,* muffins,* biscuits,* pancakes,* and waffles;* cereals containing malt; vitamin-fortified cereals*
	Flours not vitamin enriched: rice flour, cornmeal and corn flour, potato flour, soy flour, low protein wheat-starch flour; unenriched wheat, graham, and rye flours	Flours enriched with vitamins that are derived from yeast: wheat,* graham,* rye*
	Potatoes; rice; hominy grits; starchy vegetables; low protein wheat-starch pasta; popcorn	Commercial rice mixes; pasta;* noodles* and macaroni* products; crackers;* pretzels;* snack foods* and chips*
Vegetable	All except those in the "Avoid" column	Mushrooms; truffles; morels; sauerkraut; pickled vegetables
Fruit	Freshly prepared fruit juices; all fruits and fruit products except those in the "Avoid" column	Dried fruit; frozen and canned fruit juices; commercially prepared pie filling*
Soup	Homemade broth, vegetable soup, and cream soups thickened with allowed flours	Commercially prepared soup,* soup mixes,* and bouillon*
Dessert	Meringues; plain gelatin; custard; cornstarch, rice, or tapioca pudding; specially prepared desserts made with allowed flours and leavening agents	Commercially prepared desserts and mixes; cookies;* cakes;* piecrust;* pastries;* ice cream cones;* gelatin with added vitamins; puddings;* ice cream;* sherbet*
Sweets	Sugar; honey; jelly; jam; molasses; corn syrup; pure maple syrup; pure baking chocolate; pure cocoa; coconut	Flavored syrups;* chocolate and cream candies*
Miscellaneous	Salt; all spices and herbs except those in the "Avoid" column	Barbecue sauce, chili sauce; pepper; curry powder;* vinegar; catsup; mustard; bottled meat sauces; soy sauce; horseradish; pickles; seasoning mixes;* yeast tablets; beer; wine; distilled alcoholic beverages; chutney; mayonnaise; salad dressings; tabasco sauce

*Check label carefully. Avoid if ingredients include substances that may contain yeast or yeast derivatives. Since yeast spores occur naturally in the air, foods should be covered and properly refrigerated to inhibit growth.

should be avoided unless the manufacturer verifies that yeast is not the source of added vitamins. If the list of ingredients includes "leavening," avoid the product unless the manufacturer verifies that yeast is not the leavening agent. If "stabilizers," "emulsifiers," or "thickening agents" are in the list of ingredients, patients should avoid the products unless the manufacturer verifies that they do not contain vitamin-enriched flour.

Substitutions

Bakers' yeast	baking soda, baking powder
Brewers' yeast	nonalcoholic flavorings used in place of wine or liquor in foods.
Vitamins	synthetic vitamins
Vinegar	pure lemon juice

SUGGESTED FURTHER READING

Candidiasis—an epidemic or a non-disease? Environmental Nutrition Inc 1986;(Jan): S-1 and S-2.
Nonken PP, Hirsch SR. The allergy cookbook. New York: Warner Books, 1982.
Rajan VS, Giam YC. An approach to urticaria. Ann Acad Med 1983;12:74–80.

CARDIOVASCULAR DISEASE

HYPERTENSION

General Description

The dietary management of hypertension focuses on the control of weight and on the restriction of the sodium intake. A limitation of the alcoholic intake is also prescribed. Other dietary factors (i.e., calcium, potassium, fat, fiber, and fatty acids) that are thought to be implicated in hypertension may be considered as well.

Nutritional Inadequacy

The diet for hypertension is not inherently inadequate in nutrients when compared to the RDA. However, for those diets where calories are restricted to 1,200 Kcal or less, it is difficult to meet the RDA consistently. A daily multiple vitamin that provides nutrients at a level equivalent to the RDA is recommended for persons who consume 1,200 Kcal or less.

Indication and Rationale

A sustained elevation of the blood pressure is known as hypertension. Primary or essential hypertension is that elevation of blood pressure that is unrelated to any identifiable cause. The Joint National Committee on Detection, Evaluation, and Treatment of High Blood Pressure states that "The diagnosis of hypertension in adults is confirmed when the average of two or more diastolic blood pressures on at least two subsequent visits is 90 mm Hg or higher, or when the average of multiple systolic blood pressures on two or more subsequent visits is consistently greater than 140 mm Hg."[1]

Prescribed treatment regimens vary because hypertension varies in its degree of severity. Pharmacologic therapy is often employed as the sole treatment of hypertension. However, because of the attendant risks and costs of the drugs, one also should look to the use of the nonpharmacologic means of treatment, such as diet and physical exercise.[2,3] In mild hypertension, diet and physical exercise are the recognized approaches to treatment.[4] Additionally, the combination of diet therapy as an adjunct to the pharmacologic treatment of moderate to severe hypertension has been shown to enhance the effectiveness of the drug treatment and, in some cases, to reduce the quantity of the medications needed for blood pressure control.[2-6]

The precise relationship of diet to the etiology of hypertension remains controversial and is in need of further study. However, dietary changes are a major part of the nonpharmacologic treatment of existing hypertension.[2,3,6] The established means of dietary treatment include the control of weight, the reduction of excessive sodium intake, and the reduction of excessive alcoholic intake.[2,3,6-9] Additional dietary manipulations that are proposed for the treatment of hypertension include an increase in the potassium intake, an increase in the potassium to sodium ratio, an increase in the calcium intake, a decrease in the total fat intake while increasing the percentage of polyunsaturated fatty acids, and a decrease in the caffeine intake.[2,3,5,6,10,11]

Weight Control. While not all obese individuals become hypertensive, obesity does appear to be associated with hypertension. Specific characteristics of obesity (e.g., the body fat distribution pattern, the insulin level, the adipose cell morphology, and the body composition) appear to influence the likelihood of developing hypertension. Both hemodynamic and hormonal-based theories (increased insulin levels may result in increased sodium retention) have also been advanced as possible explanations for the hypertensive effects of obesity.[12-14]

Independent of other variables, the reduction of the body weight in the obese hypertensive patient has been shown to aid in the reduction of the blood pressure levels.[2-4,6,15] It has been shown that an absolute weight loss of as little as 10 pounds can decrease the blood pressure. Once the body weight is decreased it must be maintained in order for the beneficial effects on blood pressure control to continue on a long-term basis.[3]

Sodium. Individual blood pressure response to sodium restriction varies in degree from patient to patient.[2,3,6,16,17] Most persons with hypertension experience a decrease in blood pressure levels with sodium restriction and are described as "sodium sensitive."[5,6,16,17] While a reliable means of prospectively identifying sodium sensitive individuals is unavailable at the present time, there is some indication that hypertensives with a low plasma renin activity may be more responsive to sodium restriction.[5,17] A moderate sodium restriction in hypertensive patients can be of therapeutic value whether medications are used or not.[2-5,10,17] For those patients on diuretic therapy, a dietary sodium restriction lessens the risk of hypokalemia by preventing the excessive urinary loss of potassium. The antihypertensive effect of sodium restriction is particularly additive to vasodilators, to converting enzyme inhibitors, and to adrenergic inhibitors.[5,6]

Alcohol. The reduction of an excessive alcoholic intake has been shown to reduce the blood pressure.[2,6,7,9] An ethanol intake of 1 to 2 ounces daily may, in some individuals, cause an increase in the blood pressure.[2,3,6] (Two ounces by volume of ethanol would correspond to approximately 4 ounces of 100 proof spirits, or to 20 to 24 ounces of wine, or to 48 to 60 ounces of beer. See *Appendix 3* for computing the alcoholic content of other beverages.) It has been suggested that during the initial treatment of hypertension the patient abstain from alcohol, and then the blood pressure be observed closely for the effects of the reintroduction of alcohol.[2]

Other Dietary Factors. In epidemiologic studies, the observation has been made that as the dietary sodium intake rises, the dietary potassium intake falls.[2,3,6,10,18] The role of potassium in the pathogenesis of hypertension remains unclear.[6,18] The effectiveness of potassium supplementation for the purpose of lowering the blood pressure has not been proven. From the practical standpoint, a decrease in the dietary sodium (along with improving overall dietary habits) results in an increased intake of fruits and vegetables with a subsequent increase in the potassium intake. It has been suggested that this increase in the ratio of the potassium to the sodium intake in the diet may lower the blood pressure for some hypertensive individuals.[2,3,10,11]

There are varied results in the studies on the influence of dietary calcium intake on hypertension.[5,19-21] At this time, it is difficult to identify an inadequate calcium intake as a precursor to or a cause of hypertension.[5,20] However, it would be reasonable, with the presently available information, to say that an adequate calcium intake is of value to the general health of the patient and may possibly be of some benefit in the treatment tof hypertension.[2,3] Aggressive calcium loading or supplementation as a treatment for essential hypertension is not recommended.[5,6,19]

An increase in the dietary fiber intake has beneficial effects on bowel regulation and on general health. When the dietary fiber is increased, studies have reported variable effects on the lowering of the blood pressure(s). Therefore, at this time it is difficult to recommend an increased fiber intake specifically for the purpose of lowering the blood pressure.

Some studies indicate that the use of polyunsaturated fat in the place of saturated fat, as well as a decrease of the total fat intake (to 25 to 30 percent of the total calories), may lower the blood pressure in some hypertensive individuals.[3,6,22,23] The antihypertensive effect of increasing polyunsaturated fatty acids may be attributable to an increase in the linoleic acid, which acts as a precursor of vasodilatory and of natriuretic prostaglandins.[24] Clinical studies are not yet conclusive in establishing the effectiveness of altering the dietary fat intake in the treatment of hypertension.[6] However, hypertension alone is considered a major risk factor in the development of cardiovascular disease; and, when uncontrolled hypertension is coupled with lipid abnormalities, the patient's risk of cardiovascular disease increases dramatically.[25] Some antihypertensive medications (thiazides and related sulfonamides, loop diuretics, and beta-adrenergic blockers) increase the cholesterol and/or the triglycerides as a side effect.[1] In situations in which an increase in serum lipids poses a problem, the concomitant use of a low saturated fat, of a low total fat, and of a low cholesterol diet may be necessary. If serious lipid abnormalities persist even with the dietary treatment, a change in the drug therapy may be advisable.

The blood pressure rises acutely with the ingestion of caffeine.[6,26] In one study, an acute rise in the blood pressure of 5 to 15 mm mercury occurred within 15 minutes after the ingestion of 150 mg caffeine (i.e., approximately 2 to 3 cups of brewed coffee).[26] This elevation may persist for a short time. However, the chronic or the prolonged elevation of the blood pressure attributable to caffeine consumption has not been demonstrated owing to the body's development of a tolerance to the effects of caffeine.[3,6,26,27] Nonetheless, it is common practice to caution the patient against the excessive intake of caffeine and to limit the coffee consumption to less than 3 to 5 cups per day.

Goals of Dietary Management

The goal of therapy for hypertension is to sufficiently lower and maintain the blood pressure in accordance to the standards set by the Joint National Committee on Detection, Evaluation, and Treatment of High Blood Pressure.[1] When it is possible and feasible, dietary management alone may be effective enough to accomplish this goal. However, dietary modifications are valuable as an adjunct to pharmacologic therapy. One further reduces the risk of cardiovascular disease by controlling the blood pressure with dietary and/or drug treatment, because an uncontrolled elevated blood pressure is a risk factor in the development of cardiovascular disease.[25]

Dietary Recommendations

Table 6–8 presents a summary of the dietary recommendations for essential hypertension. This table includes those dietary features that are possible to quantify and that are viewed as the primary considerations of dietary management. While it may be relatively easy to make numerical recommendations for dietary restrictions, the feasibility of implementing the restrictions varies according to the individual patient. The diet as prescribed should take into consideration the individual's needs, including the life-style, the responses to treatment (particularly the sodium and the alcohol sensitivities), and the ability to follow recommendations.

While it is advisable for any hypertensive patient who is more than 115 percent of the desirable body weight to reduce weight, it may not be possible or advisable to reduce all the patients' weights to the level indicated in the Height-Weight Tables (*Appendix* 4). It has been shown that absolute weight reduction results in a lowered blood pressure in the obese hypertensive patient even when the desirable body weight is not achieved.[1] A weight loss to the level that is accompanied by a good blood pressure control should be the goal in the management of hypertension. Therefore, it may be more realistic, and equally effective, to set a weight goal for the patient that is higher than the desirable body weight listed in the tables. A weight goal that is reasonable for the patient to achieve and to maintain on a long term basis is likely to enhance both the effectiveness of and the compliance with the diet regimen. It should be noted, however, that some individuals, whose weights fall within the higher limits of normal as listed in the Height-Weight Tables, may also benefit from a moderate weight loss.

TABLE 6–8 Dietary Recommendations

Body Weight	Weight reduction if greater than 115% of the desirable weight or if greater than the usual weight even if current weight is within the limits of the Height-Weight Tables Reduce weight to a desirable weight or an intermediate goal weight at which blood pressure control is improved Continued maintenance of the appropriate weight
Sodium Intake	Recommended level by degree* of hypertension High Normal or Borderline: 90–120 mEq (2,070–2,760 mg) per day or "No Extra Salt" diet Mild: 90 mEq (2,070 mg) per day Moderate: 60–90 mEq (1,380–2,070 mg) per day. Severe: 60 mEq (1,380 mg) per day or less if feasible
Alcoholic Intake	Initial stage of treatment, abstinence is advised to assess the impact of alcohol on the blood pressure level Subsequently, limit to less than or equal to two alcoholic beverages (12 to 24 oz of beer, 4 to 8 oz of wine, $1\frac{1}{2}$ to 3 oz of liquor) per day, if blood pressure control is not worsened by the addition of alcohol to the diet

* Definitions of degree of hypertension for persons 18 years of age or older:[1]
High Normal or Borderline: 85–89 mm of mercury diastolic; 140–159 mm of mercury systolic.
Mild: 90–104 mm of mercury diastolic; and/or 160–169 mm of mercury systolic.
Moderate: 105–114 mm of mercury diastolic; and/or greater than 200 mm of mercury systolic.
Severe: Equal to or greater than 115 mm of mercury diastolic; and/or greater than 200 mm of mercury systolic.

It is difficult to quantify an acceptable level of alcohol use for all persons with hypertension. Alcohol, if used, should be limited to moderate amounts, and its effect on blood pressure control should be assessed. For some persons, the avoidance of alcohol may be advisable.

Additional dietary modifications may be of benefit to some persons with hypertension (Table 6–9). However, these modifications should be considered subsequent or secondary to caloric, to sodium, and to alcoholic restricted programs. The efficacy of such secondary considerations varies more among individual patients than does the efficacy of the preceding recommendations in Table 6–8. Also, in some of the secondary considerations, clinical evidence with which to make specific recommendations is at this time lacking or inadequate. In all dietary regimens, it is critical that one monitors the patient's response to treatment and makes the dietary adjustments accordingly. Both quantitative and qualitative changes may be needed as therapy proceeds (e.g., adding lipid restrictions or making further sodium or alcoholic limitations).

TABLE 6–9 Secondary Considerations for Treatment of Hypertension

Further sodium restriction for individuals who are sodium sensitive
Elimination of alcohol for individuals sensitive to alcohol
Increase in total potassium
Increase in potassium to sodium ratio
Maintenance of adequate dietary calcium intake
Reduction of total dietary fat
Reduction of saturated fat
Increase in polyunsaturated fat

Food Sources of Sodium

Sources of dietary sodium are (1) table salt, (2) foods to which salt or sodium compounds have been added, (3) foods that inherently contain sodium, (4) chemically softened water that contains sodium salts, and (5) some medications.

Depending on the source and the method of calculation, estimates of the sodium content of the American diet range from 260 to 656 mEq of sodium (i.e., 6 to 15 g sodium).[28] The inherent sodium content of foods and the sodium added by food manufacturers must be considered when a sodium controlled diet is prescribed. The major source of sodium in the diet is salt (40 percent sodium), commonly used in cooking, in food processing, and at the table.

Foods. The sodium that is inherent in some foods must be calculated as part of the sodium allowance. Animal foods such as meats, eggs, and dairy products, and some vegetables contain natural sodium and should be used in controlled amounts. Sodium compounds are used in food processing for various reasons; for example, sodium benzoate is a preservative used in relishes, sauces, and margarine, and sodium citrate enhances the flavor of gelatin desserts and of beverages. Although there are many low sodium products on the market, such items may be used in controlled amounts. If such a product contains no more than 10 mg of sodium per serving, it is considered to contribute negligible amounts of sodium in the diet.

Food Labeling. It is important to read labels on foods that are purchased. Federal regulations were formulated, effective July 1, 1986, by the United States Food and Drug Administration to control the terms used in sodium labeling.[29,30] These regulations define the descriptive terms that refer to the sodium content as follows:[29]

1. "Sodium-free" means less than 5 mg of sodium per serving.
2. "Very low sodium" means 35 mg of sodium or less per serving.
3. "Low sodium" means 140 mg of sodium or less per serving.
4. "Reduced sodium" means foods are processed to reduce the usual level of sodium by 75 percent.

Such information may be used to calculate the sodium content of the specific food item and to establish the use of that food in the diet.

Medications. Antacids, laxatives, cough medicines, and other medications may contain significant amounts of sodium. One should check the label or ask a local pharmacist or the manufacturer for the sodium content.

Softened Water. Drinking water, either natural or softened, may be a significant source of sodium. Patients on severe sodium restriction (less than or equal to 60 mEq per day) are advised to ask the public health department about the sodium content of the local water supply. If the content exceeds 40 parts per million (2 mEq or 40 mg of sodium per liter), it may be necessary for the patient to use distilled water for drinking and for cooking.

Sodium Calculation. Establishing the level of sodium restriction depends on the severity of the disease and on the individual response to treatment. The amount of sodium calculated by the dietitian when formulating the diet plan should be no greater than 10 percent above the level of sodium that is prescribed by the physician. However, it is acceptable for the calculated level of sodium to be more than 10 percent below the prescribed level. In most situations, one should not add extra table salt to bring the sodium intake up to the prescribed level.

Table 6–10 presents a summary of the approximate sodium values for selected foods. These values can be used as estimates in calculating different levels of sodium restrictions. The food groups are based on exchanges as used in the

Diabetes Mellitus Food Exchange List (see page 114). Exact sodium content, especially of processed or convenience foods, varies; figures represent the average values. When tailoring a diet to the individual's needs, it may be necessary to consult the food composition tables, the manufacturers' analyses, or the product labels for more specific information on the sodium content. Some foods noted in the table may be difficult or impossible to include in sodium restricted diets.

TABLE 6-10 Approximate Sodium Content of Selected Foods

Foods by Group	Approx. Portion	Approx. Sodium (mEq)
Meat		
Unsalted	1 oz	1
Salted	1 oz	3[†]
Cottage cheese (dry curd)	1/4 cup	1
Egg	1 med	3
Mild aged cheddar cheese	1 oz	8
Cottage cheese, creamed	1/4 cup	10
Ham	1 oz	12–18
Processed American cheese food	1 oz	12–15
Cold cuts	1 oz	14–18
Smoked link sausage	1 oz	18
Milk		
Whole	8 oz	5
Skim, nonfat or 1%	8 oz	6
Buttermilk (from skim milk)	8 oz	14
Starch		
Puffed ready-to-eat cereal	$1\frac{1}{2}$ cups	0–1.5
Low sodium bread	1 slice	0.5
Cooked potatoes, cereals, and other starches (unsalted) (pasta, rice, etc.)	1/2 cup	0.5
Salt-free soda crackers	six 2″ sq	6
Graham crackers	three $2\frac{1}{2}″$ sq	6
Regular bread	1 slice	5
Regular saltine crackers	six 2″ sq	11
Cooked potatoes, cereals, and other starches (salted)	1/2 cup	10[†]
Corn or wheat flake cold cereal	3/4 cup	10*
Pancake, biscuit, waffle (from mix)	1 med	10–15*
Commercial soup	1 cup	15–40*
Vegetables		
Unsalted (most kinds)	1/2 cup	Trace–1
Raw celery	3 stalks	3
Reg. canned (except tomatoes)	1/2 cup	10[†]
Reg. canned tomatoes, sauce or puree	1/4 cup	7–12
Reg. canned tomatoe juice	1/2 cup	19
Reg. vegetable juice cocktail	1/2 cup	19
Dill pickle	1 med	62
Fruit		
Most kinds, fruit or juice	1/2 cup	Trace[§]
Fat		
Cream (any weight)	1 Tbsp	Trace[§]
Vegetable oil	1 tsp	Trace[§]
Unsalted butter, margarine	1 tsp	Trace[§]
Regular mayonnaise	1 tsp	1
Regular butter, margarine	1 tsp	2
Mayonnaise type salad dressing	2 tsp	3
Green olives	9–10 small	27–30
Regular pourable salad dressing (average)	1 Tbsp	7
Blue cheese salad dressing	1 Tbsp	6–11*
Bacon	1 med strip	7
Commercial gravy or gravy mix	2 Tbsp	7
Tartar sauce	$1\frac{1}{2}$ tsp	4

TABLE 6–10 Approximate Sodium Content of Selected Foods (*continued*)

Foods by Group	Approx. Portion	Approx. Sodium (mEq)
Beverages		
Beer, liquor, or wine	12 oz, or 1½ oz, or 4 oz	0–0.5
Coffee (reg. or decaf)	8 oz	Trace
Carbonated drinks	12 oz	Trace–3
Tea, instant	8 oz	Trace
Tea, brewed	8 oz	1
Tang, orange	12 oz	1
Hawaiian punch	12 oz	2
Tonic water	8 oz	4
Club soda	12 oz	6
Instant cocoa	1 pkt	7
Tang, grape	12 oz	10
Bouillon	1 cube	41
Desserts		
Sherbet, fruit ice	1/3 cup	1
Ice cream	1/2 cup	2*
Flavored gelatin (average)	1/2 cup	2*
Low calorie instant pudding	1/4 cup	2*
Angel food cake (homemade, no ring)	1/16	3‡
Cooked pudding (mix, but not instant)	1/4 cup	4
Cookies, assorted plain	two 2″ diam.	4–10*
Pie, fruit or cream (homemade)	1/8 of 9″ pie	9–14‡
Instant pudding from mix	1/4 cup	8
Other		
Prepared mustard	1 tsp	3
Regular catsup	1 Tbsp	7
"Light" salt	1/4 tsp	10
Regular meat tenderizer	1/4 tsp	19
Garlic or onion salt	1/4 tsp	17–20*
Salt	1/4 tsp	23
Regular soy sauce	1 Tbsp	37–45*

* Actual sodium content of commercially prepared items varies with manufacturer.
† "salted" = 1/4 tsp salt per pound of meat; or 1/8 tsp salt per half cup serving potato or substitute, vegetable cereal.
‡ Wide variations depending on recipes.
§ Trace is <0.5 mEq (12 mg) sodium.

A "No Extra Salt" (NES) or "No Added Salt" diet is a noncalculated diet in which the primary objective is to limit highly concentrated sources of sodium and of added salt. The actual sodium content of a NES diet may be inconsistent and usually ranges from 90 to 150 mEq or more depending on the caloric level of the diet. Guidelines for a NES diet are:

1. Do not add salt to food at the table.

2. Use only limited amounts of salt in food preparation: no more than 1/4 tsp of salt per pound of meat; no more than 1/8 tsp of salt per serving of cooked cereal, potatoes, potato substitutes, and cooked vegetables.

3. Limit high sodium foods (see Table 6–10).

Physicians: How to Order Diet

The diet order should indicate *diet for hypertension*. It may include those parameters that the physician wishes to be addressed, such as weight control, sodium control, potassium control, and the modification of fat, alcohol, and calcium. If specific amounts of sodium or other elements are ordered, the dietitian plans a diet that does not exceed that amount by more than 10 percent.

Supplementary Information

Additional information (both patient and professional) is available on request from the sources listed below.

National Heart, Lung, and Blood Institute
Public Inquiries and Reports Branch
Building 31, Room 4A21
National Institutes of Health
Bethesda, MD 20205

The American Heart Association—consult your local affiliate or contact:

The American Heart Association
7320 Greenville Avenue
Dallas, Texas 75231

The American Dietetic Association
208 South LaSalle Street
Chicago, Illinois 60611

REFERENCES

1. The Joint Nat'l. Comm. on Detection, Evaluation, and Treatment of High Blood Pressure. The 1984 report of the Joint National Committee on Detection, Evaluation, and Treatment of High Blood Pressure. Arch Intern Med 1984;144:1045–1057.
2. Kaplan NM. Use of non-drug therapy in treating hypertension. Am J Med 1984;96:101.
3. Kaplan NM. Non-drug treatment of hypertension. Ann Intern Med 1985;102:359–373.
4. Lansford HG, Blaufox D, Oberman A, Hawkins M, Curb JD, Cutter GR, Wassertheil-Smoller S, Presse S, Babcock C, Abernethy JD, Hotchkiss J, Tyler M. Dietary therapy slows the return of hypertension after stopping prolonged medication. JAMA 1985;253:657–664.
5. MacGregor GA. Sodium is more important than calcium in essential hypertension. Hypertension 1985;7:628–637.
6. National Institutes of Health. U.S. Department of Health and Human Services. Nonpharmacologic approaches to the control of high blood pressure. Final report of the Subcommittee on Nonpharmacologic Therapy of the 1984 Joint National Committee on Detection, Evaluation, and Treatment of High Blood Pressure. National Heart, Lung and Blood Institute. Bethesda, MD. U.S. Government Printing Office, 1986 (Publication #1986–491–292:41147).
7. Clark LT. Alcohol use and hypertension. Postgrad Med 1984;75:273–276.
8. Larbi EB, Stamler J, Dyer H, Cooper H, Paul O, Shekelle RB, Lepper M. The population attributable risk of hypertension from heavy alcohol consumption. Public Health Rep 1984;99:316–319.
9. Saunders JB, Beevers DG, Paton A. Alcohol-induced hypertension. Lancet 1981;2:653–656.
10. MacGregor GA. Sodium and potassium intake and blood pressure. Hypertension 1983;5(supp III):79–84.
11. MacGregor GA. Dietary sodium and potassium intake and blood pressure. Lancet 1983;1:750–753.

12. Dustan HP. Obesity and hypertension. Ann Intern Med 1985;103:1047–1049.
13. Horan MJ, Blaustein MP, Dunbar JB, Grundt S, Kachadorian W, Kaplan NM, Kotchen TA, Simopoulos AP, Van Itallie TB. NIH report on research challenges in nutrition and hypertension. Hypertension 1985;7:818–823.
14. Lucas CP, Estigarribia JA, Darga LL, Reaven GM. Insulin and blood pressure in obesity. Hypertension 1985;7:702–706.
15. Berchtold P, Sims EAH, Horton ES, Berge M. Obesity and hypertension: epidemiology, mechanisms, treatment. Biomed Pharmacother 1983;37:251–258.
16. Bergiund G. The role of salt in hypertension. Acta Med Scand 1983;672(suppl):117–129.
17. Davidman MJ, Opsah J. Mechanisms of elevated blood pressure in human essential hypertension. Med Clin North Am 1984;68:301–320.
18. Langford HG. Potassium in hypertension—the case for its role in pathogenesis and treatment. Postgrad Med 1983;74:227–233.
19. McCarron DA. Is calcium more important than sodium in the pathogenesis of essential hypertension. Hypertension 1985;7:607–627.
20. Gruchow HW, Sobocinski KA, Barboriak JJ. Alcohol:nutrient intake, and hypertension in U.S. adults. JAMA 1985;253:1567–1570.
21. McCarron DA, Morris CD. Blood pressure response to oral calcium in persons with mild to moderate hypertension. Ann Intern Med 1985;103:825–831.
22. Iaocono JM, Dougherty RM. The role of dietary polyunsaturated fatty acids and prostaglandins in reducing blood pressure and improving thrombogenic indices. Prev Med 1983;12:60–69.
23. Smith–Barbaro PA, Pucak GJ. Dietary fat and blood pressure. Ann Intern Med 1983;98:829–831.
24. Weber PC, Scherer B, Siess W. Prostaglandins and hypertension. Adv Exp Med Biol 1984;164:269–281.
25. Kannel WB, Doyle JT, Ostfeld AM, Jenkins CD, Kuller L, Podell RN, Stamler J. Atherosclerosis Study Group. Optimal resources for primary prevention of atherosclerotic diseases—Amer Heart Assoc Report. Circulation 1984;70:157A–205A.
26. Robertson D, Hollisten AS, Kincaid D, Workman R, Goldberg MR, Rung C, Smith B. Caffeine and hypertension. Am J Med 1984;77:54–68.
27. Curatolo PW, Robertson D. The health consequences of caffeine. Ann Intern Med 1983;98:641–653.
28. Fregly MJ. Estimates on daily sodium ingestion. In: Olson RE, Broquist HP, Chichester CO, Darby WJ, Kolbye AC, Stalvey RM, eds. Nutrition review's present knowledge in nutrition. 5th ed. Washington, D.C.: The Nutrition Foundation, 1984:441.
29. Miller RW. Food labels to tell more about sodium. FDA Consumer 1984;July–Aug.:30–31.
30. Lecos C. New regulation to help sodium conscious consumers. FDA Consumer 1986;May.

HYPERLIPIDEMIA

General Description

Dietary management is the primary treatment for most types of hyperlipidemia. For persons above desirable body weight, caloric restriction is emphasized. Recommendations for the levels of the intake of fat (amount and kind), cholesterol, carbohydrate, and alcohol are determined by which lipids are elevated in the blood serum.

Nutritional Inadequacy

Diets for the management of hyperlipidemia are not inherently inadequate in nutrients as compared to the RDA. However, for diets that emphasize caloric restriction to 1,200 Kcal or less, it is difficult to meet the RDA consistently. A daily multiple vitamin supplement that provides nutrients at a level that is equivalent to the RDA is recommended for persons who consume 1,200 Kcal or less. A multiple vitamin supplement may also be warranted for persons who have food aversions or intolerances that greatly limit the variety of food choices.

Indications and Rationale

Hyperlipidemia is a general term that refers to an abnormal elevation of lipids (triglycerides and cholesterol). Hyperlipoproteinemia is an abnormal elevation of lipoproteins in the blood. Lipoproteins serve to transport cholesterol, triglycerides, and phospholipids in the blood. Some appear to be regulators of the cholesterol accumulation in the arterial wall.

The elevation of serum cholesterol or of triglycerides is of concern because of its association with the predisposition to atherosclerosis. The treatment is based on the assumption that normalization of the serum lipid values reduces the rate of atherogenesis. Normal values, however, do not necessarily indicate an absence of risk for atherosclerosis.

Diagnosis. The diagnosis of hyperlipidemia is based on the laboratory determination of the cholesterol and triglyceride concentration in the plasma. When the laboratory diagnosis is unclear, a lipoprotein analysis may be done to determine whether abnormal lipoprotein values are present and to determine the type of lipoproteinemia.

Lipoproteins are classified by their density, their composition, and their electrophoretic mobility into five classes as shown in Table 6–11.[1,2] Many constituents of lipoproteins, of cholesterol, of triglycerides, and of lipoprotein fractions are evaluated and used as screening tools for atherosclerosis.

TABLE 6–11 Classification of Lipoproteins

Classification	Major Lipid Components
Chylomicrons	Triglycerides
Chylomicron remnants	Triglycerides
Very low-density lipoprotein (VLDL)	Triglycerides
Low-density lipoprotein (LDL)	Cholesterol
High-density lipoprotein (HDL)	Phospholipids

Primary hyperlipoproteinemias are a result of genetic abnormalities and of environmental factors. Severe forms often are inheritable; a modified diet and, often, drugs are necessary for treatment. Milder forms may be the consequence of undesirable dietary practices. Modifying the diet produces a small to moderate reduction in the serum cholesterol concentration or, less frequently, normalizes the serum cholesterol value.

When a disorder of lipid metabolism occurs secondary to a particular disease such as diabetes mellitus or hypothyroidism, treatment of the underlying illness often corrects the lipid abnormality.

The dietary related hyperlipidemias most often found in medical practice are an elevated serum cholesterol value that is associated with abnormal concentrations of LDL and an elevated serum triglyceride value that results from abnormal concentrations of VLDL. Diets that are high in fat, in saturated fat, and in cholesterol tend to increase the levels of LDL. By consuming less saturated fat and cholesterol and by isocalorically substituting polyunsaturated fats the LDL levels are reduced. Diets that are high in calories, in simple carbohydrates, or in alcohol may increase the levels of VLDL. The VLDL levels usually are reduced by a weight reduction and by consuming fewer simple carbohydrates and less alcohol. The avoidance of very large meals and of high fat meals also is generally recommended.

Treatment. Lipid disorders are treated first by modification of the diet. After an average time span of 3 to 6 months, drugs may be prescribed if the dietary regulations are unsuccessful. The effects of diet and of drugs are additive, thus the dietary modification should be continued during the drug therapy. Continuation of the diet is advised even with the normalization of the blood lipids and of the lipoprotein pattern. Regular exercise and improved physical conditioning have a direct favorable effect on the serum lipids.

Cholesterol. Cholesterol is a part of the normal cell membranes and performs necessary functions in the body. Cholesterol is deposited in the lining of the arteries as atherosclerotic plaques. These deposits, if large enough, may obstruct the flow of blood. Cholesterol is synthesized from the intermediary metabolism of carbohydrate, of fats, and of proteins, and probably only a small fraction of cholesterol deposits are derived directly from dietary cholesterol.

Hypercholesterolemia can be caused by a diet that is high in cholesterol and in saturated fat as well as by hypothyroidism, by obstructive liver disease, by nephrosis, by porphyria, and by dysproteinemia. Also, hypercholesterolemia is likely to be more severe in the genetically susceptible person.

Levels of serum cholesterol that are above 200 to 230 mg per deciliter are associated with an increased risk of developing premature cardiovascular heart disease (CHD). For each one percent decrease in blood cholesterol, there can be an expected two percent decrease in CHD.[3-6] Most studies recommend dietary intervention in accordance with the following guidelines:

1. Individuals with plasma cholesterol levels above the 90 percentile (Table 6–12) should receive dietary treatment and be advised to engage in an exercise program. If there is no response to diet and to other nondrug therapy, such as exercise, the use of lipid lowering medications should be considered.

TABLE 6–12 Plasma Cholesterol (mg/dl) and Percentile Ranking[10]

Ages of Females	Percentiles				
	5	20	50	70	90
20	128	144	163	177	197
30	141	159	180	194	217
40	155	175	198	215	239
50	171	192	218	236	263
60	188	212	240	259	290
70	207	232	264	285	309
Ages of Males					
20	128	145	166	181	204
30	150	170	194	211	238
40	162	185	211	229	258
50	170	193	221	240	270
60	175	198	228	247	278
70	177	202	230	250	282

2. Individuals with plasma cholesterol levels between the 75 to 90 percentiles should receive dietary treatment and be advised to engage in an exercise program, particularly if there are associated risk factors such as diabetes, hypertension, or a family history of coronary heart disease.

As a goal, it has been recommended to encourage the reduction of the blood cholesterol level to approximately 180 mg per deciliter for adults who are under the age of 30 years and to approximately 200 mg per deciliter for individuals who are 30 years of age or older.[5,7]

Triglycerides. Triglycerides are a form of fat that is produced by the body from the conversion of any form of excess calories into fat. Simple carbohydrates are thought to be a major substrate for triglycerides. Alcohol also elevates the levels of triglycerides.[8]

Triglycerides are measured after a 12 to 14 hour fast. An abnormal level is considered at greater than or equal to 95 percent (Table 6–13).[9]

TABLE 6–13 Plasma Triglycerides (mg/dl) and Percentile Ranking[10]

Ages of Females			Percentiles		
	5	20	50	70	95
20	32	43	56	67	97
30	35	46	62	74	106
40	40	52	68	81	117
50	43	56	75	89	128
60	47	62	82	97	140
70	52	68	90	107	154
Ages of Males					
20	34	48	69	86	137
30	43	62	87	109	171
40	48	67	96	119	189
50	50	70	99	123	195
60	51	71	101	125	198
70	51	71	101	126	199

Hypertriglyceridemia has been associated with obesity, uncontrolled diabetes mellitus, excessive alcohol ingestion, renal failure, systemic lupus erythematosus, lipodystrophy, glycogen storage disease, and with the use of various medications, such as estrogens, oral contraceptives, beta-blockers, and hydrochlorothiazide.

The association of elevated serum triglycerides with coronary artery disease is not as direct as that for cholesterol, but high triglyceride levels (>200 mg/dl) appear to be a risk factor for coronary heart disease and for peripheral vascular disease, especially if other risk factors are present.

For levels greater than 500 mg per deciliter, an attempt to lower triglycerides should be made to prevent pancreatitis even if there are no cardiac risk factors present.[8]

High-Density Lipoproteins. High-density lipoproteins have been shown to have an inverse relationship with coronary heart disease. They are usually measured by their content of cholesterol, i.e., HDL cholesterol. This is sometimes referred to as a beneficial or a protective form of cholesterol.

Factors that can cause an increase in HDL cholesterol are an increased clearance of VLDL, exercise, a moderate intake of alcohol, insulin therapy for diabetes, and estrogen.

Factors that are associated with a decrease in HDL cholesterol are starvation, obesity, cigarette smoking, poorly controlled diabetes mellitus, chronic renal failure, hypothyroidism, liver disease, and the use of progesterone. Elevated levels of triglycerides are also associated with low HDL cholesterol levels.

The ratio of total cholesterol to HDL cholesterol can be used to help determine the risk factor (Table 6–14).

TABLE 6–14 Ratio of Total Cholesterol to HDL Cholesterol[4,7]

	Goal
Males	≤5.0
Females	≤4.5

Low-Density Lipoproteins. Increased plasma levels of low-density lipoproteins (LDL) have been shown to be associated with increased atherosclerosis. There is good evidence that cholesterol of dietary origin is transferred ultimately into other lipoprotein classes, especially into LDL, and contributes in this manner to total plasma cholesterol.[1] Factors that can raise LDL are a diet high in saturated fat and in cholesterol and obesity. Genetic predisposition may also play a major role in the elevation of LDL.

To calculate LDL cholesterol, one may use the following formula:[6]

$$\text{LDL cholesterol} = \text{total cholesterol} - \left(\frac{\text{triglycerides}}{5} + \text{HDL}\right)$$

Table 6–15 shows the levels of LDL cholesterol and its relationship to the risk for heart disease.

TABLE 6–15 LDL Cholesterol and Risk of Heart Disease

	Age	Moderate to High
		LDL Cholesterol
Men	20–29	≥125
	30+	≥150
Women	20–29	≥125
	30+	≥145
	40+	>155

Typing. Cholesterol, triglycerides, HDL cholesterol, LDL cholesterol, and other lipoproteins can be used for distinguishing hyperlipoproteinemias. Fredrickson's classification (Table 6–16) is the most commonly used classification scheme.[2,6] However, this type of classification is not uniformly employed and is probably not essential to the formulation of dietary and of other recommendations.

Cardiovascular Risk Factors. Risk factors are conditions and habits that have been demonstrated to be associated with an increased probability of cardiovascular disease.[7,11] Genetic factors greatly influence the risk of developing premature coronary heart disease. If one or more close relatives suffered a heart attack before the age of 60 years or has a primary form of hyperlipidemia, the

TABLE 6-16 Typing of Hyperlipoproteinemias

Fredrickson Type	Lipid Abnormality	Elevated Lipoproteins
I	Hyperchylomicronemia	Chylomicrons
IIa	Hypercholesterolemia	LDL
IIb	Combined hypercholesterolemia and endogenous hypertriglyceridemia	LDL, VLDL
III	Dysbetalipoproteinemia (broad beta pattern)	IDL (intermediate density lipoproteins)
IV	Hypertriglyceridemia	VLDL
V	Hypertriglyceridemia	VLDL, chylomicrons

likelihood of other family members to have hyperlipidemia is greater. The entire family should be screened if a primary abnormality is suspected in a patient.

The three most important treatable factors are an elevated total cholesterol, an elevated blood pressure, and an abuse of tobacco. The significance of the risk factors varies with individuals, and the presence of more than one risk factor tends to greatly increase the risk. Elevated blood pressure is a common accompaniment to hyperlipidemias. The major dietary treatment is sodium restriction, weight reduction if obesity exists, regular exercise, and reduction of excessive alcohol intake (see section on *Hypertension*).

Cigarette smoking has a profound effect on increasing the probability of premature cardiovascular disease. It deserves special attention in the prevention of cardiovascular disease and should be given a high priority in the risk factor reduction and the treatment of cardiovascular disease.

Obesity is associated with an increased incidence of coronary disease. Obesity is associated with an increased arterial blood pressure, hyperinsulinemia, an impaired glucose tolerance, a reduced HDL cholesterol, hypertriglyceridemia, and hyperuricemia. Weight loss produces corresponding changes in these parameters.

An objective of weight reduction in the person who is obese and has hyperlipidemia is the normalization of the lipid profile and the other parameters. For some individuals, this may occur with a modest reduction in weight; but for other persons, the achievement of a distinctly lean weight may be necessary. Various indices of obesity can be used. Body mass index is easily calculated (see *Appendix 7*). The percent of body weight as fat is perhaps the best, but the measurement requires rather complex procedures such as underwater weighing. Body mass can be approximated by skinfold measurements and has been helpful in the serial follow-up of patients referred to the Cardiovascular Health Clinic. The sum of axilla, tricep, and suprailium skinfolds for men and women for predicting body fat can be used. Normal values are 16 to 19 percent of body weight as fat for men and 23 to 26 percent of body weight as fat for women.[12,13]

Regular aerobic physical activity (for a minimum of 20 to 30 minutes three times per week) appears to offer some protection from the complications of cardiovascular disease as well as having a lowering effect on the total plasma cholesterol and on the LDL cholesterol levels, especially when coupled with a weight reduction.[14]

Psychological, social, cultural, and religious factors influence the risk of coronary heart disease by their effects on the kinds and the amounts of foods eaten, on the cigarette and alcohol use, and on exercise. Persons who are impatient, highly competitive, and live with a sense of time urgency are greater candidates for cardiovascular disease than persons who live in a more relaxed fashion. Stress management, relaxation skills, and biofeedback may also aid in the reduction of overall risk factors.

Other Dietary Factors Associated with Heart Disease.   There are a variety of interactions between fiber and cholesterol, from altering gastric emptying to interfering with cholesterol and triglyceride absorption. Wheat and corn bran seem to have less benefit than oat bran, pectin, and guar gum (found in fresh fruits, vegetables, and legumes). Current recommendations are neither qualitative nor quantitative. Rather, an increase in the total fiber intake is advocated. Along with the increased consumption of high fiber plant foods is a proportionately greater consumption of carbohydrate and thus a proportionately lower consumption of fat and cholesterol.

Different types of oils have been investigated for their atherogenic effects. Several studies support the theory that certain polyunsaturated fish oils can reduce the incidence of coronary heart disease.[15–17a] Particular attention has been given to the omega-3 essential fatty acids, especially eicosapentaenoic acid (EPA) and docosahexaenoic acid (DHA). EPA and DHA originate in the photoplankton that is consumed by marine fish and by shellfish, especially in oily fish (salmon, mackeral, sea herring, anchovies, mullet, trout, catfish, sardines, and smelt). The increased use of fish, perhaps one to two servings or more of fish per week, is recommended primarily because of the low total fat and saturated fat content.

There may be some undesirable side effects associated with the supplementation of the diet with fish oils. Cod liver oil is a rich source of omega-3 fatty acid, but the oil also supplies large amounts of fat soluble vitamins A and D, which may accumulate to toxic levels if taken in excess. More research is needed in this area before a safe recommendation can be made.[15–17a] In our practice, fish oils used as a supplement are not recommended except under the discretionary advice of the physician.[17b]

Although the use of monounsaturated fats, which includes olive oil, is not generally promoted, there is some evidence that monounsaturated fats may have a favorable effect on the blood lipids when substituted for saturated fats.[18]

Persons who drink alcohol in moderate amounts (one to two drinks per day) have been shown to have a lower risk for heart disease. Recent studies have tried to link alcohol to HDL levels and to examine what fraction of HDL cholesterol is increased. HDL2 is thought to be antiatherogenic while HDL3 is not related to atherosclerosis. Some studies have shown that alcohol increases HDL2 levels while other studies state that alcohol raises HDL3 levels only.[19] Despite these uncertainties, the use of alcohol is not advocated as a means of improving the blood lipid levels because of the potential for other deleterious effects from chronic daily use.

Coffee has been linked with heart disease, but studies have reported conflicting results. At the time of this publication, coffee is not considered a risk factor for atherosclerosis.

Although caffeine does not play a causal role in the development of atherosclerosis, caffeine can cause bradycardia, tachycardia, arrhythmias, and palpitations in some people. For these persons, it is wise to use decaffeinated beverages.

Onions and garlic have been said to reduce serum cholesterol, but convincing proof is lacking.

Goals of Dietary Management

The goal of dietary management, alone or in conjunction with lipid lowering medications, is to reduce any tendency to atherosclerosis and to modify its progression in patients with the disease.

Dietary Recommendations

Various approaches to dietary management have been proposed. The approach is to tailor the recommendations according to the abnormalities of the specific lipid components.

Dietary programs for each of the Fredrickson types of hyperlipidemia have been developed. Difficulties exist in the use of this approach because typing is not universally done and because the lipid profile, and therefore typing category, of an individual may change over time. The American Heart Association (AHA) advocates a three phase approach to diet planning for all lipid abnormalities (*Appendix 9*). This approach may be justified in many situations, but it can impose an unnecessary stringent restriction of cholesterol for patients with hypertriglyceridemia. There is also little evidence to support the specific restriction of sodium and the increased intake of potassium in persons who have hyperlipidemia and are normotensive. Table 6–17 presents the Mayo Clinic's modified approach to the aforementioned AHA scheme, which has been found useful in planning dietary modifications for patients.

TABLE 6–17 Guidelines for Planning Diets for Hypercholesterolemia

	Level I	Level II	Level III
Guidelines for use	Initial diet for treatment or prevention	Next step of diet when insufficient response to Level I	Next step of diet when insufficient response to Level II
Compliance issues	Requires some change in dietary habits for most persons	Requires substantial changes in dietary habits	Adherence is difficult and likely to be achieved by only highly motivated persons.
Dietary cholesterol (mg/day)	≤300	200–250	100–150
Total fat (% of Kcal)	30–35	25–30	20–25
Saturated fat (% of Kcal)	10–15	8–10	≤8

Assessment. A diet history should be taken prior to the formulation of a diet plan. The approximate intake of cholesterol, of total fat, of saturated fat, of alcohol, and of simple carbohydrate should be determined. In the clinical setting, it is generally sufficient to make an approximation of the intake. For individuals who are overweight, assessment should include a review of the weight history, the previous weight reduction efforts, and the eating related behavior.

Hypercholesterolemia. Plasma lipid abnormalities include (1) an elevation of the total cholesterol, (2) a low ratio of total cholesterol to HDL cholesterol, or (3) an elevated LDL cholesterol. When these abnormalities exist, the dietary intake of cholesterol, total fat, and saturated fat should be restricted to the extent that the patient accepts. The guidelines are based on those of the American Heart Association. The dietary intake of cholesterol should be restricted in accordance with the recommended guidelines and patient acceptance (see Table 6–17). Most dietary cholesterol comes from egg yolks, organ meat, and whole milk dairy products. Plasma cholesterol can be reduced to about 300 mg by eliminating foods that are high in cholesterol and in saturated fat (egg yolk, organ meats) by substituting soft margarine for butter, oils for shortening and lard, skim milk for whole milk, and by limiting meat portions. A further reduction to about 200 mg of cholesterol per day can be achieved by reducing the amount of animal fats consumed.

The reduction in the total fat intake necessitates a corresponding increase in the complex carbohydrate to meet the caloric needs. The carbohydrate fraction then usually contributes 45 to 60 percent of the kilocalories. Whole grain bread and cereal products and fruits and vegetables are encouraged to increase the fiber intake. The protein intake is usually 12 to 20 percent of the caloric intake.

For individuals who are overweight, weight reduction is advised (see page 188 for additional information). Regular physical activity should also be encouraged.

Calculation of the polyunsaturated fat. The saturated fat ratio is not generally necessary since an acceptable ratio is usually achieved when saturated fat is displaced by polyunsaturated fats within the total fat allowance. Currently, polyunsaturated oils are recommended in preference to those that are predominantly monounsaturated fat, such as olive oil. However, the use of monounsaturated fat should not be prohibited. Table 6–18 is the Provisional Table on the Fatty Acid and Cholesterol Content of Selected Foods compiled by the United States Department of Agriculture.[20] This appendix can be of aid in planning diets for individuals with hyperlipidemia.

Hypertriglyceridemia. When the predominant plasma lipid abnormality is the elevation of triglycerides, the very low-density lipoprotein is found to be elevated and the total cholesterol only slightly or moderately increased. This is the Fredrickson Type IV hyperlipidemia and is most often found associated with obesity and marginally or distinctly elevated levels of plasma glucose. Dietary measures should emphasize the reduction of weight and the restriction of alcohol and excess simple carbohydrates. Some modification of the fat intake and a program of regular physical activity should also be encouraged.

For persons with plasma triglycerides that are moderately elevated, the alcohol intake should be substantially reduced or eliminated. For those with greater elevations in plasma triglycerides, especially for those with triglyceride levels greater than 500 mg per deciliter, abstinence from alcohol is advised.

A weight loss to effect the reduction in triglycerides to near normal levels is recommended. For some persons, this may necessitate the achievement of a distinctly lean weight. (See page 184 for additional information on weight reduction.)

The intake of simple carbohydrates from sweeteners (table sugar, corn syrup, honey, fructose) should be restricted. However, simple carbohydrates from lactose, fructose, and sucrose that naturally occur in fruits and milk are acceptable as these comprise only 10 to 15 percent of the carbohydrate kilocalories. This restriction of simple sugar results in a decrease in the total intake of carbohydrates, especially if this measure is the means by which kilocalories are reduced. However, it is generally not necessary to specifically restrict the proportion of the kilocalories from carbohydrates.

A moderate restriction of the total fat to 30 to 35 percent of the kilocalories and of the saturated fat to 10 to 15 percent of the kilocalories may be helpful in lowering triglyceride levels in some patients. This results in a distribution of kilocalories of approximately 12 to 20 percent of the kilocalories from protein, 30 to 35 percent of the kilocalories from fat, and 45 to 60 percent of the kilocalories from carbohydrates.

For some patients, it is reasonable to encourage a cholesterol intake that is at or slightly below the average (300 to 450 mg). This precaution does not tend to correct the underlying lipid abnormality. However, it is added as a prudent modification against the evolution of vascular disease.

Hypercholesterolemia and hypertriglyceridemia. Hypercholesterolemia and hypertriglyceridemia include Fredrickson Type IIb and Type III. Guidelines for hypercholesterolemia should be used with additional restrictions of alcohol and of simple carbohydrate.

Hypertriglyceridemia in the form of chylomicrons. This is an uncommon syndrome seen mainly in children and designates Type I in the Fredrickson classification. The total fat intake should be restricted to very low levels; medium-chain triglycerides may be used as a kilocalorie source. (See section on *Fat Malabsorption*, page 136).

Physicians: How to Order Diet

The diet order should specify *low cholesterol, low saturated fat, and low simple carbohydrate* as needed. The dietitian determines the caloric level and whether or not further modifications (e.g., sodium) are necessary.

TABLE 6–18 Provisional Table on the Content of Cholesteral, Fatty Acids, and Omega = 3 Fatty Acids in Selected Foods (100 g Edible Portion, Raw)*

			Fatty Acids					
Food item	Total fat (g)	Total saturated (g)	Total monoun-saturated (g)	Total polyun-saturated (g)	18:3 (g)	20:5 (g)	22:6 (g)	Choles-terol (mg)
Finfish								
Anchovy, European	4.8	1.3	1.2	1.6	—[†]	0.5	0.9	—
Bass, freshwater	2.0	0.4	0.7	0.7	Tr[‡]	0.1	0.2	59
Bass, striped	2.3	0.5	0.7	0.8	Tr	0.2	0.6	80
Bluefish	6.5	1.4	2.9	1.6	—	0.4	0.8	59
Burbot	0.8	0.2	0.1	0.3	—	0.1	0.1	60
Capelin	8.2	1.5	3.8	1.5	0.1	0.6	0.5	—
Carp	5.6	1.1	2.3	1.4	0.3	0.2	0.1	67
Catfish, brown bullhead	2.7	0.6	1.0	0.8	0.1	0.2	0.2	75
Catfish, channel	4.3	1.0	1.6	1.0	Tr	0.1	0.2	58
Cisco	1.9	0.4	0.5	0.6	0.1	0.1	0.3	—
Cod, Atlantic	0.7	0.1	0.1	0.3	Tr	0.1	0.2	43
Cod, Pacific	0.6	0.1	0.1	0.2	Tr	0.1	0.1	37
Croaker, Atlantic	3.2	1.1	1.2	0.5	Tr	0.1	0.1	61
Dogfish, spiny	10.2	2.2	4.2	2.7	0.1	0.7	1.2	52
Dolphinfish	0.7	0.2	0.1	0.2	Tr	Tr	0.1	—
Drum, black	2.5	0.7	0.8	0.5	Tr	0.1	0.1	—
Drum, freshwater	4.9	1.1	2.2	1.2	0.1	0.2	0.3	64
Eel, European	18.8	3.5	10.9	1.4	0.7	0.1	0.1	108
Flounder, unspecified	1.0	0.2	0.3	0.3	Tr	0.1	0.1	46
Flounder, yellowtail	1.2	0.3	0.2	0.3	Tr	0.1	0.1	—

TABLE 6-18 Provisional Table on the Content of Cholesteral, Fatty Acids, and Omega = 3 Fatty Acids in Selected Foods (100 g Edible Portion, Raw)*
(continued)

Food item	Total fat (g)	Total saturated (g)	Total monoun-saturated (g)	Total polyun-saturated (g)	18:3 (g)	20:5 (g)	22:6 (g)	Choles-terol (mg)
Finfish (*continued*)								
Grouper, jewfish	1.3	0.3	0.3	0.4	Tr	Tr	0.3	49
Grouper, red	0.8	0.2	0.1	0.2	—	Tr	0.2	—
Haddock	0.7	0.1	0.1	0.2	Tr	0.1	0.1	63
Hake, Atlantic	0.6	0.2	0.2	0.1	Tr	Tr	Tr	—
Hake, Pacific	1.6	0.3	0.3	0.6	Tr	0.2	0.2	—
Hake, red	0.9	0.2	0.3	0.3	—	0.1	0.1	—
Hake, silver	2.6	0.5	0.7	0.9	0.1	0.2	0.3	—
Hake, unspecified	1.9	0.5	0.6	0.5	—	0.1	0.4	—
Halibut, Greenland	13.8	2.4	8.4	1.4	Tr	0.5	0.4	46
Halibut, Pacific	2.3	0.3	0.8	0.7	0.1	0.1	0.3	32
Herring, Atlantic	9.0	2.0	3.7	2.1	0.1	0.7	0.9	60
Herring, Pacific	13.9	3.3	6.9	2.4	0.1	1.0	0.7	77
Herring, round	4.4	1.3	0.8	1.5	0.1	0.4	0.8	28
Mackerel, Atlantic	13.9	3.6	5.4	3.7	0.1	0.9	1.6	80
Mackerel, chub	11.5	3.0	4.7	3.0	0.3	0.9	1.0	52
Mackerel, horse	4.1	1.2	1.4	0.9	Tr	0.3	0.3	41
Mackerel, Japanese horse	7.8	2.5	2.4	2.3	0.1	0.5	1.3	48
Mackerel, king	13.0	2.5	5.9	3.2	—	1.0	1.2	53
Mullet, striped	3.7	1.2	1.1	1.1	0.1	0.3	0.2	49
Mullet, unspecified	4.4	0.3	1.3	1.5	Tr	0.5	0.6	34
Ocean perch	1.6	0.3	0.6	0.5	Tr	0.1	0.1	42
Perch, white	2.5	0.6	0.9	0.7	0.1	0.2	0.1	80
Perch, yellow	0.9	0.2	0.1	0.4	Tr	0.1	0.2	90
Pike, northern	0.7	0.1	0.2	0.2	Tr	Tr	0.1	39
Pike, walleye	1.2	0.2	0.3	0.4	Tr	0.1	0.2	86
Plaice, European	1.5	0.3	0.5	0.4	Tr	0.1	0.1	70
Pollock	1.0	0.1	0.1	0.5	—	0.1	0.4	71
Pompano, Florida	9.5	3.5	2.6	1.1	—	0.2	0.4	50
Ratfish	1.2	0.3	0.4	0.1	Tr	Tr	0.1	—
Rockfish, brown	3.3	0.8	0.8	1.0	Tr	0.3	0.4	—
Rockfish, canary	1.8	0.4	0.5	0.6	Tr	0.2	0.3	34
Rockfish, unspecified	1.4	0.2	0.3	0.6	Tr	0.2	0.3	—
Sablefish	15.3	3.2	8.1	2.0	0.1	0.7	0.7	49
Salmon, Atlantic	5.4	0.8	1.8	2.1	0.2	0.3	0.9	—
Salmon, chinook	10.4	2.5	4.5	2.1	0.1	0.8	0.6	—
Salmon, chum	6.6	1.5	2.9	1.5	0.1	0.4	0.6	74
Salmon, coho	6.0	1.1	2.1	1.7	0.2	0.3	0.5	—
Salmon, pink	3.4	0.6	0.9	1.4	Tr	0.4	0.6	—
Salmon, sockeye	8.6	1.5	4.1	1.9	0.1	0.5	0.7	—
Saury	9.2	1.6	4.8	1.8	0.1	0.5	0.8	19
Scad, Muroaji	8.7	2.8	2.2	2.6	0.1	0.5	1.5	47
Scad, other	0.5	0.1	0.1	0.1	—	Tr	Tr	27
Sea bass, Japanese	1.5	0.4	0.3	0.5	Tr	0.1	0.3	41
Seatrout, sand	2.3	0.7	0.8	0.4	Tr	0.1	0.2	—
Seatrout, spotted	1.7	0.5	0.4	0.3	Tr	0.1	0.1	—
Shark, unspecified	1.9	0.3	0.4	0.8	—	Tr	0.5	44
Sheepshead	2.4	0.6	0.7	0.5	Tr	0.1	0.1	—
Smelt, pond	0.7	0.2	0.1	0.3	—	0.1	0.2	72
Smelt, rainbow	2.6	0.5	0.7	0.9	0.1	0.3	0.4	70
Smelt, sweet	4.6	1.6	1.2	1.0	0.3	0.2	0.1	25
Snapper, red	1.2	0.2	0.2	0.4	Tr	Tr	0.2	—
Sole, European	1.2	0.3	0.4	0.2	Tr	Tr	0.1	50
Sprat	5.8	1.4	2.0	1.5	—	0.5	0.8	38
Sturgeon, Atlantic	6.0	1.2	1.7	2.1	Tr	1.0	0.5	—
Sturgeon, common	3.3	0.8	1.6	0.5	0.1	0.2	0.1	—
Sunfish, pumpkinseed	0.7	0.1	0.1	0.2	Tr	Tr	0.1	67
Swordfish	2.1	0.6	0.8	0.2	—	0.1	0.1	39
Trout, arctic char	7.7	1.6	4.6	0.9	Tr	0.1	0.5	—

TABLE 6–18 Provisional Table on the Content of Cholesteral, Fatty Acids, and Omega = 3 Fatty Acids in Selected Foods (100 g Edible Portion, Raw)* (*continued*)

	Fatty Acids							
Food item	Total fat (g)	Total saturated (g)	Total monoun-saturated (g)	Total polyun-saturated (g)	18:3 (g)	20:5 (g)	22:6 (g)	Choles-terol (mg)
Finfish (*continued*)								
Trout, brook	2.7	0.7	0.8	0.9	0.2	0.2	0.2	68
Trout, lake	9.7	1.7	3.6	3.4	0.4	0.5	1.1	48
Trout, rainbow	3.4	0.6	1.0	1.2	0.1	0.1	0.4	57
Tuna, albacore	4.9	1.2	1.2	1.8	0.2	0.3	1.0	54
Tuna, bluefin	6.6	1.7	2.2	2.0	—	0.4	1.2	38
Tuna, skipjack	1.9	0.7	0.4	0.6	—	0.1	0.3	47
Tuna, unspecified	2.5	0.9	0.6	0.5	—	0.1	0.4	—
Whitefish, lake	6.0	0.9	2.0	2.2	0.2	0.3	1.0	60
Whiting, European	0.5	0.1	0.1	0.1	Tr	Tr	0.1	31
Wolffish, Atlantic	2.4	0.4	0.8	0.8	Tr	0.3	0.3	—
Crustaceans								
Crab, Alaska king	0.8	0.1	0.1	0.3	Tr	0.2	0.1	—
Crab, blue	1.3	0.2	0.2	0.5	Tr	0.2	0.2	78
Crab, Dungeness	1.0	0.1	0.2	0.3	—	0.2	0.1	59
Crab, queen	1.1	0.1	0.2	0.4	Tr	0.2	0.1	127
Crayfish, unspecified	1.4	0.3	0.4	0.3	Tr	0.1	Tr	158
Lobster, European	0.8	0.1	0.2	0.2	—	0.1	0.1	129
Lobster, northern	0.9	0.2	0.2	0.2	—	0.1	0.1	95
Shrimp, Atlantic brown	1.5	0.3	0.3	0.5	Tr	0.2	0.1	142
Shrimp, Atlantic white	1.5	0.2	0.2	0.6	Tr	0.2	0.2	182
Shrimp, Japanese (kuruma) prawn	2.5	0.5	0.5	1.0	Tr	0.3	0.2	58
Shrimp, northern	1.5	0.2	0.3	0.6	Tr	0.3	0.2	125
Shrimp, other	1.3	0.4	0.3	0.3	Tr	0.1	0.1	128
Shrimp, unspecified	1.1	0.2	0.1	0.4	Tr	0.2	0.1	147
Spiny lobster, Caribbean	1.4	0.2	0.2	0.6	Tr	0.2	0.1	140
Spiny lobster, southern rock	1.0	0.1	0.2	0.3	Tr	0.2	0.1	—
Mollusks								
Abalone, New Zealand	1.0	0.2	0.2	0.2	Tr	Tr	—	—
Abalone, South African	1.1	0.3	0.3	0.2	Tr	Tr	Tr	—
Clam, hardshell	0.6	Tr	Tr	0.1	Tr	Tr	Tr	31
Clam, hen	0.7	0.2	0.1	0.1	—	Tr	Tr	—
Clam, littleneck	0.8	0.1	0.1	0.1	Tr	Tr	Tr	—
Clam, Japanese hardshell	0.8	0.1	0.1	0.2	—	0.1	0.1	—
Clam, softshell	2.0	0.3	0.2	0.6	Tr	0.2	0.2	—
Clam, surf	0.8	0.1	0.1	0.2	Tr	0.1	0.1	—
Conch, unspecified	2.7	0.6	0.5	1.1	Tr	0.6	0.4	141
Cuttlefish, unspecified	0.6	0.1	0.1	0.1	Tr	Tr	Tr	—
Mussel, blue	2.2	0.4	0.5	0.6	Tr	0.2	0.3	38
Mussel, Mediterranean	1.5	0.4	0.4	0.3	—	0.1	0.1	—
Octopus, common	1.0	0.3	0.1	0.3	—	0.1	0.1	—
Oyster, eastern	2.5	0.6	0.2	0.7	Tr	0.2	0.2	47
Oyster, European	2.0	0.4	0.2	0.7	0.1	0.3	0.2	30
Oyster, Pacific	2.3	0.5	0.4	0.9	Tr	0.4	0.2	—
Periwinkle, common	3.3	0.6	0.6	1.1	0.2	0.5	Tr	101
Scallop, Atlantic deepsea	0.8	0.1	0.1	0.3	Tr	0.1	0.1	37
Scallop, calico	0.7	0.1	—	0.2	Tr	0.1	0.1	—
Scallop, unspecified	0.8	0.1	0.1	0.3	Tr	0.1	0.1	45
Squid, Atlantic	1.2	0.3	0.1	0.5	Tr	0.1	0.3	—
Squid, short-finned	2.0	0.4	0.4	0.7	Tr	0.2	0.4	—
Squid, unspecified	1.1	0.3	0.1	0.4	Tr	0.1	0.2	—
Fish Oils								
Cod liver oil	100	17.6	51.2	25.8	0.7	9.0	9.5	570
Herring oil	100	19.2	60.3	16.1	0.6	7.1	4.3	766
Menhaden oil	100	33.6	32.5	29.5	1.1	12.7	7.9	521
MaxEPA, concentrated fish body oils	100	25.4	28.3	41.1	0	17.8	11.6	600
Salmon oil	100	23.8	39.7	29.9	1.0	8.8	11.1	485

TABLE 6–18 Provisional Table on the Content of Cholesteral, Fatty Acids, and Omega = 3 Fatty Acids in Selected Foods (100 g Edible Portion, Raw)* (*continued*)

Food item	Total fat (g)	Total saturated (g)	Total monoun-saturated (g)	Total polyun-saturated (g)	18:3 (g)	Choles-terol (mg)
Beef						
Chuck, blade roast, all grades, separable lean and fat, raw	23.6	10.0	10.8	0.9	0.3	73
Ground, regular, raw	27.0	10.8	11.6	1.0	0.2	85
Round, full cut, choice grade, separable lean and fat, raw	17.5	7.4	7.8	0.7	0.2	66
Separable fat from retail cuts, raw	70.9	31.0	32.4	2.6	1.0	99
T-Bone steak, choice grade, lean only, raw	8.0	3.2	3.4	0.3	Tr	60
T-Bone steak, choice grade, separable lean and fat, raw	26.1	11.2	11.7	1.0	0.3	71
Cereal Grains						
Barley, bran	5.3	1.0	0.6	2.7	0.3	0
Corn, germ	30.8	3.9	7.6	18.0	0.3	0
Oats, germ	30.7	5.6	11.1	12.4	1.4	0
Rice, bran	19.2	3.6	7.3	6.6	0.2	0
Wheat, bran	4.6	0.7	0.7	2.4	0.2	0
Wheat, germ	10.9	1.9	1.6	6.6	0.7	0
Wheat, hard red winter	2.5	0.4	0.3	1.2	0.1	0
Dairy and Egg Products						
Cheese, Cheddar	33.1	21.1	9.0	0.9	0.4	105
Cheese, Roquefort	30.6	19.3	8.5	1.3	0.7	90
Cream, heavy whipping	37.0	23.0	10.7	1.4	0.5	137
Milk, whole	3.3	2.1	1.0	0.1	0.1	14
Egg yolk, chicken, raw	32.9	9.9	13.2	4.3	0.1	1,602
Fats and Oils						
Butter	81.1	50.5	23.4	3.0	1.2	219
Butter oil	99.5	61.9	28.7	3.7	1.5	256
Chicken fat	99.8	29.8	44.7	20.9	1.0	85
Duck fat	99.8	33.2	49.3	12.9	1.0	100
Lard	100	39.2	45.1	11.2	1.0	95
Linseed oil	100	9.4	20.2	66.0	53.3	0
Margarine, hard, soybean	80.5	16.7	39.3	20.9	1.5	0
Margarine, hard, soybean and soybean (hydrog)	80.5	13.1	37.6	26.2	1.9	0
Margarine, hard, soybean (hydrog.) and palm	80.5	17.5	31.2	28.2	2.3	0
Margarine, hard, soybean (hydrog.) and cottonseed	80.5	15.6	36.1	25.3	2.8	0
Margarine, hard, soybean (hydrog.) and palm (hydrog.)	80.5	15.1	32.0	29.8	3.0	0
Margarine, liquid, soybean (hydrog.), soybean, and cottonseed	80.6	13.2	28.1	35.8	2.4	0
Margarine, soft, soybean (hydrog.) and cottonseed	80.4	16.5	31.3	29.1	1.6	0
Margarine, soft, soybean (hydrog.) and palm	80.4	17.1	25.2	34.6	1.9	0
Margarine, soft, soybean, soybean (hydrog.) and cottonseed (hydrog.)	80.4	16.1	30.7	30.1	2.8	0
Mutton tallow	100	47.3	40.6	7.8	2.3	102
Rapeseed oil (Canola)	100	6.8	55.5	33.3	11.1	0
Rice bran oil	100	19.7	39.3	35.0	1.6	0
Salad dressing, comm., blue cheese, reg.	52.3	9.9	12.3	27.8	3.7	17
Salad dressing, comm., Italian, reg	48.3	7.0	11.2	28.0	3.3	0
Salad dressing, comm., mayonnaise, imitation, soybean, w/o cholesterol	47.7	7.5	10.5	27.6	4.6	0
Salad dressing, comm., mayonnaise, safflower & soybean	79.4	8.6	13.0	55.0	3.0	59

TABLE 6–18 Provisional Table on the Content of Cholesteral, Fatty Acids, and Omega = 3 Fatty Acids in Selected Foods (100 g Edible Portion, Raw)* (*continued*)

Food item	Fatty Acids					
	Total fat (g)	Total saturated (g)	Total monoun- saturated (g)	Total polyun- saturated (g)	18:3 (g)	Choles- terol (mg)
Fats and Oils (*continued*)						
Salad dressing, comm., mayonnaise, soybean	79.4	11.8	22.7	41.3	4.2	59
Salad dressing, comm., mayonnaise-type	33.4	4.7	9.0	18.0	2.0	26
Salad dressing, comm., Thousand Island, reg.	35.7	6.0	8.3	19.8	2.5	0
Salad dressing, home recipe, French	70.2	12.6	20.7	33.7	1.9	0
Salad dressing, home recipe, vinegar and soybean oil	50.1	9.1	14.8	24.1	1.4	0
Shortening, household, lard and veg. oil	100	40.3	44.4	10.9	1.1	56
Shortening, household, soybean (hydrog.) & cottonseed (hydrog.)	100	25.0	44.5	26.1	1.6	0
Shortening, special-purpose, for bread, soy (hydrog.) & cottonseed	100	22.0	33.0	40.6	4.0	0
Shortening, special-purpose, for cake mixes, soybean (hydrog.) and cottonseed (hydrog.)	100	27.2	54.2	14.1	1.1	0
Shortening, special-purpose, heavy- duty, frying, soybean (hydrog.)	100	18.4	43.7	33.5	2.4	0
Soybean lecithin	100	15.3	10.9	45.1	5.1	0
Soybean oil	100	14.4	23.3	57.9	6.8	0
Soybean oil (hydrog.) & cottonseed oil	100	14.9	43.0	37.6	2.8	0
Soybean oil (partially-hydrog.)	100	14.9	43.0	37.6	2.6	0
Spread, margarine-like, about 60% fat, Soybean (hydrog.) & palm (hydrog.)	60.8	14.1	26.0	18.1	1.6	0
Spread, margarine-like, about 60% fat, soybean (hydrog.), palm (hydrog.), and palm	60.8	13.5	24.1	20.4	1.6	0
Tomatoseed oil	100	19.7	22.8	53.1	2.3	0
Walnut oil	100	9.1	22.8	63.3	10.4	0
Wheat germ oil	100	18.8	15.1	61.7	6.9	0
Fruits						
Avocados, California, raw	17.3	2.6	11.2	2.0	0.1	0
Raspberries, raw	0.6	Tr	Tr	0.3	0.1	0
Strawberries, raw	0.4	Tr	Tr	0.2	0.1	0
Lamb and Veal						
Lamb, leg, raw (83% lean, 17% fat)	17.6	8.1	7.1	1.0	0.3	71
lamb, loin, raw (72% lean, 28% fat)	27.4	12.8	11.2	1.6	0.5	71
Veal, leg round with rump, raw (87% lean 13% fat)	9.0	3.8	3.7	0.6	0.1	71
Legumes						
Beans, common, dry	1.5	0.2	0.1	0.9	0.6	0
Chickpeas, dry	5.0	0.5	1.1	2.3	0.1	0
Cowpeas, dry	1.9	0.6	0.1	0.8	0.3	0
Lentils, dry	1.2	0.2	0.2	0.5	0.1	0
Lima beans, dry	1.4	0.3	0.1	0.7	0.2	0
Peas, garden, dry	2.4	0.4	0.1	0.4	0.2	0
Soybeans, dry	21.3	3.1	4.4	12.3	1.6	0
Nuts and Seeds						
Beechnuts, dried	50.0	5.7	21.9	20.1	1.7	0
Butternuts, dried	57.0	1.3	10.4	42.7	8.7	0
Chia seeds, dried	26.3	10.5	7.3	7.3	3.9	0
Hickory nuts, dried	64.4	7.0	32.6	21.9	1.0	0
Soybean kernels, roasted and toasted	24.0	3.2	5.6	12.7	1.5	0
Walnuts, black	56.6	3.6	12.7	37.5	3.3	0
Walnuts, English/Persian	61.9	5.6	14.2	39.1	6.8	0
Pork						
Pork, cured, bacon, raw	57.5	21.3	26.3	6.8	0.8	67
Pork, cured, breakfast strips, raw	37.1	12.9	16.9	5.6	0.9	69

TABLE 6–18 Provisional Table on the Content of Cholesteral, Fatty Acids, and Omega = 3 Fatty Acids in Selected Foods (100 g Edible Portion, Raw)* (*continued*)

Food item	Total fat (g)	Total saturated (g)	Total monoun-saturated (g)	Total polyun-saturated (g)	18:3 (g)	Choles-terol (mg)
Pork (*continued*)						
Pork, cured salt pork, raw	80.5	29.4	38.0	9.4	0.7	86
Pork, fresh, ham, raw	20.8	7.5	9.7	2.2	0.2	74
Pork, fresh, jowl, raw	69.6	25.3	32.9	8.1	0.6	90
Pork, fresh, leaf fat, raw	94.2	45.2	37.2	7.3	0.9	110
Pork, fresh, separable fat, raw	76.7	27.9	35.7	8.2	0.7	93
Poultry						
Chicken, broiler fryers, flesh and skin, giblets, neck, raw[§]	14.8	4.2	6.1	3.2	0.1	90
Chicken, dark meat, w/o skin, raw[§]	4.3	1.1	1.3	1.0	Tr	80
Chicken, light meat, w/o skin, raw[§]	1.7	0.4	0.4	0.4	Tr	58
Chicken, skin only, raw[§]	32.4	9.1	13.5	6.8	0.3	109
Turkey, flesh, with skin, roasted[§]	9.7	2.8	3.2	2.5	0.1	82
Vegetables						
Beans, Navy, sprouted, cooked	0.8	Tr	Tr	0.5	0.3	0
Beans, pinto, sprouted, cooked	0.9	0.1	Tr	0.5	0.3	0
Broccoli, raw	0.4	Tr	Tr	0.2	0.1	0
Cauliflower, raw	0.2	Tr	Tr	Tr	0.1	0
Kale, raw	0.7	Tr	Tr	0.3	0.2	0
Leeks, freeze-dried, raw	2.1	0.3	Tr	1.2	0.7	0
Lettuce, butterhead, raw	0.2	Tr	Tr	0.1	0.1	0
Radish seeds, sprouted, raw	2.5	0.7	0.4	1.1	0.7	0
Seaweed, spirulina, dried	7.7	2.6	0.7	2.0	0.8	0
Soybeans, green, raw	6.8	0.7	0.8	3.8	3.2	0
Soybeans, mature seeds, sprouted, cooked	4.5	0.5	0.5	2.5	2.1	0
Spinach, raw	0.4	Tr	Tr	0.1	0.1	0

*With permission from: Weihrauch JL. USDA provisional table on the content of cholesterol, fatty acids, and other fat components in selected foods. Nutrient Data Research Branch, Nutrition monitoring division, Human Nutrition Information Service 1986. HNIS-PT-103.

[†] Dashes (—) denote lack of reliable data for nutrient known to be present.

[‡] Tr = trace (less than 0.05 g per 100 g of food).

[§] Contains trace amounts of 20:5, 22:5, and 22:6.

REFERENCES

1. Mahley RW. Atherogenic hyperlipoproteinemia. Med Clin North Am 1982;66:375–402.

2. The dietary management of hyperlipoproteinemia. A handbook for physicians and dietitians. (DHEW Publication No. [NIH] 80-110). Bethesda, MD. U.S. Department of HEW, 1980.

3. Schaefer EJ, Levy RI. Pathogenesis and management of lipoprotein disorders. Engl J Med 1985;312:1300–1310.

4. Castelli WP. Cardiovascular disease and multifactorial risk: challenge of the 1980s. Am Heart J 1983;106:1191–1200.

5. National Institutes of Health Consensus Conference. Lowering blood cholesterol to prevent heart disease. JAMA 1985;253:2080–2086.

6. Hoeg JM, Gregg RE, Brewer HB. An approach to the management of hyperlipoproteinemia. JAMA 1986;255:512–521.

7. Kannel WB, Doyle JT, Ostfeld AM. Optimal resources for primary prevention of atherosclerotic diseases. Circulation 1984;70:153–205.

8. National Institute of Health. Treatment of hypertriglyceridemia. JAMA 1984; 251:1196–1200.

9. Nutrition Committee and the Council of Arteriosclerosis of American Heart Association: Recommendations for treatment of hyperlipidemia in adults. Circulation 1984;69:1064A–1090A.

10. Ellefson RD, Palumbo PJ. Mayo Clinic Reference Values. Plus Personal Communications, 1977.

11. Grundy SM, Bilheimer D, Blackburn H. Rationale of the diet-heart statement of American Heart Association. Circulation 1982;65:839A–854A.

12. Jackson AS, Pollock ML. Generalized equations for predicting body density of men. Br J Nutr 1978;40:497–504.

13. Jackson AS, Pollock ML, Ward A. Generalized equations for predicting body density of women. Med Sci Sports Exerc 1980;12:175–182.

14. Tran ZV, Weltman A. Differential effects of exercise on serum lipid and lipoprotein levels seen with changes in weight. JAMA 1985;254:919–924.

15. Nestel PJ. Fish oil attenuates the cholesterol induced rise in lipoprotein cholesterol. Am J Clin Nutr 1986;43:752–757.

16. Dyerberg J. Linolenate-derived polyunsaturated fatty acids and prevention of atherosclerosis. Nutr Rev 1986;44:125–133.

17a. Herold PM, Kinsella JE. Fish oil consumption and decreased risk of cardiovascular disease: A comparison of findings from animal and human feeding trials. Am J Clin Nutr 1986;43:566–598.

17b. Ballard-Barbash R, Callaway CW. Marine fish oils: Role in prevention of coronary artery disease. Mayo Clin Proc 1987;62:113–118.

18. Grundy SM. Comparison of monounsaturated fatty acids and carbohydrates for lowering plasma cholesterol. N Engl J Med 1986;314:745–748.

19. Haskell WL, Camargo BA, Williams PT, Varanizan KM, Krauss RM, Lindgren FT, Wood PD. The effect of cessation and resumption of moderate alcohol intake in serum high-density-lipoprotein subfractions. N Engl J Med 1984;310:805–810.

20. Weihrauch JL. USDA provisional table on the fatty acid and cholesterol content of selected foods. Nutrient Data Research Branch, Nutrition Monitoring Division, Human Nutrition Information Service 1984. HNIS/PT-101.

CARDIAC SURGERY

General Description

The dietary progression for postoperative cardiac surgery patients is similar to that progression for other types of surgery. The diet is also controlled in sodium.

Nutritional Inadequacy

The dietary precautions for cardiac surgery patients are not inherently inadequate in nutrients as compared to the Recommended Dietary Allowance (RDA). However, with an actual intake or with weight reduction diets of 1,200 Kcal or less, it is difficult to meet the RDA consistently. A daily multiple vitamin supplement that provides nutrients at a level that is equivalent to the RDA is recommended for persons who consume 1,200 Kcal or less or for those who have food aversions or intolerances that greatly limit the variety of their food choices.

Indications and Rationale

Sodium is controlled as a precaution against congestive heart failure. The degree and the duration of the sodium restriction varies with the type of surgery and with the response of the patient. The patient follows the diet postoperatively until his or her dismissal from the hospital or for several weeks after the dismissal. (See section on *Hypertension* for the calculation of sodium controlled diets for adults.) The diet is then advanced to a lesser degree of sodium restriction and is followed for several weeks or longer. Then most patients may resume their usual dietary practices. Table 6–19 summarizes the general types of heart surgery and the level of sodium restriction that is usually prescribed.[1]

TABLE 6–19 Cardiac Surgery and Dietary Sodium Restriction*

Surgical Procedure	Sodium Level and Progression
Repair of complex forms of congenital heart defects	Begin with 20 mEq sodium; advance to 90 mEq of sodium or a no extra salt diet
Prosthetic valve replacement	Begin with 20 mEq sodium; advance to 90 mEq of sodium or a no extra salt diet
Repair of simpler forms of congenital heart defects (e.g., atrial septal defect, isolated pulmonary stenosis)	Begin with sodium restriction (levels range from 20–90 mEq at discretion of physician); advance to usual diet
Coronary artery bypass grafting	Begin with sodium restriction (levels range from 20–90 mEq at discretion of physician); advance to usual diet

*It may be appropriate for persons who have had surgery related to coronary artery disease to follow a diet also intended for control of serum lipids and weight

Postsurgical cardiac patients may experience complications of gastrointestinal distress and of decreased appetite. Medications such as Persantine and Ascriptin, as well as the cardiotonic, diuretic, and antibiotic drug groups, have a tendency to result in nausea and intolerance to many foods, which makes it difficult to achieve recommended kilocalorie and protein intake.

Monitoring of dietary intake and the nutritional plan of care needs close attention during hospitalization in order to assist patients in choosing a varied and an adequate intake within the limits of the prescribed dietary modifications.

Some patients may benefit from adjustments in their meals such as small frequent feedings. Cold items are often more acceptable (i.e., cottage cheese and fruit plates, milk drinks, fruits and juices, and ice cream). Meat, potatoes, and vegetables are added gradually as tolerated.

For children, there are two levels of sodium restriction (Table 6–20), which include strict (1 mEq of sodium per 100 Kcal) and mild (4 mEq of sodium per

TABLE 6–20 Caloric Intake and Suggested Sodium Control for Children Having Cardiac Surgery

Suggested Kilocalorie Intake (Kcal)	Control of Sodium (mEq)*,†	
	Strict	Mild
less than 1,000	less than 10	less than 40
1,000–1,500	10–15	40–60
greater than 1,500	15–25	60–90

*The diet should not exceed the upper limit of sodium allowed in each group. The food exchange list for sodium control (see page 235) may be used.
†Exceptions: When calculating the sodium intake, children under 10 kg of weight are permitted up to 10 mEq sodium daily on the Strict Sodium Restricted Diet, children 20 kg and over in weight may have up to 90 mEq sodium on the Mild Sodium Restricted Diet.

100 Kcal). These levels correspond to the 20 mEq and 90 mEq of sodium restricted diets for adults.[2] The diet is based on the total number of kilocalories necessary for the child to maintain a normal weight. Generally, the hospitalized child does not require the same number of kilocalories that a healthy, more active child does. Table 6–21 may be used to estimate the caloric needs.

TABLE 6–21 Estimation of Caloric Needs for Children Having Cardiac Surgery

Body Weight (kg)	Suggested Kilocalorie Intake (Kcal)
less than 10	100/kilogram body weight
10–20	1,000 + 50 for each kilogram body weight over 10
greater than 20	1,500 + 20 for each kilogram body weight over 20

Physicians: How to Order Diet

The diet order should *specify the initial level of sodium.* This is automatically continued throughout each stage of the postoperative series (clear liquid, full liquid, and soft diets). Requests for instruction in the home diet should also indicate the level of sodium restriction. The physician should discuss the duration of the diet modifications with the patient. For adults, begin with 20 mEq of sodium and advance to 90 mEq of sodium or no extra salt, or begin with 90 mEq of sodium and advance to the usual diet. For children, begin with strict sodium restriction and advance to mild sodium restriction, or begin with mild sodium restriction and advance to the usual diet.

REFERENCES

1. Kern LS, O'Brien P. The Fontan procedure. Heart Lung 1985;14:457–467.
2. Peterson CR. Dietary counseling for patients admitted for coronary artery bypass graft. J Am Diet Assoc 1976;68:158–159.

CONGESTIVE HEART FAILURE

General Description

The diet for congestive heart failure is restricted in sodium. The diet is restricted more stringently for more severe degrees of failure. Occasionally, fluids are restricted as well.

Nutritional Inadequacy

The dietary management of congestive heart failure is not inherently inadequate in nutrients as compared to the Recommended Dietary Allowance (RDA). However, with actual intake or with weight reduction diets of 1,200 Kcal or less, it is difficult to meet the RDA consistently. A daily multiple vitamin supplement that provides nutrients at a level that is equivalent to the RDA is recommended for persons who consume 1,200 Kcal or less or for those who have food aversions or intolerances that greatly limit the variety of their food choices.

Indications and Rationale

Congestive heart failure is a condition of impaired heart function that may be a complication of any form of heart disease.[1] It is characterized by a decreased blood flow to the kidneys and a retention of both sodium and of water.[2,3]

Edema of the lower legs, shortness of breath on exertion, and episodes of shortness of breath at night (nocturnal dyspnea) are common manifestations of congestive failure.

To minimize the sodium and the fluid retention, the hospitalized patient who is in severe cardiac failure is often given a diet that contains 45 mEq or less of sodium per day. For the patient who is in moderate failure, a 90 mEq or less sodium diet may be specified. Potassium supplementation may be needed if diuretics have induced a potassium depletion. The selection of high potassium foods may not be adequate to correct such deficits. Fluids may be restricted if hyponatremia occurs.

The work load of the heart is decreased by caloric restriction and by small feedings. Most patients prefer small feedings, possibly because larger amounts increase the cardiac work load. Larger feedings may induce dyspnea as a result of gastric distension. Caffeine is avoided because it may increase the heart rate and favor the occurrence of a dysrhythmia.

Physicians: How to Order Diet

The diet order should indicate a specific *level of sodium* (20, 45, or 90 mEq of sodium) or a *no extra salt* diet (no more than 120 mEq of sodium). The physician should specify the level of the fluid restriction if necessary.

REFERENCES

1. Bernard MA, Jacobs DO, Rombeau JL. Cardiac failure. In: Bernard MA, Jacobs DO, Rombeau JL, eds. Nutritional and metabolic support of hospitalized patients. Philadelphia: WB Saunders, 1986;129–145.
2. Zeman FJ. Cardiovascular System. In: Zeman FJ, ed. Clinical nutrition and dietetics. Lexington, Mass: Collamore Press, 1983;311–313.
3. Poindexter SM, Dear WE, Dudrick SJ. Nutrition in congestive heart failure. Nutr Clin Prac 1986;1:83–88.

MYOCARDIAL INFARCTION

General Description

The dietary program for patients in the coronary care unit routinely consists of the control of sodium, cholesterol, kilocalories, and the restriction of caffeine-containing beverages.

Nutritional Inadequacy

The dietary precautions that follow myocardial infarction are not inherently inadequate in nutrients as compared to the Recommended Dietary Allowance (RDA). However, for Phase I diets and those diets that may emphasize caloric restriction to 1,200 Kcal or less, it is difficult to meet the RDA consistently. A daily multiple vitamin that provides nutrients at a level that is equivalent to the RDA is recommended for persons who consume 1,200 Kcal or less. A multiple vitamin may also be warranted for persons who have food aversions or intolerances that greatly limit the variety of their food choices.

Indications and Rationale

The diet is modified primarily as a precautionary measure, rather than as therapy, for patients who have sustained a myocardial infarction.[1]

During the first several days or weeks after a myocardial infarction, the patient may experience congestive heart failure. The control of sodium in the diet lessens the cardiac work load, is a precaution against congestive failure, and favors the control of hypertension if that is a factor.[2,3]

A cardiac arrhythmia, which is a particular hazard during this time, may possibly be provoked by caffeine. Therefore, caffeine-containing beverages are restricted.[2,3]

For severely compromised patients, large meals may interfere with breathing by distending the stomach and may increase the metabolic rate (postprandial thermogenesis), thus increasing the cardiac work load.[3,4] The patient with an uncomplicated myocardial infarction should tolerate light meals in the post-infarction period without undue hemodynamic stress.

If the patient is obese and his or her diet is intended for longer term use and is limited to a certain caloric level, then the diet served in the coronary care unit should not exceed that caloric level. This policy facilitates nutritional education of the patient at the time of dismissal and emphasizes the importance of long-term weight control.

Usually, the patient is aware that the infarction may have been the consequence of atherosclerotic plaques of the coronary arteries. Thus, the patient may be fearful of foods that are high in cholesterol or in saturated fats for several days or for weeks after the post-infarction period. The control of cholesterol and of saturated fats during the immediate post-infarction time is reasonable to lessen the apprehensions of the patient and to facilitate future dietary compliance. Cholesterol and fat modification is prudent even though the atherosclerotic process evolved only after many years of interaction between genetic and dietary factors.

General Dietary Recommendations

The dietary recommendations vary according to the recovery phase of the patient and are organized into three phases. The length of each stage varies according to the extent of the infarct and the protocol of the coronary care unit.

Phase I (inpatient)

Stage I. The diet is low in sodium (≤90 mEq) and in cholesterol with a consistency of full liquids or of a soft diet during the first 24 hours. The meals are small. Caffeine-containing beverages, such as coffee and tea, are not permitted. Decaffeinated coffee or tea may be served.

Stage II. The diet continues to be low in sodium (≤90 mEq) and in cholesterol and is restricted in caffeine. The caloric needs are assessed with a view toward the dismissal diet.

Stage III. The diet is individualized according to the need for the long-term control of the sodium (<90 mEq), the cholesterol, the saturated fat, the caffeine, and the weight (see sections on *Hypertension,* page 71, *Hyperlipidemia,* page 80, and *Obesity,* page 184).

Phase II (outpatient)

The current Cardiovascular Rehabilitation Program at the Mayo Medical Center is currently 8 weeks in duration. The dietary guidelines that are given in the hospital are reviewed, reinforced, and modified with each patient. The patient returns at 3, 6, and 9-month intervals for the evaluation of serum lipids and for dietary and exercise compliance.

Physicians: How to Order Diet

The diet order should indicate *postmyocardial infarction dietary precautions.* Additional dietary modifications should be specified.

REFERENCES

1. Jones RJ. Dietary management in the coronary care unit (questions and answers). JAMA 1977;237:2645.
2. Hemzacek KI. Dietary protocol for the patient who has suffered a myocardial infarction. J Am Diet Assoc 1978;72:182–185.
3. Christakis G, Winston M. Nutritional therapy in acute myocardial infarction. J Am Diet Assoc 1973;63:233–238.
4. Bagatell C, Heymsfield S. Effect of meal size on myocardial oxygen requirements: Implications for postmyocardial infarction diet. Am J Clin Nutr 1984;39:421–426.

DIABETES MELLITUS

General Description

The diets that are used as part of the management of diabetes mellitus are controlled in kilocalories, protein, fat, and carbohydrates. Additional dietary considerations include consistency in the timing of meals, in the distribution of kilocalories and/or carbohydrates among the meals, and in the control of the intake of kilocalories, saturated fat, and cholesterol. The nature of the specific dietary recommendations and the importance of additional considerations varies with the type of diabetes mellitus and with the total medical management program.

Nutritional Inadequacy

The diet that is recommended for diabetes mellitus is adequate in nutrients when compared to the Recommended Dietary Allowance (RDA). However, for diets of 1,200 Kcal or less, it is difficult to meet the RDA consistently. A daily multivitamin supplement is recommended for persons who consume diets of 1,200 Kcal or less.

Indications and Rationale

Diabetes is a heterogeneous disease with no single cause and with no standard treatment. It is necessary to individualize the care of each person according to the nature and severity of the disease.

The following is a summary of the classification of diabetes and other categories of glucose intolerance.[1] All categories are associated with hyperglycemia; but the cause, severity, and other clinical characteristics vary. Almost all persons with diabetes have either noninsulin-dependent diabetes or insulin-dependent diabetes.

Insulin-Dependent Diabetes Mellitus (IDDM). Insulin-dependent diabetes accounts for 10 to 15 percent of persons with diabetes and usually appears before the age of 40, but may develop at any age. Classic symptoms include polydipsia, polyphagia, and polyuria. A sudden onset of these symptoms is the norm, with a progression to ketoacidosis and coma in a short period of time if untreated. Insulin-dependent diabetes is associated with a total or near total loss of the capacity of the beta cells to secrete insulin. Insulin therapy, rather than the use of oral hypoglycemic agents, is required to prevent ketosis. Conventional insulin therapy usually consists of one or two injections daily of an intermediate or a mixture of intermediate and regular insulin. The diet therapy emphasizes good nutrition with modifications of the diet to reduce the risk of atherosclerotic complications. Special modifications are tailored to the specific insulin program.

Intensive Insulin Therapy for IDDM is a program of treatment that is intended for individuals with unstable patterns of glycemia who are ready to comply with a relatively elaborate mode of treatment. The plasma glucose level in the nondiabetic is maintained within relatively narrow limits by the secretion of larger amounts of insulin during and immediately after meals and by the secretion of a low level of insulin from the pancreas between meals and at night. Intensive Insulin Therapy seeks to imitate this pattern of delivery of insulin by an injection of rapidly acting (regular) insulin before meals and by an injection of longer acting (ultralente) once daily. The premeal injections of regular insulin are adjusted according to the level of the capillary plasma glucose level, which is determined prior to the injection. Insulin pumps deliver regular insulin continuously via a catheter, which is placed subcutaneously, and are programmed to deliver a bolus of insulin before each meal.

A weight gain commonly follows the initiation of intensive insulin therapy for IDDM because of the diminished glycosuria and its associated caloric wastage. Therefore, the caloric allowance may require an adjustment downward. If changes in meal size or in composition are made, the program of Intensive Insulin Therapy provides mechanisms for adjusting the premeal dose of regular insulin. With intensive insulin therapy usually only 15 g of carbohydrate (or one starch exchange) is needed for a bedtime snack. Usually midmorning and midafternoon snacks are not necessary with intensive insulin therapy.

Noninsulin-Dependent Diabetes Mellitus (NIDDM). Noninsulin-dependent diabetes accounts for 85 to 90 percent of persons with diabetes. Although it usually develops in the middle-aged, overweight individual, occasionally it occurs in those persons who are under age 40 and not overweight. The onset is gradual, characterized by subtle symptoms, and is usually detected by screening blood tests. Persons having noninsulin-dependent diabetes have some pancreatic insulin production and do not require injected insulin to prevent ketosis. However, the person with NIDDM may use oral hypoglycemic agents or insulin for the correction of symptomatic or persistent hyperglycemia. Mild ketosis may develop under special circumstances, such as in episodes of infection or of stress. Many obese individuals have a resistance to both endogenous and injected insulin.

In the obese individual with NIDDM, the glucose tolerance improves with weight loss. Control of the total caloric intake is the most important dietary measure in NIDDM. Often, glucose values improve remarkably within days after a low kilocalorie diet is begun, and further improvement results with the correction of obesity. Further modification of the diet may be recommended in an attempt to reduce the risk of atherosclerotic complications.

Secondary Diabetes Mellitus. Diabetes may occur as the result of pancreatitis, surgical removal of the pancreas, Cushing's disease, pheochromocytoma, and pharmacologic doses of glucocorticoids (e.g., Prednisone) or other diabetogenic hormones or drugs. Diabetes may resolve if the primary disorder or the cause is corrected. Dietary recommendations are dependent on the treatment modality, whether the diabetes is controlled by diet alone or by diet in conjunction with insulin.

Impaired Glucose Tolerance (IGT). Persons with impaired glucose tolerance are generally asymptomatic. The fasting blood glucose levels are normal or slightly elevated, and the oral glucose tolerance or postprandial plasma glucose levels are abnormal. Subtypes of IGT are nonobese IGT, obese IGT, and IGT that is associated with conditions that include pancreatic disease, diabetogenic hormones or drugs, and insulin receptor abnormalities. IGT may occur during administration of central parenteral nutrition. For some individuals, IGT may represent a stage in the development of IDDM or NIDDM. Diet therapy emphasizes the correction of obesity, if present.

Gestational Diabetes Mellitus (GDM). Gestational diabetes is defined as the glucose intolerance that begins or is recognized during pregnancy. Persons with diabetes who become pregnant are not included in this category. GDM is associated with increased perinatal complications and with an increased risk for the progression to diabetes within 5 to 10 years after parturition. The causes of GDM are not completely understood, but may be due, in part, to insulin resistance. Good glycemic control is recommended during pregnancy. Diet therapy emphasizes good nutrition with a controlled intake of calories for an appropriate weight gain. Specific recommendations for a diet during pregnancy are discussed on page 12.

Goals of Dietary Management

The goals of dietary management for diabetes mellitus are (1) a nutritionally adequate intake with a caloric intake that is appropriate for the achievement and/or the maintenance of a desirable weight, (2) the prevention of hyperglycemia and of hypoglycemia, and (3) the reduction of the risk of atherosclerosis. Whether dietary measures can significantly delay or prevent long-term complications of diabetes is not known. Tables 6–22 and 6–23 list priorities for meal planning. The priorities listed are of equal importance within each group.

Dietary Recommendations

Weight Reduction and/or Maintenance of Desirable Weight. The adult with insulin-dependent diabetes is usually lean and should receive sufficient kilocalories to maintain a desirable body weight. Additional kilocalories and nutrients are warranted for periods of increased requirements (e.g., pregnancy and lactation), as in the nondiabetic individual. Those who are overweight may benefit from a weight reduction.

The majority of individuals with noninsulin-dependent diabetes are overweight. Since obesity is associated with the cellular resistance to insulin action, a weight reduction helps to correct this resistance and may even result in a

TABLE 6–22 Priorities for Dietary Management of Insulin-Dependent Diabetes Mellitus (IDDM)

Higher Priority	Lower Priority
1. Consume adequate kilocalories to maintain desirable weight. 2. Keep the timing of meals and the composition of the diet consistent from day to day, with the carbohydrate content fairly evenly divided from meal to meal. 3. Avoid large amounts of simple carbohydrates. 4. Plan for a bedtime snack to prevent nocturnal hypoglycemia; take midmorning and midafternoon snacks, if needed, to match the food intake to the peak insulin action. 5. Plan for food to be taken to correct hypoglycemic episodes. 6. Plan for food to be taken for periods of increased physical activity and during illness. 7. Make modifications in the diet for hypertension, hyperlipidemia, and/or renal insufficiency, if present.	1. If obese, follow a low kilocalorie diet to reduce weight, then a kilocalorie-controlled diet to maintain a desirable weight (persons with IDDM are usually not obese).

return of the plasma glucose levels to the normal range. A kilocalorie restricted diet and regular exercise are of primary importance in achieving a desirable weight. Weight control may also reduce the individual's risk for cardiovascular disease through the reduction of blood lipids and the improved management of hypertension.

The desirable or the goal weight for the person with NIDDM is the same as for other obese persons. (See *Obesity, Determination of Desirable Weight,* page 188.) Standard height-weight tables can be used as an initial guide. However, other factors, such as the individual's weight history and the current and the past medical history, should be considered. There is evidence that the insulin resistance is related to the fat cell morphology and the pattern of body fat distribution.[2] Therefore, some individuals whose weight is within the standards of the height-weight tables may achieve an improved plasma glucose control through weight reduction. Individuals who are morbidly obese may normalize their plasma glucose levels at weights that are substantially greater than the statistical norms.

Meal Timing and Consistency in Composition of Meals. For persons taking insulin, keeping the number of meals, the scheduled times for eating, and the composition of meals relatively consistent from day to day is important. The food intake should be synchronized with the prescribed insulin program. It is recommended that individuals who receive conventional insulin therapy consume three meals per day spaced 4 to 5 hours apart and a bedtime snack. A consistent distribution of kilocalories, protein, and carbohydrate among the main meals helps to prevent large glucose excursions and to curtail hypoglycemia. If there is a consistent tendency toward glycosuria or toward hypoglycemia at a given time of day, adjustments in the timing and the size of the meals and the snacks may improve glycemic control and thus avoid the need for changing from a simple to a more complex insulin regimen. Somewhat more flexibility in the timing and the meal size is possible with intensive insulin therapy. If insulin is not used, the timing and the composition of the meals are less crucial.

TABLE 6–23 Priorities for Dietary Management for Noninsulin-Dependent Diabetes Mellitus (NIDDM)

Noninsulin-Dependent Diabetes Mellitus (NIDDM) Managed by Diet	Noninsulin-Dependent Diabetes Mellitus (NIDDM) Managed by Diet and Oral Hypoglycemic Agents	Noninsulin-Dependent Diabetes Mellitus (NIDDM) Managed by Diet and Insulin

High Priority

1. If obese, follow a low kilocalorie diet to reduce weight, then a kilocalorie-controlled diet to maintain a desirable weight. 2. Avoid large amounts of simple carbohydrates. 3. Make modifications in the diet for hypertension, hyperlipidemia and/or renal insufficiency, if present.	1. If obese, follow a low kilocalorie diet to reduce weight, then a kilocalorie-controlled diet to maintain desirable weight. 2. Avoid large amounts of simple carbohydrates. 3. Make modifications in the diet for hypertension, hyperlipidemia, and/or renal insufficiency, if present. 4. Keep the timing of the meals and the composition of the diet consistent from day to day with the carbohydrate content evenly divided from meal to meal. 5. Plan a bedtime snack to prevent nocturnal hypoglycemia when a long acting oral hypoglycemic agent (i.e., chlorpropamide, glyburide, Diaβeta) is used.	1. If obese, follow a low kilocalorie diet to reduce weight, then a kilocalorie-controlled diet to maintain a desirable weight. 2. Avoid large amounts of simple carbohydrates. 3. Keep the timing of the meals and the composition of the diet consistent from day to day, with the carbohydrate content of the diet fairly evenly divided from meal to meal. 4. Plan a bedtime snack to prevent nocturnal hypoglycemia; midmorning and midafternoon snacks, if needed, to match the food intake to the peak insulin action. 5. Plan for food to be taken to correct hypoglycemic episodes. 6. Plan for food to be taken for periods of increased physical activity or during illness. 7. Make modifications in the diet for hypertension, hyperlipidemia, and/or renal insufficiency, if present.

Lower Priority

1. Keep the timing of the meals and the composition of the diet consistent from day to day with the carbohydrate content evenly divided from meal to meal.	1. Take midmorning or midafternoon snacks if between meal intervals are extended or if there is a history of hypoglycemia. 2. Plan for food to be taken for periods of increased physical activity. 3. Plan a bedtime snack to prevent nocturnal hypoglycemia when a short acting oral hypoglycemic agent (i.e., acetohexamide, tolbutamide, tolazamide, glipizide) is used.	

Kilocalories. See *Nutritional Assessment,* page 3, for the methods that are used for the estimation of the caloric needs. For persons who require a weight reduction see *Obesity,* page 184, for the determination of the caloric level and the recommended rate of weight loss.

Distribution of Kilocalories. The recommended distribution of kilocalories is 12 to 20 percent of kilocalories as protein, 20 to 35 percent of kilocalories as fat, and 45 to 60 percent of kilocalories as carbohydrate.[2]

The protein requirements of individuals with diabetes are not different from other individuals. The amount of protein in the diet meets, and may exceed, the Recommended Dietary Allowance (RDA) of 0.8 g per kilogram of body weight. The percentage of kilocalories from protein may be as much as 20 percent in diets of 1,200 Kcal or less and may decrease to 12 percent at higher caloric levels.

There is no known advantage associated with a protein intake that is in excess of the RDA. In fact, high levels of protein intake may be disadvantageous for the person with diabetes.[3] Many high protein foods in the American food supply are also high in fat. Inordinate emphasis on high protein food choices may result in a higher intake of fat and a corresponding decrease in the percentage of kilocalories from carbohydrate. The person with IDDM is vulnerable to renal complications (diabetic nephropathy) that may progress to chronic renal failure. This process may possibly accelerate with a high protein diet.[4] For the person who has only a slight elevation of creatinine levels (perhaps 2 mg per deciliter), it is prudent to keep the protein level at approximately the RDA (0.8 g per kilogram of body weight). Further reductions in the protein intake may be necessary with the progression of renal disease (see page 235).

The person with diabetes is at an increased risk of premature atherosclerosis.[5] Recommendations for the fat intake are consistent with the guidelines of the American Heart Association. (See page 37). Generally, it is recommended that the total fat intake be limited to 30 percent or less of the total kilocalories, that polyunsaturated fats be used in preference to saturated fats, and that cholesterol be limited to 300 mg or less. For persons with hypercholesterolemia, further reductions in total fat and cholesterol is warranted. (See page 80.) For persons who otherwise have a low risk of cardiovascular disease and have blood cholesterol levels less than the 75th percentile, the usual admonishments regarding cholesterol and saturated fat restriction may be liberalized. Generally, for the very elderly person with diabetes and for those with surgery- or steroid-induced diabetes, there is less emphasis on cholesterol and fat restrictions. Also, for some persons, the restriction of fat may need to be liberalized to obtain compliance with the total management plan.

Carbohydrates generally constitute 45 to 60 percent of the total kilocalories. Higher levels of carbohydrate do not impede good glycemic control[6] and generally allow a corresponding decrease in the fat levels, which may be advantageous in reducing blood lipids and the risk of atherosclerosis.[5,7] An increased use of plant fibers from whole grain bread and cereal products, legumes, fruits, and vegetables is encouraged.

The Food Exchange Lists for Diabetes, see page 114, can be used for meal planning.

Restriction of Simple Carbohydrates. Simple carbohydrates are defined as monosaccharides and disaccharides. Lactose, sucrose, and fructose are those that are most prevalent as an inherent constituent of usual foods. The most widely used sweeteners (table sugar, corn syrup, and honey) are composed almost exclusively of sucrose and fructose.

It has been common practice to limit the intake of simple carbohydrate, particularly from sweeteners, in the diet of persons with diabetes on the premise that simple carbohydrates are quickly absorbed and cause a rapid postprandial rise in the plasma glucose concentrations. Recent research, which suggests that some complex carbohydrates produce greater plasma glucose excursions than foods predominantly composed of simple carbohydrates, has prompted reevaluation of long standing assumptions.[8] However, more evidence is necessary before radical changes can be recommended.

At the present, the recommendation remains that simple carbohydrates be limited to 10 to 15 percent of the total kilocalories, as they provide suboptimal nutritional value, and an excess consumption may impede weight control efforts. The excessive use of simple carbohydrates also has the potential to elevate the blood triglyceride levels.

Glycemic Effects of Carbohydrates. The effect of carbohydrates on the plasma glucose levels are not as clear-cut as once believed. Recent scientific reports[8–10] have focused attention on the differences in the plasma glucose response to simple sugars (mono- and disaccharides) and to complex carbohydrates (polysaccharides). While the studies have challenged current concepts and practices, they have not provided final answers.

Factors that have been said to lower the glycemic response by delaying the digestion and/or the absorption of food include (1) a whole or a compact food, (2) the fibrous coatings on food such as legumes, (3) raw foods, (4) natural substances that act as antinutrients, such as pectins, phytates, tannins, or starch-protein and starch-lipid combinations, and (5) the fiber content, particularly of guar and pectin. Carbohydrate eaten at one meal may delay the carbohydrate digestion in the next meal. Carbohydrate eaten over several hours as compared to carbohydrate eaten over a short period of time tends to reduce the glycemic response. Carbohydrates eaten separately or as part of a meal may have different plasma glucose responses. Individuals often respond differently to various carbohydrates.

At this time, there is insufficient information to make a precise appraisal of the glycemic response of foods, especially when they are eaten as part of a mixed meal. Current recommendations, based on those of the American Diabetes Association,[11] are to place more emphasis, when possible, on the use of carbohydrate-containing foods that produce the smallest rise in the plasma glucose level and less emphasis on those that are associated with higher glycemic responses. The consumption of a modest amount of sucrose is acceptable, contingent on the maintenance of metabolic control. In addition, regular plasma glucose level monitoring can be an effective tool to assess individual responses to foods. Further research is necessary before major changes can be made in the Food Exchange Lists.

Fiber. The role of dietary fiber in the treatment of diabetes is not clear. Studies[8] have suggested that an increase in the intake of dietary fiber can lead to a decrease in plasma glucose levels and glycosuria and a reduction in the insulin requirements. High fiber intakes have also been associated with decreased cholesterol and triglyceride levels.[12] Four factors appear to influence the effectiveness of fiber.[8,12]

1. The type of fiber is a factor. Guar and pectin are two major types of soluble fibers that are associated with delayed gastric emptying and a longer intestinal transit time. They appear to have the greatest effect in lowering the plasma glucose and the serum cholesterol levels. Insoluble fibers (wheat, bran,

and whole grain products) are associated with a shortened intestinal transit time, but do not appear to have an immediate effect on the plasma glucose or the serum cholesterol levels.

2. The presence of food is a factor. Soluble fibers have a greater effect when mixed with food.

3. The carbohydrate content of the diet is a factor. The effect of fiber is enhanced if given as part of a high complex carbohydrate diet.

4. The preparation or the form is a factor. The effect of fiber is greater if the fiber sources are in whole or in raw form.

The palatability of a high fiber diet is a major problem since large amounts are required for a significant effect. The gastrointestinal side effects of flatulence, fullness, increased bowel movements, and nausea are intolerable for some persons. In addition, the long-term effects of high fiber diets on calcium, iron, zinc, and other trace mineral absorption are not known.[6]

Current recommendations encourage a moderate increase in the dietary fiber intake through emphasis on the use of whole grains, legumes, and fresh or lightly cooked fruits and vegetables. More research is necessary before a very high fiber diet can be routinely recommended.[10,11]

For persons with gastroparesis or with other disorders of autonomic function,[13] see the dietary management of delayed gastric emptying, page 148.

Sweeteners. The use of common sweeteners, which includes table sugar and honey, that are composed of simple carbohydrates is discouraged. The use of artificial, alternative, or substitute sweeteners is not advocated. However, there is a demand for acceptable substitute sweeteners because of the widespread use of sweeteners in the Western diet.

Although none of the available sweeteners can be recommended without reservation, the dietitian can advise individuals on the appropriateness of the use of sweeteners after considering the characteristics of the desired sweetener, the individual's glycemic control, caloric contribution, and the safety of the desired amount of the sweetener.

Alternative sweeteners can be classified as nutritive or as non-nutritive. Nutritive sweeteners are identical in the caloric value by weight to sucrose (table sugar).[14] Nutritive sweeteners include fructose, corn syrups, dextrose, sorbitol, mannitol, xylitol, and maltitol.[14–17] (See *Appendix 10*).

Persons with diabetes should restrict their intake of nutritive sweeteners because of the sweeteners' caloric content and its potential to cause a significant elevation in the plasma glucose levels. Sorbitol can be converted in some measure to glucose as it is partially absorbed. Under circumstances of good glycemic control in IDDM, fructose has less impact on the plasma glucose levels than has dietary glucose. Therefore, good glycemic control should be achieved before these sweeteners are used.[12,15] If used in substantial amounts, as in a candy bar or to sweeten a dessert, these sweeteners should be included as part of a mixed meal and their caloric contribution considered part of the total caloric intake. It is important to remind the overweight person that the caloric value of nutritive sweeteners and of sucrose are essentially identical. Even though a smaller amount of some sweeteners, such as fructose, can be used, the decreased quantity may not result in a significant kilocalorie savings. Sorbitol is commonly present in "sugarless" gum; for most persons using gum in moderation, the caloric contribution and the glycemic effect is probably not significant. Used in larger amounts, sorbitol may cause diarrhea because of its incomplete absorption in the small intestine.

Non-nutritive sweeteners are characterized by an intensely sweet taste. Some contain kilocalories, but generally non-nutritive sweeteners are used in such small quantities that they do not make a significant contribution to the caloric intake.[14] The two non-nutritive sweeteners that are currently available in the United States are aspartame and saccharin. Cyclamate, Thaumatin, and Stevioside are available in other countries. Acesulfame-K is in the process of passing qualification tests for marketing.[14,17] (See *Appendix 10*).

The American Diabetes Association states that there is no indication for diabetic individuals to avoid the use of saccharin in moderate amounts.[18] Still, there is considerable question in regards to the safety of saccharin in general.

From clinical studies, aspartame demonstrates no effect on diabetes control. The American Diabetes Association has approved the use of foods that contain aspartame for persons with diabetes.[19,20] The recommended safe limit for aspartame is 50 mg per kilogram of body weight per day. (Twenty mg of aspartame is approximately equal in taste to 4 to 5 g of sucrose, and due to its concentrated sweet flavor, only small quantities need to be used.) Equal, the commercially available form of aspartame, is also known as NutraSweet. One g ($\frac{1}{4}$ tsp) is equal in sweetness to 4 to 5 g (1 tsp) of sucrose. There is little information on the effects of aspartame during pregnancy. Currently, the advice is to avoid any artificial or substitute sweeteners during pregnancy.

Dietetic Foods. Foods that are for special dietary use are widely available and are of interest to persons with diabetes because of the reduced caloric and/or sugar content. A person with diabetes should be taught to read the nutrition labels in order to recognize the energy and the nutritional value of such dietetic products. (See *Appendix 8*, for a definition of the terminology that is used with dietetic foods).

A dietetic product that contains less than 20 Kcal per serving may be used as a "free food" at meals or at snacks. "Free Foods" should be limited to a total of 20 Kcal per meal or to a total of 60 Kcal maximum that are distributed throughout the day.

Foods that are represented as useful in the diet of a diabetic must be accompanied by a nutrition label and by the statement "Diabetics: This product may be useful in your diet on the advice of a physician." The use of dietetic products, such as dietetic candy, cookies, chocolate, and ice cream, that are of high caloric density and contain sorbitol or mannitol are generally discouraged. *Appendix 10* presents information on nutritive and non-nutritive sweeteners. *Appendix 8* discusses food labeling.

Alcoholic Beverages. For the person with diabetes, the alcoholic intake should be limited because alcohol is high in kilocalories, it tends to be both ketogenic and hypoglycemic, and it tends to promote hypertriglyceridemia.

For the lean, insulin-taking diabetic who is in good glycemic control, a moderate alcoholic intake generally has little perceptible effect on the state of the diabetes. But if meals are delayed or omitted, ketogenesis and hypoglycemia may result. It is recommended that alcohol be consumed with food.

Persons who take the sulfonylurea oral agent chlorpropamide (Diabinese) should be warned about the possible disulfiram (Antabuse) effect of the drug. Persons taking chlorpropamide may experience flushing, nausea, tachycardia, and abdominal discomfort after drinking alcohol.[21]

For the person who consumes a low kilocalorie diet, alcohol should be used infrequently, if at all, because of its high caloric content. If alcohol is used only occasionally and in moderation ($\leq$2 standard drinks/week), and the plasma glucose level is in good control, it may be practical and reasonable to permit the use of alcohol without the substitution for other foods or to consider its caloric contribution into the initial calculation of the meal plan. (See *Appendix 3* for the caloric content of alcoholic beverages).

Although the metabolism of alcohol does not permit its classification as protein, fat or, carbohydrate, alcohol is sometimes considered as a substitute for fat exchanges. Using alcohol in this fashion should not be encouraged, however, as it does not have the same nutritional or metabolic characteristics, and it would be misleading and falsely reassuring to the person to consider it as such. Furthermore, diets for diabetics are generally planned with a modest number of fat exchanges to achieve the desired distribution of kilocalories in fat, carbohydrate, and protein. For these reasons, it is often not feasible to make such substitutions. Recommendations for the use of alcohol are left to the discretion of the physician and the dietitian.

Modifications of the Standard Diet for Diabetes

Dietary Recommendations During Illness. The stress of illness, injury, or surgery can raise the plasma glucose levels and increase the insulin requirements. In insulin-dependent diabetes mellitus, ketosis may occur if the insulin dose is not appropriately adjusted and if there is not an adequate amount of carbohydrate given. Persons who do not require insulin are less likely to develop ketoacidosis, but may develop hyperosmolar nonketotic coma if excessive glycosuria occurs and if an adequate amount of water is not consumed.

If the person is too ill to consume regular foods, a combination of soft and easily digested foods or liquids that give approximately the same amount of carbohydrate as the regular meal plan should be consumed.

If nausea or vomiting are present or the person is not able to consume usual foods, the carbohydrate content of the meal plan can be replaced by using sugar-containing liquids. Table 6–24 indicates the amount of available carbohydrate from one exchange from each food group.

TABLE 6–24   Available Carbohydrate*

Food Groups	Grams of Available Carbohydrate from One Exchange
Meat	5.0
Fat	0.5
Skim Milk	17.0
Starch	17.0
Vegetables*	6.0
Fruits	15.0

*Available carbohydrate is the proportion of macronutrients that can be converted into glucose by the body (100% of carbohydrate, 60% of protein, 10% of fat)

For hospitalized patients who receive clear liquid diets, a precise calculation of the available carbohydrate is not necessary since stress, trauma, and intravenous glucose are likely to alter the insulin requirement. Postoperatively, the diabetic liquid diet is similar to the regular clear and full liquid diets. As the patient's appetite improves, the composition and the caloric level of the diet more closely resemble a diabetic diet.

Hypoglycemia. Hypoglycemia in diabetes may occur as a consequence of the action of insulin or of oral hypoglycemic agents. Symptoms tend to occur when the plasma glucose level falls below 45 to 55 mg per deciliter, although the exact level may vary. Hypoglycemic episodes are usually termed "insulin reactions" although these episodes may also occur with the oral agents. A hypoglycemic episode is more likely to occur if a meal is delayed or incompletely consumed or if there is increased exercise. To prevent nocturnal hypoglycemia, a bedtime feeding is recommended for all persons who take insulin or an oral hypoglycemic agent. Between meal feedings should be included if the span between meals is more than 5 hours. There is no risk of hypoglycemia in the diabetic person who does not receive insulin or oral hypoglycemic agents.

The initial symptoms of a hypoglycemic episode are mainly the results of epinephrine or catecholamine release. These symptoms include feelings of apprehension and anxiety, rapid heartbeat, and cold perspiration.[22] Fortunately, these symptoms ordinarily awaken the person if they occur during sleep. If the person's cardiac status is such that a dysrhythmia may be provoked by a catecholamine excess, such as during the period that follows a myocardial infarction, a hypoglycemic episode could have serious or even fatal consequences. In a long-term diabetic, there may be a deterioration of the function of the autonomic nervous system so that epinephrine-related symptoms are blunted or absent, and symptoms that result from impaired brain function may be the first clue that hypoglycemia is occurring. The brain and the other parts of the nervous system use only glucose for fuel. With prolonged or severe hypoglycemia, cerebral function is disturbed, which results in confusion, a change in personality, and finally coma or seizures.[22] Hypoglycemic episodes pose a particular threat of stroke for those with limited cerebral circulation.

Although plasma glucose levels may rise well above hypoglycemic levels within 5 to 15 minutes after the ingestion of food, symptoms of hypoglycemia may persist for longer periods, particularly the cerebral symptoms. It is important to give enough food to correct the hypoglycemia, but resist giving excessive amounts of food when the symptoms do not resolve promptly. During the next several hours there may be an appearance of excessive lability if the patient takes larger-than-needed amounts of food and has a resultant hyperglycemia. In general, the administration of 10 to 15 g of a simple carbohydrate is sufficient, but may need to be repeated if the symptoms do not abate within about 15 minutes. It is particularly important that the person who is vulnerable to insulin reactions take precautions to avoid such episodes while driving a car. A particularly hazardous time is the hour before the evening meal when the person may be driving home from work. If the person has not eaten in the previous 2 hours, the taking of a fruit exchange before getting behind the wheel of a car is often a reasonable precaution.

Exercise. Along with diet and insulin, a regular exercise program can aid in the management of diabetes. It may improve glucose homeostasis in the non-insulin-dependent diabetic and may lower insulin requirements in the insulin-dependent diabetic. Frequent monitoring of the blood glucose levels is helpful in predicting plasma glucose levels before, during, and after exercise.

The plasma glucose response to exercise in the insulin-dependent diabetic is variable. It depends upon the level of metabolic control before exercise and the level of insulin at the time of exercise. Exercise usually decreases the plasma glucose levels in the moderately well controlled diabetic. In the poorly controlled ketotic diabetic (plasma glucose > 300 mg/dl), exercise may actually increase the glucose levels, free fatty acids, and ketone bodies.[23]

In the noninsulin-dependent diabetic, plasma glucose levels normally decrease following exercise, but may increase in those diabetics with more severe hyperglycemia (plasma glucose > 300 mg/dl). Since many individuals with noninsulin-dependent diabetes are overweight, regular exercise may be a useful adjunct to diet. Both exercise and weight reduction independently enhance insulin sensitivity and decrease very low-density lipoproteins and low-density lipoprotein cholesterol levels.

For individuals taking insulin, hypoglycemia commonly occurs during or following exercise and requires adjustments in insulin and diet. Suggested dietary guidelines to prevent hypoglycemia during exercise appears in Table 6–25.

TABLE 6–25 Dietary Guidelines During Exercise[23,24]

Plasma Glucose Level Prior to Exercise	Recommended Intake of Carbohydrate for Moderate Exercise
<80 mg/dl	20–50 g prior to exercise then 10–15 g/hr
80–180 mg/dl	10–15 g/hr
180–300 mg/dl	none needed for 1 hr of exercise

The recommended foods are fruit and starch exchanges. Overeating prior to exercise with the intent to prevent hypoglycemia is common and can be avoided. Individuals need to monitor their plasma glucose levels and adapt these guidelines to their personal needs.

Liberalized Diabetic Diet. A liberalized diet, (termed at Mayo Clinic as the "Diabetic Diet—No Kilocalorie Restriction,") is used for persons with a mildly impaired glucose tolerance who are at an appropriate weight, but who may benefit from a moderate restriction of simple carbohydrates and an improvement in eating habits; for those who need a diabetic diet, but have a poor food intake; or for those persons with diabetes who cannot or will not follow the exchange system. (Such individuals may include cancer patients who have significant eating problems, the elderly, and those who have impaired sight or a learning disability.)

The principles of the "Diabetic Diet—No Kilocalorie Restriction" appear in Table 6–26.

TABLE 6–26 Diabetic Diet—No Kilocalorie Restriction

(1) This diet does not use food exchanges or measurements.
(2) The diet should be varied and nutritionally balanced. It should meet the normal nutritional needs of the person.
(3) Sugar and foods high in sugar should be avoided. (See *Foods to Avoid,* page 114.)
(4) Dietetic foods with a significant caloric content should be avoided.
(5) Meals and snacks should be eaten at regular intervals with each meal consistent in quantity.

Diabetes and Chronic Renal Failure. In the presence of impaired renal function secondary to diabetic nephropathy, modifications in the dietary protein, sodium, potassium, and/or fluid allowances are often necessary.

As renal failure progresses, the principles of the diabetic diet may need to be adjusted. The features of the renal diet take priority, especially when very low protein levels are necessary. (See *Dietary Management* of *Chronic Renal Failure,* page 218.)

The decrease in protein requires a corresponding increase in fat and carbohydrate. Low protein products can be used as a source of kilocalories. To assure adequate kilocalories, simple carbohydrates such as sugar, jellies, and sweetened fruit may also have to be included. If simple carbohydrates are consumed, they should be measured carefully and distributed evenly throughout the day to minimize the fluctuation in the plasma glucose levels. The rationale for incorporating simple sugars into the diet must be clearly explained to the patient to ensure compliance. Consistency in the timing and the composition of meals and the use of additional food for increased exercise to prevent hypoglycemic reactions remain necessary.

The renal exchange list should be used in planning the diet for individuals with diabetes and renal failure. (See *Dietary Management of Chronic Renal Failure,* page 218).

Diabetes and Pregnancy. The diet for pregnancy follows the same basic principles as the standard diabetic diet and also includes the necessary requirements for pregnancy.

Of all pregnancies, 0.1 to 0.5 percent are in women who have been previously diagnosed as having diabetes, an additional 2.5 percent of pregnant women develop gestational diabetes.[25] Gestational diabetes is defined as an abnormal glucose tolerance test that is noted during the course of the pregnancy. All women should be screened at 24 to 28 weeks of gestation. If the plasma glucose levels of the gestational diabetic cannot be kept under 105 mg per deciliter by the diet alone, insulin therapy may be started. Sulfonylureas are contraindicated during pregnancy.

Good control of the plasma glucose levels during pregnancy is critical both to the health of the mother and of the fetus. Studies have shown that perinatal infant mortality rates drop to near normal ranges for those patients who demonstrate good glycemic control (i.e., 80 to 100 mg/dl fasting and before meals) during their pregnancy.[25] An increase in the plasma glucose levels during the first 6 to 8 weeks after conception increases the chances of fetal malformations. An increase in the plasma glucose levels later on in the pregnancy is associated with macrosomia, fetal hypoglycemia, and respiratory distress syndrome.

The caloric level of the diet is based on the number of kilocalories that are required to maintain the person's pre-pregnancy weight with an increase of approximately 300 Kcal per day to achieve a total weight gain of 7 to 13.6 kg (15 to 30 lb). The rate of weight gain during pregnancy should be carefully monitored and similar to that desired for nondiabetic pregnant women. (See page 14.) A weight loss during the pregnancy is contraindicated because of the need for adequate fetal nutrition and also because of the increased incidence of maternal ketonurea with very low kilocalorie diets.[25] The fetus acts as a "glucose sink," by constantly removing glucose from the maternal circulation. This renders the woman vulnerable to hypoglycemia before meals and to ketosis. Between meal feedings minimize the fluctuations in plasma glucose levels and help prevent ketosis. The caloric allotment is divided into three meals and three snacks—a midmorning, a midafternoon, and a bedtime snack. Regularity of meals and exercise are advised to prevent wide fluctuations in the plasma glucose levels. Alcohol, artificial sweeteners, and caffeine are not recommended. For further information regarding the diet in pregnancy, see page 12.

Diet Following Gastroplasty for Weight Reduction. For persons with diabetes who have undergone gastroplasty for weight reduction, the dietary plan for gastroplasty is ordinarily satisfactory during the first few months. The person is restricted to a very small volume of food at each meal because of the limited gastric capacity. Between meal snacks may be necessary. The diet can be gradually modified toward the standard diabetic diet recommendations. See *Gastroplasty* for weight reduction, page 193, for further information.

Tube Feeding for the Person with Diabetes. Diabetic persons on tube feeding should be provided with adequate kilocalories and protein to meet their nutritional requirements. Kilocalories should not be spared in order to achieve optimal plasma glucose levels. Rather, insulin regulation and glucose monitoring should be used to achieve glycemic control. In the hospital, continuous feedings are suggested for optimal glycemic control. These continuous feedings help slow gastric emptying and delay and perhaps reduce the peak glucose response. If continuous feedings are not possible, an intermittent feeding schedule with a small volume at a slow rate is recommended. See *Enteral Nutrition,* page 261, for further information.

Physicians: How to Order Diet

The diet order should indicate *diabetic diet.* If weight reduction is desired, the diet order should indicate *diabetic, weight reduction diet.* The dietitian determines the appropriate caloric level and the other characteristics of the diet based on the previous discussion. If additional therapeutic modifications, such as full liquid or sodium restriction, are desired, they should be indicated in the diet order.

Community Support Programs

The dietitian should be aware that there are many community support programs and associations available to the person with diabetes. These support systems can provide both up to date information as well as peer support.

The American Diabetes Association
National Service Center
1660 Duke Street
Alexandria, VA 22314

The American Dietetic Association
208 South LaSalle Street
Chicago, IL 60611

The American Diabetes Association of Minnesota
3005 Ottawa Avenue South
Minneapolis, MN 55416

The National Diabetes Information Clearinghouse
Box NDK
Bethesda, MD 20205

Juvenile Diabetes Foundation
23 East 26 Street
New York, NY 10010

Canadian Diabetes Association
Suite 601
123 Edward Street
Toronto, Ontario
Canada M5G 1E2

FOOD EXCHANGE LISTS[26-30]

The following list is adapted from the 1986 American Diabetes Association and the American Dietetic Association (ADA) Exchange Lists for Meal Planning.[31] However, several modifications to the ADA Exchange Lists were made in order to include a more comprehensive listing of foods as well as their gram weights. This detailed information is intended as a reference for the dietitian and not necessarily for patient instruction. For patient education, the following exchange list may be simplified, condensed, or modified depending on the goals of the dietary management, the need for other dietary restrictions, and the abilities of the patient. Table 6–27 summarizes the amount of carbohydrate, protein, and fat in one serving from each exchange list.

TABLE 6–27 Summary of Nutrients in One Serving from Each Exchange List

Exchange List	Carbohydrate (g)	Protein (g)	Fat (g)	Kilocalories (Kcal)
Meat				
Lean	—	7	3	55
Medium–fat	—	7	5	75
High–fat	—	7	8	100
Milk				
Skim	12	8	trace	80
Low-fat	12	8	5	120
Whole	12	8	8	150
Starch or Bread	15	3	trace	80
Vegetable	5	2	—	25
Fruit	15	—	—	60
Fat	—	—	5	45

Group 1–Foods to Avoid

Foods that contain large amounts of sugar generally should be avoided or used in limited amounts.*

Candy	Honey	Pudding[†]
Candy bars	Jam	Sugar
Cake[†]	Jelly	Sugar coated cereals
Chewing gum	Marmalade	Sweet rolls
Cookies[†]	Molasses	Sweetened condensed milk
Custard[†]	Pastries	Sweetened fruit
Granola	Pies	Sweetened soft drinks
Granola type bars		Sweetened yogurt
		Syrup

---

*Sugar-containing foods may be recommended for some circumstances, particularly as a caloric source for persons with chronic renal failure or a severely restricted intake because of illness and for treatment of hypoglycemia.
†Exceptions are listed under *Special Occasion Foods,* see page 120.

Group 2–"Free" Foods

The foods listed under "Use as Desired" are relatively free of kilocalories and do not need to be calculated in the meal plan.

The foods listed under "Use in Limited Amounts" contain less than 20 Kcal per serving. They do not need to be calculated in the meal plan unless the total sum of their use exceeds 20 Kcal per meal or a total of 60 Kcal maximum that is distributed throughout the day. Artificially sweetened foods and beverages are limited because of a general restriction on the quantity of artificial sweeteners used rather than their caloric contribution.

Beverages

Use as Desired

Coffee
Decaffeinated coffee
Tea
Water
Club Soda
Carbonated water
Mineral water
Tonic water, sugar-free

Use in Limited Amounts

Artificially sweetened beverages

Condiments and Seasonings

Use as Desired

Salt
Pepper
Herbs
Spices
Flavoring extracts
Mustard
Horseradish
Dill Pickles
Lemon juice
Lime juice
Vinegar
Fat-free butter flavoring
Worstershire or soy sauce

Use in Limited Amounts

Barbecue sauce (1 Tbsp)
Cocktail sauce (1 Tbsp)
Dietetic jam or jelly (2 tsp)
Ketchup (1 Tbsp)
Pancake syrup, sugar-free (2 Tbsp)
Salad dressing, low kilocalorie (2 Tbsp)
Taco sauce (1 Tbsp)
Whipped topping, low kilocalorie (1 Tbsp)

Other Foods

Use as Desired

Plain, unflavored gelatin
Fat-free bouillon or broth

Use in Limited Amounts

Unsweetened cocoa powder (1 Tbsp)
Artificially sweetened, flavored gelatin
Artificial sweetener
Gum, sugar-free (2–3 sticks)
Hard candy, sugar-free (2–3 pieces)
Unsweetened cranberries ($\frac{1}{2}$ cup)

116 / MAYO CLINIC DIET MANUAL

Group 3—Meat Exchanges

Meat should be weighed after cooking and after the bone, skin, and excess fat have been removed. The use of meats from the lean and the medium fat categories is encouraged.

Measure or Weight	Gram Weight	Lean Meat: 7 g protein; 3 g fat; 55 Kcal
1 oz	30	Beef: baby beef (very lean), chipped beef, chuck, flank steak, tenderloin, plate ribs, plate skirt steak, round (bottom, top), all rump cuts, lean spareribs, tripe, ground (more than 90% lean), USDA good or choice cuts
1 oz	30	Pork: leg (whole rump, center shank), tenderloin, ham (canned, cured, boiled), Canadian bacon
1 oz	30	Veal: leg, loin, rib, shank, shoulder
1 oz	30	Poultry (meat without skin): chicken, turkey, cornish hen, guinea hen
1 oz	30	Wild game: venison, rabbit, squirrel, pheasant, goose (without skin)
1 oz	30	Fish: any fresh or frozen
1 oz	30	Herring (uncreamed or smoked)
1/4 cup	30	Tuna, mackerel (canned in water)
1 oz (2 medium)	30	Sardines, drained
2 oz (1/3 cup)	30	Clams, crab, lobster (fresh or canned in water)
3 oz (6 medium)	90	Oysters
2 oz (8)	50	Scallops (Bay)
2 oz (5–6 medium)	60	Shrimp
1/4 cup	60	Egg substitutes, fat-free
3 whites	90	Egg whites
1 oz	30	Cheeses (low fat that contain 3 g fat or less/oz)
1/4 cup	45	Cottage cheese: any
2 Tbsp	10	Parmesan cheese (grated)
1 oz	30	Low fat luncheon meat (containing 3 g fat or less/oz or greater than 90% lean)

Measure or Weight	Gram Weight	Medium-fat Meat: 7 g protein; 5 g fat; 73 Kcal
1 oz	30	Beef: roasts and steaks, ground (more than 80% lean), corned beef (canned), rib eye
1 oz	30	Lamb: leg, rib, sirloin, loin (roast and chops), shank, shoulder
1 oz	30	Pork: loin (all tenderloin cuts), shoulder arm (picnic), shoulder blade, Boston butt
1 oz	30	Poultry: chicken and turkey (with skin); ground turkey; capon; domestic duck or goose (well drained of fat)
1 oz	30	Veal, cutlet (ground or cubed, unbreaded)
1 oz	30	Liver, heart, kidney, sweetbreads
1 oz	30	Cheese: mozzarella, ricotta, Neufchatel, farmer cheese
1 oz	30	Low-fat luncheon meats (containing 3 to 5 g fat/oz or 85–90% lean)
1/4 cup	30	Tuna (canned in oil, drained), salmon (canned, drained)
1	50	Egg
4 oz	120	Tofu

Measure or Weight	Gram Weight	High-fat Meat: 7 g protein; 8 g fat; 100 kcal These meats are high in fat and kilocalories and, therefore, should be used only occasionally.
1 oz	30	Beef: brisket, corned beef (brisket), ground (less than 80% lean), chuck (ground commercial), roasts (rib), steaks (club and rib) USDA Prime
1 oz	30	Pork: spareribs, loin (back ribs), ground, country-style ham, deviled ham, sausage
1 oz	30	Lamb, breast, ground
1 oz	30	Veal, breast
1 oz	30	Cheese: all regular, including American, Blue, Cheddar, Monterey, Swiss
2 Tbsp	30	Cheese spreads
1 slice $4\frac{1}{2}$ in by 1/8 in ($1\frac{1}{2}$ oz)	45	Cold cuts
1 oz	30	Sausage: Polish, Italian, Bratwurst, Knockwurt, smoked
1 small ($1\frac{1}{2}$ oz)	45	Frankfurter, turkey or chicken (beef, pork, or combination—omit 1 fat)
2 Tbsp	30	Peanut butter (omit 2 fats)

Meat Alternatives

If these foods are used as a substitute for meat (as in a vegetarian diet) the carbohydrate content needs to be accounted for as indicated below.

Measure or Weight	Gram Weight	Meat Alternative	Exchange Value
1 cup	220	Beans (cooked): Butter	1 lean meat + 2 starch
2/3 cup	100	Lima	1 lean meat + 1 starch
1/2 cup	60	Pinto	1 lean meat + 2 starch
1 cup	200	Red	1 lean meat + 2 starch
1/3 cup	70	Soy	1 lean meat + 1/2 starch
1 cup	200	White	1 lean meat + 1 starch
$3\frac{1}{2}$ oz	100	Garbanzo beans or chick peas (canned)	1 lean meat + 1 starch + 1 fruit
2/3 cup	100	Lentils (cooked)	1 lean meat + 1 starch
2/3 cup	100	Peas (cooked): Black eyed	1/2 lean meat + 1 starch
1 cup	200	Split	1 lean meat + 2 starch + 1 vegetable
1/4 cup (25 nuts)	30	Nuts and Seeds: Peanuts	1 med fat meat + 2 fat + 1 vegetable
1 oz (3 Tbsp)	30	Pumpkin seeds	1 high fat meat + 1 fat + 1 vegetable
1 oz (3 Tbsp)	30	Sesame seeds	1 med fat meat + 2 fat
1 oz (1/4 cup)	30	Soybean nuts	2 lean meat + 1/2 vegetable
1 oz (3 Tbsp)	30	Squash seeds	1 high fat meat + 1 fat + 1 vegetable
1 oz (3 Tbsp)	30	Sunflower or safflower seeds	1 high fat meat + 1 fat + 1 vegetable
1/4 cup	30	Wheat germ (toasted)	1 lean meat + 1 starch

Group 4—Milk Exchanges

Measure	Gram Weight	Nonfat Fortified Milk: 8 g protein; 12 g carbohydrate; trace fat; 80 Kcal
1 cup	240	Skim or nonfat milk
1/3 cup	25	Powdered milk (nonfat dry, before adding liquid)
1/2 cup	120	Canned, evaporated skim milk
1 cup	240	Buttermilk made from skim milk
1 cup	240	Yogurt make from skim milk (plain, unflavored)
		1% Fat Fortified Milk (1 nonfat milk + 1/2 fat exchange): 8 g protein; 12 g carbohydrate; 2.5 g fat; 102 Kcal
1 cup	240	1% milk
1 cup	240	Low-fat buttermilk
		2% Fat Fortified Milk (1 nonfat milk + 1 fat exchange): 8 g protein; 12 g carbohydrates; 5 g fat; 120 Kcal
1 cup	240	2% milk
1 cup	240	Yogurt made from 2% milk (plain, unflavored)
1/2 cup	120	Canned evaporated 2% milk
		Whole Milk (1 nonfat milk + 2 fat exchanges): 8 g protein; 12 g carbohydrate; 8 g fat; 150 Kcal
1 cup	240	Whole milk
1/2 cup	120	Canned, evaporated whole milk
1 cup	240	Buttermilk made from whole milk
1 cup	240	Yogurt made from whole milk (plain, unflavored)

Group 5—Starch Exchanges

Each serving from the starch group contains 3 g protein, 15 g carbohydrate, trace fat, 80 Kcal

Measure	Gram Weight	Bread
1/2	30	Bagel, small
2	25	Breadsticks, crisp − 4 in long by 1/2 in diameter
1/2 cup	20	Croutons (plain or herb seasoned)—no fat added
1/2	30	English muffin, small
1/2	35	Frankfurter bun
1/2	35	Hamburger bun
1/2	30	Pita bread, thin—6 in in diameter
1	30	Plain dinner roll, small
1 slice	25	Raisin bread (unfrosted)
1 slice	25	Rye or pumpernickel bread
1	30	Tortilla, 6 in in diameter
1 slice	25	White, including French and Italian
1 slice	25	Whole wheat
4 Tbsp	20	Dried bread crumbs

Measure	Gram Weight	Cereal
1/2 cup	30	Bran cereals, flakes, chex
1/3 cup	25	Other bran cereals
1/2 cup	100	Cooked cereal
1/2 cup	100	Grits, cooked
3 Tbsp	20	Grape-Nuts
$1\frac{1}{2}$ cups	20	Puffed cereal, unfrosted
3/4 cup	20	Other ready-to-eat, unsweetened cereal
1 Biscuit or 1/2 cup	25	Shredded Wheat

Measure	Gram Weight	Other Starches
1/2 cup	100	Barley or bulgur, cooked
$2\frac{1}{2}$ Tbsp	20	Cornmeal, dry
$2\frac{1}{2}$ Tbsp	25	Cornstarch
3 Tbsp	20	Flour
1/2 cup	100	Pasta: spaghetti, noodles, macaroni (cooked)
3 cups	20	Popcorn (popped, without oil)
$1\frac{1}{2}$ cups	20	Popcorn (popped in oil)
1/3 cup	75	Rice, brown or white (cooked)
$2\frac{1}{2}$ Tbsp	20	Tapioca

Measure	Gram Weight	Crackers
10	18	Animal Crackers
3	20	Arrowroot
3	35	Graham, $2\frac{1}{2}$ in square
3/4	22	Matzoth, 4 in by 6 in
5	20	Melba toast, $3\frac{3}{4}$ in by 2 in
24	20	Oyster
25	20	Pretzels, $3\frac{3}{8}$ in long by 1/8 in in diameter
3	20	Rye wafers, 2 in by $3\frac{1}{2}$ in
2	20	Rice cakes
6	20	Saltines

Measure	Gram Weight	Starchy Vegetables
1/3 cup	70	Beans, peas (dried, cooked)
1/4 cup	50	Baked beans (canned, no pork)
1/2 cup	80	Corn
1 small	100	Corn on the cob, 3 to 4 in long
1/2 cup	100	Lima beans
2/3 cup	130	Parsnips
1/2 cup	100	Peas, green
1/2 cup	75	Lentils (cooked)
1/2 cup	75	Plantain
1 small	100	Potato, baked or boiled
1/2 cup	100	Potato, mashed
1 cup	200	Pumpkin
1/2 small	50	Sweet potato, baked
1/3 cup	100	Yam (canned or fresh), sweet potato (canned), plain
3/4 cup	150	Squash, winter (acorn, butternut, buttercup, hubbard)

Measure	Gram Weight	Prepared Foods (omit 1 fat exchange)
1	35	Biscuit, 2 in in diameter
1/2 cup	30	Chow mein noodles
1	50	Corn bread, 2 in cube
1	40	Corn muffin, 2 in in diameter
6	25	Crackers, round butter type
6	30	Whole wheat crackers
1	40	Muffin, plain, small
2	45	Pancakes, 4 in diameter (from mix)
10	45	Potatoes, French fried, $2-3\frac{1}{2}$ in long
1/4 cup	45	Stuffing, bread (prepared)
2	20	Taco shell, 6 in diameter
1	40	Waffle, 5 in diameter

Measure	Gram Weight	Special Occasion Foods. (Many of the following foods contain added sugar and fat. They should be eaten only occasionally, in limited amounts, and with other foods.)
1/16 of 10-in cake (1½ in)	45	Angel food cake, plain
1/12 cake or 3″ square	50	Cake, no icing (omit 1 additional starch and 2 fat)
1/16 of 10-in cake (1½ in)	35	Cake, sponge
1	30	Croissant, small—5 in by 2 in (omit 2 fat exchanges)
2 small	25	Cookies 1¾ in (omit 1 fat exchange)
1	30	Doughnut, plain cake (omit 1 fat exchange)
5	20	Gingersnaps, 1¾ in by 1/8 in
1/2 cup	140	Gelatin, sweetened (commercial flavored)
1/4 cup	30	Granola (omit 1 fat exchange)
1 small	25	Granola bar (omit 1 fat exchange)
1/2 cup	70	Ice cream (omit 2 fat exchanges)
1/2 cup	60	Ice milk (omit 1 fat exchange)
2	25	Ice cream cone (cone only)
1/4 cup	75	Pudding
1/3 cup	65	Sherbet
1 oz	30	Snack chips, all varieties (omit 2 fat exchanges)
2	20	Shortbread cookies, 1½ in by 1/4 in (omit 1 fat exchange)
5	20	Vanilla wafers, about 1¾ in by 1/8 in
1/3 cup	75	Yogurt, frozen fruit

Group 6—Vegetable Exchanges

Each serving from the vegetable group contains 2 g protein, 5 g carbohydrate, and 25 Kcal. One exchange is 1/2 cup (100 g) cooked vegetable or juice; or 1/2 to 1 cup raw (unless another amount is given).

Artichoke (medium globe)	Green pepper (1 large)	Tomatoes
Asparagus (5–7 sprouts)	Jicama	raw (1 large)
Bamboo shoots	Kale	cherry (6)
Bean sprouts	Kohlrabi (2/3 cup)	paste (2 Tbsp)
Beets	Leeks (2 medium)	sauce (1/4 cup)
Beet greens	Mustard greens	stewed (1/2 cup)
Broccoli	Okra	Tomato juice
Brussel sprouts	Onions	Turnips
Carrots	Pea pods or Snow peas	Turnip greens
Chard greens	Rutabaga	Vegetable juice cocktail
Collard greens	Sauerkraut	Water chestnuts (5)
Dandelion greens	Spinach	
Eggplant	String beans, green or yellow	

The following vegetables have little protein, fat or carbohydrate. One to two cups may be considered "free" and used without substitution in the meal plan.

Alfalfa sprouts	Endive	Rhubarb
Cabbage	Escarole	Romaine
Cauliflower	Green onion	Summer squash
Celery	Hot peppers	Watercress
Chicory	Lettuce	Zucchini
Chinese cabbage	Mushrooms	
Cucumber	Radishes	

Group 7—Fruit Exchanges

Each serving from the fruit group contains 15 g carbohydrate and 60 Kcal. Fruit may be fresh, unsweetened canned, cooked, frozen, or dried. Juice-packed fruits should be drained; the juice should be counted separately.

Measure	Gram Weight		Measure	Gram Weight	
1 small	100	Apple, 2 in diameter	1/2 small	120	Nectarine, 3 in diameter
1/2 cup	120	Apple juice			
1/2 cup	120	Applesauce	1	130	Orange, $2\frac{1}{2}$ in diameter
1/2 cup	120	Apple cider	1/2 cup	120	Orange juice
4 medium	135	Apricots, fresh	3/4 cup	165	Orange sections in-
7 halves	25	Apricots, dried			cluding mandarin
1/2 cup or 4 halves	100	Apricots, canned	$2\frac{1}{2}$ ounces	75	Papaws
			1/2 medium	150	Papaya
1/2 cup	120	Apricot nectar	or 1 cup		
1/2	60	Banana, 9 in long	3 medium	60	Passion fruit
3/4 cup	100	Blackberries	1 medium	140	Peach, $2\frac{3}{4}$ in diameter
3/4 cup	100	Blueberries	2 halves	25	Peach, dried
1/4 or 1 cup chunks	160	Cantaloupe, 6 in diam- eter	1/2 cup	135	Peaches, canned
			1/2 cup	120	Peach nectar
12	80	Cherries, large, sweet	1 small	100	Pear
1/2 cup	120	Cherries, canned	1 half	20	Pear, dried
1/3 cup	100	Cranberry juice cock- tail	1/2 cup	120	Pears, canned
			1/2 cup	120	Pear nectar
$1\frac{1}{4}$ cup	300	Cranberry juice cock- tail (low kilocalorie)	2 medium	50	Persimmon, native
			3/4 cup	120	Pineapple, fresh
2 large	20	Dates	1/3 cup	100	Pineapple, canned
2	75	Figs, fresh 2 in	1/2 cup	120	Pineapple juice
1 large	20	Figs, dried	1/2 cup or 3	100	Plums, canned
1/2 cup	125	Fruit cocktail	2	100	Plums, 2 in diameter
1/2 medium	125	Grapefruit	1/2 medium	80	Pomegranates
1/2 cup	120	Grapefruit juice	1 medium	150	Prickly pear
3/4 cup	155	Grapefruit sections	3 medium	25	Prunes
15 small	90	Grapes	1/3 cup	80	Prune juice
1/3 cup	90	Grape juice	2 Tbsp	20	Raisins
1 medium	100	Guava	1 cup	125	Raspberries
1/8 medium or 1 cup chunks	170	Honeydew	$1\frac{1}{4}$ cup	190	Strawberries
			1 medium	175	Tangelo
			2 medium	135	Tangerine, $2\frac{1}{2}$ in diam- eter
1 large	100	Kiwi			
5 medium	95	Kumquats	1/2 cup	120	Tangerine juice
1/2 small	90	Mango	$1\frac{1}{4}$ cup	190	Watermelon

Group 8—Fat Exchanges

Each serving from the fat list contains 5 g fat, and 45 Kcal.

Measure	Gram Weight	Predominantly Polyunsaturated
1 tsp	5	Margarine: soft, tub (made with safflower, sunflower, or corn oil)
1 Tbsp	15	Diet margarine (made with safflower, sunflower, or corn oil)
1 tsp	5	Oil (Safflower, sunflower, corn, soybean, cottonseed, or sesame oil)
2 Tbsp	30	Nondairy cream substitute*
1 Tbsp	15	French or Italian style salad dressing*
2 Tbsp	30	Reduced kilocalorie salad dressing*
1 tsp	5	Mayonnaise*
2 tsp	10	Mayonnaise-type salad dressing*
1 Tbsp	15	Reduced kilocalorie mayonnaise*
$1\frac{1}{2}$ tsp	10	Tartar sauce
6 whole	8	Almonds
5 halves	7	Pecans
4 halves	8	Walnuts
2 tsp	5	Pumpkin seeds
1 Tbsp without shells	7	Sunflower seeds

Measure	Gram Weight	Predominantly Monounsaturated Fats
1 tsp	5	Margarine (any containing soybean, cottonseed, or partially hydrogenated vegetable oil as first ingredient—check label)
1 tsp	5	Olive oil
1 tsp	5	Peanut oil
9–10 medium	35–40	Green olives
5 large	25	Ripe olives
2 medium	10	Brazil nuts
5	10	Hazel nuts
20 small, 10 large	10	Peanuts
20	10	Pistachio nuts

Measure	Gram Weight	Predominantly Saturated Fats
1/8	30	Avocado, 4 in in diameter
1 tsp	5	Butter
1 tsp	5	Bacon fat
1 strip	10	Bacon, crisp
2 Tbsp	30	Sour cream
3 Tbsp	45	Half and half or light cream
1 Tbsp	15	Cream, heavy whipping
2 Tbsp	30	Other nondairy cream substitutes
1 Tbsp	15	Cream cheese
2 Tbsp	30	Gravy
1 tsp	5	Lard or shortening
1/4 oz	7	Salt pork
4 large or 6 small	8	Cashews
3 large whole, or 4 medium	8	Macadamia nuts

*Made with safflower, sunflower, corn, soybean, cottonseed, or sesame oil.

REFERENCES

1. National Diabetes Data Group. Classification and diagnosis of diabetes mellitus and other categories of glucose intolerance. Diabetes 1979;28:1039–1057.
2. Arky R, et al. Examination of current dietary recommendations for individuals with diabetes mellitus. Diabetes Care 1982;5:59–61.
3. Epstein F. Dietary protein intake and the progressive nature of kidney disease. N Engl J Med 1982;307:652–657.
4. Bergstrom J. Discovery and rediscovery of the low protein diet. Clin Nephrol 1984;21:29–35.
5. Scott DW, Gorry GA, Gotto AM. Diet and coronary heart disease: the statistical analysis of risk. Circulation 1981;63:516–518.
6. Nuttall FQ. Diet and the diabetic patient. Diabetes Care 1983;6:197–207.
7. National Research Council, National Academy of Sciences. Toward healthful diets. 1980 Stock No. ISBN 0-309-03077-3.
8. Crapo P. Theory vs fact: the glycemic response to foods. Nutr Today 1984;19:6–11.
9. Diabetes Care and Education Dietetic Practice Group. Diabetes mellitus and glycemic responses to different foods: a summary and annotated bibliography. 1985.
10. Franz M. Glycemic effects of carbohydrates. Diabetes Educator 1985;11:69–70.
11. American Diabetes Association. Glycemic effects of carbohydrates policy statement. Diabetes Care 1984;7:607–608.
12. Crapo P. The nutritional therapy of non-insulin dependent (type II) diabetes. Diabetes Educator 1983;9:13–19.
13. Yang R, Arem R, Chan L. GI tract complications of diabetes mellitus: pathophysiology and management. Arch Intern Med 1984;144:1251–1256.
14. Wylic-Rosett J. Alternative sweeteners for diabetics. Cardiovasc Rev Rep 1982;3:1386–1394.
15. Lapworth D, Hallburg J. Counseling diabetics in the use of substitute sweeteners. Diabetes Educator 1985;11:55–59.
16. Lecos C. Sweetness minus calories controversy. FDA Consumer 1985;19:18–23.
17. O'Sullivan D. New sweeteners gain ground in Europe. Chem Eng News 1983(Jan 24):29.
18. ADA policy statement—saccharin. Diabetes Care 1979;2:380.
19. Council on Scientific Affairs of the American Medical Association of the Am Med Association. Aspartame: review of safety issues. JAMA 1985;254:400–402.
20. Horwitz D, Nehrling JB. Can aspartame meet our expectations. J Am Diet Assoc 1983;83:142–146.
21. Franz M. Diabetes mellitus: considerations in the development of guidelines for the occasional use of alcohol. J Am Diet Assoc 1983;83:147–152.
22. Cryer PE, Gerich JE. Glucose counterregulation, hypoglycemia, and intensive insulin therapy in diabetes mellitus. N Engl J Med 1985;313:232–241.
23. Schiffrin A, Parikh S. Accommodating planned exercise in type I diabetic patients on intensive treatment. Diabetes Care 1985;8:337–342.
24. Diabetes and exercise. Diabetes Care and Ed Newsletter 1985;7.
25. Nelson RL. Diabetes and pregnancy: primary care. 1983;10:225–240.
26. United States Department of Agriculture. Composition of foods. Agricultural Handbook 1976–1984:1–12.
27. Pennington JA, Church HN. Bowes and Church's food values of portions commonly used. 14th ed. Philadelphia: JB Lippencott, 1985.
28. Leveille GA, Zabik ME, Morgan KJ, Agee DH. Nutrients in foods. Cambridge, MA: The Nutrition Guide, 1983.
29. Cinnamon PA, Swanson MA. Everything about exchange values for foods. 3rd ed. Moscow, Id: University Press of Idaho, 1981.
30. Alli C, Crapo P. The bitter debate. Diabetes Forecast 1985;35:34–37.
31. American Diabetes Association and American Dietetic Association. Exchange lists for meal planning. Alexandria, VA and Chicago, IL. 1986.

ANOREXIA NERVOSA AND BULIMIA

General Description

The dietary recommendations for patients with eating disorders include a kilocalorie level that meets the current energy needs. For the patient with anorexia nervosa, relatively small, gradual increments are made in the kilocalorie level. For patients with bulimia, the recommended kilocalorie level may be constant through the course of the treatment. For both anorexia nervosa and bulimia, it is essential that a diet plan consider individual needs. Education that regards the normal nutritional needs and the physiologic effects of starvation and refeeding is also a critical component of the treatment. Management often requires long-term nutritional counseling of the patient.

Nutritional Inadequacy

The initial kilocalorie recommendations in anorexia nervosa may be low, which results in all the nutrients being less than the Recommended Dietary Allowance (RDA). As the kilocalorie level is increased with the treatment, the diet meets the RDA for all nutrients.

The dietary recommendations in bulimia are designed to meet the RDA for all nutrients.

Indication and Rationale

Anorexia Nervosa. Anorexia nervosa occurs chiefly in adolescent girls shortly after menarche.[1,2] The problem may begin just before puberty or later in adolescence and is less common after the age of 20. Anorexia nervosa occurs ten times more frequently in girls than in boys. The disorder is characterized by self-imposed dieting, refusal to eat, hyperactivity, and extreme loss of weight. Psychological characteristics include misperception of the body image with the patient seeing herself as being fatter than she is, the fear of becoming fat, and the denial of fatigue.[3] The physiologic accompaniments consist of the somatic changes associated with starvation, notably a lowered basal metabolic rate and a reduced gonadotropin production that results in the cessation of menses in girls.[2,4]

A primary form of anorexia nervosa in which relentless pursuit of thinness is the driving motivation has been differentiated from atypical forms in which patients are concerned about weight loss, but may use it as a means of controlling others.[3] Often dieting begins as a reaction to obesity. Sometimes atypical forms are associated with the major psychiatric illnesses of depression and of schizophrenia. These forms occur chiefly in the postadolescent age group.

Treatment of the patient may involve care by a pediatrician, an internist, a psychiatrist, or a general physician and collaboration with a dietitian. Communication among the practitioners and a coordinated approach to treatment are essential. The family may also benefit from therapy and/or from support groups. In the hospital setting, teamwork is especially important to assure consistency in treatment.[5,6]

Requirements for medical treatment vary greatly and depend on the age of the patient, the duration and the severity of starvation, and the degree of dehydration or of other complications. The diet history, the presence of bulimia and of vomiting, and the abuse of medications (which includes laxatives and diuretics) influence the approach to treatment. Restoring the normal physiologic function by the correction of changes that are associated with starvation is the initial aim of the treatment. Too rapid a reversal of the hypometabolic state by rapid refeeding may cause excessive peripheral edema. Some edema is to be expected during the refeeding and should not be cause for alarm. Nearly all patients should be able to resume an oral intake of small amounts of regular food. This approach is much preferable to liquid food substitutes given orally or to tube feeding, because the aim is for the patient to resume normal eating habits.

Patients often react to the changes associated with refeeding by the fear that they are becoming fat. An explanation of the physiologic changes that are associated with starvation[2,7] and a careful explanation of the treatment are essential before treatment is begun. The long-term goal, beyond restoring normal eating patterns, is for the patient to become an effective, independently functioning individual.

The treatment of patients with anorexia nervosa, particularly the primary form, can be exceedingly difficult and time consuming. Hospitalization, which includes long-term intensive psychotherapy that is coordinated with nutritional rehabilitation, is often necessary.[5] Some patients require only a brief hospitalization and others can be managed entirely as outpatients. The treatment principles are no different for hospitalized patients than for those who are outpatients. Hospitalization is required when medical complications warrant it or when eating behaviors are severely out of control. Principles involve the restoration of a satisfactory nutritional state, preferably through the patient's own efforts, and the restoration of an adequate weight and of normal eating patterns.

During the initial phase of hospitalization, the intravenous restoration of fluids and of electrolytes may be required. In our institution a program of oral intake that is supported by peripheral parenteral nutrition is preferred if the nutritional status is precarious. Central parenteral nutrition and tube feedings are avoided.

The treatment goals are set with the patient, and there should be flexibility in implementing the program. The setting of a series of goal weights that are acceptable to the patient is often useful. These weights may be based on the patient's history and, for adolescents, on the standard growth charts. At first, dependence on the therapist and on the program is fostered; in time there is a gradual movement toward greater responsibility and autonomy for the patient.

Clinical judgment dictates whether dietary instruction should be avoided entirely. Some patients, especially children, respond best when the external pressure to eat is removed and the normal drive to eat is allowed to reassert itself. In other instances, specific advice about meal plans and food choices is helpful in initially structuring the dietary guidelines and in resolving decisions about eating. Care must be taken not to reinforce the compulsive rituals and the preoccupation with food that exists in many patients. Principles, rather than rigid plans, should be conveyed.[8]

Bulimia. Bulimia (ravenous appetite) is the term commonly applied to the syndrome that involves binge-eating, vomiting, and purging.[9] Patients who present with bulimia may be overweight, normal in weight, or underweight. The patients manifest a wide range of psychopathologic features. Anorexia nervosa and bulimia can coexist; bulimia may be a sequel of anorexia nervosa.

The treatment for bulimia is not as well established as the treatment for anorexia nervosa. Many approaches have been advocated and include individual and group psychotherapy and psychopharmacologic treatment. No treatment has yet proven reliably effective. This is not surprising because of the diversity among bulimic patients. Several principles are basic to the treatment of bulimic patients, although the implementation of these may not necessarily stop the binge-eating and purging behaviors. The principles include an education about the physiologic changes due to fasting and refeeding and about the nutritional and the health consequences of bulimic behavior. For some patients, bulimia begins after a period of dieting to lose weight. After the onset of bulimia, binge-eating may be more frequent after meal skipping or undereating at preceding meals. Periods of deprivation should be avoided. Guidelines about kilocalorie needs and food choices are often helpful. The undesirable behaviors often are minimized by regulating eating habits and by structuring daily routines. When the binge-purge pattern is severely out of control and the complications, such as hypokalemia from vomiting and laxative abuse, have ensued, hospitalization is needed. Metabolic derangements are corrected in the hospital. Psychiatric hospitalization can provide a structured environment to interrupt and prevent the harmful eating and purging behaviors.

Goals of Dietary Management

The goal of dietary treatment in anorexia nervosa is to aid the patient in reestablishing a normal eating pattern.[8] While this is also the ultimate goal in bulimia, the initial goal is for the patient to gain control of the binge-eating episodes. The diet helps in achieving the goals initially by resolving decisions about eating and later by providing guidelines for appropriate food choices.

The dietary recommendations and the techniques for their implementation were developed for outpatient treatment; however, the same principles apply to hospitalized individuals.

Experience has suggested that there is a variety of eating patterns among patients with anorexia nervosa or bulimia. This variability in the diet patterns makes it essential to tailor the diet to each patient's specific needs.[10]

Several specific areas need to be included in the formulation of a dietary treatment plan that reflects the needs of each patient with anorexia nervosa or bulimia. The first is a detailed diet history, which helps to identify the particular areas that will require the greatest amount of attention during the treatment. It also provides an opportunity for the dietitian to become acquainted with the patient and to begin developing the rapport that is necessary for working together successfully. The history taking is followed by determining the kilocalorie content of the initial diet, by designing a diet plan, by increasing the kilocalorie content of the diet, by identifying the weight gain expectations, and by formulating the maintenance diet plan.

Dietary Recommendations: Anorexia Nervosa

Diet History. The initial diet history forms the basis for the dietary management of the patient with anorexia nervosa from the design of the initial dietary guidelines to those of the weight maintenance diet. It should identify, as accurately as possible, the patient's eating pattern before the reduction of the food intake and the evolution of the present practices. The current kilocalorie and protein intake should be estimated along with the current eating pattern, which includes meal and snack frequency and content. Family eating patterns, which include where and with whom the patient eats, should be determined. Food likes, dislikes, preferences, and aversions need to be identified; true food dislikes must be differentiated from aversions that have resulted from recent dietary manipulations. The kind, the frequency, and the duration of physical activity also needs identification.

Kilocalorie Content of Initial Diet. When a patient's food supply has been insufficient to meet the energy needs for some time, the body adjusts to a lower level of metabolism in order to conserve energy. As a result, the basal or resting energy requirement is reduced. In severely malnourished patients, the basal metabolic rate may be more than 40 percent below that predicted using the Mayo Clinic Nomogram or the Harris-Benedict equation.

Generally, basal energy requirement can be estimated by using the Nomogram (see *Appendix 6*). However, because of the lowered basal metabolic rate that results from starvation, the calculated basal kilocalorie requirement overestimates the actual basal kilocalorie needs. Therefore, a diet planned at the calculated basal level usually results in a stopping or at least a slowing weight loss.

In severely malnourished patients, it may be helpful to determine the actual kilocalorie expenditure by measuring oxygen consumption. Such measurements can be used to guide the planning of the initial diet. Occasionally, a series of oxygen consumption measurements can be made and the increasing metabolic rates can be regarded as an indicator of improvement in the physiologic function. However, this degree of precision is not essential in formulating an initial kilocalorie prescription or a follow-up.

To determine the kilocalorie content of the initial diet, the calculated basal kilocalorie requirement is compared with the kilocalorie estimate of the current diet that is obtained in the initial diet history. If the basal kilocalories are 250 to 300 Kcal more than the current kilocalorie intake, the patient probably will not accept more than the estimate of the basal kilocalories. If the discrepancy is less, an addition of 250 to 300 Kcal to the basal kilocalories may be appropriate. If an estimate of the current kilocalorie intake cannot be made, an initial prescription that is equal to the basal kilocalorie requirement is appropriate. If the kilocalorie content of the initial diet is set too high, the patient may feel overwhelmed rather than challenged; the consideration of motivation and of readiness to accept diet instructions is essential. Usually, the initial goal is to stop the weight loss while beginning to establish regularity in the eating pattern.

Often the patient is reluctant to start following the diet because he or she fears that eating and weight gain will become uncontrollable and excessive. Providing an explanation of the energy relationship to the individual's own kilocalorie needs, as well as the reassurance that the diet will be monitored, may help to give the individual the confidence to try what is suggested.

Diet Plan Design. The priority in designing the diet plan is that the diet be of an appropriate nutrient composition as well as an appropriate kilocalorie content. The dietitian should discuss with the patient the body's need to have nutrients for growth, for development, and for maintenance and how these needs can be met by food. The initial and progressive diets are designed to include foods from each of the basic food groups, with portions being increased as kilocalorie increases are made. Supplementary vitamins are rarely necessary since vitamin deficiencies are infrequent among patients with anorexia nervosa and since the prescribed maintenance diet contains sufficient vitamins. In most cases, the need for eating a varied diet must be emphasized frequently. The diet plan should respect and reflect the patient's likes and dislikes.

Initially, weighing meats and measuring the other foods in the diet is recommended to ensure that adequate portions are being taken. If the portion sizes are determined in relation to the patient's present desire for food, adequate intake usually will not be achieved. In the initial stages of treatment, the definition of portions also gives the patient greater confidence that overeating will not occur than if the portion sizes were estimated. As eating becomes more comfortable for the individual, estimating the food portions is encouraged.

The meal plan, which depends on the patient's preferences, should include three meals with or without snacks. Abdominal distention, which is attributable to the presence of increased bulk in the gastrointestinal tract, and slowed gastric emptying often result in the feelings of fullness. The patient recognizes that more has been eaten than in the past. This contributes to the initial discomfort that is felt after eating the prescribed diet. The reasons for this discomfort should be discussed with the patient so that it is understood that such initial discomfort is normal and that the capacity for food will increase and less discomfort will be experienced with time as the diet is consistently eaten. In contrast to low kilocalorie weight reduction diets, the bulk content of meals should not be excessive in the initial stages because of the easy filling and discomfort that is experienced.

The dietary plan is presented as a minimum guideline, and it is emphasized that the patient may eat more of any of the foods, or eat foods that are not on the diet as long as the prescribed diet is eaten. Yet most patients are not comfortable in modifying the prescribed diet until they have gained confidence in using it and feel assured that they are not gaining too rapidly.

It is helpful to provide the specific written dietary guidelines based on the food exchange lists. Also it is useful to expand the food exchange lists to include desserts and sweets and a favorite foods list that includes special recipes, fast foods, and convenience foods, with an indication of the food exchange value of these foods. Written instructions should contain a daily meal plan and a sample menu, which can be completed by the patient and the dietitian at the initial consultation. This approach allows the diet to be viewed by the patient as the guideline for normal nutritional needs.

Keeping a food record is useful for most patients. The dietitian should rely on the food records for general trends and patterns, rather than for specific information, although some patients keep very detailed records. Record keeping can be discontinued as soon as eating becomes comfortable and spontaneous. In the hospital, the food intake should be monitored through kilocalorie counts or through close observation of the food intake within the context of a well supervised environment.

While constipation is a frequent concern, it is usually not a problem once the quantity of food that is eaten increases and a more regular pattern of eating is established. Diarrhea may, in fact, occur during the initial stages as the kilocalorie intake increases.

Diet Progression. The progression of the kilocalorie content of the diet is highly individual. The increases should present a challenge while being realistic. In general, increments of 200 Kcal per week can be made during the early stages of treatment with greater increases as eating becomes more comfortable. The increase in the number of kilocalories should be made slowly. This allows time for the psychological changes, which are needed for the acceptance of the weight gain. With some patients, the kilocalorie content of the diet may not be changed for several weeks if efforts need to be directed toward difficult changes in other areas such as eating patterns or expanding the variety of foods eaten.

Weight Gain Expectations. In general, as long as progress continues to be made (initially by stopping the weight loss followed by consistent increases in the weight), dietary treatment is considered to be satisfactory. Usually, one cannot expect the patient to gain a specific number of pounds each week. The patient must be reassured that the weight gain, which results from the rehydration of refeeding, does not represent a rapid accumulation of body fat and will resolve spontaneously if the prescribed diet is continued. A long-term goal weight should be set considering the previous weight history or growth pattern and the weight the patient will accept. The goal weight can be renegotiated as the treatment progresses.

Diet Plan for Weight Maintenance. Dietary guidelines should be designed for weight maintenance when the patient reaches her goal weight. The goal weight is determined individually based on the knowledge of the previous growth history. It is the weight at which normal physiologic functions are presumed to occur. Menstruation often returns at this weight. However, there can be a delay of months or years after the goal weight is attained before this function is resumed. Sometimes a lower weight is selected as an initial goal with re-evaluation when the initial goal is reached.

Food records during this phase are again useful because they offer reassurance to the patient that the food intake is appropriate. Also, such records, along with the patient's weight response, enable the dietitian to evaluate the appropriateness of the kilocalorie level of the maintenance diet. Because of variations in activity, this level for weight maintenance may require adjustment.

Dietary Recommendations: Bulimia

The principles of dietary treatment used for patients with anorexia nervosa can be adapted for patients with bulimia. The specific areas that need consideration in the bulimia treatment program are similar to those in the anorexia nervosa program with the following additional considerations.

Diet History. During the initial diet history, the factors that trigger the eating binges should be identified, as well as when and how frequently the binges occur. Also, the occurrence of fasting should be noted along with the frequency and duration. It is useful to determine what foods usually are eaten during an eating binge and what a patient identifies as an eating binge.

Information in these areas is helpful in acquainting the dietitian with the patient and in defining the areas that will need the greatest attention during the coming weeks of nutrition education.

Kilocalorie Content of Initial Diet. The kilocalorie content of the initial diet should be set at a level that the patient can accept and that results in weight stabilization. It is important not to set the kilocalorie level of the initial diet too high so that the patient is fearful that weight gain will result and may be tempted to purge or fast. Likewise, the kilocalorie level should not be so low as to impose too great a restriction on the food intake, which results in further binge-eating. It should be a compromise that the patient can accept and that results in weight stabilization. Emphasis during the initial stages usually is not to change weight, but to establish more acceptable eating patterns.

The kilocalorie level of the initial diet can be set by determining the basal kilocalories by means of the Harris-Benedict equation or the Mayo Clinic Nomogram for present weight (see *Appendix 6*). A diet planned at this level usually results in a weight stabilization or a slow weight loss. If the patient is very active, a kilocalorie allowance for activity should be added. The addition of kilocalories for activity equal to 10 to 15 percent of the basal kilocalories is generally sufficient. Usually this kilocalorie level is also acceptable to the patient.

Diet Plan Design. In designing the diet, the priorities are similar to those in anorexia nervosa. The regularity of eating three meals each day is important. Uncontrolled eating binges are often minimized by maintaining a regular diet pattern and eating adequately at meals. Also, the use of snacks needs to be carefully considered. Some patients feel that snacks trigger a binge; others feel that they need snacks to help prevent the overwhelming hunger that may occur between meals and that results in triggering a binge. Fasting, skipping meals, and eating inadequate amounts at meals may contribute to the occurrence of binges.

Food records are helpful, but they need to include a notation of the times of the binges, the kinds of foods eaten, and the relapses of vomiting.

Weight Gain or Loss. Generally the kilocalorie level of the diet does not change during the treatment. When the patient has regulated the dietary intake and begins to feel more confident with the ability to control eating behaviors while keeping weight relatively stable, the kilocalorie level of the diet can be re-evaluated. If body weight is inappropriate, a realistic goal may be set. A daily kilocalorie level of less than 1,200 Kcal or one that results in greater than a one pound loss per week is perhaps too restrictive and may reinitiate binge-eating, fasting, and purging.

Diet Plan for Weight Maintenance. A weight maintenance diet should be designed at a suitable time. The kilocalorie level of this diet can be determined by the basal kilocalories for the height, age, sex, and goal weight with the addition of an appropriate increment for the activity. A goal weight, which is physiologically appropriate, should be set. The previous growth history is a useful guide. Setting a goal weight that is too low may result in a less than comfortable intake of kilocalories for weight maintenance, which may again initiate a binging, purging, and/or fasting cycle.

Follow-up support and nutrition counseling needs to carry through into this phase also.

Physicians: How to Order Diet

The diet order should indicate diet for *anorexia nervosa* or *bulimia*. The dietitian determines the content and the kilocalorie level according to the previously outlined principles.

REFERENCES

1. Lucas AR, Duncan JW, Piens V. The treatment of anorexia nervosa. Am J Psychiatry 1976;133:1034–1038.
2. Lucas AR, Callaway CW. Anorexia nervosa and bulimia. In: Berk JE, ed. Bockus Gastroenterology. 4th ed. Philadelphia: WB Saunders, 1985:4416.
3. Bruch H. Eating disorders: obesity and anorexia nervosa. New York: Basic Books, 1973.
4. Berkman JM. Anorexia nervosa: the diagnosis and treatment of inanition resulting from functional disorders. Ann Intern Med 1945;22:679–691.

5. Andersen AE. Practical comprehensive treatment of anorexia nervosa and bulimia. Baltimore: Johns Hopkins Press, 1985.
6. Lucas AR, Huse DM. Behavioral disorders affecting food intake: anorexia nervosa and bulimia. In: Shils ME, Young VR, eds. Modern nutrition in health and disease. 7th ed. Philadelphia: Lea and Febiger (in press, 1987).
7. Keys A, Brovek J, Henschel A, Mickelsen O, Taylor HL. The biology of human starvation. Vol. 1 and 2. Minneapolis: University of Minnesota Press, 1950.
8. Huse DM, Lucas AR. Dietary treatment of anorexia nervosa. J Am Diet Assoc 1983;83:687–690.
9. Kirkley BG. Bulimia: clinical characteristics, development and etiology. J Am Diet Assoc 1986;86:468–475.
10. Huse DM, Lucas AR. Dietary patterns in anorexia nervosa. Am J Clin Nutr 1984;40:251–254.

GASTROINTESTINAL DISEASES AND DISORDERS

ABDOMINAL GAS AND FLATULENCE

General Description

Dietary management focuses on the avoidance of foods that are likely to increase abdominal gas and flatulence or those foods the individual finds through trial to increase abdominal gas and flatulence. Behaviors that increase the swallowing of air may also be identified and avoided.

Nutritional Inadequacy

The diet is not inherently inadequate in nutrients when compared to the Recommended Dietary Allowance (RDA). However, individual intake should be assessed and supplemented accordingly.

Indications and Rationale

Five gases (nitrogen, oxygen, hydrogen, carbon monoxide, and methane) make up 99 percent of bowel gas.[1-4] These gases may be derived from two sources, which include swallowed air and gas that is produced within the intestinal tract. Increased intestinal motility may also contribute to symptoms by decreasing the time available for the absorption of gases in the intestinal tract.

Nitrogen and oxygen are present in the atmosphere and usually enter the gastrointestinal tract in swallowed air. Ingestion of air is usually responsible for gas in the esophagus and stomach. It is not clear what fraction of swallowed air, if any, passes into the small bowel. Most swallowed air is regurgitated and usually does not enter the small bowel. However, a horizontal position may interfere with the normal eructation of stomach gas and increase the likelihood of gas passing into the duodenum.[3]

Hydrogen, carbon dioxide, and methane are produced in the intestine and comprise the bulk of flatus. Hydrogen is formed in the colon by the action of colonic bacteria on fermentable substrate. Carbon dioxide may be produced in the upper intestinal tract when fatty acids, which are released during the digestion of dietary fats, and gastric hydrochloric acid are neutralized by bicarbonate.

Like hydrogen, carbon dioxide is also produced in the colon by the action of bacteria on fermentable intestinal contents. Methane is produced in the colon by bacteria, but its production is not related to the ingestion of particular foods. The tendency to produce methane appears to be a familial trait.

Normally, gas is reabsorbed through the colonic wall as it passes through the intestine. If colonic motility is disturbed for any reason, bloating and distention may result in abdominal pain.

Complaints of gas usually take one of three forms: (1) excessive belching, (2) abdominal pain or bloating, and (3) excessive passage of flatus.

Excessive Belching. Swallowed air (aerophagia) usually is responsible for belching. Persons with chronic repetitive belching often precede each belch with a swallowing or an aspirating maneuver that causes air to enter the esophagus. Aerophagia is usually the result of a habit. In some persons, eructation primarily occurs during or immediately after meals.[5] For these persons, habits that are associated with eating and drinking and that result in frequent repetitive swallowing increase the amount of air that is swallowed (Table 6–28). Anxiety may also increase aerophagia. Foods that include air as part of their natural structure or that have air added in their preparation may also contribute to swallowed air.

Abdominal Discomfort and Bloating. Abdominal discomfort and bloating, often described by the patient as "too much gas," are frequently encountered gastrointestinal complaints. Many patients with these complaints have no signs of excessive gas production, but they appear to have an abnormality of intestinal motility that results in the disruption of the passage of gas through the bowel.[2-4] In addition, these patients may sense discomfort with intestinal gas volumes that are well-tolerated by most people. Thus, symptoms that are produced by disordered motility and by a heightened pain response to gut distension seem to be misinterpreted as a feeling of increased gas, when in actuality the total intestinal gas volume may be normal.

Excessive Flatus. Most patients who pass excessive flatus excrete gases that are formed in the colon.[3,4] Swallowed air does not contribute appreciably to rectal gas. Also, the carbon dioxide formed in the duodenum is absorbed as it passes through the small bowel and does not contribute to flatus excretion. The excessive production of colonic gas may result from malabsorptive disorders or the ingestion of foods that contain nonabsorbable carbohydrates. In patients with malabsorptive disorders, food constituents such as lactose, which are normally digested and absorbed in the small bowel, are delivered to the colon where they undergo fermentation by the colonic bacteria.

Normal subjects without malabsorptive disorders may also produce large quantities of gas. Certain carbohydrates that cannot be completely digested by enzymes in the small intestine pass unabsorbed into the colon where bacteria readily ferments them into hydrogen. Such nonabsorbable carbohydrates are found in whole wheat products and a variety of fruits, vegetables, and grains. It has also been shown that the artificial sweetener sorbitol may result in intestinal gas production.[6]

Goals of Dietary Management

The goal of dietary management is to reduce symptoms to a level that the individual finds tolerable.

Dietary Recommendations

The general approach to otherwise healthy persons who complain of gas is to assure them that increased gas, per se, is not harmful. Patients should be educated to restrict foods and behaviors that may contribute to gas formation. More specific treatment depends on the source of gas (see Table 6–28).

TABLE 6–28 Factors that Contribute to Abdominal Gas and Flatulence

Foods that may contribute to gas production (avoid on a trial basis)	Dried beans, dried peas, baked beans, soybeans, lima beans, lentils, cabbage, radishes, onions, broccoli, Brussels sprouts, cauliflower, cucumbers, sauerkraut, kohlrabi, rutabaga Prunes, apples, raisins, bananas Whole wheat products, such as whole wheat bread, bran cereals, bran muffins High lactose foods: milk, ice cream, ice milk, and cream (see page 165 for additional information on lactose) The artificial sweeteners sorbitol and mannitol, which are found in some "dietetic" candies and sugar-free gums High fat foods, such as fried foods, fatty meats, rich cream sauces, gravies, pastries
Sources of swallowed air	Frequent, repetitive swallowing that may be caused by ill-fitting dentures, chewing gum or tobacco, sucking on hard candy, or sipping beverages Eating rapidly and "gulping" food and beverages "Drawing" on straws, narrow-mouthed bottles, cigars, cigarettes, and pipes Foods that contain air such as carbonated beverages and whipped cream
Habits that may cause retention of gas	Reclining after eating Lack of regular exercise Stress

Excessive Belching. The treatment of chronic repetitive belching should consist of an explanation of the cause and the benign nature of the symptoms.[2–5] Belching can usually be managed by avoiding foods and behaviors that contribute to air swallowing.[2]

Abdominal Discomfort and Bloating. The treatment of abdominal pain and of bloating should include a discussion of the role of emotions in the disturbance of the gut motility.[2–4] Since bowel distension from even normal volumes of gas may cause pain in persons with functional abdominal pain, it is often helpful to attempt to reduce the quantity of accumulating gas. Patients should be advised to avoid foods and behaviors that may contribute to swallowed air, because a fraction of the aspirated air may enter the stomach, and to maintain habits that minimize the retention of gas. Restricting foods that contribute to gas production may greatly relieve the patient's symptoms.

Excessive Flatus. If malabsorption has been ruled out, most patients who complain of excess flatus usually benefit by restricting or eliminating gas-producing foods.[3,4] Patients should be advised to omit foods one at a time on a trial basis until they reach a level of gas excretion that is tolerable. They should also be advised against the unnecessary omission of foods, which may result in nutritional deficiencies. If milk products or wheat products are omitted, foods with similar nutrient content should be substituted. Persons who are trying to increase their fiber intake can minimize gas production by increasing the fiber intake gradually over a period of several weeks.[7]

The effect of exercise on flatulence has not been systematically studied. However, regular exercise is often found to be helpful and should be encouraged as it may relieve abdominal distention and intestinal gas.

Physicians: How to Order Diet

The diet order should indicate *diet to relieve abdominal gas.*

REFERENCES

1. Krause MV, Mahan LK. Nutritional care in intestinal diseases. In: Krause MV, Mahan LK, eds. Food, nutrition and diet therapy. 7th ed. Philadelphia: WB Saunders, 1984:439.
2. Levitt MD. Role of gas in functional abdominal pain. South Med J 1984;77:962–963.
3. Levitt MD, Bond JH. Intestinal gas. In: Sleisenger MH, Fordtran JS, eds. Gastrointestinal disease: pathophysiology, diagnosis, management. 3rd ed. Philadelphia: WB Saunders, 1983:222.
4. Levitt MD, Bond JH. Flatulence. Ann Rev Med 1980;31:127–137.
5. Roth JLA. The symptom patterns of gaseousness. Ann NY Acad Sci 1968;150:108–124.
6. Hyams JS. Sorbitol intolerance: an unappreciated cause of functional gastrointestinal complaints. Gastroenterol 1983;84:30–33.
7. Marthinsen D, Fleming SE. Excretion of breath and flatus gases by humans consuming high fiber diets. J Nutr 1982;112:1133–1143.

ESOPHAGEAL REFLUX

General Description

Basic guidelines are given to reduce and/or to prevent esophageal reflux symptoms. The use of specific dietary regimens depends on individual patient tolerances to all aspects of medical management.

Nutritional Inadequacy

Dietary modifications for esophageal reflux do not result in a diet that is inherently inadequate in nutritional value when compared to the Recommended Dietary Allowance (RDA).

Indications and Rationale

Esophageal reflux refers to the regurgitation of gastric contents into the esophagus. The most common symptom is heartburn (substernal pain or discomfort). Usually, esophageal reflux is a mild condition that can be managed medically. However, chronic reflux may lead to esophagitis and subsequently to ulceration, to hemorrhage, and to stricture, which may even necessitate surgical treatment.

The esophagus ordinarily is protected from reflux of gastric contents by the contraction of the lower esophageal sphincter. It is generally believed that the lower esophageal sphincter is incompetent in persons with chronic esophageal reflux. The mean sphincter pressure tends to be lower in these persons, so that the likelihood of reflux is increased.[1-4]

Changes in the lower esophageal sphincter pressure normally occur in response to hormonal, to mechanical, to drug, and to dietary factors. Some of the factors that reduce this pressure and therefore increase the chances of reflux are cigarette smoking, alcohol, a high-fat meal, chocolate, and carminatives (peppermint and spearmint oils, garlic, onions, cinnamon, etc.)[2-4] Persons with esophageal reflux tend to experience discomfort with the ingestion of citrus and tomato juices. These foods have not been found to consistently decrease the lower esophageal sphincter pressure, but have a direct irritating effect on inflamed esophageal mucosa.[2] Some persons associate reflux symptoms with spicy foods. Spices are not believed to affect the esophageal mucosa or the lower esophageal sphincter pressure, but are often eaten with high fat or tomato-based foods.

Coffee, decaffeinated coffee, and caffeine have been implicated in esophageal reflux owing to changes in the lower esophageal sphincter pressure and in the increased gastric acid secretion. However, recent studies have shown that coffee produces symptoms primarily through irritation of already damaged esophageal mucosa rather than through actual changes in the lower esophageal sphincter pressure or the acid secretion.[1,5]

Other factors that predispose to reflux are hiatal hernia, obesity, recumbent body position, and increased intra-abdominal pressure.[1-3,5] Nocturnal reflux may be reduced by elevating the head of the bed and by avoiding late evening snacks. Obesity and garments that constrict may increase intra-abdominal pressure. The regression of symptoms is likely to accompany a weight loss. Large meals should be avoided, since they may increase the gastric pressure on the lower esophageal sphincter.

Table 6–29 summarizes the management of esophageal reflux. The management may include the use of several medications to treat or to correct reflux.[1,3,5,7,8]

TABLE 6–29 Pharmaceutical Management of Esophageal Reflux

Category	Action	Example
Antacids	Neutralize gastric acid and increase lower esophageal sphincter pressure	Maalox
Cholinergic agents	Increase lower esophageal sphincter pressure and improve esophageal acid clearance	Bethanechol (Urecholine)
Dopamine antagonists	Increase lower esophageal sphincter pressure and improve abnormal gastric emptying	Metoclopramide (Reglan)
Histamine H_2 receptor blockers	Decrease gastric acid production	Cimetidine (Tagamet)
Alginate antacids	Produce viscous solutions, which act as a mechanical barrier on surface of the gastric pool	Gaviscon

Goals of Dietary Management

Dietary management is aimed at minimizing symptoms associated with reflux, such as heartburn, and reducing the risk of esophagitis and its sequela.

Dietary Recommendations

Dietary recommendations can be summarized as follows:[1-8]
1. Achieve and maintain a desirable body weight.

2. Avoid very large meals; the use of midmorning and midafternoon snacks permits a reduction in the size of the usual meals.

3. Avoid eating meals or snacks for at least 2 hours before lying down.

4. Avoid or limit the intake of foods and of beverages that decrease the lower esophageal sphincter pressure, such as alcohol, chocolate, high fat foods (limit fried foods, high fat meats, cream sauces, gravies, margarine, butter, cream, oil, salad dressings), and carminatives (e.g., oils of peppermint and spearmint, garlic, onion).

5. Limit the intake of foods and of beverages that can be irritating to damaged esophageal mucosa to a level that is tolerated by the individual. These foods and beverages include citrus fruit and juices, tomato products, pepper, herbs, spices, coffee (regular and decaffeinated), and all carbonated beverages.

6. Encourage the intake of foods that do not affect the lower esophageal sphincter pressure, such as protein foods with a low fat content (e.g., lean meats, skim or 1% milk, cheeses and yogurt made from skim milk) and carbohydrate foods with a low fat content (e.g., fruits, breads, crackers, cereals, potatoes, rice, noodles, and vegetables prepared without added fat).

Other Recommendations

Other important anti-reflux recommendations include the elevation of the head of the bed, the avoidance of constricting garments, and the avoidance of smoking.

Physicians: How to Order Diet

The diet order should indicate *anti-esophageal reflux diet or diet for hiatal hernia*. The dietitian modifies the diet according to the previously identified guidelines and the tolerances of the patient.

REFERENCES

1. Richter JE, Castell DO. Drugs, foods and other substances in the cause and treatment of reflux esophagitis. Med Clin North Am 1981;65:1223–1234.
2. Whelan G. Management of gastro-esophageal reflux. Aust NZ J Med 1982;12:90–96.
3. Richter JE, Castell DO. Gastroesophageal reflux: pathogenesis, diagnosis, and therapy. Ann Intern Med 1982;97:93–103.
4. Chernow B, Castell DO. Diet and heartburn. JAMA 1979;241:2307–2308.
5. Narab F, Texter EC. Gastroesophageal reflux: pathophysiologic concepts. Arch Intern Med 1985;145:329–333.
6. Cohen S. Pathogenesis of coffee-induced gastrointestinal symptoms. N Engl J Med 1980;303:122–123.
7. Jamieson GG, Beauchamp G, Duranceau AC. The physiological basis for the medical management of gastroesophageal reflux. Surg Clin North Am 1983;63:841–850.
8. Castell DO. Medical therapy for reflux esophagitis: 1986 and beyond. Editorial. Ann Intern Med 1986;104:112–114.

FAT MALABSORPTION

General Description

The restricted fat diet consists of a lowering of the individual's usual intake of visible fat and the fat that is found within food. The level of fat restriction may be either relative to current intake and to tolerance, or absolute and according to the physician's order.

Supplementation with medium chain triglyceride fat may be indicated in some situations. The rationale for the use of medium chain triglycerides and guidelines for incorporating them into the diet are given.

Nutritional Inadequacy

This diet is adequate in all nutrients if a proper amount and variety of food are consumed by the patient. The fat content of meat is sufficient to provide the required amount of linoleic acid.

Indications and Rationale

Several disorders can interfere with the normal processes for the utilization of dietary fat. Dietary fats are composed primarily of long chain triglycerides, which have a carbon chain length that is greater than 14 carbon atoms. The restriction of fat is likely to be indicated in the treatment of maldigestion, malabsorption, and disorders that involve the transport and the utilization of fat.

Maldigestion. Maldigestion occurs when there is a defect in the intraluminal breakdown of fat. Causes of maldigestion include disorders that affect gastric, pancreatic, and biliary function.

Pancreatic lipase is responsible for the hydrolysis of most dietary fat. Lipase insufficiency can occur in pancreatitis, cystic fibrosis, pancreatic cancer, and after a resection of the pancreas. It should be noted that pancreatic reserves are large. As much as 80 percent of pancreatic function can be lost without interfering with fat breakdown and subsequent malabsorption.[1]

Bile acids are responsible for the emulsification of fatty acids into micelles for absorption. Hepatobiliary disease may result in an insufficient production of bile acids or an obstruction to bile flow. Ileal disease or resection decreases the area that is available for the active absorption of bile acids and decreases the bile salt pool. Also, bacterial overgrowth in the small intestine can result in deconjugation of bile salts. Diminished bile acids lessen the emulsification of fatty acids into micelles with a subsequent decrease in the absorption of fat.[1]

Malabsorption. Malabsorption occurs with conditions that alter the structure and the function of the small bowel mucosa. Celiac sprue or Crohn's disease are examples. The restriction of gluten in sprue and the use of steroids in Crohn's disease may be sufficient to correct the malabsorption.

Patients with short bowel syndrome (SBS) have malabsorption that is related to a decrease in the mucosal surface and a decrease in the transit time. Recommendations for nutritional therapy depend on the location and the extent of the resection and the condition of the remaining bowel. The degree of fat restriction for patients with SBS is currently uncertain. In some studies, fat restriction has failed to benefit patients with less than 150 cm of jejunum that ends in a stoma,[2] whereas other studies substantiate the need for fat restriction to control stomal output and electrolyte losses.[3,4] Patients with a short bowel attached to the colon, however, may experience diarrhea because of the cathartic effect of unabsorbed fat and bile salts delivered to the colon. Such patients could benefit from a fat restriction to reduce diarrhea and to lessen the likelihood of hyperoxaluria.[5,6]

Transport. Defects in the lymphatic transport of fat, as found in intestinal lymphangiectasia, chyluria, chylous ascites, and chylothorax, result in the abnormal drainage of lymph into the intestinal lumen, the urinary tract, the peritoneal spaces, or the pleura respectively. There is a loss of chylous lymph, which contains chylomicrons that are derived from dietary fat. A restriction in long chain triglycerides aids in the management of these disorders by decreasing chylomicron formation and lymph flow. Medium chain triglycerides are rapidly absorbed by the portal route rather than through the lymph system as with long chain triglycerides and can be used to supplement the diet.[7]

Utilization

A diet that is very low in fat is recommended in the management of conditions where the utilization of fat is impaired, such as in Type I hyperlipoproteinemia and Refsum's disease. Type I hyperlipoproteinemia, or hyperchylomicronemia, is the result of a defect in the catabolism of chylomicrons by lipoprotein lipase. The clinical features include eruptive xanthomas, hepatosplenomegaly, and pancreatitis. Dietary treatment is directed at alleviating the symptoms and at minimizing the chylomicron formation by the restriction of fat to 30 g or less for adults and 15 g or less for children under age 12. See page 423, for a further description of the dietary management.

Refsum's disease results from a deficient capacity to degrade and to utilize specific fatty acids. In Refsum's disease, the genetic deficiency of α-oxidase results in the accumulation of phytanic acid in the blood and in the tissues with a subsequent peripheral neuropathy and cerebellar ataxia. Phytanic acid is a branched chain fatty acid known to be solely of dietary origin. A dietary restriction of phytanic acid has been found effective in ameliorating the progression of this disease.[8]

Medium Chain Triglycerides

Medium chain triglyceride oil (MCT oil) is derived from coconut oil through a process of fractionation and of re-esterification of the medium chain fatty acids with glycerol. MCT oil contains fatty acids primarily of eight to ten carbon atoms, whereas usual dietary fats contain fatty acids of 16 to 18 carbon atoms. At room temperature, MCT oil is a thin, clear, light yellow, odorless liquid with a bland taste.

MCT are available in two principle forms, MCT oil and formulas that contain MCT oil (see page 434). MCT oil provides 8.3 Kcal per gram. One Tbsp (15 ml) weighs 14 g and provides 116 Kcal.

MCT oil is a special purpose food for use as supportive nutritional therapy. It may be used in addition to a fat restricted diet or for nearly the total replacement of fat. The primary purposes for the use of MCT oil are to increase the caloric value and to improve the palatability of a low fat diet.

The rationale for the use of MCT is based on the differences in digestion, in absorption, in transport, and in catabolism between MCT and long chain triglycerides (LCT). Although MCT are rapidly hydrolyzed by pancreatic lipase, absorption can occur before hydrolysis. Bile salts and micelle formation are not required for the dispersion or the absorption of MCT. MCT are transported across the mucosal cell more rapidly than LCT. MCT do not enter the lymph system, but are transported through the portal venous system as albumin bound free fatty acids. They are not incorporated into chylomicrons and, therefore, do not require lipoprotein lipase for oxidation. MCT may be used as a dietary supplement in most disorders in which a fat restricted diet is indicated.

In addition, the metabolism of MCT under circumstances of carbohydrate restriction produces ketone bodies. These products of fat metabolism have an anticonvulsant effect. Although many drugs that have anticonvulsant actions are now available, a ketogenic diet that incorporates MCT remains a part of the treatment for seizure disorders.[9] See also page 423 for a description of ketogenic diets.

MCT is contraindicated in individuals who are prone to ketosis and to acidosis (such as insulin-dependent diabetic patients) and in patients with cirrhosis with or without portacaval shunt. In the former, the ketogenic properties of MCT aggravate any tendency toward metabolic acidosis. In cirrhosis, with or without portacaval shunt, the blood levels of MCT increase owing to the reduced hepatic clearance. Increased levels result in a syndrome that resembles hepatic encephalopathy. This syndrome includes hyperventilation, hyperammonemia, hyperlactacidemia, and disturbed electroencephalogram findings.

The amount of MCT oil that is used should be small at first and then gradually increased to the desired level. Unpleasant side effects, such as nausea, vomiting, abdominal pain, abdominal distention, and diarrhea, may occur with the rapid introduction of MCT into the diet or the intake of excessively high levels of MCT. Some of the side effects may be related to the hyperosmolar solution that is produced by rapid hydrolysis of MCT. Although the mechanisms are not clearly understood, it may be that the interaction between LCT and MCT or the additive effects cause increased malabsorption and diarrhea when MCT are added to a diet already high in LCT or when excessively large amounts of MCT are incorporated into the diet.

Divided doses of no more than 15 to 20 ml (3 to 4 tsp) at any one time are usually well-tolerated. The total daily supplementation should be individualized and based on the clinical situation and the therapeutic and the nutritional need. Although divided doses of up to 100 ml of MCT may be administered in a 24-hour period, the current practice is for the medium and the long chain fatty acid content of the diet not to exceed 35 to 40 percent of the total kilocalories.

The main problem that relates to patient compliance is that of palatability. This can usually be resolved by a variety of methods:

1. Add MCT to beverages by combining 1 tsp (~5 g) of MCT for each 4 oz of skim milk, juice, or carbonated beverage. Flavoring may be added, such as sugar, vanilla, lemon, maple, coffee, or strawberry, if desired.

2. Use MCT in cooking and baking. MCT can be substituted in equal amounts for other fats. Moderately low heat (150 to 160° C or 300 to 325° F) should be used when frying foods to prevent the thermal breakdown of MCT. Recipes are available for baked goods.

3. Use MCT as a dressing or spread. MCT can be made into acceptable vegetable dressings and sandwich spreads.

4. Special recipes are available from the manufacturer. Write for "Recipes Using MCT Oil and Portagen," Mead Johnson and Company, Evansville, IN 47721.

MCT oil is a nonprescription item that is available from pharmacies. A physician's prescription along with the Federal Registry Number (87-0365-03) of MCT can help secure third party reimbursement for this rather expensive item.

Goals of Dietary Management

The goals of dietary management are the remission of clinical symptoms while providing caloric and nutritional adequacy.

Dietary Recommendations

Except for the following modifications, the fat restricted diet is based on a general, well-balanced diet.

Foods with a high fat content are reduced. The total amount of fat in the daily diet may be relative (based on symptomatic response) or absolute (according to physiologic necessity).

No differentiation is made between saturated and unsaturated fat in the diet.

Medium chain triglycerides can be incorporated into the daily diet. Supplementation should be individualized and based upon the clinical situation and the therapeutic and the nutritional need. Current practice is for the medium and the long chain fatty acid content of the diet not to exceed 35 to 40 percent of the total kilocalories.

Physicians: How to Order Diet

The diet order should indicate *low fat diet* or *low fat diet with MCT*. If the level of fat is not specified, the dietitian determines the appropriate amounts.

REFERENCES

1. Friedman HI, Nylund B. Intestinal fat digestion, absorption, and transport. Am J Clin Nutr 1980;33:1108–1139.
2. McIntyre PB, Fitchew M, Lennard-Jones JE. Patients with a high jejunostomy do not need a special diet. Gastroenterology 1986;91:25–33.
3. Greenberger NJ. The management of the patient with the short bowel syndrome. Am J Gastroenterol 1978;70:528–540.
4. Mitchell A, Watkins RM, Collin J. Surgical treatment of the short bowel syndrome. Br J Surg 1984;71:329–333.
5. Andersson H, Isaksson B, Sjogren B. Fat-reduced diet in the symptomatic treatment of small bowel disease: metabolic studies in patients with Crohn's disease and in other patients subjected to ileal resection. Gut 1974;15:351–359.
6. Cummings JH. Short chain fatty acids in the human colon. Gut 1981;22:763–779.
7. Christophe A, Matthys F, Verdonk G. Chylous-fluid triglycerides and lipoproteins in a patient with chylothorax on a diet of butter or medium-chain triglyceride. Arch Int Physiol Biochem 1980;88:B17–18.
8. Steinberg D. Phytanic acid storage disease (Refsum's Disease). In: Stauburg JB, Wyngaarden JB, Fredrickson DS, Goldstein JL, Brown MS, eds. The metabolic basis of inherited disease. 5th ed. New York: McGraw Hill, 1983:731.
9. Bach AC, Babayan VK. Medium-chain triglycerides: an update. Am J Clin Nutr 1982;36:950–962.

FIBER AND RESIDUE CONTROL

High Fiber Diet

General Description

The diet emphasizes the use of whole grain bread and of cereal products, legumes, nuts, fruits, and vegetables in order to increase the intake of dietary fiber. The calculated dietary fiber content of the high fiber diet is 25 to 50 g per day (or approximately 14 g per 1,000 Kcal). The *General Hospital Diet* (page 43), which includes a variety of foods, provides approximately 10 to 20 g of dietary fiber per day.

Nutritional Inadequacy

A high fiber diet is nutritionally adequate when compared to the Recommended Dietary Allowance (RDA) as long as a balanced selection of food items is chosen. High fiber intakes have been associated with a loss of some trace elements in the stool (calcium, iron, and zinc); however, this has not been found to be of nutritional significance.[1]

Indications and Rationale

Fiber is commonly referred to as roughage, bulk, non-nutritive residue, or unavailable carbohydrate. In the past, many food composition tables have reported fiber content as "crude" rather than "dietary." Crude fiber is defined as the residue of plant materials that is left after sequential extraction with dilute acid and dilute alkali and consists primarily of cellulose, some hemicellulose, and lignin.[2] Dietary fiber is defined in physiologic terms as all food residue that is partially or completely resistant to hydrolysis by digestive enzymes, i.e., cellulose, hemicellulose, lignins, pectins, gums, and nondegradable animal tissues (mucopolysaccharides and crustacean exoskeleton).[2-4] The term dietary fiber is preferred because it more accurately represents the total fiber content of the food item. However, the methodology for determining dietary fiber is not without its faults. New techniques are currently being developed and used, but they have not been applied to all the food items included in this text.[2,3] Therefore, the most widely accepted and the complete sources of dietary fiber content are used.[5,6] When appropriate, it is recommended that future literature be used to supplement the tables that are provided.

High fiber diets are useful in the treatment of chronic constipation.[1] Fiber increases the stool volume and decreases the intracolonic pressure and the intestinal transit time.[7] For most persons with chronic constipation and for some with diverticulosis or irritable bowel syndrome, an increased intake of fiber may lead to more regular bowel habits and to the partial relief of symptoms.[7] Although the evidence is less conclusive, an increased intake of fiber also appears to benefit some persons with diarrhea. An increased intake of fiber tends to normalize the intestinal transit time. That is, the transit time becomes slower for persons with a rapid transit time.[8] An increased intake of high fiber foods also is encouraged for those who have spinal cord injuries to aid in bowel training.

Epidemiologic evidence has also implicated a low consumption of dietary fiber in the etiology of a number of diseases, such as colon cancer and diverticulitis.[7-9] The role of dietary fiber in health and disease control is discussed in other areas of the diet manual.

The goal of a high fiber diet is to increase the consumption of dietary fiber to greater than what is usual for the individual. Generally, this is to greater than 25 g per day. The consumption of greater than 50 g of dietary fiber does not improve bowel function further.[1,9] The use of wheat and cereal bran is the preferred or the primary method of increasing dietary fiber.[4,8] An intake of other types of high fiber foods is helpful also. In most cases, food preparation techniques may change the fiber structure, but do not significantly change the fiber content.[9]

Initially, a high fiber diet may produce some unpleasant effects, such as increased flatulence and borborygmus.[7] These symptoms are likely to be less of a problem with gradual increases in intake of high fiber foods and often resolve with time as the person becomes accustomed to the diet.

Goals of Dietary Management

Nutritional therapy is generally directed towards the provision of a nutritionally adequate diet and to the normalization of bowel function.

Dietary Recommendations

The diet plan seeks to increase the intake of fiber to greater than what was usual for the individual. A high fiber intake is generally considered to consist of 25 to 50 g of dietary fiber per day. This can be accomplished by (1) including 1/4 to 1/2 cup (1/2 to 1 oz) of bran daily; (2) increasing the consumption of whole grain breads, cereals, flours, and other whole grain products; and (3) increasing the consumption of vegetables and fruits, especially those with edible skins, seeds, and hulls. Table 6–30 presents the dietary fiber content of selected foods. It can be helpful for evaluating the current dietary fiber intake as well as for planning a high fiber diet.

Patients should also be advised to increase their intake of high fiber foods gradually in order to minimize gastrointestinal discomforts. If intolerance occurs, the individual should also be advised to try various sources of fiber in order to identify which foods are best tolerated. Better tolerance and improved symptoms can be expected if foods rich in fiber are consumed at each meal, eaten at regular times, and eaten with meals that are fairly equal in size. Adequate fluid intake (eight or more cups each day) is important in establishing better utilization of increased fiber consumption. A regular exercise program is also helpful in promoting bowel regularity and health.

Physicians: How to Order Diet

The diet order should indicate *high fiber diet*.

Restricted Fiber Diet

General Description

The restricted fiber diet restricts the intake of whole grain bread and cereal products and of fiber foods such as fruits, vegetables, nuts, seeds, legumes, hulls, and fibrous skins. The degree of fiber restriction is more liberal than that achieved by the low residue diet. According to calculations made from the hospital diet, the plan provides 10 to 15 g per day (or 5.5 g per 1,000 Kcal).

Nutritional Inadequacies

The diet is not inherently inadequate in nutrients when compared to the Recommended Dietary Allowance (RDA). However, the individual's food intake should be assessed and supplemented accordingly.

TABLE 6-30 Dietary Fiber Content of Selected Foods[5,6]

	Grams Per Serving				
	0.5 or less	0.5–1.0	1.1–2.0	2.1–3.0	3.0 or greater[‡]
FRUIT[*†]	banana cherries coconut (shred) currants (dried) dates fruit juice plums (ckd) pomegranate prunes raisins watermelon rhubarb (raw)	apricots apple (raw, dried) applesauce cantaloupe cranberries (raw) grapefruit grapes kiwifruit mango nectarine orange peach pineapple plums (raw) rhubarb (ckd) tangerine	blueberries coconut (fresh) currants (raw) gooseberries papaya pear strawberries	blackberries boysenberries pears (dried)	elderberries (5) guava (5) raspberries
VEGETABLES[*†]	bamboo shoots bean sprouts cabbage celery endive mushrooms onions parsley radishes summer squash vegetable juice water chestnuts watercress	asparagus beans (string) carrots beets broccoli (raw) cauliflower cucumber eggplant greens (ckd) beet collard dandelion kale mustard	artichoke broccoli (ckd) Brussels sprouts pumpkin sauerkraut chicory (raw)		

*Based on the content of one diabetic exchange for each item listed.
†Includes all forms (raw, dried, cooked) for fruits and vegetables except where noted.
‡Actual dietary fiber content listed in parentheses.

TABLE 6–30 Dietary Fiber Content of Selected Foods[5,6]

	Grams Per Serving				
	0.5 or less	0.5–1.0	1.1–2.0	2.1–3.0	3.0 or greater[‡]
VEGETABLES (continued)		spinach swiss chard turnip green pepper kohlrabi okra rutabaga soybean sprouts spinach (raw) tomato turnips			

STARCHES*§	Cornflakes
	corn grits
	cream of wheat, rice,
	  and corn
	farina
	graham crackers
	maltomeal
	potato chips
	potatoes
	puffed cereals
	Rice Krispies
	saltines
	spaghetti
		granola
		oatmeal (ckd)
		spaghetti & macaroni
		  from whole wheat
		  flour
		white bread
		white flour
		white rice
		white roll or bun
			black-eyed peas
			brown bread
			brown rice
			Cheerios
			Grapenuts
			green peas
			popcorn
			Ralston (cooked cereal)
			sesame seed kernels
			soybeans
			split peas
			Total
			Wheat Chex
				40% Branflakes
				bulgur
				parsnips
				Raisin Bran
				Rykrisp
				Shredded Wheat
				wheat germ
					All-Bran (13)
					Bran Buds (12)
					100% Bran (9)
					bran muffin (3.5)
					dried kidney beans (5)
					dried navy beans (5)
					dried peas (5)
					lentils (3.1)
					wheat bran (4)

noodles
macaroni
Special K
sweet potatoes

Wheat flakes
Wheaties
whole wheat bread
whole wheat roll or bun
whole wheat flour (100%)
whole wheat flour (85%)
winter squash

MEAT SUBSTI-TUTES*

peanut butter
peanuts
pumpkin seeds
soybeans
sunflower seed kernels
squash seeds

FATS AND OILS*

nuts,
almonds
brazil
cashews
hazelnuts
macadamia
pecan
pistachio

avocado
walnuts

*Based on the content of one diabetic exchange for each item listed.
†Includes all forms (raw, dried, cooked) for fruits and vegetables except where noted.
‡Actual dietary fiber content listed in parentheses.
§All refer to foods in their cooked or usually consumed form.

Indications and Rationale

A restricted fiber diet may be used as a transition from a low residue diet to a general diet. This diet is often used during the resolution of exacerbations of inflammatory bowel disease (Crohn's disease or ulcerative colitis, see page 158), of radiation enteritis, or of partial bowel obstruction.

Goals of Dietary Management

The goal of this diet is to reduce the fecal volume to a level that does not distend the bowel and aggravate the disease process, while providing a more normal food intake and nutritional adequacy.

Dietary Recommendations

A restricted fiber diet contains less than 25 g of dietary fiber each day.[1,9] This level can be accomplished by the consumption of refined grain products (avoid whole grain products), of fruits and vegetables without skins, hulls, or seeds, and by avoiding nuts, seeds, and legumes. Table 6–30 presents the dietary fiber content of selected foods.

Physicians: How to Order Diet

The diet order should indicate *restricted fiber diet*. If the diet is used as a transition diet, the dietitian assists the patient with food selections in the establishment of tolerances and of nutritional adequacy.

Low Residue Diet

General Description

The diet consists of foods that are very low in dietary fiber. Foods that are omitted include those of moderate and of high fiber content as well as those foods that are believed to increase the fecal residue despite the low content of fiber. The calculated dietary fiber content of the low residue diet is less than 8 g per day (or 3.5 g per 1,000 Kcal).

Nutritional Inadequacy

The diet may be low in a number of nutrients. It is intended to be used for a short time period only. If the long-term use of a low residue diet is indicated, supplementation with either a multivitamin, a monomeric or a polymeric formula, or parenteral nutrition should be considered (see page 273).

Indications and Rationale

The diet may be used during acute exacerbations of inflammatory bowel disease (Crohn's disease, ulcerative colitis) or of diverticulitis and in partial obstruction. It is also used pre- and postoperatively for intestinal surgery. It allows the bowel to rest by minimizing the fecal volume while still allowing the patient to consume food.

The term "residue" refers to unabsorbed dietary constituents, sloughed cells from the gastrointestinal tract, and intestinal bacteria.[3,10,11] Some foods, such as milk and the connective tissue of meats, are low in dietary fiber, but may contribute to stool volume, particularly in individuals with altered gastrointestinal capabilities. The restriction of these so-called residue-producing foods is based more on tradition and is not well-documented in the literature.[11-13]

Goals of Dietary Management

The goal of the low residue diet is to allow the bowel to rest by minimizing the fecal volume and to allow the patient to consume food. Nutrition therapy is directed towards establishing a tolerance to food. Therefore, the diet is intended to be used for a short time period only and as a transition from a liquid diet to foods more moderate in fiber content.

Dietary Recommendations

A low residue diet can be accomplished by (1) consuming refined grain products (avoid whole grain products); (2) avoiding potatoes, legumes, seeds, and nuts (use rice and pasta products made from refined flour); (3) avoiding whole fruits and vegetables (use fruit and vegetable juices, except prune juice); (4) avoiding meat and shellfish with tough connective tissue; and (5) limiting the use of milk or foods that contain milk (ice cream, pudding, cottage cheese, other cheese, strained creamed soups, etc.) to 2 cups (or the equivalent) or less each day.

Physicians: How to Order Diet

The diet order should indicate *low residue diet*. If certain foods such as milk and milk products do not need to be restricted, the diet order should indicate *low residue diet with fruits, vegetables, and milk products as tolerated*. If a more restricted diet is preferred, one should employ commercial formulas with monomeric nutrient sources.

REFERENCES

1. Smallwood R. Bran and bowel habit. Med J Aust 1984(Sept 29):447–449.
2. Lanza E, Butrum RR. A critical review of food fiber analysis and data. J Am Diet Assoc 1986;6:732–740.
3. Hellendoorn EW. Dietary fiber or indigestible residue? Am J Clin Nutr 1981;34:1437–1439.
4. Selvendran RR. The plant cell wall as a source of dietary fiber: chemistry and structure. Am J Clin Nutr 1984;39:320–327.
5. Paul AA, Southgate DAT. McCance and Widdowson's the composition of foods. 4th ed. New York: Elsevier/North Holland Biomedical Press, 1978.
6. Human Nutrition Information Service, United States Government Printing Office. Composition of Foods. Washington, DC, United States Department of Agriculture, 1982–1984.

7. Achord JL. Dietary fiber and the gastrointestinal tract. Curr Concepts Gastroenterol 1981(Summer):10–18.

8. Anderson JW. Health implications of wheat fiber. Am J Clin Nutr 1985;41:1103–1112.

9. Eastwood MA, Passmore R. A new look at dietary fiber. Nutr Today 1984(Sept/Oct):6–11.

10. Beyer PL, Flynn MA. Effects of high- and low-fiber diets on human feces. J Am Diet Assoc 1978;72:271–277.

11. Kramer P. The meaning of high- and low-residue diets (editorial). Gastroenterology 1964;6:649–652.

12. Watts JH, Graham DCW, Jones F, et al. Fecal solids excreted by young men following the ingestion of dairy foods. Am J Diag Dis 1963;4:364–375.

13. Weinstein L, Olson RE, Van Itallie TB, et al. Diet as related to gastrointestinal function. JAMA 1961;11:935–941.

DELAYED GASTRIC EMPTYING

General Description

The management of delayed gastric emptying is aimed at the modification of the composition, consistency, size, and frequency of feedings to a level that the individual can tolerate. This can be accomplished by serving small quantities of liquid to soft foods at frequent intervals. The diet should be planned according to individual tolerances. If oral feedings are not tolerated, enteral or parenteral feedings may be necessary.

Nutritional Inadequacy

The nutritional adequacy of the diet depends on the type of diet the patient can tolerate. The full liquid diet is inadequate in most nutrients. The individual's food intake should be closely assessed, and the nutritional adequacy of the diet can be improved through the use of liquid dietary supplements. If the diet fails to meet the Recommended Dietary Allowance (RDA) for all nutrients, a multivitamin supplement should be ordered.

Indications and Rationale

Mechanical Obstruction. Normal gastric emptying may be disrupted by either mechanical obstruction or altered gastric motility. Anatomical obstruction, attributable to pyloric stenosis, peptic ulcer disease, gastric polyps, or gastric carcinoma, causes increased resistance at the gastric outlet. The result is gastric retention, initially of indigestible solids, then later of digestible solids and liquids.[1-3] Mechanical obstruction is almost always managed by surgical intervention.[4,5]

Gastric Motility Dysfunction. Many clinical situations are associated with gastric retention without evidence of structural outlet obstruction. All of these conditions appear to be linked by abnormalities of gastric motor function, which presents as gastric stasis.[3,6] The term "gastroparesis" has been used to designate this disorder of gastric emptying. A number of disorders that may impair gastric motility are summarized in Table 6–31.

The usual manifestations may include some combination of nausea, vomiting, early satiety, abdominal pain, postprandial abdominal bloating and dis-

TABLE 6–31 Conditions that May be Associated with Impaired Gastric Motility[1,2,6,8–13]

Transient Delayed Gastric Emptying	*Drugs*
Postoperative ileus	Anticholinergics
Acute viral gastroenteritis and other infections	Tricyclic antidepressants
Hyperglycemia	Levodopa
Diabetic ketoacidosis	Opiates (e.g., morphine)
Hypokalemia and other electrolyte imbalances	β-adrenergic agonists
	Alcohol
	Nicotine

Chronic Gastric Stasis	
Diabetes mellitus: autonomic neuropathy	Muscular dystrophies
Collagen—vascular diseases	Central and peripheral neurologic disorders
Acid peptic diseases	Postgastric surgery (e.g., vagotomy, gastric resection, fundoplication)
Achlorhydria and atrophic gastritis (with or without pernicious anemia)	Idiopathic pseudo-obstruction
Caloric deprivation (e.g., starvation, anorexia nervosa)	

tention, anorexia, weight loss, and, at times, bezoar formation.[1–3,7] Symptoms may be of varying degrees of severity.

Some gastroparetic states are acute or transient, such as those associated with certain metabolic abnormalities (which include hyperglycemia, ketoacidosis, and electrolyte imbalances), with postoperative ileus, and with viral gastroenteritis.[2,6] In these conditions, gastric retention usually resolves or improves as the acute illness abates. Prolonged or chronic gastric retention is often associated with a number of metabolic and endocrine states, some postgastric surgeries, neurologic conditions, connective tissue diseases, and such gastric disorders as gastroesophageal reflux and ulcer disease. In some cases, gastroparesis may be idiopathic. In addition, certain pharmacologic agents cause delayed gastric emptying.

Different mechanisms and regions of the stomach are involved in the emptying of the solid and the liquid components of gastric contents.[2,14–16] Gastric emptying of liquids is determined by slow sustained contractions in the fundus and in the proximal body of the stomach. Gastric emptying of solids is determined by vigorous peristaltic contractions in the antrum or in the distal part of the stomach. In the process of emptying, the two functions that are necessary are the antral peristaltic contractions of grinding and mixing (trituration), which reduce solids to the near liquid form that is required for emptying, and the propulsive forces of the fundus, which push the stomach contents into the duodenum.

If the stomach has lost its ability to triturate solids into the size that is necessary for emptying or its ability to generate a gastroduodenal pressure gradient that can push chyme out of the stomach, across the pylorus, and into the duodenum, gastric stasis or gastric retention results.

Motility disorders that are confined to the distal portion of the stomach result in delayed emptying of solids, but normal emptying of liquids.[2] Distal gastric dysfunction would preclude the breakdown of solids, but the functioning proximal stomach retains the capacity to generate the gastroduodenal pressure gradient that is required for the emptying of liquids. Fundic motility disorders, on the other hand, may delay the emptying of both solids and liquids. Although adequate trituration of solids occurs, the stomach contents do not empty properly because of the impaired gastroduodenal pressure gradient.

Nondigestible solids, such as plant fibers, are impervious to breakdown by antral contractions and, therefore, are not emptied with liquids and digestible solids.[2,15] These solids are retained in the stomach until the rest of the meal is emptied. After the liquids and the digestible solids are digested, powerful contractions sweep the nondigestible solids out of the stomach and down the small intestine to the colon by a special mechanism called the migrating motor complex. Disruption of this motor activity may lead to the retention of indigestible material in the stomach and to the possible formation of fibrous bezoar.[3,14]

The rate at which the stomach empties is influenced by the physical nature and the composition of the gastric contents, i.e., solid or liquid state, the original size of the solids, osmolality and nutrient composition.[2,3,14,15] Liquids leave the stomach most rapidly. Solids leave the stomach much more slowly, therefore allowing for the reduction in size to the consistency required for emptying. Osmolality and nutrient composition affect the gastric emptying by the action of specific small bowel receptors on neural or hormonal pathways. Fluids of high osmolality have slower emptying rates than do isotonic liquids, which allows for the gradual adjustment of their osmolality to isotonicity in the upper intestine. Although protein, carbohydrate, and fat all slow gastric emptying, fat is a more potent inhibitor. The fatty acid chain length determines the degree of inhibition, with longer chain lengths causing the greatest delay in emptying.

The treatment of delayed gastric emptying includes (1) the elimination of the cause (e.g., drugs) or the treatment of the underlying disorder (e.g., uncontrolled diabetes) if one can be documented; (2) the manipulation of the diet; and (3) the employment of drugs to improve motility.[2,6] Metoclopramide, the most commonly used drug for this problem, has a central antiemetic effect as well as prokinetic properties. Surgery, however, has limited indications in gastroparesis.[3,17]

Goals of Dietary Management

The dietary management of gastric retention is aimed at finding a diet that the individual is capable of digesting, at allowing symptomatic relief, and at providing adequate nutrition. The purpose of the dietary modifications for obstruction is to provide foods that can pass by the partial obstruction. Small feedings are provided to prevent excessive distention. In delayed gastric motility, the diet is manipulated to find the composition, consistency, and volume of food that the patient can triturate and empty without nausea, pain, distention, and bezoar formation.

Dietary Recommendations

Mechanical Obstruction. The degree of obstruction determines the type of diet the patient can tolerate. A full liquid diet (see page 45) can be used if the obstruction is nearly complete. Emphasis is also placed on smaller and more frequent feedings. A mechanical soft diet (see page 48) may be tolerated in the instances of a lesser obstruction. If the obstruction is complete, enteral feeding below the obstruction or parenteral nutrition may be used.

Gastric Motility Dysfunction. The role of the diet in the treatment of gastric motor disorders has not been clearly defined. In general, patients with gastric motility disorders tolerate solid foods poorly. Patients with mild disturbances of gastric emptying (as is commonly observed with diabetic, postsurgical, or idiopathic gastroparesis) may tolerate small, frequent meals of soft foods that are low in fat. Since these patients have a tendency to develop bezoars, low fiber foods are also advised. The dietitian should work with the patient to find the degree of consistency (or particle size) and the level of fat that is tolerated by the individual. These patients may also require periodic gastric lavage to remove nondigestible foods. Depending on the patient's tolerance, a variable number of kilocalories may need to be derived from liquids.

Patients with more severe gastroparesis may be unable to triturate and empty solid food, but may still be capable of emptying fluids. In these patients, blenderized diets or commercial liquid formula diets may be used. Small amounts of isotonic formula at frequent intervals may be tolerated. Monomeric formulas tend to be poorly tolerated owing to their hyperosmolality.

If the patient is unable to tolerate liquid oral feedings, jejunal feedings may be necessary. A continuous slow infusion by pump is preferable to gravity feeding in order to prevent distention, nausea and vomiting, and dumping syndrome. Feeding into the duodenum is contraindicated since duodenal contents tend to reflux back into the stomach, and duodenal motor abnormalities are commonly associated with gastric motor disorders. In patients unable to tolerate oral or enteral feedings owing to intestinal motility disorders, parenteral nutrition may be necessary.

Physicians: How to Order Diet

This diet may be ordered as *diet for gastric retention*. The dietitian consults with the physician and the patient regarding tolerances and follows the guidelines that were previously discussed in the chapter.

REFERENCES

1. Fisher RS. Gastroduodenal motility disturbances in man. Scand J Gastroenterol 1985;20:59–68.
2. Minami H, McCallum RW. The physiology and pathophysiology of gastric emptying in humans. Gastroenterology 1984;86:1592–1610.
3. Roch E, Malmud L, Fisher RS. Motor disorders of the stomach. Med Clin North Am 1981;65:1269–1289.
4. Malagelada JR. Disorders of gastric emptying. In: Bayless TM, ed. Current therapy in gastroenterology and liver disease, 1984–1985. Philadelphia: BC Decker, 1984:95.
5. Alpers DH. Dietary management and vitamin-mineral replacement therapy: In: Sleisenger MH, Fordtran JS, eds. Gastrointestinal disease: pathophysiology, diagnosis, management. 3rd ed. Philadelphia: WB Saunders, 1983:1819.
6. McCallum RW. Gastric emptying disorders. Drug Ther 1986;April:41–76.
7. Rogers AI. Gastric emptying disorders. Compr Ther 1985;11:20–25.
8. Saltzman MB, McCallum RW. Diabetes and the stomach. Yale J Biol Med 1983;56:179–187.
9. Stanghellini V, Malagelada JR. Gastric manometric abnormalities in patients with dyspeptic symptoms after fundoplication. Gut 1983;24:790–797.
10. Yang R, Arem R, Chan L. Gastrointestinal tract complications of diabetes mellitus. Pathophysiology and management. Arch Intern Med 1984;144:1251–1256.
11. Steen LE, Oberg L. Familial amyloidosis with polyneuropathy: roentgenological and

gastroscopic appearance of gastrointestinal involvement. Am J Gastroenterol 1983;78:417–420.

12. Wright RA, Clemente R, Wathen R. Diabetic gastroparesis: an abnormality of gastric emptying of solids. Am J Med Sci 1985;289:240–242.

13. Abell TL, Lucas AR, Brown ML, Malagelada JR. Gastric electrical dysrhythmias in anorexia nervosa. Gastroenterology 1985;88:1300.

14. Schiller LR. Motor function of the stomach. In: Sleisenger MH, Fordtran JS, eds. Gastrointestinal disease: pathophysiology, diagnosis, management. 3rd ed. Philadelphia: WB Saunders, 1983:521.

15. Malagelada JR, Miller LJ. The gut response to a meal and its hormonal control. In: Bouchier IAD, Allan RN, Hodgson HJF, Keighley MRB, eds. Textbook of gastroenterology. London: Balliere Lindall, 1984:345.

16. Feldman M. Nausea and vomiting. In: Sleisenger MH, Fordtran JS, eds. Gastrointestinal disease: pathophysiology, diagnosis, management. 3rd ed. Philadelphia: WB Saunders, 1983:160.

17. Lindor KD, Malagelada JR. Symposium on upper gastrointestinal motility disorders. Gastric motor disorders. Gastric motor disorders: an overview. South Med J 1984;77:943–946.

GLUTEN SENSITIVITY: CELIAC SPRUE AND DERMATITIS HERPETIFORMIS

General Description

The diet eliminates gluten, which is the protein that is found in wheat, oats, rye, and barley. Even very small amounts of gluten must be eliminated from the diet. The widespread use of gluten-containing grain products in commercially processed foods and the difficulties in ascertaining the presence of gluten in many foods can make strict adherence problematic.

Nutritional Inadequacy

A gluten-free diet is not nutritionally inadequate; however, when malabsorption is present, appropriate vitamin and/or mineral supplements should be prescribed. A calcium supplement is recommended if the patient is also lactose intolerant and is not able to consume or tolerate adequate amounts of lactase treated dairy products.[1]

Indications and Rationale

Celiac Sprue. Celiac sprue is also termed gluten-sensitive enteropathy, nontropical sprue, gluten-induced enteropathy, and idiopathic steatorrhea. Several mechanisms, which include a disorder of immunologic function, have been postulated to explain the toxicity of gluten.[2,3] The disease is characterized by atrophy of villi of the small intestinal mucosa, especially of the duodenum and of the proximal jejunum, and by malabsorption, which usually results in steatorrhea and in diarrhea.[4] Although diarrhea is the most common complaint, it is not always present.[5] Malabsorption of protein, fat and fat soluble vitamins, vitamin B_{12} or folate, iron, calcium, and of other nutrients can occur. Weight loss, anemia, and bone pain, the latter a manifestation of osteomalacia, can also result.[6] However, the clinical presentation of celiac disease is highly variable and emphasizes the subtleties that are involved in the diagnosis of malabsorption syndromes. Although studies clearly implicate gluten, particularly the glia-din fraction, as the etiologic agent that is involved, the exact pathogenic mechanism is unknown.[7]

The diagnosis is confirmed by demonstrating the characteristic lesion of a flat jejunal mucosa with the loss of normal villi[8] and by the subsequent relief of symptoms with a gluten-free diet.

Once gluten is removed from the diet, symptoms gradually improve over a period of several weeks or months.[9] There may be continuing difficulties with fat malabsorption, with lactose intolerance, and with subsequent osteomalacia because of incomplete recovery.[10] Initially, a high kilocalorie, high protein diet and a nutritional supplement may be necessary until the mucosa responds and absorption improves.

Gluten-sensitive enteropathy should be considered a chronic disease that is controlled by diet. An asymptomatic state depends on the lifelong maintenance of a gluten-free diet. Patients should be cautioned against ingesting gluten once they start to gain weight and to feel better. The ingestion of gluten damages the mucosa and causes recurrent symptoms, although several weeks may lapse before the symptoms are observed. An assessment of dietary adherence is critical in determining whether the recurrent symptoms are related to sprue or to another unrelated problem.

Failure to respond to a gluten-free diet is not common, but it may occur because of diffuse intestinal ulceration, severe secondary lactase deficiency, or concurrent disease, such as pancreatic insufficiency[8] or intestinal lymphoma.[11] Collagenous sprue is an extremely rare entity and is characterized by a lack of response to dietary therapy.[8]

Dermatitis Herpetiformis. Dermatitis herpetiformis is a chronic inflammatory disease of the skin that is characterized by a pruritic, blistering rash and is accompanied in the majority of patients by a jejunal lesion that is similar to that of sprue. Gastrointestinal symptoms may be present, but more often are not. Both the histologic appearance of the jejunum and of the skin lesions respond to gluten withdrawal and relapse with a challenge of gluten.[12] Therefore, the long-term adherence to a gluten-free diet is recommended.

Goals of Dietary Management

The goals of dietary management are the remission of clinical symptoms, the normalization of absorptive function, and the regeneration of mucosal villi.

Dietary Recommendations

The avoidance of gluten is paramount and should be considered lifelong. Gluten is a protein that is found only in the grains of wheat, oats, rye, and barley (Table 6–32). Although abstaining from these grains appears to be direct and simple, strict dietary adherence is difficult for most patients. Gluten-containing grains and products that are made from them are a staple in Western diets. The widespread use of emulsifiers, thickeners, and other additives derived from gluten-containing grains in commercially processed foods further complicates the strict adherence to a gluten-free diet. It is necessary for patients to read food labels carefully and to avoid products that list questionable ingredients that cannot be verified as gluten-free by the manufacturer. The uninten-

TABLE 6–32 Sources of Gluten*

Food Groups	Foods that Contain Gluten	Foods that may Contain Gluten	Foods that do not Contain Gluten
Beverage	Cereal beverages (e.g., Postum), malt, Ovaltine, beer and ale	Commercial chocolate milk; cocoa mixes; other beverage mixes; dietary supplements	Coffee; tea; decaffeinated coffee; carbonated beverages; chocolate drinks made with pure cocoa powder; wine; distilled liquor
Meat and meat substitutes		Meat loaf and patties, cold cuts and prepared meats, stuffing, breaded meats, cheese foods and spreads; commercial souffles, omelets, and fondue; soy protein meat substitutes	Pure meat, fish, fowl, egg, cottage cheese, and peanut butter
Fat and oil		Commercial salad dressing and mayonnaise, gravy, white and cream sauces, nondairy creamer	Butter, margarine, vegetable oil
Milk	Milk beverages that contain malt	Commercial chocolate milk	Whole, low-fat, and skim milk; buttermilk
Grains and grain products	Bread, crackers, cereal, and pasta that contains wheat, oats, rye, malt, malt flavoring, graham flour, durham flour, pastry flour, bran, or wheat germ; barley; millet; pretzels; communion wafers[13,14]	Commercial seasoned rice and potato mixes	Specially prepared breads made with wheat starch,[†] rice, potato, or soybean flour or cornmeal; pure corn or rice cereals; hominy grits; white, brown, and wild rice; popcorn; low protein pasta made from wheat starch

Category	Foods Allowed	Foods to Avoid	Commercial foods (investigate)
Vegetable	All fresh vegetables; plain commercially frozen or canned vegetables		Commercial seasoned vegetable mixes; commercial vegetables with cream or cheese sauce; canned baked beans
Fruit	All plain or sweetened fruits; fruit thickened with tapioca or cornstarch		Commercial pie fillings
Soup	Soup thickened with cornstarch, wheat starch, or potato, rice or soybean flour; pure broth	Soup that contains wheat pasta; soup thickened with wheat flour or other gluten-containing grains	Commercial soup, broth, and soup mixes
Desserts	Gelatin; custard; fruit ice; specially prepared cakes, cookies, and pastries made with gluten-free flour or starch; pudding and fruit filling thickened with tapioca, cornstarch, or arrowroot flour	Commercial cakes, cookies and pastries; commercial dessert mixes	Commercial ice cream and sherbet
Sweets			Commercial candies, especially chocolates
Miscellaneous‡	Monosodium glutamate; salt; pepper; pure spices and herbs; yeast; pure baking chocolate or cocoa powder; carob; flavoring extracts; artificial flavoring		Ketchup; prepared mustard; soy sauce; commercially prepared meat sauces and pickles; vinegar; flavoring syrups (syrups for pancakes or ice cream)

*The terms "commercially prepared" and "commercial" are used to refer to partially prepared foods purchased from a grocery or food market and to prepared foods purchased from a restaurant.

†Wheat starch may contain trace amounts of gluten. Avoid if not tolerated.

‡Medications may contain trace amounts of gluten.[15] A pharmacist may be able to provide information on the gluten content of medications.

tional consumption of gluten is a common cause of recurrence of symptoms. Other reasons patients fail to maintain a strict gluten-free diet are the boredom with the taste of alternatives to wheat breads, crackers, and pasta and the limited availability of appropriate foods when eating away from home. Patients should be encouraged to use gluten-free bread replacements to maintain adequate carbohydrate and kilocalorie intake.

Initially, a high kilocalorie and a high protein diet should be recommended, especially if weight loss and if specific deficiencies owing to malabsorption are pronounced. The kilocalorie and the protein recommendations may be normalized as the absorption improves. Supplemental vitamins and minerals may also be indicated initially, but may not continue to be necessary as absorption improves.

For some patients, lactose and fat may need to be initially restricted because of secondary lactase deficiency and fat malabsorption. Dairy products and fats should be reintroduced into the diet gradually since a degree of lactose intolerance and malabsorption may continue indefinitely for some patients. (See page 165 for additional information on lactose intolerance).

Physicians: How to Order Diet

The diet order should indicate *gluten-free diet*. The need for secondary restrictions, such as lactose and fat, should also be indicated according to the individual patient tolerance.

Food Labeling

Gluten-containing grains are widely used in the preparation of foods. A thorough review of the list of ingredients on the label reveals obvious sources of gluten. The patient should be alert to less obvious food sources of gluten such as pasta products, cold cuts, commercial soups and salad dressings, sauces, and instant cereal beverage mixes. The labels on commercial breads should also be reviewed since some products include wheat flour. The following ingredients that are listed on food labels may or may not contain gluten:

cereal	hydrolyzed vegetable protein
cereal additive	modified food starch
emulsifier	stabilizer
flavoring	starch
hydrolyzed plant protein	vegetable protein

If one of the aforementioned ingredients is listed on the label, the absence of gluten should be verified with an up to date product list, or the patient should be advised to call or write to the company to request information on the gluten content. When the ingredients are not listed on the label, the manufacturer should be contacted for the complete ingredient information.

Substitutions for Wheat Flour

Most patients find special cookbooks helpful. Recipes can be modified by the following substitutions.

For baking, 1 cup of wheat flour may be replaced by:

1 cup of wheat starch
1 cup of corn flour
1 scant cup of fine cornmeal
3/4 cup of coarse cornmeal
5/8 cup (10 Tbsp) of potato flour
7/8 cup (14 Tbsp) of rice flour
1 cup of soy flour plus 1/4 cup of potato flour
1/2 cup of soy flour plus 1/2 cup of potato flour

For thickening, 1 tablespoon of wheat flour may be replaced by:

1/2 Tbsp of cornstarch, potato flour, rice starch, or arrowroot starch
2 Tbsp of quick-cooking tapioca

Patient Support Groups

American Celiac Society
45 Gifford Avenue
Jersey City, NJ 07304

Gluten-Intolerance Group
Elaine I. Hartsook, R.D.
26604 Dover Court
Kent, WA 98031

National Celiac-Sprue Society
Eleanor McAlester
5 Jeffrey Road
Wayland, MA 01778

Midwest Gluten Intolerance Group
5660 Rebecca Lane
Minnetonka, MN 55345

REFERENCES

1. Skinner S, Martens RA. Good nutrition without lactose. In: Skinner S, Martens RA, eds. The milk sugar dilemma: living with lactose intolerance. East Lansing, MI: Medi-Ed Press, 1985:42.
2. Auricchio S, DeRitus G, DeVincenzi M, Silano V. Toxicity mechanisms of wheat and other cereals in celiac disease and related enteropathies. J Pediatr Gastroenterol Nutr 1985;4:923–930.
3. Shiner M. Present trends in celiac disease. Postgrad Med 1984;60:773–778.
4. Trier JS. Celiac sprue. In: Sleisenger MH, Fordtran JS, eds. Gastrointestinal disease: pathophysiology, diagnosis, management. 3rd ed. New York: WB Saunders, 1983:1050.
5. Mann JG, Brown WR, Kern F. The subtle and valuable clinical expressions of gluten-induced enteropathy. Amer J Med 1970;48:357.
6. Winick M. Gastrointestinal diseases that affect nutrition: sprue. In: Winick M, ed. Nutrition and gastroenterology. New York: Wiley-Interscience Publications, 1980:96.
7. Kottgen, E, Volk B, Kluge F, Gerok W. Gluten, the causative agent of gluten-sensitive enteropathy. Biochem Biophys Res Commun 1982;109:168–173.
8. Greenberger NJ, Winship DH. Gastrointestinal disorders. Small intestine. In: Myers

J, Rogers DE, eds. Gastrointestinal disorders: a pathophysiologic approach. 2nd ed. Chicago: Year Book Medical Publishers, 1980:128.

9. Rawcliffe P, Rolph R. How is sprue treated? In: Rawcliffe P, Rolph R, eds. The gluten-free diet book. New York: Arco Publishing, 1985:17.
10. Gitnick G. Lactose tolerance test. In: Rubinstein M, ed. Practical diagnosis gastrointestinal and liver disease. Boston: Houghton Mifflin, 1979:250.
11. Cooper BT, Holmes GKT, Cooke WT. Lymphoma risk in celiac disease of later life. Digestion 1982;12:89–92.
12. Renuala T, Kosnai I, Karpati S, Kuitunen P, Torok E, Savilahi E. Dermatitis herpetiformis: jejunal finding and skin response to gluten-free diet. Arch Dis Child 1984;59:519–522.
13. Scotta MS, DeGiacomo C, Maggiore G, Siena S, Ugazio A. Eucharistic problems for celiac patients. N Engl J Med 1982;307:898.
14. Jackson HT. More on eucharistic problems for patients with celiac disease. N Engl J Med 1983;308:287–288.
15. Patel DG, Krough CM, Thompson WG. Gluten in pills: a hazard for patients with celiac disease. Can Med Assoc J 1985;133:114–115.

INFLAMMATORY BOWEL DISEASE

General Description

Recommendations for inflammatory bowel disease are variable and dependent on the nutritional status of the individual, the location and the extent of the disease, and the nature of the surgical or medical management.

Nutritional Inadequacy

Dietary modifications for inflammatory bowel disease are based on individual food tolerances. Each person's diet should be assessed for nutritional adequacy and supplemented to provide the Recommended Dietary Allowance (RDA) for nutrients. Extra supplementation may be necessary to correct additional needs that are attributable to malabsorption and to increased requirements.

Indications and Rationale

Inflammatory bowel disease is a general term that primarily refers to two distinct disease processes, which are chronic ulcerative colitis and Crohn's disease. Chronic ulcerative colitis (CUC) is an idiopathic, inflammatory disorder that is confined to the mucosa of the large intestine. The process may involve the rectum alone (ulcerative proctitis) or may involve the entire large intestine (pancolitis). Involvement is generally uniform; it begins in the rectum and spreads proximally in a continuous fashion. Crohn's disease, or regional enteritis, on the other hand, may involve the small or the large intestine, or both, and its distribution is segmental. As opposed to CUC, Crohn's is a transmural process and as such is more commonly associated with stricture formation, with fistulous tracts, and with abscesses. The pathology of the two diseases may be indistinguishable. Generally, CUC is marked by mucosal inflammation, crypt distortion, and crypt abscesses with shallow ulcer formation. Crohn's is characterized by mucosal inflammation, which progresses to deep linear ulceration and to transmural involvement with granuloma formation. The major symptoms of inflammatory bowel disease include abdominal pain, diarrhea, intestinal bleeding, protein loss, and fever. These symptoms respectively result in nutritional wasting owing to a decreased intake from anorexia, an increased loss of nutrients from maldigestion and malabsorption, and an increase in requirements owing to fever. Malnutrition occurs with chronic disease. Fluid and electrolyte imbalances occur with acute exacerbations.

Medical therapy is mainly geared at the symptomatic control and the treatment of the complications, because currently no medical cure exists for either disease process. Sulfasalazine (Azulfidine) and corticosteroids (Prednisone) are successful in the management of acute exacerbations, yet neither has been effective in the maintenance of a remission in Crohn's disease. Azulfidine has been successful in this regard in CUC. A newer preparation that employs 5-Aminosalicylic Acid will soon be available for use, yet it falls under the same limitations as previously mentioned. The judicious use of anticholinergics and of antidiarrheal agents, e.g., Lomotil or Imodium, also have a role in the symptomatic care. Surgery is curative in CUC, and newer ileostomy alternatives (see subsequently) make this approach more acceptable to the younger population. Crohn's, however, tends to recur following the surgical resection of the affected segments in the majority of patients. For this reason, one is more conservative in the treatment of Crohn's disease, reserving surgery for truly refractory disease or for significant complications such as obstruction, abscess, fistulae, or bleeding. Patient education and psychological support are important aspects in the management for patients with inflammatory bowel disease.

Goals of Dietary Management

The nutritional goals are to replace the nutrient losses that are associated with the inflammatory process, to correct the body deficits, and to provide sufficient nutrients to achieve energy, nitrogen, fluid, and electrolyte balance. Dietary recommendations should also be designed to avoid aggravating symptoms.

Dietary Recommendations

A nutritional assessment should be performed to determine the patient's nutritional status and to estimate the patient's needs (see page 3). The approach to nutritional therapy must take into account the intestinal function, the site and the extent of the disease process (Figure 6–1), and the anticipated medical and surgical treatment.

Inflammation of the Large Bowel. During the acute phase, diarrhea, tenesmus, and frequent bowel movements are a problem. Pharmacologic agents are used to control symptoms. The extent of diet control is dependent on the severity of symptoms. The patient who suffers from severe abdominal cramps and diarrhea and who is rapidly becoming dehydrated needs hospitalization and bowel rest. Oral intake may increase the amount of liquid that is presented by the small intestine to the colon and may consequently aggravate diarrhea. "Bowel rest" is accomplished by forbidding the oral intake of both food and fluid, although one can expect only diminution, not abolition, of peristaltic and of secoratory activity. Parenteral nutritional support is used to provide the nutritional and the fluid needs for patients who require bowel rest. This support can

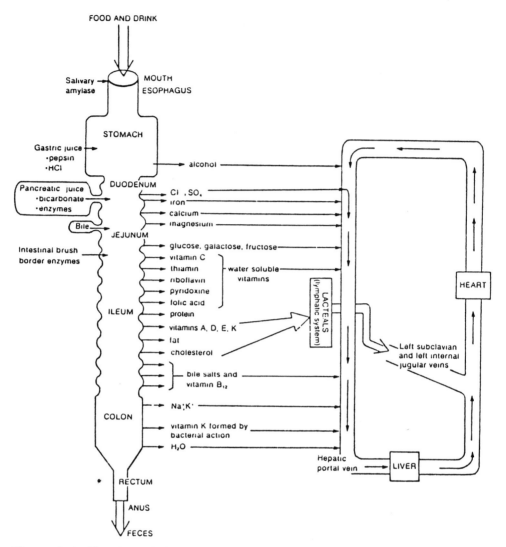

Figure 6–1 The site and the extent of the disease process and the effect on nutrient absorption. Reprinted with permission from Krause MV, Mahon LK. Food nutrition and diet therapy. Philadelphia: WB Saunders, 1984:86.

be administered peripherally for short-term management or centrally if the course is fulminating and the therapy is likely to be more extended. As the patient improves and the number of bowel movements decrease, oral intake can be initiated. Transitional feedings can commence with monomeric or with polymeric enteral formulas, and they can be provided via tube or, with a well-motivated patient, taken orally. Progression can continue as tolerated to a minimal residue diet, to a low fiber diet, and, as symptoms subside, to a regular diet that includes fiber to a degree that the patient feels is tolerable. The restriction of fiber for chronic colitis is based on anecdotal experience, and there are no good studies to demonstrate that fiber has a deleterious effect. For the patient with chronic colitis who is asymptomatic, the intake of fiber should not be limited if fiber does not induce symptoms. Because lactose intolerance is common, the initial selection of food should avoid lactose. Tolerance for lactose can be established, once symptoms abate, by either laboratory testing or by subjective trial. If intolerance exists, lactase may be added to the milk. Although it seems prudent to limit the intake of spices, their exact effect on the colon has not been studied. The patient's food preferences should be encouraged and not limited because of the spice content. In general, limiting dietary choices is discouraged.[1,2]

Inflammation of the Small Bowel. Acute and chronic Crohn's disease is similar to acute and to chronic colitis, with some exceptions. For acute flares with evidence of obstruction, all oral feeding is stopped and nasogastric suction and intravenous nutritional support is initiated. If either the complete or the partial obstruction does not respond to medical management, surgical resection of the stenotic segment is indicated. Because Crohn's disease has a high rate of recurrence, attempts at preventing resection should be carried out vigorously. New approaches to induce a remission include bowel rest and attempts to improve general nutritional status. Parenteral nutritional support and the use of monomeric enteral diets are still being evaluated for their exact role in the management of Crohn's disease.[3,4]

The dietary management for Crohn's disease is similar to the nutritional therapy guidelines for colitis. In colitis, the focus is on maintaining fluid and electrolyte balance. However, patients with ileitis additionally experience selective malabsorption of other nutrients that is directly proportional to the site and to the extent of small bowel involvement or resection. Therefore, the diet should be planned with this in mind. (See the section on short bowel, page 163). Initial feedings should be minimal in residue. If there is no sign of a stricture, the diet can be progressed, as tolerated, to a low fiber diet and, as symptoms subside, to a regular diet. There may be indications for modifying the diet to be restricted in fat, in lactose, and possibly in oxalates. Additional vitamin and mineral supplementation may be necessary for vitamin B_{12}, folate, calcium, magnesium, and zinc because of increased losses that are attributable to malabsorption or to a decreased dietary intake.

Colostomy. A colostomy may be constructed when a segment of large bowel is removed because of disease or obstruction. Dietary management depends on the colostomy site because the output from the stoma is proportional to the length of the remaining bowel (Figure 6–2). Patients with colostomies in the

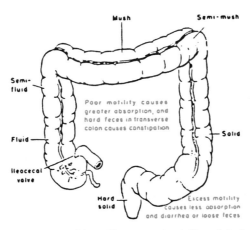

Figure 6–2 The colostomy site and its effect on output. Reprinted with permission from Krause MV, Mahon LK. Food nutrition and diet therapy. Philadelphia: WB Saunders, 1984:698.

transverse or in the descending colon often achieve control of colonic function so that they have relatively little loss of fluid secretions from the stoma and can control evacuation by daily irrigation. Cecostomies or colostomies in the ascending colon have a more liquid stool output, therefore, a greater loss of fluid and electrolytes. Most patients with colostomies can return to a normal diet after surgery. Dietary modification is based solely on individual tolerance. Restriction should be limited only to those foods that produce annoying side effects for the individual, such as gas or loose stools.[5] The patient may feel greater comfort and may find caring for the ostomy easier by following the guidelines in Table 6–33.

TABLE 6–33 Dietary Guidelines for Colostomy and Ileostomy

1. Eat meals at regular times, three or more times daily.
2. Chew food well to avoid a blockage at the stoma site.
3. Drink adequate amounts of fluid.
4. Avoid gaining excessive weight, which may affect the stoma function.
5. Limit foods that may produce excessive gas and loose stools and those foods that may not be completely digested or that produce undesirable bulk.

Gas Forming and/or Odor Producing Foods*

asparagus	broccoli	cauliflower	onions
baked beans	Brussel sprouts	eggs	parsnips
cabbage	fish	beer or carbonated beverages	

Foods that May Produce Loose Stools*

baked beans	excessive coffee	red wine
beer	heavily spiced foods	spinach
broccoli	hot beverages or soups	large meals
chocolates	licorice	dried beans
prune juice		

Foods that Are Not Completely Digested*

celery	mushrooms	relishes
coconut	nuts	salad greens
coleslaw	peas	seeds
corn	popcorn	skins
membrane on orange	raisins or dried fruit	
	pineapple	

*Do not abandon foods without a fair trial. Test a small amount of the suspected food one at a time to establish tolerance. This list has been developed largely from anecdotal accounts and should be regarded only as an initial guideline. Because of the nature of the ostomy and of the remaining gastrointestinal tract, the foods that alter function may not be the same as those that produce the same affect in the unaltered gastrointestinal tract.

Ileostomy. An ileostomy is usually fashioned when the entire colon and rectum is removed. The consistency of output is more liquid than that from a colostomy. Although more water, sodium, and other minerals are lost, fluid and electrolyte balance may eventually be achieved, depending upon the length of remaining gut and upon the adaptation that results with increased absorption. As with patients with colostomies, dietary restrictions should be based solely on the individual's intolerances.[5] The patient with an ileostomy may also benefit from the general guidelines in Table 6–33.

Ileal Pouch (Kock Pouch). The ileal pouch is an alternative form of ileostomy that allows for continence and frees the patient from wearing a stomal appliance. A pouch is created from the ileum and serves as an internal reservoir for the collection of feces. In addition, a valve, which is constructed from the intestine, allows continence. On the abdominal wall, a stoma is created through which a catheter is placed, and the pouch is drained. Patients eventually evacuate their pouches two to four times daily. Dietary management is directed towards supporting pouch function as well as providing a balanced, nutritious diet. The patient should be encouraged to drink adequate amounts of fluids. The maintenance of hydration allows the consistency of fecal matter to be more liquid, thereby facilitating evacuation. Prune, grape, or other fruit juices can also provide a laxative effect. Foods that remain undigested and that plug the catheter should be individually identified and avoided. Modifying eating habits and avoiding foods that produce gas (see section on *Abdominal Gas and Flatulence*) also aid in patient comfort.[6] Table 6–33 can be used as a guideline in planning the diet for a patient with an ileal pouch.

Ileo-Anal Anastomosis (J Pouch). The ileo-anal anastomosis is an alternative to an ileostomy. This surgical procedure removes the diseased colon and part of the rectum, yet preserves the anal sphincter by stripping off only the involved mucosa. The ileum is pulled through the rectal muscular tube and is attached to the anus. This preserves anal continence and allows for a more normal pattern of evacuation. A small reservoir or J pouch is made at the end of the ileum and serves to store fecal matter and to control bowel evacuation. A temporary ileostomy is made at the time of surgery to protect the pouch and to allow time for healing. After 2 to 3 months, the ileostomy is closed and bowel continuity is established. The dietary management for patients with ileo-anal anastomosis is directed toward managing the temporary ileostomy and achieving bowel control. The consistency and the frequency of bowel movements varies from patient to patient. To increase the consistency of the stool, patients may wish to avoid those foods that tended to loosen the stool during the temporary ileostomy. Fresh fruits and vegetables and their juices may also have a laxative effect. Patients may find that eating the main meal midday and avoiding large quantities of fluids in the evening result in fewer bowel movements during the night.[7]

Short Bowel Syndrome. The symptoms and the consequences of the short bowel syndrome depend on the site and the extent of the small bowel that is removed, on the presence of the ileocecal valve, and on the condition of the remaining gut as well as whether or not there is colon continuity. It is important to remember that the short bowel syndrome can result from surgical resection, from extensive disease, or from a combination of both. Significant ileal resection or disease can result in the malabsorption of carbohydrate, protein, and fat, and thus can result in malnutrition. The malabsorption of fat results from the loss of the section of intestine that is responsible for absorption of fat and bile salts. Bile salt malabsorption can result in either bile salt depletion through stomal loss or in the passage of bile salts into the colon. Depletion through stomal loss results in further steatorrhea, as the lack of bile salts limits the micelle formation and consequently fat digestion and absorption are impaired. Colonic deconjugation of bile salts results in increased water and electrolyte secretion, thus causing watery diarrhea. In this setting, resins, such as cholestyramine, that are capable of binding bile salts may be given to help control diarrhea, yet these may further aggravate malabsorption.

Calcium and magnesium deficiency can occur due to the binding of calcium and of magnesium in malabsorbed stool fat,[8] to inadequate dietary intake, or to both. One frequent complication is calcium-oxalate nephrolithiasis in patients with colonic continuity.[9] An increased urinary oxalate excretion occurs because of an increased colonic uptake of oxalate, because calcium is bound to fat and is no longer available to bind oxalate in the colon and to prevent its absorption. Stone formation is also enhanced by dehydration owing to the increased intestinal fluid loss or the decreased intake. Because the small bowel is the site of vitamin and mineral absorption, nutritional deficiencies are likely. The steatorrhea of short bowel syndrome may result in the malabsorption of fat soluble vitamins. Vitamin B_{12} deficiency may occur if the site for absorption, the terminal ileum, is impaired or resected. The dietary intake of vitamins, such as vitamins C and folate, may be reduced due to the restriction of the fruit and the vegetable intake or their intolerance. Supplemental calcium, in amounts of 500 or more mg per day of elemental calcium, helps prevent both oxalate nephrolithiasis and calcium deficiency. The latter deficiency may be manifested as osteomalacia. Magnesium deficiency is common, but oral magnesium preparations contribute to diarrhea. Iron therapy given orally (or by injection if not tolerated orally) is helpful to correct anemia. Hence, routine multiple vitamin-mineral supplementation is indicated.[10]

Nutritional support influences bowel function significantly. Parenteral support is indicated if the patient cannot take adequate nutrients or if the oral diet aggravates symptoms. The loss of ability to secrete digestive enzymes follows prolonged bowel rest. Villi growth is stimulated by the presence of food. Therefore, it is preferable to return to oral feedings as soon as possible, even in small amounts, rather than to depend on prolonged parenteral feeding. Enteral nutritional support that uses nutritional formulas may be helpful as either a sole source of nutrition or as a supplement to the food intake (see section on *Enteral Nutrition*). Selection of the appropriate formula is based on the individual's digestive and absorptive capabilities.

The dietary management for patients with short bowel syndrome should take all of the aforementioned factors into account. Most patients initially require fat restriction. Depending on the severity of malabsorption, the patient may also benefit from the use of medium chain triglyceride fat (see page 138). In the presence of colonic continuity, dietary sources of oxalate should be limited for the prevention of urolithiasis. Modifications in lactose and in fiber can be made according to individual tolerance. There is current evidence that fiber may enhance gut function by promoting gut hypertrophy.[11] Vitamins and minerals should be supplemented according to the intake and to the capability of absorption.

Patients with short bowel syndrome may experience a secretory-type diarrhea that approaches two or more liters daily with a high electrolyte content. The management of fluid and of electrolyte deficits may be difficult. Recently, the use of oral rehydration solutions has been successfully used to manage high output diarrhea. The mechanism is based upon the coupled absorption of glucose and of sodium. If the glucose absorption is not damaged in the small intestine, the intake of glucose activates the mechanisms for absorption of sodium and water with the glucose, which results in the reversal of net water secretion and in the correction of diarrhea. Originally, such oral rehydration solutions were successfully used to manage the hydration of cholera victims. More recently, such therapy has been successfully applied to patients with short bowel syndrome and pseudo-obstruction and to patients who receive home parenteral nutrition and continue to have a high intestinal output.[12,13] See *Appendix 11* for examples of oral rehydration solutions. The amounts and the rate of oral intake depend on the degree of dehydration and of diarrhea. In general, the intake should match the output.

Physicians: How to Order Diet

The diet order should reflect the underlying disorders (diet for *chronic ulcerative colitis, Crohn's disease, colostomy, ileostomy, Kock pouch, ileo-anal anastomosis (J-pouch), or short bowel syndrome*, etc.). The dietitian plans the nutritional program according to the aforementioned guideline.

REFERENCES

1. National Foundation for Ileitis and Colitis, New York. Questions and answers about diet and nutrition in ileitis and colitis.
2. Cobden I. Management of acute colitis. Compr Ther 1984;10:36–42.
3. Morain C, Segal AW, Levi AJ. Elemental diet as primary treatment of acute Crohn's disease: a controlled trial. Br Med J 1984;288:1859–1862.
4. Mueller JM, Keller HW, Erasmi H, Pichlmaier H. Total parenteral nutrition as therapy in Crohn's disease—a prospective study. Br J Surg 1983;70:40–43.
5. Thawley C, Stadnik L. Nutrition information for ostomates. Wilmington medical center cancer program. National Cancer Institute Grant No. 2R18CA22071. 1980.
6. Cox BG, Wentworth AA. The ileal pouch procedure—a new outlook for the person with an ileostomy. Mayo Comprehensive Cancer Center. National Cancer Institute Contract No. 45120-B, 1977.
7. Division of colon and rectal surgery, Mayo Clinic. Ileo-anal anastomosis procedure. 1984.
8. Hessov I, Hasselblad C, Fasth S, Hultén L. Magnesium deficiency after ileal resections for Crohn's disease. Scand J Gastroenterol 1983;18:643–649.
9. Mandell I, Krauss E, Millan JC. Oxalate induced acute renal failure in Crohn's disease. Am J Med 1980;69:628–632.
10. Weser E. Nutritional aspects of malabsorption: short gut adaptation. Am J Med 1979;67:1014–1020.
11. Ecknauer R, Sircar B, Johnson LR. Effect of dietary bulk on small intestine morphology and cell renewal in the rat. Gastroenterology 1981;81:781–786.
12. MacMahon RA. The use of the World Health Organizations and rehydration solution in patients on home parenteral nutrition. JPEN 1984;8:720–721.
13. Mann GV. Diarrhea. Am J Clin Nutr 1975;28:804.

LACTOSE INTOLERANCE

General Description

Lactose is the primary carbohydrate in milk. Lactose restriction limits milk and milk products according to individual tolerance.

Nutritional Inadequacy

The diet may be low in calcium, in riboflavin and in vitamin D, depending upon the extent of lactose restriction and of age-related nutrient requirements. The Recommended Dietary Allowance (RDA) for all the aforementioned nutrients can be met through the use of lactase enzyme-treated milk and milk products. If these treated products are not used, supplementation may be indicated. In particular, the need for calcium supplementation should be considered for children, adolescents, postmenopausal women,[1] and for women who are at risk for developing osteoporosis. Calcium supplementation is generally contraindicated for individuals with hypercalcemia, hypercalciuria, or with a history of calcium-containing urolithiasis. The current practice is to recommend calcium supplements, usually calcium carbonate, to meet or to slightly exceed the RDA. (See *Appendix 12* for the calculation of the calcium content of foods and of supplements.) Vitamin D supplementation is necessary only if the individual has an inadequate exposure to sunlight. Vitamin D supplements should not exceed the RDA. Supplementary riboflavin is rarely indicated because of its availability from other foods.

Indications and Rationale

Lactase deficiency can be defined as a lowered level of intestinal lactase activity. Lactose intolerance is the condition of intestinal symptoms that follows the ingestion of lactose in a subject with lactase deficiency. It should be noted that a lactase-deficient subject may tolerate small amounts of milk without having symptoms, thus, the person is lactose tolerant. This same person may develop symptoms following an intake of greater quantities of lactose, and at that level of intake the person is considered lactose intolerant.[2] Lactase deficiency is generally not a debilitating disorder, but it can cause uncomfortable and unpleasant symptoms. It is, in fact, a "normal" condition, as the majority of people in the world have lactase deficiency. Lactose intolerance varies in degree among individuals who are affected and rarely signifies complete or total intolerance.

In the individual with sufficient lactase, lactose is hydrolyzed by the intestinal enzyme, lactase, into glucose and galactose. If the amount of the enzyme is insufficient to hydrolyze the lactose ingested, some undigested lactose remains in the intestine. Through osmotic effect, the undigested lactose causes water to be drawn into the digestive tract, which results in intestinal symptoms. The undigested lactose passes into the large bowel where it is fermented by normal colonic bacteria to form lactic acid and hydrogen. Symptoms of lactose intolerance include abdominal cramping, flatulence, and diarrhea and may occur shortly after the ingestion of lactose or a number of hours later. The severity of symptoms depends upon the amount of lactose that is ingested and the degree of intolerance to lactose.

The diagnosis of lactase deficiency can be determined by (1) a diet history that relates the intake of milk and of milk products to the symptoms, (2) a trial of a lactose-restricted diet and an observation of the elimination of the symptoms, (3) a hydrogen breath test to measure the hydrogen in the expired air following the metabolism of lactose (see page 511 for the discussion of diet in the preparation for a hydrogen breath test), (4) a small bowel biopsy to measure the lactase activity, and (5) a lactose tolerance test. The lactose tolerance test is performed by measuring the blood glucose levels following the ingestion of a lactose load. In the adult, an increase in the blood glucose that is less than 20 mg per deciliter after a 50 g lactose load is stongly suggestive of lactase deficiency.

The prevalence of lactase deficiency is high in many non-Caucasian populations, which includes blacks, orientals, Greeks, Jews, Mexicans, American Indians, and Aborigines. This is a primary intolerance with no history or signs of underlying intestinal disease.

Secondary lactase deficiency can occur in those with acute or chronic diseases that involve malabsorption, such as tropical or celiac sprue, or in those who have had small bowel or gastric surgery. Periods of disuse of the intestinal tract, such as is encountered with the extended use of central parenteral nutrition, may cause atrophy of the small intestine and hence lactase deficiency. The recovery from such functional impairment usually can be accomplished through the gradual resumption of the dietary intake over a period of several weeks.

Goals of Dietary Management

The goals of dietary management are to provide a nutritionally adequate diet and to minimize or to reduce symptoms to a level that the patient finds tolerable.

Dietary Recommendations

The tolerance of lactose varies among individuals. The following guidelines may be helpful for individuals who are suspected of or who are diagnosed as having lactase deficiency.

1. Initially consume a lactose-free diet. Establish the tolerance level by gradually adding small amounts of lactose-containing foods.

2. Most people can tolerate 5 to 8 g of lactose at a given time or the amount in 1/2 cup of milk.

3. Small amounts of lactose that are within the individual's tolerance level generally can be taken on several occasions throughout the day.

TABLE 6–34 Lactose Content of Foods

Lactose-Free Foods	Low Lactose Foods (0 to 2 g/serving)	
Broth-based soups	1/2 cup	Milk treated with lactase enzyme
Plain meat, fish, poultry, peanut butter	1/2 cup	Sherbet
Breads that do not contain milk, dry milk solids, or whey	1–2 oz	Aged cheese
Cereal, crackers	1 oz	Processed cheese
Fruit, plain vegetables		Butter or margine
Desserts made without milk, dry milk solids, or whey		Comercially-prepared foods containing dry milk solids or whey
Tofu and tofu products, such as tofu-based ice cream substitute		Some medications and vitamin preparations may contain a small amount of lactose. Generally, the amount is very small and is tolerated well.

High Lactose Foods (5 to 8 g/serving)			
1/2 cup	Milk (whole, skim, 1%, 2%, buttermilk, sweet acidophilus)	1/2 cup	White sauce
1/8 cup	Powdered dry milk (whole, nonfat, buttermilk—before reconstituting)	1/2 cup	Party chip dip or potato topping
		3/4 cup	Creamed or low fat cottage cheese
1/4 cup	Evaporated milk	1 cup	Dry cottage cheese
3 Tbsp	Sweetened condensed milk	3/4 cup	Ricotta cheese
3/4 cup	Heavy cream	2 oz	Cheese food or cheese spread*
1/2 cup	Half and Half	3/4 cup	Ice cream or ice milk
1/2 cup	Sour cream	1/2 cup	Yogurt†

*Lactose content is higher than that of aged cheese and of processed cheese because of the addition of whey powder and of dry milk solids.
†Yogurt may be tolerated better than foods with similar lactose content because of hydrolysis of lactose by bacterial lactase found in the culture.

4. Lactose is generally tolerated if it is taken along with food rather than taken alone as a beverage or as a snack.

5. Yogurt may be better tolerated than milk, since the bacterial lactase that is found in the yogurt culture hydrolyzes lactose, in addition to the hydrolysis that occurs in the intestinal tract.[3,4] However, tolerance to yogurt may vary with different brands and processing methods.

6. Lactase enzyme is available as Lactaid and may be added to the milk 24 hours in advance of ingestion. In addition, a tablet form is available that can be ingested just prior to eating a meal that contains lactose. Depending on the degree of intolerance, 1/2 to 3 tablets may be used.

7. Special commercially-prepared low lactose foods, including ice cream and cottage cheese, are available in some supermarkets and in some areas.

8. Lactobacillus acidophilus milk is not better tolerated than regular milk.[5,6]

Table 6–34 presents the lactose content of foods.

Physicians: How to Order Diet

The diet order should indicate *lactose-restricted diet*. The dietitian plans the diet according to the aforementioned guidelines and modifies the diet according to the needs and the tolerances of the patient.

REFERENCES

1. Metabolic bone disease as a result of lactase deficiency. Nutr Rev 1979;37:72–73.
2. Newcomer AD, McGill DB. Clinical importance of lactase deficiency. N Engl J Med 1984;310:42–43.
3. Kolars JC, Levitt MD, Mostafi Aouji DA, Savaiano DA. Yogurt—an autodigesting source of lactose. N Engl J Med 1984;310:1–3.
4. In vivo digestion of yogurt lactose by yogurt lactase. Nutr Rev 1984;42:216–217.
5. Newcomer AD, Park P, O'Brien PC, McGill DB. Response of patients with irritable bowel syndrome and lactase deficiency using unfermented acidophilus milk. Am J Clin Nutr 1983;38:257–263.
6. Savaiano DA, Abdiehak Abou El Anouar DA, Smith DE, Levitt MD. Lactose malabsorption from yogurt, pasteurized yogurt, sweet acidophilus milk, and cultured milk in lactase-deficient individuals. Am J Clin Nutr 1984;40:1219–1223.

PEPTIC ULCER DISEASE

General Description

Guidelines are given to avoid extreme elevations of gastric acid secretion. Generally, only slight modifications in the patient's usual diet are recommended.

Nutritional Inadequacy

Dietary modifications for pepic ulcer disease do not result in a diet that is inherently inadequate in nutrients when compared to the Recommended Dietary Allowance (RDA).

Indications and Rationale

Various bland and ulcer diets with progressive levels of intake have historically been used in the treatment of peptic ulcer disease (gastric and duodenal ulcers). In some instances, the rationale for these diets has been physiologically inappropriate and the food restrictions have been unwarranted. There is evidence that a bland or an ulcer diet is no more effective than a general diet in speeding the rate of ulcer healing and in reducing gastric acid secretion. Controlled trials in patients with a duodenal ulcer have shown that these diets do not hasten the remission of symptoms nor prevent recurrences.[1] However, bland and ulcer diets probably are not detrimental to most persons if they are used for a short time and may be of psychological benefit to some. Prolonged adherence to these regimens is not necessary.

Rough or coarse food has previously been excluded from bland diets on the presumption that it irritates the gastric mucosa. This effect has not been found to be true.[2]

Milk has been an important part of ulcer diets because it was believed to buffer gastric contents. While it is true that milk, in addition to many other foods, has a transient buffering effect, it tends to be a strong secretagogue, largely owing to its calcium and protein content. It has been found that whole, low-fat, and non-fat milk each produce a significant increase in mean gastric-acid secretion 2 to 3 hours after ingestion.[3] Since milk has only a transient buffering effect on gastric acid that is followed by a sustained rise in acid secretion, frequent milk ingestion for ulcer treatment is not encouraged.[4]

Spices, condiments, and fruit juices, although frequently producing dyspepsia, have not been shown to impair ulcer healing.[4] The spices most often implicated are black pepper, chili powder, and red pepper. Cocoa has also been cited as a gastric irritant.[2] The restriction of spices and of other foods should be determined by individual tolerances.

It is rational to recommend a restriction of stimulators of gastric acid secretion, which include regular coffee, other sources of caffeine, and decaffeinated coffee.[5] For many people, coffee is a cause of dyspepsia. The effect of coffee can be attenuated by consuming it with food.[4] A restriction of the consumption of coffee and of other beverages that are strong secretagogues should be encouraged.

Alcohol is thought to damage the gastric mucosa. During treatment for gastric ulcers, patients should be advised to minimize their alcoholic intake.[6]

Small volume, frequent feedings have not been found to be more effective than three meals per day in the long-term treatment of peptic ulcer disease. In fact, some authorities advise against extra feedings because they increase acid secretion[4,7] and may unduly complicate the patient's eating pattern.[8] However, some patients claim a relief of symptoms with frequent feedings, especially during the acute stages.

Goals of Dietary Management

The goals of dietary management are to avoid the hypersecretion of gastric acid and the direct irritation of gastric mucosa, which may delay the healing of the ulcer and the resolution of symptoms.

Dietary Recommendations

Limit or avoid coffee, decaffeinated coffee, caffeine-containing beverages, and alcoholic beverages. Also limit or avoid spices and foods that are not tolerated.

Physicians: How to Order Diet

The diet order should indicate *peptic ulcer precautions*.

REFERENCES

1. Baron JH, Wastell C. Medical treatment. In: Wastell C, ed. Chronic duodenal ulcer. London: Butterworth, 1972:126.
2. American Dietetic Association. Position paper on bland diet in the treatment of chronic duodenal ulcer disease. J Am Diet Assoc 1971;59:244–245.
3. Ippoliti AF, Maxwell V, Isenberg JI. The effect of various forms of milk on gastric acid secretion. Ann Intern Med 1976;84:286–289.
4. Soll AH, Isenberg JI. Duodenal ulcer. In: Sleisinger MH, Fordtran JS, eds. Gastrointestinal disease: pathophysiology, diagnosis, management. 3rd ed. Philadelphia: WB Saunders, 1983:655.
5. Cohen S, Booth GH, Jr. Gastric acid secretion and lower-esophageal-sphincter pressure in response to coffee and caffeine. N Engl J Med 1975;293:897–899.
6. Richardson CT. Gastric ulcer. In: Sleisinger MH, Fordtran JS, eds. Gastrointestinal disease: pathophysiology, diagnosis, management. 3rd ed. Philadelphia: WB Saunders, 1983:681.
7. Stapleton JF. Update in gastroenterology. Med Times 1981;109:31–34.
8. Center for Ulcer Research Education. Grossman MI, ed. Peptic ulcer: a guide for the practicing physician. Chicago: Yearbook Medical Publishers, 1981:82–83.

POSTGASTRECTOMY DUMPING SYNDROME

General Description

The dietary management of dumping syndrome is aimed at reducing the volume and the osmotic effect of food that enters the proximal small bowel, thereby preventing small bowel distention and late hypoglycemia. This can be achieved by (1) limiting the intake of mono- and disaccharides, (2) consuming small frequent meals, and (3) limiting fluids with meals. Because symptoms vary greatly in severity and duration, the diet should be individualized and modified according to the patient's symptoms.

Nutritional Inadequacy

The modifications for dumping syndrome do not result in a diet that is inherently inadequate in nutrients when compared to the Recommended Dietary Allowance (RDA). However, each individual's diet should be assessed for nutritional adequacy because of the variation in food tolerances. The long-term restriction of important nutrients may warrant supplementation (e.g., a calcium supplementation for the restriction of milk because of lactose intolerance).

Indications and Rationale

Dumping syndrome may develop as a complication of a total or subtotal gastrectomy or of any surgical procedure that removes, disrupts, or bypasses the pyloric sphincter.[1-3] As many as 20 to 40 percent of patients suffer from dumping symptoms immediately after surgery, but symptoms usually decrease with time; 5 to 10 percent of patients may suffer persisting disability because of dumping.[4] Occasionally, symptoms of dumping may appear for the first time after a period of months or years after surgery.

Dumping syndrome can be divided into early and late phases.[1,3-7] The intensity and duration of symptoms vary considerably with the individual, but there are common characteristics. The early phase occurs 15 to 30 minutes postprandially and is characterized by the gastrointestinal symptoms of epigastric fullness, abdominal cramps, vomiting, and/or diarrhea and the vasomotor symptoms of tachycardia, postural hypotension, sweating, weakness, flushing, and/or syncope. However, patients commonly experience the intestinal symptoms without the associated vasomotor phenomena or, conversely, may experience only vasomotor symptoms.

Most of the symptoms of the early phase are related to rapid gastric emptying with consequent distention of the jejunum. The hypertonicity of the jejunal contents produces a rapid and significant influx of fluid as the hyperosmolar content is diluted. The syndrome may be aggravated by the consumption of meals that are high in simple carbohydrate, and which increase the osmolality of the gastric contents and meals with large volumes of liquids, which enhance the rate of transfer of food from the stomach.[5] Symptoms of fullness, cramps, and vomiting can be attributed to the rapid jejunal filling. Diarrhea is attributable to the rapid entry of hypertonic liquids into the small intestine, thereby overwhelming its absorptive capacity and resulting in the passage of large volumes of unabsorbed material into the colon.[5]

Like the gastrointestinal symptoms, the vasomotor abnormalities can be evoked by the rapid filling of the jejunum with hypertonic material. This can cause a combination of autonomic reflexes, hemoconcentration that is secondary to a rapid osmotic shift of plasma fluid into the bowel lumen with a subsequent fall in the blood volume, and an excessive release of vasoactive hormones, all of which may account for many of the vasomotor symptoms.

The late phase occurs about 2 hours postprandially and is associated with symptoms that have been attributed to hypoglycemia, i.e., perspiration, hunger, nausea, anxiety, tremors, and/or weakness.[2] The late phase is seen much less frequently than the symptoms of early dumping.

The medical treatment of dumping syndrome consists almost entirely of dietary management.[2,3,5,7,8] Drug therapy is usually not effective, and surgical intervention may be necessary in severe cases.

Goals of Dietary Management

The goals of dietary management are to provide a nutritionally adequate diet and to reduce symptoms to a level that the patient finds tolerable. This can be achieved through manipulations and restrictions that are designed to normalize gastric emptying, thereby controlling the volume and the osmolality of food that enters the jejunum.[4,5,9-11]

Dietary Recommendations

Early satiety and the desire to ameliorate symptoms frequently result in a decreased food intake and a subsequent weight loss after gastric surgery. Kilocalories should be adjusted to meet the patient's needs with an increase of complex carbohydrate, protein, and fat to provide sufficient kilocalories. Table 6–35 presents the recommendations for postgastrectomy dumping syndrome.

TABLE 6–35 Dietary Recommendations for Postgastrectomy Dumping Syndrome

1. Small frequent meals are recommended to decrease the jejunal distention that is caused by the rapid emptying of a large meal.
2. Mono- and disaccharides should be kept to a minimum to prevent the formation of hyperosmolar intestinal contents. Sugar, honey, syrup, and foods with added sugar should be avoided initially and may need long-term limitation.
3. Tolerance to milk and to other lactose-containing products should be established by a gradual introduction into the diet.
4. Fluids should not be taken with meals, but may be taken 45 to 60 minutes before or after meals. Initially, it may be helpful to limit the volume of fluids to 4 oz per serving. The restriction of fluids is necessary to retard gastric emptying. Hypertonic liquids are emptied most rapidly.
5. Food should be eaten slowly in a relaxed setting. Lying down for 15 to 30 minutes after meals may help to decrease the rate of gastric emptying by reducing the effect of gravity.

Several months following gastrectomy, the patient's nutritional status should be assessed to determine whether or not malabsorption and/or dietary restriction are having adverse effects. Mild anemia is a common finding, generally developing several years after a partial or total gastrectomy.[4,5,10] The cause may be multifactorial and its presence should be assessed by monitoring serum iron, B_{12}, and folate levels. An inadequate intake as well as gastrointestinal blood loss may be contributing factors. Serum albumin should be monitored to determine whether maldigestion-malabsorption of protein and/or inadequate protein intake are causing protein malnutrition.

The vast majority of symptoms resolve or improve with time.[3,10,12] Increased food tolerance encourages the patient to begin liberalizing the diet. Only a few persons need to maintain the restrictions for extended periods of time. Most persons are able to identify their own levels of tolerance with guidance from the dietitian. Additional modifications of diet may be necessary for persons with malabsorption.

Physicians: How to Order Diet

The diet order should indicate *diet for postgastrectomy dumping syndrome*. The dietitian plans the diet according to the previously mentioned guidelines and modifies the diet according to the needs and tolerances of the patient.

REFERENCES

1. Herrington JL. Postgastrectomy syndromes. In: Bayless TM, ed. Current therapy in gastroenterology and liver disease, 1984–1985. Philadelphia: BC Decker, 1984:69.
2. Stabile BE, Passaro E. Duodenal ulcer: a disease in evolution. Curr Probl Surg 1984;21:1–79.
3. Cooperman AM. Postgastrectomy syndromes. Surg Annu 1981;13:139–161.
4. Smith FW, Jeffries GH. Late and persistent postgastrectomy problems. In: Sleisenger MH, Fordtran JS, eds. Gastrointestinal disease: pathophysiology, diagnosis, management. Philadelphia: WB Saunders, 1973:822–828.
5. Meyer JH. Chronic morbidity after ulcer surgery. In: Sleisenger MH, Fordtran JS, eds. Gastrointestinal disease: pathophysiology, diagnosis, management. 3rd ed. Philadelphia: WB Saunders, 1983:757–779.
6. Venobles CW, Wheldon EJ, Cranage JD. Adverse effects of gastric surgery for peptic ulceration. J R Coll Physicians Lond 1980;14:173–177.

7. Spiro HM. Postgastrectomy and post-vagotomy syndrome. In: Clinical gastroenter-ology. 3rd ed. New York: MacMillan, 1983:434.
8. Maniel JJ. Gastric emptying disorders. In: Nord HJ, Brady PJ, eds. Critical care gastroenterology. New York: Churchill Livingstone, 1982:123.
9. Williamson J. Physiological stress. Nutritional care for patients having surgery, trauma or burns. In: Krause MV, Mahan LK, eds. Food, nutrition, and diet therapy. 7th ed. Philadelphia: WB Saunders, 1984:689.
10. Alpers DH, Clouse RE, Stenson WF. Restrictive diets. In: Alpers DH, Clouse RE, Stenson WF, eds. Manual of nutritional therapeutics. 1st ed. Boston: Little, Brown and Company, 1983:279–328.
11. Goodhart RS, Shils ME. Appendix A-24. In: Goodhart RS, Shils ME, eds. Modern nutrition in health and disease. 6th ed. Philadelphia: Lea and Febiger, 1980:1294–1296.
12. Ralphs DNL. The dumping syndrome. Br J Clin Pract 1981;35:291–293.

HEPATOBILIARY DISEASE

HEPATIC ENCEPHALOPATHY

General Description

Protein, sodium, and fluid intakes are restricted according to individual needs.

Nutritional Inadequacy

The nutritional adequacy of diets for hepatic encephalopathy is similar to that of other protein-controlled diets. Potential amino acid deficiencies exist in diets that provide less total protein than the Recommended Dietary Allowances (RDA) of 0.8 g of protein per kilogram of body weight. To counter this risk, approximately 75 percent of the total protein intake should be high biologic value protein or complementary vegetable proteins. If the patient follows the diet for more than several weeks or has been previously malnourished, vitamin supplementation may be beneficial. Diets of 50 g of protein or less per day provide inadequate calcium, iron, phosphorous, thiamine, riboflavin, niacin, and folic acid by RDA criteria. Therefore, a daily multivitamin that includes folic acid is recommended. Natabec Rx is currently the preferred vitamin preparation because it provides 1 mg of folic acid and all other recommended vitamins in one tablet.

Indications and Rationale

Hepatic encephalopathy or coma is a potential and serious complication of advanced liver disease. It is seen in the presence of hepatic decompensation that is secondary to acute liver failure or in chronic liver disease with or without spontaneous or surgical portal systemic shunts.[1] Hepatic encephalopathy is associated with changes in conciousness, behavior, and neurologic status. Symptoms may include mild personality changes, apathy, slurred speech, disrupted sleep rhythms, asterixis, confusion, and drowsiness that progresses to coma. In chronic encephalopathy, symptoms may advance slowly, but are usually only episodic, and recovery to the premorbid state is common.

The cause of hepatic encephalopathy is unknown, but precipitating factors that are coupled with chronic liver disease have been identified. The three proposed general mechanisms that lead to hepatic coma[2] are (1) an accumulation of various toxins owing to impaired hepatic function (ammonia is the leading candidate), (2) an altered plasma amino acid composition (decreased ratio of branched chain to aromatic amino acids), and (3) an increase in serum and brain neuroinhibitory substances (increased gamma-aminobutyric acid [GABA] levels and augmented density of cerebral GABA receptors).[3]

A widely accepted concept is that hepatic encephalopathy is closely associated with increased levels of blood ammonia.[2,4] This increase can be caused by a decreased production of urea that results from impaired liver function, by an increased bacterial production of ammonia in the intestine from available nitrogenous substrates (dietary protein, gastrointestinal hemorrhage), by enterohepatic circulation of urea, by renal failure (the increased availability of urea for enterohepatic circulation), and by constipation (the increased ammonia production and the prolonged transit time, which allows increased absorption). Other proposed causes of hepatic encephalopathy include infection (increased catabolism of body protein coupled with abnormal ammonia metabolism), sedative abuse, diuretic overuse that causes fluid and electrolyte imbalances, anesthesia and surgery, elevated levels of blood mercaptans (methionine metabolites), and altered branched chain amino acid to aromatic amino acid ratio and its effect on neurotransmitter synthesis.[2,4] Acute hepatic encephalopathy in the absence of pre-existing liver disease usually is seen in conjunction with acute viral hepatitis or with drug-induced liver damage. The medical management of hepatic encephalopathy is aimed at the identification and the treatment of precipitating factors.[5] A fundamental principle of therapy is the removal of sources of excess ammonia.

Ammonia is a product of protein metabolism; therefore, dietary protein is generally restricted. However, sufficient protein and caloric intake are necessary to maintain nitrogen balance. Severe protein restriction is not always necessary and may actually be harmful by promoting the catabolism of lean body tissue. Metabolic abnormalities that are associated with liver disease (hyperglucagonemia and hyperinsulinemia) coupled with the needs for tissue repair may actually increase protein requirements for cirrhotic and for encephalopathic individuals.

Recent studies have explored the advantages of using nonmeat sources of dietary protein in the treatment of hepatic encephalopathy.[5-7] Vegetable and dairy products contain lower amounts of ammonia, methionine, and aromatic amino acids and have a higher branched chain amino acid content than meat protein. Branched chain amino acids are not catabolized by the liver, but are taken up preferentially by extrahepatic tissues. The metabolism of branched chain amino acids is not dependent on liver function, as is the case with other amino acids. Vegetable proteins also contain lower amounts of ammonia and of mercaptans. Compliance with vegetable protein diets is difficult because of anorexia and of early satiety (a frequent condition of hepatic encephalopathy), which precludes the ingestion of the increased volume of food that is needed to assure nutritional adequacy of the diet. A recent publication did not find significant differences regarding mental status, nitrogen balance, and plasma amino acids when a diet that consists of vegetable protein was compared with a diet that consists of animal protein.[8] The study also found that compliance to the regimen was more difficult for the vegetable protein diet. Although dairy protein sources have not been shown conclusively to be more advantageous than meat protein, it seems reasonable to use dairy protein sources to the extent that they are accepted by the patient. Oral supplementation or tube feeding of formulas that are high in branched chain amino acids and are low in aromatic amino acids have also been proposed.[2,5,8]

The sodium intake is often restricted because of the presence of edema and ascites. The fluid intake is often restricted because of associated renal failure and ascites.

Goals of Dietary Management

Nutritional therapy is generally directed at clinical manifestations of the disease rather than the etiology.[10] The goals of dietary management are to maintain adequate nutrition, to prevent the catabolism of body protein tissue, to control edema and ascites, and to prevent or to ameliorate symptoms of hepatic encephalopathy to the greatest possible extent.

Dietary Recommendations

The diet should be individualized according to the needs of each patient. Protein intake may be restricted to 0.25 g, 0.50 g, or perhaps, 0.75 g per kilogram of edema-free body weight in the early stages of hepatic encephalopathy or for patients who have compensated, but advanced, liver disease. To avoid muscle catabolism, the total protein content of the diets for hepatic encephalopathy should not be less than 35 to 50 g of protein per day.[2,4,5,10] Dairy protein sources (milk and cheese) should be used in preference to meat. Vegetable protein sources can be used to the degree the patient accepts them.

For patients whose symptoms are resistant to treatment with conventional low protein diets, the use of a high branched chain or low aromatic amino acid formula may be indicated.[9,10] The formula may be decreased as the oral intake of a low protein diet increases. There is a limited benefit to oral supplementation with the formula for patients who are able to take more than 50 g per day of protein from food.[9]

The caloric intake should be sufficient to prevent the catabolism of body protein for energy. Caloric needs are generally not unusually high unless the patient is extremely restless or agitated. Many patients are anorexic and drowsy and may have difficulty consuming enough kilocalories.

The sodium intake may be restricted to 20 mEq or less if ascites is present. A sodium intake of 90 mEq or less is appropriate if ascites and edema are not present and if the patient is not in a positive sodium balance, therefore retaining fluid. However, a rapid gain in weight may indicate that some fluid is being retained and that the sodium level may need to be reduced to 40 mEq or less.

The fluid intake is variable. It is controlled carefully in relation to the urinary output, changes in weight, and serum electrolyte values.

The diet for hepatic encephalopathy should be planned with the use of the exchange list for protein, for sodium, and for potassium control. (See page 235. The potassium controls can be disregarded.)

Physicians: How to Order Diet

The diet order should indicate (1) the *specific level of protein*. The most common levels are 0.25 g, 0.50 g, and 0.75 g per kilogram of edema-free body weight; (2) the *specific level of sodium*. The most common levels are 20, 40, and 90 mEq. If there is a positive sodium balance the level given should be able to put the patient into a negative sodium balance; and (3) the *specific level of fluid*. The dietitian calculates the caloric needs.

REFERENCES

1. Fraser CL, Arieff AI. Hepatic encephalopathy. N Engl J Med 1985;313:865–873.
2. Bernardini P, Fischer JE. Amino acid imbalance and hepatic encephalopathy. In: Darby WJ, Broquist HP, Olson RE, eds. Annual review of nutrition, Vol. 2. Palo Alto: Annual Reviews, 1982;419.
3. Schafer DF, Jones EA. Hepatic encephalopathy and the gamma-aminobutyric acid neurotransmitter system. Lancet 1982;1:18–20.
4. Mezey E. Liver disease and protein needs. In: Darby WJ, Broquist HP, Olson RE, eds. Annual review of nutrition, Vol. 2. Palo Alto: Annual Reviews, 1982;21.
5. Crossley IR, Williams R. Progress in the treatment of chronic portosystemic encephalopathy. Gut 1984;25:85–98.
6. Uribe M, Márquez MA, Ramos GG, Ramos-Uribe MH, Vargas F, Villalobas A, Ramos C. Treatment of chronic portal-systemic encephalopathy with vegetable and animal protein diets: a controlled crossover study. Dig Dis Sci 1982;27:1109–1116.
7. Misra P. Hepatic encephalopathy IV: Symposium on acute medical illness. Med Clin North Am 1981;65:209–226.
8. Shaw S, Warner TM, Lieber CS. Comparison of animal and vegetable protein sources in the dietary management of hepatic encephalopathy. Am J Clin Nutr 1983;38:59–63.
9. Skipper A. Specialized formulas for enteral nutrition support. J Am Diet Assoc 1986;86:654–658.
10. Jacobs DO, Boraas MC, Rombeau JL. Enteral nutrition and liver disease. In: Rombeau JL, Caldwell MD, eds. Clinical nutrition Vol I: enteral and tube feeding. Philadelphia: WB Saunders, 1984:376.

LIVER TRANSPLANT

General Description

Liver transplantation has recently proved to be an effective treatment for patients with end-stage liver disease.

Many patients with liver failure have the signs and the symptoms of protein-calorie malnutrition that are related to the effects of liver disease.[1] Nutritional intervention is dependent upon the type and the extent of the liver disease (see sections on *Hepatobiliary Disease*) and its impact on the nutritional status as identified through nutritional assessment (see sections on *Nutritional Assessment*). The optimum nutritional intake by oral feeding, by enteral tube feeding, or by the parenteral route is essential to support successful liver transplantation. Table 6–36 describes the dietitian's role during the three phases of liver transplantation, which are pre-transplant, immediate post-transplant, and follow-up.

TABLE 6–36 Dietitians' Role—Liver Transplantation

Pre-transplant
   Nutritional Assessment: Anthropometric measurements, biochemical data, dietary history, and evaluation of nutrient intake
   Nutritional Intervention: Modify diet, provide specialized nutritional support to optimize intake according to disease state and patient's nutritional status
   Low Bacteria Diet: Implement in anticipation of transplant

Immediate Post-Transplant
   Monitor Nutritional Status: Biochemical data, nutrient intake, anthropometrics
   Nutritional Intervention: Central Parenteral Nutrition, (CPN) (initiate within 12 to 36 hr post-transplant), oral diet (initiate within 48 to 72 hr post-transplant)—high protein, high kilocalorie as can be achieved, low bacteria diet. When oral food intake achieves 1,500 Kcal, decrease CPN; consider enteral tube feeding or oral supplements when oral intake is inadequate
   Nutrition Education: Begin in anticipation of dismissal

Outpatient Follow-up 6 wk, 3 mo, 6 mo, and annually post-transplant.
   Nutritional Assessment: Biochemical data, anthropometrics
   Evaluation of Nutrient Intake: One- to three-day food intake records (kilocalories, protein, fat, sodium)

REFERENCE

1. Henir DJ, Jenkins RL, Bistrian BR, Blackburn GI. Nutrition in patients undergoing orthotopic liver transplant. JPEN 1985;9:695–700.

Low Bacteria Diet

General Description

When the decision is made to proceed with liver transplantation, a low bacteria diet is initiated in the pre-transplant period. It is continued in the post-transplantation phase whenever selective bowel decontamination measures are in effect.

The diet (Table 6–37) restricts foods that contain gram-negative bacteria and some yeasts. Food handling and food preparation practices (Table 6–38) that minimize bacterial contamination are recommended. Practices that are likely to promote bacterial growth are also to be avoided. Individuals who must con-

TABLE 6–37 Low Bacteria Diet

Food Groups	Allow	Avoid*
Meat	All	All cheese and cottage cheese products
Fat	Butter, margarine, oil	None
Milk	All	None
Starch	All	None
Vegetables	All cooked vegetables	All raw vegetables (including salads and garnishes)
Fruit	Fresh fruit washed and peeled; fruit juices; canned & frozen fruit	Fresh fruit with peels that are consumed (grapes, cherries, berries, etc.)

*Avoid all foods that are kept heated or at room temperature for long periods of time (soups, gravies, sauces, and combination foods) when eating in restaurants.

TABLE 6–38   Low Bacteria Food Preparation and Handling Practices*

Practice careful handwashing prior to all food preparation

Defrost frozen foods in the refrigerator or microwave rather than at room temperature

Serve foods soon after preparation; avoid holding heated and room temperature foods for long periods of time

Properly store leftovers (cover and freeze or refrigerate quickly); use refrigerated leftovers within 2 days of preparation

*Individuals who must follow a low-bacteria diet beyond hospitalization should be informed of appropriate food selection and preparation practices for home and restaurant dining.

tinue a low bacterial diet beyond hospitalization are informed of appropriate food selection and preparation practices.

Nutritional Inadequacy

The diet is similar to the general hospital diet and is not inherently inadequate in nutrients as compared to the Recommended Dietary Allowance (RDA). A daily multiple vitamin supplement, which provides nutrients at a level that is equivalent to the RDA, is recommended for persons who consume diets of 1,200 Kcal or less or for those with food aversions or intolerances that greatly limit the variety of food choices. During the transition from central parenteral nutrition to oral intake, vitamins and minerals at levels that meet the RDA are provided parenterally.

Indications and Rationale

A low bacteria diet, in conjunction with selective bowel decontamination measures, is initiated pre-transplant and is continued into the post-transplant period. The low bacteria diet and the prophylactic administration of antibiotics reduce gram-negative and fungal flora in the gastrointestinal tract.[1–4] The risk of bacterial and of fungal infection for the immunosuppressed patient is thereby reduced during the early post-transplant course.

Physicians: How to Order Diet

The diet order should indicate *low-bacteria diet*. Additional dietary modifications that may be necessary (e.g., sodium restriction) should also be indicated. The dietitian determines the appropriate caloric level and the other characteristics of the diet based on nutritional assessment, patient tolerance, and discussion with the physician.

REFERENCES

1. Wiesner RH, Hermans P, Rakela J, Perkins J, Washington J, DiCecco S, Krom RAF. Selective bowel decontamination to prevent gram-negative bacterial and fungal infection following orthotopic liver transplantation. Transplantation Proc 1987;xix:2420–2423

2. Remington JS, Schimpff SC. Occasional notes: please don't eat the salads. N Engl J Med 1981;304:433–435.

3. Alar SN, Cheney CL. The use of sterile and low-microbial diets in ultra-isolation environments. JPEN 1983;7:390–397.

4. Washington J. Personal Communication. Mayo Clinic Laboratories, 1985.

COPPER METABOLISM

General Description

A goal of medical management of hepatobiliary disease that affects copper metabolism is the achievement of a negative copper balance. A copper-restricted diet may be used as an adjunct to copper chelating medications. Copper is widely distributed in foods and does not occur exclusively in particular groups of foods. Foods have been categorized as high, moderate, or low in copper content. A low copper diet (less than 2 mg of copper per day) can be achieved by restricting foods with a high copper content; a very low copper diet (less than 1 mg of copper per day) can be achieved by restricting foods with a high and a moderate copper content.

Nutritional Inadequacy

The low copper diet is not so restrictive that it imposes the danger of nutritional inadequacy. However, a very low copper diet greatly limits the variety of foods and may, therefore, increase the risk of nutritional imbalance. The diet of persons on a very low copper diet should be carefully evaluated. If the use of a vitamin-mineral supplement is warranted, it should be free of copper.

Patients who are taking D-penicillamine may be at risk for a vitamin B_6 deficiency because of the possible antipyridoxine effect of the drug. It is standard practice to use 25 mg daily of vitamin B_6 for patients who are on D-penicillamine therapy.

Indications and Rationale

A copper-restricted diet may be indicated in the treatment of Wilson's disease, of primary biliary cirrhosis (PBC), and of primary sclerosing cholangitis (PSC). These disorders are associated with the excessive accumulation of copper in various tissues.

Wilson's disease (hepatolenticular degeneration) is an inherited disorder of copper metabolism that is characterized by the abnormal transport and storage of copper.[1] Copper accumulates primarily in the liver, brain, kidney, and cornea and has a toxic effect on these tissues. The primary metabolic defect is in the liver, where copper accumulates in lysosomes as the disease progresses. A block of lysosomal copper excretion may explain the decrease in biliary copper excretion. Also, there is a decrease in the incorporation of copper into the ceruloplasmin, which is the main mechanism for copper transport. Symptoms include hepatic, neurologic, and psychiatric dysfunction.

Long-term therapy consists primarily of the use of a copper chelating agent such as D-penicillamine to keep the patient in a negative copper balance. If the treatment with D-penicillamine alone does not achieve negative copper balance, a low or very low copper diet may be an appropriate adjunct. Treatment usually improves neurologic and hepatic function. Furthermore, treatment of asymptomatic patients with Wilson's disease with D-penicillamine and diet usually prevents the occurrence of signs and of symptoms.

Primary biliary cirrhosis (PBC) is also associated with the excessive storage of copper. Excessive concentrations of copper are found in the liver, in the spleen, and in the kidney, but not, as in Wilson's disease, in the brain. PBC is a chronic

TABLE 6–39   Copper Content of Foods*[6-8]

Food Groups	High (>0.2 mg/portions commonly used[†])	Moderate (0.1 to 0.2 mg/portions commonly used[†])	Low (0.1 mg/portions commonly used[†])
Meat and Meat Substitutes	Lamb; pork; pheasant; quail; duck; goose; salmon; all organ meats including liver, heart, kidney, brain; all shellfish, including oysters, scallops, shrimp, lobster, clams, and crab; meat gelatin; soy protein meat substitutes; tofu; all nuts and seeds	All other fish; turkey; peanut butter; chicken	Beef; cheese; cottage cheese; eggs; cold cuts and frankfurters that do not contain pork, turkey, or organ meats
Fats and Oils	Avocado	Olives	All Others
Milk	Chocolate; cocoa		All other dairy products; milk flavored with carob
Starch	Dried beans including soybeans, lima beans, baked beans, garbanzo beans, pinto beans; dried peas; lentils; millet; barley; wheat germ; bran breads and cereals; granola; soy flour; soy grits; fresh sweet potatoes	Whole wheat bread; potatoes in any form; pumpkin; melba toast; whole wheat crackers; parsnips; winter squash; green peas; instant oatmeal; instant ralston; some ready-to-eat dry cereals (check labels); dehydrated and canned soups	All others
Vegetables	Mushrooms; broccoli	Bean sprouts; beets; spinach; summer and winter squash; tomato juice and other tomato products	All others, including fresh tomatoes
Fruits	Nectarines; dried fruits including raisins, dates, and prunes (Dried fruits are permitted if dried at home)	Mango; pears; pineapple; papaya; orange juice; cranberry juice cocktail; grape juice	All others
Desserts	Desserts that contain significant amounts of any foods high in copper		All others
Sugar and sweets	Chocolate; cocoa	Licorice; carbonated beverages; syrups	All others including jams, jellies, and candies made with allowed fruits; carob; flavoring extracts
Miscellaneous	Brewers Yeast	Ketchup	
Beverages[‡]	Instant breakfast beverages; mineral water[†]; alcohol[§]	Postum, and other cereal beverages	All others including fruit-flavored beverages; lemonade

* Data that are available on the average copper content of foods vary greatly. There is disagreement on the copper content of the usual American diet, with estimates that range from 1 mg of copper a day to 2 to 5 mg a day. The concentration of copper in foods is affected by many factors, including soil conditions, geographic location, species, diet, processing method, and contamination in processing. The exact copper content of the foods is difficult to verify. It is estimated that avoidance of high copper foods results in a diet of approximately 2 mg/day; avoidance of both high and moderate copper foods results in a diet of approximately 1 mg/day. For practical purposes, the diets are designed to limit foods that tend to have a higher copper content than other foods, and not to achieve a specific level of copper in the diet.

† Portions commonly used are those that are generally accepted as typical portion sizes in various nutrient data source manuals.

‡ A water sample from the patient's home water supply should be analyzed for copper content. Demineralized water should be used if the water contains more than 100 μg per liter.

§ Although not necessarily high in copper, alcoholic beverages are discouraged because of their action as a hepatotoxin.

disease of unknown cause characterized by a progressive destruction of the intrahepatic bile ducts, which leads eventually to cirrhosis. The initial clinical findings are usually pruritus and jaundice.

Primary sclerosing cholangitis (PSC) is a chronic hepatobiliary disease that is associated with inflammation and fibrosis of the bile ducts inside and outside of the liver.[2] Under these circumstances, excess copper accumulates in the liver cells of some patients. The symptoms of PSC are similar to those of PBC. For both disorders, neither a definitive cause nor a curative treatment have been identified.

Initial treatment efforts for PBC and for PSC were limited to efforts to deplete the liver stores of copper and to alleviate symptoms. The original rationale for the use of D-penicillamine in PBC and in PSC is that these diseases were associated with elevated hepatic copper stores as in Wilson's disease.[3] D-penicillamine has been shown to be effective in the treatment of Wilson's disease. However, three controlled trials for PBC and one for PSC in the use of D-penicillamine have shown no beneficial effect of this agent over a placebo in either disease. Currently, copper-restricted diets are not routinely used in the treatment of PBC and of PSC.[4,5] However, current recommendations for the treatment of PBC and PSC may, in some circumstances, include a low copper diet (less than 2 mg of copper per day). Since the efficacy of this therapeutic approach has not been established in either disease, any decision that regards such an approach should be made in conjunction with a physician.

Goals of Dietary Management

The restriction of copper is not routinely advised for patients with Wilson's disease, PBC, or PSC. If D-penicillamine alone does not achieve a negative cop per balance, a copper-restricted diet may be indicated. The diet is considered adjunctive to D-penicillamine.

Dietary Recommendations. A diet very low in copper (less than 1 mg/day) allows only foods of low copper content. All the foods that are listed as having moderate or high copper content should be avoided.

A diet that is low in copper (less than 2 mg/day) allows foods of low and moderate copper content. Foods of high copper content should be avoided. Table 6–39 presents the copper content of foods.

Physicians: How to Order Diet

The diet order should indicate *low copper diet* (avoidance of high copper foods) or *very low copper diet* (avoidance of moderate and high copper foods).

REFERENCES

1. Dobyns WB, Goldstein NP, Gordon H. Clinical spectrum of Wilson's disease (hepatolenticular degeneration). Mayo Clin Proc 1979;54:35–42
2. Alberti-Flor JJ, Avent GR, Dunn GD. Primary sclerosing cholangitis. South Med J 1985;78:173–177.
3. James OF. D-penicillamine for PBC. Gut 1985;26:109–113.
4. Smithgall JM. The copper controlled diet: Current aspects of dietary copper restriction in management of copper metabolism disorders. J Am Diet Assoc 1985;35:609–611.

5. Kaplan MM. Primary biliary cirrhosis. N Engl J Med 1987;316:521–528.
6. Leveille GA, Zabik ME, Morgan KJ. Nutrients in foods. Cambridge, MA: The Nutrition Guild, 1983.
7. Hook L, Brandt IK. Copper content of some low-copper food. J Am Diet Assoc 1966;49:202–203.
8. Pennington JAT, Church HN. Bowes and Church's food values of portions commonly used. 14th ed. Philadelphia: JB Lippincott, 1985.

HYPOGLYCEMIA

General Description

For hypoglycemia that results from islet cell tumors and other neoplasms, idiopathic hypoglycemia of childhood, and ketotic hypoglycemia, food is given at frequent intervals in amounts that are necessary to prevent symptoms. Sugars need not be specifically avoided and are particularly useful for the rapid correction of symptoms.

For reactive hypoglycemia, if this is fully documented, the meal plan can be that for diabetes. Large amounts of sucrose and of other simple carbohydrates should be avoided. If three regular meals are not well-tolerated, smaller feedings at intervals of 2 to 3 hours may, by trial, be tolerated better.

Nutritional Inadequacy

There are no nutritional inadequacies inherent in the dietary recommendations for hypoglycemia.

Indications and Rationale

Hypoglycemia may result from many causes; classifications have been published.[1,2] Only those categories that involve dietary factors are discussed here.

Hypoglycemia that occurs with islet cell tumors and with some extrapancreatic tumors is elicited by the deprivation of food and tends to become progressively more severe with an increasing duration of fasting. The treatment is surgical. Trials of diet as definitive therapy are inappropriate. While the patient awaits the arrangements for surgery or if surgery has not succeeded in removing the tumor, feedings should be given often enough to prevent symptoms. Although a gain in weight is not necessarily characteristic of such patients, obesity could become a problem if large, frequent feedings are used to prevent symptoms for a substantial period. The carbohydrate and the protein content of the diet should be emphasized, since fat is largely ineffective in correcting hypoglycemia and would contribute additional kilocalories. Sugars rapidly correct symptoms and need not be avoided. Carbohydrates that are more slowly absorbed than sugar may be preferable for preventing symptoms, since they may extend the intervals between feedings.

Idiopathic hypoglycemia of infancy and ketotic hypoglycemia occur in infants and in children up to about 5 years of age. Food appropriate for the child's age should be given in frequent feedings. Again, sugars need not be specifically avoided. Ketotic hypoglycemia tends to resolve spontaneously, but idiopathic hypoglycemia of infancy may require subtotal pancreatectomy or drugs, such as diazoxide.

Hypoglycemia that occurs 1 to 3 hours after a meal and resolves spontaneously can be termed "reactive hypoglycemia." "Reactive hypoglycemia" is a diagnosis often made mistakenly in persons with anxiety or with panic attacks to explain different symptoms that occur throughout the day but have some relation to meals.[3,4] Commonly, the anxious patient feels somewhat better on a high protein diet that is designated for hypoglycemia. The patient considers partial relief of the symptoms to confirm the diagnosis of "hypoglycemia", whereas the real cause of the symptoms is anxiety, and the apparent response to the diet may be the result of suggestion. The symptoms of anxiety and of hypoglycemia are qualitatively similar, since both are mediated by the release of epinephrine.

The diagnosis of reactive hypoglycemia that is severe enough to cause significant symptoms can be established if plasma glucose levels of less than 40 mg per deciliter after ordinary meals are associated with symptoms of epinephrine release, such as tachycardia and feelings of apprehension and of anxiety. Symptoms should either spontaneously abate in an hour or less or be relieved promptly, consistently, and completely by the ingestion of carbohydrate. A rapid decrease in the glucose concentration itself does not provoke epinephrine release and cannot be invoked as a cause for symptoms if the glucose level is well above 40 mg per deciliter at the time of symptoms. Plasma glucose levels of less than 40 mg per deciliter may occur in normal, asymptomatic persons during the course of the oral glucose tolerance test. Epinephrine-release symptoms that coincide with the nadir of the plasma glucose concentration in the glucose tolerance test is only circumstantial evidence that symptoms that occur after ordinary meals are hypoglycemic in origin, since the glucose tolerance test is a challenge to glucose homeostasis in excess of that posed by ordinary meals.

A recent study[5] of patients who regarded themselves as having "reactive hypoglycemia" showed that the symptoms that follow the ingestion of glucose coincided with the low point of the blood glucose no more than one might expect by chance. There was no significant difference in insulin, glucose, or glucagon levels between those subjects who had symptoms and those without. When the subjects were given a standard test meal, no significant hypoglycemia occurred, although some of the subjects had characteristic symptoms. These findings suggest that one should be very skeptical of the diagnosis of reactive hypoglycemia unless one can demonstrate that blood sugar levels are significantly and consistently low at the time of symptoms during the course of an ordinary day with ordinary meals. One should not rely on the glucose tolerance test alone for the diagnosis.[5]

Documented reactive hypoglycemia with significant symptoms is rare. The disorder sometimes occurs in persons who have had gastric surgery, but the symptoms of "dumping" (see page 170) should be clearly distinguished from those of hypoglycemia. Hypoglycemia that occurs at the fourth hour or later in the glucose tolerance test has been said to predict the later occurrence of diabetes, although this is not clearly established.

The dietary management of reactive hypoglycemia consists of avoiding simple carbohydrates. If several larger feedings of protein, fat, and slowly absorbed carbohydrate are followed by distress, small feedings may be tried. The frequency of feedings may need to be increased to provide the necessary caloric intake. The restriction of slowly absorbed carbohydrate generally does not relieve symptoms. The meal plans for diabetes offer a reasonable general guide to diet planning in reactive hypoglycemia (see page 182).

Goals of Dietary Management

The goal of dietary management is to minimize the patient's symptoms or to reduce them to a level that the patient finds tolerable.

Physicians: How to Order Diet

The diet order should indicate *diet for reactive hypoglycemia*. If the disorder is indicated, the dietitian determines the appropriate modifications according to the guidelines given and to the tolerances of the patient.

REFERENCES

1. Service FJ. Hypoglycemias. Compr Ther 1976;2:27–31.
2. Fajans SS, Floyd JC Jr. Fasting hypoglycemia in adults. N Engl J Med 1976;294:766–772.
3. Gastineau CF. Is reactive hypoglycemia a clinical entity? Mayo Clin Proc 1983;58:545–549.
4. Nelson RL. Hypoglycemia: fact or fiction? Mayo Clin Proc 1985;60:844–850.
5. Hogan MJ, Service FJ, Sharbrough FW, Gerich JE. Oral glucose tolerance test compared with a mixed meal in the diagnosis of reactive hypoglycemia: a caveat on stimulation. Mayo Clin Proc 1983;58:491–496.

OBESITY

General Description

The management of obesity includes an individualized assessment of the need for weight loss and the determination of appropriate weight goals. The treatment may include dietary, exercise, behavior and/or psychological intervention; emphasis on a particular treatment modality is dependent upon individual circumstances. In general, dietary recommendations include a moderate caloric restriction and modifications in the meal pattern and in the selection of foods.

Nutritional Inadequacy

Diets that are recommended for a weight reduction are not inherently inadequate as compared to the Recommended Dietary Allowance (RDA). However, for diets of 1,200 Kcal or less, it is difficult to meet the RDA consistently. A daily multiple vitamin supplement that provides nutrients at a level that is equivalent to the RDA is recommended for persons who consume diets of 1,200 Kcal or less. High potency or "therapeutic" vitamin and mineral supplements are rarely indicated. A multiple vitamin supplement may also be warranted for persons who have food aversions or intolerances that greatly limit the variety of food choices.

Indications and Rationale

Obesity is not a single disorder, but rather a heterogeneous group of disorders that are associated with varying types and degrees of risk for morbidity and for mortality.[1,2] Management decisions should be based on the evaluation of risk and the consideration of contributing and predisposing factors. The salient questions in the management of obesity are what risks does obesity pose to an individual (i.e., who has a medical need for weight loss), how much weight should an individual lose, and how should the weight loss be accomplished.[2]

The causes of obesity in most persons are unknown. Excess energy intake relative to expenditure is simply a statement of the conditions that are required for the deposition of lipids in the adipocytes and not the cause of the caloric imbalance. Although the underlying causes of obesity have not been clearly elucidated, consideration of predisposing factors and of attendant circumstances promote the formulation of a potentially more effective treatment plan.

There have been numerous attempts in the past to classify human obesities,[2] but these schemes have not been shown to be practical from a clinical standpoint. Progress is being made in characterizing persons with obesity;[2] however, newer concepts promise a more rational and differentiated approach to the prevention and the intervention in the future and provide a useful guide for the evaluation and the treatment now. The types of data of interest include personal and demographic data, developmental patterns, family history, energy balance, body composition and fat distribution, psychological and behavioral measures, endocrine and metabolic measures, and complications and associated conditions.[2]

Personal and Demographic Data. Personal and demographic data include age, sex, education, occupation, and socioeconomic status. It has been estimated that as much as a third of the variance in body weight can be accounted for by socioeconomic factors.[3] In the United States, in general, the higher the socioeconomic level, the lower the prevalence of obesity, especially for women. In other societies, particularly in nonindustrialized societies, the pattern is generally reversed.

Developmental Patterns. Developmental data include the age of onset of obesity, the identifiable circumstances that are associated with the onset of obesity, and the maximum and minimum adult weight.[3] The individual's personal history of weight gain and loss and of associated events (such as puberty, pregnancy, forced inactivity, and psychological factors) may give some indications of the pathophysiologic mechanisms that are involved and provides information that is important in determining appropriate weight goals. Periods of rapid and substantial weight gain that are then sustained at any age, but particularly during early or late childhood, suggest hyperplasia of fat cells.[4] Individuals with hyperplastic obesity can reduce their fat cell size yet remain overweight because of large fat cell numbers.[4] This is probably of greater social and psychological consequence than the health risk since the reduction in fat cell size tends to correct most metabolic abnormalities.[5] In addition, persons who have been overweight for a prolonged period of time may have increased muscle mass, which is described as a "weight-lifter effect."[6] Individuals who have historically been lean and then gain weight with life-style and activity changes are probably at a greater risk for health consequences, even with a lesser amount of excess weight, especially if the weight gain is centrally distributed and the individual has co-existing medical conditions that are affected by obesity (e.g., diabetes, hyperlipidemia, hypertension, or a family history of these disorders).

Family History. A review of the individual's family background should consider the prevalence of obesity and of medical conditions that are associated with obesity (diabetes, hyperlipidemia, and hypertension). Recent research suggests that there is a significant genetic component for obesity.[7] The occurrance of truly morbid obesity (arbitrarily defined as 100 percent or 100 lb above the height-weight table norms) in individuals who have absolutely no family history of obesity is rare. Such individuals probably deserve more thorough evaluations for other factors such as endocrine and central nervous system abnormalities or severe psychiatric disturbances. There is evidence that cardiovascular risks of obesity cluster in families with associated conditions such as hyperlipidemia, noninsulin-dependent diabetes mellitus, and hypertension.[8] A family history of these conditions carries a different prognostic significance than if family members tend to live into old age without obesity-related complications, in spite of being heavier than average.

Energy Balance. Both caloric expenditure and caloric intake should be considered. Caloric expenditure can be estimated by the use of the Mayo Clinic nomogram or Harris-Benedict equation (see *Nutritional Assessment,* page 7). Indirect calorimetry measurements of the resting metabolic rate may be useful for some individuals, particularly for those who have been unsuccessful despite persistent attempts to restrict their caloric intake or for those who have severe misconceptions regarding caloric needs. The caloric intake and, perhaps, the meal pattern affect the metabolic rate. Very low kilocalorie diets result in a reduction in the metabolic rate that is greater than can be accounted for by a loss of weight.[9] This is an adaptation to periods of semi-starvation that is thought to be mediated by the reduced adrenergic autonomic nervous system activity and potentiated by the reduced conversion of thyroxine (T_4) to triiodothyronine (T_3). These changes may account for many of the symptoms that are experienced by patients on low and very low kilocalorie diets, including cold intolerance, postural hypotension, and gastrointestinal motility disturbances.[9] Recent evidence suggests that skipping meals is associated with lower resting metabolic rates than eating three or more times daily.[10] Persons with "night-eating syndrome" who skip breakfast, eat little or no food at lunch, and consume a large percentage of their caloric intake in the evening often have resting metabolic rates 5 to 10 percent below predicted.[10] A history of exercise patterns is useful in determining the contribution of physical activity to the caloric expenditure and in assessing the overall contributions of inactivity to the development of obesity.

An assessment of the caloric intake can include an approximation of the total caloric intake and should include the daily meal-snack pattern, the day-to-day variations in the intake, the frequency of very low kilocalorie diets and of binge eating, the variety of foods that are eaten with particular attention to the proportion of the intake that is contributed by fat, sugar, and alcohol, and the circumstances that are associated with changes in the eating behavior, such as psychological factors. Very low kilocalorie diets or the perception of frequent restriction and deprivation increase the likelihood of periods of rebound, uncontrolled overeating, a phenomena known as restrained eaters' syndrome.[11] A preference for calorically dense, highly palatable foods is variable, but an intake of these foods may enhance the likelihood of consuming excess kilocalories through a variety of mechanisms, including decreased gastric distention with smaller volumes of calorically concentrated foods and the overriding of satiety indicators. Frequent snacking and binge eating may be part of an individual's means of dealing with boredom, anxiety, or stress. The role of diet in the etiology of obesity remains unclear. Reports of eating habits and of food choices of obese and nonobese persons have provided conflicting data, but, on the whole, have not substantiated the view that the obese have major differences in food choices or in eating patterns[12] or in responsiveness to environmental stimuli.[13] Nonetheless, an assessment of dietary intake, of pattern, and of influencing factors can guide the recommendations for treatment.

Body Composition. Measurements of height and weight are important for obvious reasons. Standard height-weight tables can serve as an initial reference; however, their usefulness is limited. Of greater importance in establishing goals for the individual patient are other assessment data, such as developmental pattern, family history and complications or associated conditions. An estimation of percent body fat (see *Nutritional Assessment,* page 3) may be useful for determining the degree of obesity and the weight goals for some patients. The concept of body composition also includes the measures of fat cell size and the number and pattern of fat distribution. A measurement of fat cell size is not practical in the clinical setting. However, the developmental pattern may suggest the likelihood of increased fat cell numbers. There is evidence of regional differences in adipocyte metabolism, including responsiveness to lipolytic stimuli.[14] The distribution of fat that has been described as central, abdominal, truncal, or upper body obesity is associated with a greater risk of noninsulin-dependent diabetes, glucose intolerance, hyperinsulinemia, hyperlipidemia, and coronary artery disease than lower body, hip and thigh, or gynecoid distribution patterns.[5,15] A fat distribution pattern can be documented with measurements of the waist or the hip circumference and expressed as the waist-hip ratio.[15]

Psychological and Behavioral Measures. There is no consistent psychological profile among obese persons,[16] and there is not unanimity of opinion as to the best means of assessing these variables. In the clinical setting, it is often practical only for the physician or for the dietitian to make subjective determinations of psychologically related behavior patterns and of the patient's motivation and confidence in his or her ability to influence or to improve his or her situation.

Complications and Associated Conditions. Disorders clearly associated with obesity include noninsulin-dependent diabetes, hypertension, hyperlipidemia, hyperuricemia, and some types of cancers.[17] Cancers of the colon, the rectum, and the prostate are more common in obese males than in lean males. In obese females, there is a higher mortality from cancer of the gallbladder, the biliary ducts, the breast (postmenopausal), the uterus (cervix and endometrium), and the ovaries.[17] Obesity may be a complicating factor in severe cardiopulmonary disorders, such as sleep apnea, and musculoskeletal impairments, such as degenerative joint disease and chronic low back pain. Complications with general anesthesia and following some types of surgery are more common among very obese persons.

Although rare, there is a variety of conditions or syndromes associated with obesity.[2] These include some endocrine disorders, such as Cushing's disease, insulin-producing tumors, and hypogonadal syndromes (Klinefelter's syndrome, Kallmann's syndrome), and some chromosomal and congenital anomalies, such as Prader-Labhart-Willi syndrome, Laurence-Moon-Bardet-Biedl syndrome, and Down syndrome. Obesity is also associated with central nervous system lesions from trauma or from surgical injury, tumors (such as craniopharyngiomas and metastatic tumors) and infiltrative lesions (such as leukemias, histiocytosis X, and sarcoidosis), and post-viral encephalopathies (Kleine-Levin syndrome). Syndromes associated with obesity and/or abnormal fat distribution include steatopygia, partial lipoatrophy with secondary lipohypertrophy (Barraquer-Simmons disease) and Madelung's Neck or Launois-Bensaudi syndrome. The dietary treatment of these unusual syndromes has not proven effective, and one can question whether the major efforts at treatment are appropriate.

Obesity is associated with the use of a number of medications including corticosteroids (prednisone), the tranquilizers diazepam (Valium) and chlordiazepoxide (Librium), many of the tricyclic antidepressants including amitriptyline (Elavil), and the antipsychotic drug lithium.[18] Because of the catabolic effect of corticosteroids on lean body tissue, only a very modest caloric restriction should be imposed to avoid worsening the nitrogen balance. In some circumstances, especially if weight loss is imperative, the discontinuation of psychotherapeutic medications should be considered.

Determination of Desirable Weight. The term desirable weight is used throughout this text to indicate a weight that is likely to be accompanied by a benefit to an individual's health. The desirable weight is not necessarily congruent with the ideal weight or the statistical norms that are promulgated by the standard height-weight tables. Rather, the desirable weight is intended to suggest an appropriate or a goal weight that is based on the individual's health status. Both patients and health professionals are attuned to the custom of identifying a particular goal that can be measured in pounds. Although this is an almost universal practice, it is not critical to the achievement of the objectives of weight reduction.

Although height-weight tables are of limited usefulness, they can serve as a reference point.[19] However, weight-for-height tables have serious limitations when applied to individuals. These tables fail to distinguish the "metabolically obese, normal weight individual" from the "metabolically normal, obese individual," and they do not provide a reference for the naturally lean.[19]

The determination of desirable weight should include the consideration of developmental pattern, the family history, the body composition, the fat distribution, and the complications and associated conditions. Weight goals may vary substantially among seemingly similar individuals. For example, in a man who weighs 230 lb, the desirable goal weight could justifiably be greater if he had weighed 200 lb during an athletic career or if he had been obese since adolescence and had a healthy, long-lived family background than if he had been 170 lb as a young adult and had gained weight with decreasing physical activity and life style changes, had hypertension, and had a family medical background that included glucose intolerance and premature coronary heart disease. In the former situation a goal of 200 lb might be appropriate; in the latter situation, a much lower weight goal would be appropriate.

Goals of Dietary Management

The goal of dietary management is to reduce body fat to a level that is accompanied by an improvement in health or is consistent with a reduced risk of complications. Individual goals should be based on functionally important indicators, such as plasma glucose, lipids, and blood pressure, rather than arbitrary weight tables or the rate or degree of weight loss. The treatment should be directed at establishing habits and practices related to food choices, eating behaviors, and physical activity patterns that are conductive to the long-term maintenance of weight loss.

Recommendations

The treatment of obesity includes dietary modifications, physical activity, and behavioral and/or psychological intervention.[20]. Treatment modalities should be adapted to the circumstances of each patient. No single approach is appropriate for all obese persons. The emphasis that is placed on diet, exercise, and behavioral and/or psychological interventions varies among individuals. Drug therapy for weight reduction is rarely of benefit. The success of anorectic drugs has been variable and generally temporary; some risks are associated with their use. Surgery for weight reduction is addressed on page 192.

Dietary Recommendations. Dietary intervention may include qualitative modifications in food selection, alteration of the meal-snack pattern, and quantitative recommendations for a specific kilocalorie-restricted diet. Emphasis on one or more of these aspects is dependent on individual circumstances and previous dietary patterns.

Relatively high complex carbohydrate, low fat diets, which also tend to be higher in fiber and volume, may be associated with increased satiety and generally form the basis for dietary recommendations. Although complete restriction of alcohol and of high sugar and/or high fat foods is not necessary, it is generally recommended that they be reduced or used only infrequently.

The use of non-nutritive sweeteners is not advocated, but some patients may find them useful (see page 107). Dietetic foods are not universally advocated or prohibited; their utility depends on the caloric content and the use in the individual's diet.

For some patients, emphasis should be placed on the redistribution of the caloric intake. A regular structured meal pattern is more conducive to the voluntary control of intake than is an erratic pattern or frequent snacking. Persons who experience episodes of binge eating may benefit from a more equitable distribution of kilocalories throughout the day, especially if deprivation is antecedent to binge eating. For persons with night-eating syndrome and who consume the vast majority of kilocalories in the evening, emphasis should be placed on establishing a three-meal-per-day pattern and gradually increasing physical activity rather than on further restriction of the caloric intake while maintaining a night-eating pattern.

For most individuals, a moderate caloric restriction that is equal to or near to (perhaps, approximately 10 percent above or below) the measured or estimated resting metabolic rate (at present weight) is recommended. This caloric level is sufficient for an average weight loss of $1/2$ to $1\frac{1}{2}$ lb per week, depending on the activity level. No single proportion of kilocalories from protein, fat, and carbohydrate is recommended. The distribution recommended for diabetes (see page 114) can serve as a guide. The *Food Exchange Lists* for diabetes (see page 114) with modifications for the occasional use of desserts, sweets, or alcohol or other tools for meal planning (see page 119) can be used.

A moderate caloric restriction is less likely than very low kilocalorie diets to be associated with undesirable metabolic adaptations, including a reduction in the resting metabolic rate, alterations in the appetite control, and with negative nitrogen balance, electrolyte imbalances, and changes in fluid balance.[9] Furthermore, it appears that repeated caloric deprivation leads to an enhanced capacity for physiologic adaptation, especially of the metabolic rate when caloric deprivation (i.e., dieting) is experienced again. Overeating or binge eating following caloric deprivation (i.e., the restrained eaters syndrome) compounds the problems that are posed by the reduction of the metabolic rate and may contribute greatly to the cyclically up and down weight pattern that is experienced by many dieters.[21]

The use of very low kilocalorie diets (diets of 800 Kcal or less per day) is not advocated for general use. They should be restricted to extreme circumstances in which rapid weight loss is necessary to ameliorate other life-threatening conditions. Diets that are severely restricted in kilocalories, especially carbohydrates, frequently result in ketosis, diuresis, dehydration, and significant losses in sodium, potassium, calcium, phosphorous, magnesium, and other essential elements.[9] Electrolyte imbalances and cardiac dysrhythmias are a hazard during the use of very low kilocalorie diets and especially during refeeding.[9] If life-threatening circumstances warrant the use of a very low kilocalorie diet, it should be administered only under the supervision of a physician who is knowledgeable about the regimen's risks and management.

Low kilocalorie diets (diets of 1,200 Kcal or less, or less than approximately 50 or 60 percent of the total calories that are needed for weight maintenance) do not pose the immediate hazards of very low kilocalorie diets, but they are associated with undesirable metabolic adaptations. And, like very low kilocalorie diets, low kilocalorie diets have not demonstrated convincingly that they result in long-term success.[9]

Weight-reduction diets variously called "Mayo Diet," "Mayo Clinic Two-Week Diet" or "Mayo Clinic Egg Diet" have had periodic popularity. In general, these diets are relatively low in carbohydrates and high in protein with varying levels of fat and of kilocalories. They advocate the use of a specific combination of foods, such as grapefruit, eggs, and spinach. These diets did not originate at the Mayo Clinic and are neither used nor recommended by the Mayo Clinic.

Physical Activity. Physical activity has the obvious benefit of increasing the caloric expenditure. Furthermore, increasing physical activity from sedentary to moderate levels is not accompanied by a compensatory increase in the caloric intake and may act to some degree to suppress the appetite.[22,23] The greatest increase in caloric expenditure is with activities that use large muscle groups, that are rhythmic and aerobic in nature, and that can be maintained continuously for a period of time, such as walking, swimming, cycling, running, and endurance game activities. An activity of low to moderate intensity that is maintained for 30 minutes or more, 3 to 5 days per week, is generally recommended for both increased caloric expenditure and improved cardiorespiratory function.[24] For physically deconditioned persons, increases in activity should be made gradually. Substantive, rapid changes from the usual activity patterns are discouraged. Those persons who are beginning an exercise program, who are over 35 years of age, and who are deconditioned or who have a major risk factor for cardiovascular disease should consult with their physicians. Persons with restricted mobility, such as might result from a degenerative joint disease or arthritis, should consult with a physician or physical therapist to plan an exercise program. In addition to a formal exercise program, increases in life-style activities and the physical actions that are required for daily living, such as walking and climbing stairs, may contribute to maintaining weight loss.

Behavior Modification and Psychological Intervention. Behavioral approaches are aimed at altering eating, exercise, and life-style habits to promote weight control.[25] Techniques and emphasis vary with the individual. Behavioral approaches can take the form of any or all of the following procedures. Records can be kept by the patient of factors that might be related to the urge to eat, such as mood, time of day, varieties of food available, activity, and emotional or situational forces. These records then may enable the identification of situations that may have been associated with inappropriate eating. Common examples include watching television, reading a newspaper or book, or seeing or smelling easily available food. Snack-type foods in an already opened package might provoke eating, whereas food that requires preparation might be much less tempting.

Once such factors are identified, efforts to control or to avoid them can be made. Modifications of eating techniques, such as the cultivation of small bite sizes, the avoidance of rapid eating, or laying down the fork or spoon between bites, might be helpful. A controlled intake of foods that are highly desired by the patient may be helpful rather than abstinence, which may ultimately result in binges. A conscious effort can be made by the patient to minimize the discouragement and the guilt, which may follow binges or which may result from his perception of his appearance or other personal characteristics, through techniques such as positive self-statements, imagery, and the setting of reasonable goals.[20,26]

Physicians: How to Order Diet

The diet order should indicate *weight reduction*. The dietitian makes recommendations according to the preceding guidelines. If a specific treatment approach, a caloric level, or a weight goal has been previously established in discussions with the patient, the diet order should indicate this information.

REFERENCES

1. Callaway CW, Greenwood MRC. Introduction to the workshop on methods for characterizing human obesity. Int J Obes 1984;8:477–480.
2. Callaway CW, Greenwood MRC. Methods for characterizing human obesities: a progress report. In: Hirsch J, Van Itallie TB, eds. Recent advances in obesity research: IV. London: John Libbey, 1985:138–143.
3. Stunkard AJ. The social environment and the control of obesity. In: Stunkard AJ, ed. Obesity. Philadelphia: WB Saunders, 1980:438–462.
4. Sjöström L. Fat cells and body weight. In: Stunkard AJ, ed. Obesity. Philadelphia: WB Saunders, 1980:72–100.
5. Krotkiewski M, Björntorp P, Sjöström L, Smith U. Impact of obesity on metabolism in men and women. J Clin Invest 1983;72:1150–1162.
6. Gastineau CF. Weight loss on restricted calorie diets. In: Spittell JA, ed. Clinical medicine. Philadelphia: Harper and Row, 1986:1–7.
7. Stunkard AJ, Sorensen TIA, Hanis C, Teasdale TW, Chakrabortz R, Schull WJ, Schulsinger F. An adoption study of human obesity. N Engl J Med 1986;314:193–198.
8. Brunzell JD. Are all obese patients at risk for cardiovascular disease? Int J Obes 1984;8:571–578.
9. Callaway CW. Unproven, but popular approaches in treating obesity: metabolic con-

sequences. In: Frankle RT, Dwyer J, Moragne L, eds. Dietary treatment and prevention of obesity: A satallite symposium, Fourth International Congress on Obesity. London: John Libbey, 1985:11–19.

10. Callaway CW, Pemberton C. Relationship of basal metabolic rates to meal-eating patterns. Unpublished Observations presented at 4th International Congress on Obesity, October 5–8, 1983, New York.

11. Herman CP, Polivy J. Restrained eating. In: Stunkard AJ, ed. Obesity. Philadelphia: WB Saunders, 1980:208–225.

12. Mahoney MJ. The obese eating style: bites, beliefs, and behavior modification. Addict Behav 1975;1:47–53.

13. Rodin J. Current status of the internal-external hypothesis for obesity. What went wrong? Am Psychol 1981;36:361–372.

14. Smith U. Regional differences in adipocyte metabolism and possible consequences in vivo. In: Hirsch J, Van Itallic TB, eds. Recent advances in obesity research: IV. London: John Libbey, 1985:33–36.

15. Kalkhoff RK, Hartz AH, Rupley D, Kissebah AH, Kilber S. Relationship of body fat distribution to blood pressure, carbohydrate tolerance, and plasma lipids in healthy obese women. J Lab Clin Med 1983;102:621–627.

16. Johnson SF, Swenson WM, Gastineau CF. Personality characteristics in obesity: relation of MMPI profile and age of onset of obesity to success in weight reduction. Am J Clin Nutr 1976;29:626–632.

17. National Institutes of Health Concensus Development Conference Statement. Health implications of obesity. Ann Intern Med 1985;103:147–151.

18. Blundell JE. Pharmacologic adjustment of the mechanisms underlying feeding and obesity. In: Stunkard AJ, ed. Obesity. Philadelphia: WB Saunders, 1980:182–207.

19. Callaway CW. Weight standards: their clinical significance. Ann Intern Med 1984;100:296–298.

20. Weinsier RL, Wadden TA, Ritenbaugh C, Harrison GG, Johnson FS, Wiulmore JH. Recommended therapeutic guidelines for professional weight control programs. Am J Clin Nutr 1984;40:865–872.

21. Polivy J, Herman CP. Dieting and binging. A causal analysis. Am Psychol 1985;40:193–201.

22. Woo R, Garrow JS, Pi-Sunyer FX. Voluntary food intake during prolonged exercises in obese women. Am J Clin Nutr 1982;36:478–484.

23. Woo R, Garrow JS, Pi-Sunyer FX. Effect of exercise on spontaneous calorie intake in obesity. Am J Clin Nutr 1982;36:470–477.

24. Pollock ML. The recommended quantity and quality of exercise for developing and maintaining fitness in healthy adults: position statement of the American College of Sports Medicine. Med Sci Sports Exerc 1978;10:8–10.

25. Wilson GT. Behavior modification and the treatment of obesity. In: Stunkard AJ, ed. Obesity. Philadelphia: WB Saunders, 1980:325–344.

26. Stunkard AJ, Berthold HC. What is behavior therapy? A very short description of behavioral weight control. Am J Clin Nutr 1985;41:821–823.

GASTROPLASTY

General Description

Gastroplasty, which is performed for weight loss, alters the alimentary tract to reduce the amount of food that is consumed. As with other surgical procedures that alter the integrity of the stomach, changes in the texture and the volume of food are necessary postoperatively. More restrictions are necessary in the early postoperative period, and the transition to more usual types of food is made gradually. Long-term changes in the quantities of food that are consumed and in the eating habits must be made for weight loss to be achieved and to be maintained. Table 6–40 highlights the potential problems that follow gastroplasty and suggests dietary modifications for the problem's prevention or alleviation.

TABLE 6–40 Potential Problems Following Gastroplasty and Suggested Dietary Modifications

Potential Problems	Suggestions
Nausea and vomiting	If nausea and vomiting occur after eating a new food, wait several days before trying it again. It may be necessary to eat more liquid or pureed foods temporarily. Eating too fast, eating too much, or insufficient chewing may also cause nausea or vomiting.
Pain in shoulder or upper chest area	The patient should be advised to stop eating if pain occurs during eating and to try to eat later after the pain has resolved.
Dehydration	Dehydration may occur with inadequate fluid intake, especially if there is persistent nausea, vomiting, or diarrhea. At least 6 cups of fluid daily are recommended.
Constipation	Constipation may occur temporarily during the first postoperative month, but generally resolves with the adaptation to changes in the volume of food. The regular use of fruits and fruit juices reduces the risk of recurrent constipation.
Blockage of the stoma	The stoma may be temporarily blocked if foods with large particle size are eaten without thorough chewing. If symptoms of pain, nausea, and vomiting persist, a physician should be contacted.
Rupture of the staple line	Rupture of the staple line is unlikely. The patient should be advised to avoid eating an excessive quantity of food at one time.
Stretching of the stomach pouch	The risk of stretching the stomach pouch can be reduced by avoiding eating large portions of food at one time and by modifying the texture of foods only gradually in the early postoperative weeks. Most surgical techniques now incorporate bands of material that are placed around the stoma to prevent stretching of this opening.
Weight gain or no further weight loss	A careful diet history should be taken. Potential sources of excess kilocalories include the excessive use of high kilocalorie beverages and snacks.

Nutritional Inadequacy

Since the quantity of food that is consumed is often greatly reduced, there is the potential for nutritional inadequacies. Many patients have difficulty consuming adequate amounts of protein. This problem is particularly pronounced in the first few months that follow surgery, but may continue long-term.[1,2] Such surgery often results in an intolerance to meat and to some meat substitutes. A dislike of or an intolerance to milk, which is a major source of protein for most patients initially following gastroplasty, increases the likelihood of inadequate protein intake. Commercially prepared nutritional supplements (see page 261) may be advisable.

Because the caloric intake is very low and food choices are limited, it is difficult for the individual to be assured of an adequate intake of vitamins and minerals. Clinical signs of deficiencies have been documented in some populations following gastroplasty.[1-3] A liquid or chewable multiple vitamin supplement should be taken by these patients daily. Evidence of iron deficiency may require larger amounts of iron in the form of a liquid preparation in addition to the vitamin.

Indications and Rationale

The surgical treatment of severe obesity may be justified when there is a greatly increased risk of disease and of disability. However, surgical procedures pose a risk that necessitates the careful evaluation of all candidates.

Criteria for patient selection include a body weight that is in excess of the average desirable weight by 100 lb or by 100 percent, the presence of a high risk for developing serious medical conditions that are related to obesity, a history of repeated failure in attempts to lose weight by standard nonsurgical means, and the ability to tolerate the operative trauma and the anesthesia.[4] In addition, patients should be less than 55 years of age. Additional considerations are necessary for pediatric patients. Because of the risk of retarded growth attributable to prolonged nutritional inadequacies, gastroplasty is generally contraindicated in pediatric patients.

Gastroplasty has been replacing the earlier intestinal bypass procedures done for weight loss.[5-7] It is often termed "gastric stapling," since staples are used in the procedure. While there are a number of modifications of this operation, the common features include the construction of a small pouch with a capacity of 1 to 2 oz in the upper part of the stomach with an exit (stoma) that is approximately 10 mm in diameter that allows food to pass into the remainder of the stomach. The small size of the pouch limits the amount of food or fluid that can be consumed at a time. The small exit and the consequent slow emptying of the pouch require the patient to eat three to six small meals per day and allow eating intervals of no less than perhaps 5 to 30 minutes. Eating patterns must be planned with these limitations in mind. The patient is encouraged to cultivate and to maintain habits of eating that limit caloric consumption and yet provide sufficient amounts of essential nutrients, particularly protein. Hunger is often minimal, but the urge to eat leads many patients to test the capacity of their gastric pouch with inappropriate amounts and varieties of foods.

A rapid weight loss during the early postoperative period may represent, in considerable part, a loss of lean body mass.

Modifications in Texture and Consistency

The diet should progress from liquids to purees, then to soft foods, and finally to a general diet.

A clear liquid diet (see page 45) is the first step of the diet progression and is followed by a full liquid diet according to usual postoperative diet progressions (see page 52). The third step of the progression is pureed foods (blended solid food or prepared baby food), which, like liquids, are thought to cause very little distention of the small stomach pouch. The length of time for an advancement to solid foods depends on individual tolerances. Although this varies with each individual, by 12 weeks after surgery most people are eating ordinary solid food, provided they have learned to chew all food to a pureed consistency before swallowing. Following this 12-week period, chewing food thoroughly continues to be important.

The narrow opening from the pouch into the main portion of the stomach can easily be blocked with chunks or small pieces of food. A blockage of this passage prevents food from leaving the pouch and can cause vomiting. Rarely, an obstructed stoma requires endoscopic removal of the offending food.

Volume of Food

The patient should be advised to eat only about 1 to 2 oz (2 to 4 Tbsp or 12 tsp) of food per meal in the beginning and to stop eating or drinking when they are full. Initially, the small pouch holds only 2 oz of food at a time. However, the opening can be stretched by repeatedly challenging it with quantities of food that are larger than the pouch can hold, thus defeating the purpose of the surgery. Within the first several months or more after the surgery, the patient is able to gradually eat slightly larger amounts of food.

Liquids create a "full" feeling, but may speed emptying of the pouch and, therefore, reduce the effectiveness of the surgery. It is important that the patient eat food rather than drink beverages at mealtime. Liquids should be taken between meals. An adequate fluid intake, usually at least 6 cups per day, is encouraged to reduce the risk of dehydration.

Frequency and Duration of Meals

The patient should take small bites of food and eat or drink slowly. Approximately 20 to 30 minutes should be planned initially for each meal. Three to six frequent meals are better tolerated than infrequent meals.

Liquids

The patient should be advised to take liquids between meals. An initial guide is to sip 1 cup over a 1/2- to 1-hr period. The patient should stop sipping liquids within 45 to 60 minutes of mealtimes.

Food Intolerances

After gastroplasty, certain foods may be difficult to tolerate because they tend to cause nausea, pain, discomfort, vomiting, or blockage of the opening of the stomach. Generally, foods high in fats, foods high in fiber, and foods that are difficult to chew thoroughly should be avoided. Some people who have had a gastroplasty have found foods such as fried foods, tough meats, hamburger, meats with gristle, highly seasoned and spicy foods, fibrous vegetables (dried beans, peas, celery, corn, cabbage), raw vegetables, mushrooms, orange and grapefruit membranes, whole grain bread or cereals, bran, coconut, dried fruit, seeds, skins, pickles, nuts, granola, popcorn, and carbonated beverages difficult to tolerate.

Food intolerances vary with the individual. Through trial and error, the patient may demonstrate a tolerance to some of these foods. Any food that causes discomfort should not be eaten.

Patient and Family Education

Because of the extent and the duration of changes in eating patterns that are necessary following gastroplasty, a detailed explanation of the nature and the effects of the surgery is imperative prior to the procedure. Additional education and counseling is often necessary during hospitalization to reinforce dietary principles. Because most patients make alterations in the dietary recommendations according to individual tolerances (some of which may have adverse nutritional consequences) and because of the risk of nutritional inadequacies previously noted, diet records should be reviewed periodically.

Physicians: How to Order Diet

The diet order should indicate *diet following gastroplasty*. The dietitian makes recommendations according to the preceding guidelines.

REFERENCES

1. Graney AS, Smith LB, Hammer KA. Gastric partitioning for morbid obesity: postoperative weight loss, technical complications and protein status. J Am Diet Assoc 1986;86:630–635.
2. Raymond JL, Schipke CA, Becker JM, Lloyd RD, Moody FG. Changes in body composition and dietary intake after gastric partitioning for morbid obesity. Surgery 1986;99:15–18.
3. Crowley LV, Seay J, Mullin G. Late effects of gastric bypass for obesity. Am J Gastroenterol 1984;79:850–860.
4. Van Itallie TB, Bray GA, Connor WE, Faloon WW, Kral JG, Mason EE, Stunkard AJ. Guidelines for surgery for morbid obesity. Am J Clin Nutr 1985;42:904–905.
5. Hocking MP, Kelly KA, Callaway CW. Vertical gastroplasty for morbid obesity: clinical experience. Mayo Clin Proc 1986;61:287–291.
6. Mason EE, Printen KJ, Blommers TH, Lewis JW, Scott DH. Gastric bypass in morbid obesity. Am J Clin Nutr 1980;33:395–405.
7. Andersen T, Backer OG, Stokholm KH, Quaade F. Randomized trial of diet and gastroplasty compared with diet alone in morbid obesity. N Engl J Med 1984;310:352–356.

ONCOLOGIC AND HEMATOLOGIC DISEASE

CANCER

General Description

Anorexia, maldigestion, malabsorption, and mechanical difficulties in mastication and swallowing are common factors that make protein-calorie malnutrition a common problem in patients with advancing cancer. The dietitian should seek to provide foods that can be consumed in quantities that are sufficient to meet protein and kilocalorie needs, to correct nutritional deficits, and to minimize weight loss. Suggestions on how this may be accomplished are given.

Indications and Rationale

The maintenance of an adequate nutritional status may reduce the complications from oncologic therapy and should contribute to the patient's sense of well-being. For these reasons, nutritional care is an important part of the supportive management of the patient with cancer.

Nutritional Effects of Cancer

Protein-calorie malnutrition is the single most common secondary diagnosis in patients with cancer. It tends to be severe in patients with tumors of the head and neck, stomach, pancreas, lung, colon, and ovary and less pronounced in patients with breast cancer.[1] Clearly the presence of malnutrition with cancer is a poor prognostic sign.[2-5] Malnutrition adversely affects not only tissue function and repair but also humoral and cellular immunocompetence and can cause changes in drug metabolism through alterations in liver function.[6] Thus, malnutrition can interfere with the delivery of oncologic therapy and prolong and enhance the severity of the side effects of the therapy. Malnourished patients do not tolerate surgery, chemotherapy, or radiation therapy as well as those in a better nutritional state.[5,6] In this weakened state, cancer patients are particularly susceptible to infections. Thus, the cachexia may become more threatening to life than the local effects of the cancer.

Cancer cachexia presents clinically with anorexia, alterations in taste sensation, weight loss, muscle wasting, and malnutrition, which results in a decline in general physical and mental functions. The pathogenesis of the anorexia-cachexia syndrome is incompletely understood. Metabolic by-products of tumor metabolism may directly cause anorexia or early satiety or may do so secondarily by an effect on the hypothalamic function.[7-9] In some cases, the anorexia may be more likely the result of early satiety than of an impaired perception of hunger.[9] Substances such as anorexins, asthenins, and cachectins (whose structures are of a protein nature and have been identified in some detail) are released by tumors.[9] These substances may be major factors in causing symptoms of anorexia, weakness, and weight loss. Cachectin may be similar to or identical with a tumor necrosis factor and may have an antitumor activity. While causing a form of cachexia, it seems that cachectin does not exert its effects simply through starvation since parenteral hyperalimentation in some trials could not reverse the progression of cachexia.[10] Tumor metabolites may also be responsible for the abnormalities of sensations of taste and of smell that have been observed in persons with cancer.[7,8,11,12]

Patients may have a heightened or a decreased sensitivity for sweet taste. The taste thresholds for salty and for sour foods are often increased and that for bitter foods, decreased. The decreased threshold for bitter taste (urea as a test substance) is often responsible for the aversion to meat that is frequently experienced by patients with cancer.

Psychological stresses that are associated with cancer may contribute to anorexia.[7,13,14] Even in the absence of true depression, the presence of pain, lack of sense of well-being, discouragement, and anxiety about the treatment of the disease or its prognosis may cause emotional stress, which diminishes the enjoyment of eating. A conditioned aversion to eating certain foods may develop if patients experience nausea or other discomforts, perhaps as a consequence of radiation therapy or chemotherapy, during or after eating these foods.[14] Such aversions may persist long after the therapy has been completed. Nutritional deficiencies or excesses may result if patients avoid foods they consider as contributing to the genesis of the cancer or if they consume larger quantities of allegedly beneficial foods.

Although a decreased intake of nutrients appears to be the dominant cause of wasting, it cannot entirely explain the progressive weight loss that often occurs despite an apparently adequate intake. Other mechanisms that have been suggested include an abnormal adaptation to starving with an increased rather than a decreased metabolic rate, parasitization of the host tissues by the growing tumor, and derangements in intermediary metabolism.[1,2,5,15,16] In general, a tumor burden is thought to be too small to act as a metabolic drain of sufficient magnitude to produce host wasting. However, the presence of a tumor could induce derangements in the metabolism of carbohydrate, fat, and protein, which may cause an increase in energy requirements.

Nutritional Effects of Cancer Therapies

Besides the effects of the tumor itself, the various modalities that are used in the treatment of cancer may also have an adverse effect on nutritional status.[17,18] The malnutrition that results from treatment assumes even more importance when one realizes that many cancer patients are already debilitated from their disease. Antitumor therapies may produce only mild, transient, nutritional disturbances, such as mucositis from chemotherapy, or may lead to severe, permanent, nutritional problems, as in small bowel resection, or to disabilities in chewing or in swallowing after head and neck surgery.

Surgical Therapy

Radical surgery of the head and neck region may lead to significant malnutrition by altering the normal route of nutritional intake. Although some of these changes are temporary, many patients have permanent difficulty with chewing, swallowing, and risk of aspiration. The inadequate caloric intake resulting from postprandial symptoms that often follow a resection of the esophagus or the stomach, such as gastric stasis or dumping syndrome, is usually of greater importance than the malabsorption that may result following the surgery (see section on *Postgastrectomy Dumping Syndrome*).

The nutritional sequelae of intestinal resection are directly related to the site and extent of resection and to the individual functions of the various segments.[19] The ability of various segments of the small intestine to increase their absorptive capabilities over a period of several months prevents major clinical problems after small bowel resection unless the bowel resection is massive, a situation in which malabsorption becomes a major problem in nutritional management. Colon surgery is usually well-tolerated from a nutritional standpoint. The large water and electrolyte losses in the early postoperative period decrease rapidly soon after surgery.

Weight loss that is secondary to anorexia and malabsorption is common in patients with pancreatic cancer. Some degree of nutritional repletion prior to surgery is desirable, but not always feasible. Pancreatectomy may lead to pancreatic endocrine and/or exocrine insufficiency, which may result in diabetes and in significant malabsorption. The administration of pancreatic enzymes and histamine H_2 receptor blockers and the optimal use of insulin may lessen, but not entirely correct, the trends toward malnutrition that result from malabsorption and insulin-dependent diabetes. Conventional dietary restrictions for diabetes may need to be liberalized by the inclusion of sugars or sugar-containing foods to achieve adequate caloric intake.

Chemotherapy

Chemotherapeutic agents may contribute to malnutrition through a variety of direct and indirect mechanisms, including anorexia, nausea, vomiting, mucositis, organ injury (toxicity), and learned food aversions.[1,20,21] These agents affect normal cells as well as malignant tissues and are most active on rapidly proliferating cells such as the epithelial cells of the alimentary tract. The degree to which gastrointestinal functions are affected depends on the particular chemotherapy agent drug dosage, the duration of the treatment, the rates of metabolism, and the individual's susceptibility. Mucositis is a major gastrointestinal toxicity and may be greatly enhanced when radiation therapy is given concurrently with chemotherapy. Mucositis can affect any part of the alimentary tract and may lead to ulceration, bleeding, and malabsorption. The renewal rate of the alimentary tract mucosa is rapid so that the mucositis from chemotherapy is usually short-lived.

Nausea and vomiting commonly accompany the administration of many antitumor drugs and may even occur in anticipation of chemotherapy.[22] Indirect effects of chemotherapy that may contribute to malnutrition include fungal infections of the gastrointestinal tract and learned food aversions.[13] Candidiasis of the gastrointestinal tract is not an uncommon occurrence during chemotherapy, especially in patients with leukemias and lymphomas. Candidiasis in the oral cavity, pharynx, or esophagus can produce oral discomforts and dysphagia.

Weight gain is common in women who undergo adjuvant chemotherapy for breast cancer. It is not clear, however, whether the weight gain is a direct effect of chemotherapy.[23,24]

Radiation Therapy

The complications of radiation vary according to the region of the body that is radiated, to the dose, fractionation, length of time, and the field size of the radiation that is administered, to associated antitumor therapy such as surgery or chemotherapy, and to the patient's nutritional status at the initiation of radiation.[19,21] Complications may develop acutely during radiation or become chronic and progress even after radiation has been completed.[25] When the salivary glands are in the field of radiation, saliva production decreases in conjunction with an increase in viscosity. In addition to causing mouth dryness and impaired swallowing, the decrease in salivation causes an alteration in the composition of the oral bacteria flora, which, in turn, promotes caries formation. Secondary infection, such as candidiasis, may also develop. For some, the thick, scant secretions may create a feeling of nausea.[26]

The mucosa of the alimentary tract is sensitive to radiation exposure and responds with mucositis, erythema, and edema, which can produce a sore mouth or throat, painful ulcerations, bleeding, or even chronic radiation ulcer. Radionecrosis of oral tissue may result from the combination of trauma and infection that is superimposed on highly-radiated tissues. Trismus can occur from tumor infiltration or postradiation fibrosis.

Damage of the microvilli of the taste cells often results in suppressed or heightened taste sensation or in loss of taste sensation, which is described as "mouth blindness." Bitter and acid tastes are most often impaired, salty and sweet tastes are less influenced. In most patients, a gradual return of taste occurs within 2 to 4 months of completion of therapy, but may take up to 1 year. These symptoms have a profound effect on the desire and ability to eat and may combine to create a potentially serious situation, since the patients are often already anorectic and undernourished. Unless nutritional intervention is provided, the majority of patients lose weight during radiation therapy.[26]

Patients with tumors of the esophagus, like those with cancer of the oral cavity, are often in a marginal nutritional state at the start of radiation therapy because of impaired swallowing and, perhaps, because of habits of tobacco and alcohol use. Fatigue during eating, attributable to shortness of breath and anorexia, often contributes to a weight loss in patients with cancer of the lung. Radiation to the thoracic area induces esophagitis with its accompanying sore throat and dysphagia. This usually disappears following the cessation of therapy. Tumor necrosis, however, may result in delayed complications such as ulceration with possible fistula or sinus tract formation or obstruction owing to fibrosis and stricture.

Abdominal or pelvic radiation may result in altered intestinal function. Patients who receive upper abdominal radiation often experience nausea and vomiting, and those who receive radiation to the lower abdomen often experience diarrhea. Damage to the intestinal mucosa can produce malabsorption of fat, protein, carbohydrate, and other nutrients, as well as fluid and electrolyte deficiencies. Acute radiation enteritis usually disappears following therapy. However, late effects of abdominopelvic radiation occur in a small percentage of patients. The effects may occur months to years after the completion of radiation therapy and may be manifested as intestinal obstruction, fistula formation, or chronic enteritis.

Goals of Dietary Management

Nutritional support of the cancer patient must be individualized. Nutritional therapy should be undertaken with the overall prognosis of the patient clearly in mind so that the aggressiveness of dietary intervention (supportive, adjunctive, definitive) can be appropriately adjusted. All patients with nutritional problems should have frequent dietary consultation and should be helped to understand that nutrition is an intricate part of the total management of their disease. The dietary modifications depend on the extent to which the patient is experiencing anorexia, taste alterations, easy satiation, nausea, weight loss, and consequences of treatment.

Dietary Recommendations

Some general considerations in designing a diet for the cancer patient follow.

1. A detailed diet history can be obtained to determine past food preferences and eating habits, present caloric and protein intake, specific food intolerances, taste abnormalities distribution of feedings throughout the day, number of times the patient eats each day, who does the cooking, and whether the patient eats alone. Consideration should be given to nutritional side effects from past or current treatment.

2. Information obtained in the diet history should be carefully considered in the formulation of the diet. Table 6–41 outlines the potential nutritional problems of cancer therapy with suggested dietary approaches to help meet nutritional needs.[28-32]

3. The diet plan should be specific in the number of kilocalories and the amount of protein that is needed each day. Because the effect of cancer on metabolism is only partially understood, it is not possible to be precise about the minimum intake of kilocalories and protein that would be sufficient to meet the needs of cancer patients. Furthermore, the energy sources (carbohydrate and fat) and the quantity and the quality of protein that would promote nitrogen balance cannot yet be stated.[27] For these reasons, the recommendations for the daily kilocalorie and protein intake should be monitored and adjusted according to individual patient response.

4. If the patient has been losing weight, the first realistic goal of nutritional intervention may be to prevent a further loss of weight.

5. If the patient is nauseated from the underlying cancer, radiation, or chemotherapy, the use of an antiemetic drug, such as prochlorperazine (Compazine) from the phenothiazine class of drugs, may be very helpful. The drug should be given 30 to 60 minutes before planned meals. Likewise, if pain hinders eating, the systematic administration of analgesics may enhance the patient's willingness and desire to eat.

6. The necessity of changing lifetime meal and snack patterns should be frankly explained to the patient. For example, the patient who was conditioned to omitting snacks or desserts to avoid gaining weight before the diagnosis of cancer should be told that this routine is no longer appropriate. Eggs should no longer be avoided because of their cholesterol content.

7. Recommendations should take into account the patient's strength and ability to prepare food. If the patient is alone part of the day, ways to make food available should be suggested.

8. The patient should be given dietary guidelines in writing and should be gently encouraged to eat the suggested foods in the recommended amounts. However, the patient should not be excessively pressured by friends or by relatives concerning poor nutritional intake. Such action may create more anxiety and become counter productive.

9. Food should fill the diet prescription whenever possible. Sometimes supplementation with high kilocalorie, high protein liquid feedings is necessary. Monomeric diets should be used only if specifically indicated, as in situations of malabsorption.

10. A multiple vitamin supplement should be given to patients who are not able to ingest a well-balanced diet or who have specific deficiencies.

The patient's progress should be evaluated at regular intervals to determine whether the nutritional state is improving. Follow-up also offers a means of support and of reinforcement, so that the diet prescription can be advanced or modified in response to treatment.

If efforts at oral feeding fail or are impossible, the use of alternate feeding

TABLE 6–41 Potential Nutrition Problems of Cancer and Cancer

Problem	Frequent small meals	High protein high Kcal supplements	Avoid strong odors	Cool or room temperature foods	Increase Kcal content of foods	Increase fluid intake	Increase fiber intake
Loss of appetite and early satiety	X	X	X	X	X		
Diarrhea	X			X		X	
Nausea and vomiting	X		X	X		X	
Chewing & swallowing difficulties (sore mouth or throat)	X	X		X	X	X	
Constipation						X	X
Abdominal gas							
Dry mouth	X	X				X	

methods such as tube feeding or central parenteral nutrition (CPN) may be necessary. The use of aggressive nutritional support is beneficial for many patients who undergo therapy and who have a high probability of positive response to therapy. However, the use of nutritional support for the terminal cancer patient may be of questionable benefit. More appropriate are suggestions for oral

Therapy with Suggested Dietary Approaches[28–32]

Decrease fiber intake and roughage	Limit high fat foods	Avoid gas forming foods	Regular exercise if tolerated	Avoid liquids at mealtime	Select soft moist foods, add sauce, gravy	Avoid highly seasoned foods	Comments
	X		X	X			Pleasant mealtime atmosphere. A glass of wine or beer before meals, if allowed, may stimulate appetite.
X	X	X		X		X	Clear liquids helpful. Limit beverages containing caffeine, alcohol, and lactose.
	X			X		X	Clear, cool beverages recommended. Eat and drink slowly. Activity after a meal can stimulate vomiting.
X					X	X	Citrus fruits and juices, tomatoes, and other acidic foods may aggravate a sore throat or mouth. Cooked or canned vegetables and fruits may be easier to eat than raw or fresh ones.
			X				8 to 10 glasses of liquids each day. Balanced diet with additional servings of fruits, vegetables, and whole grain products.
X	X	X	X				Avoid eating rapidly, "gulping" beverages, "drawing" on straws, or sipping beverages frequently. It may be necessary to avoid high lactose foods and the artificial sweetners sorbitol and mannitol.
					X		Hard candy, preferably sugar-free, may be used throughout the day to keep the mouth moist. Sip liquids with meals or use artificial saliva.

feedings as tolerated and the provision of emotional support. For the end-stage patient, the pleasurable aspects of eating should be emphasized with less concern for quantity and nutrient content.

Obesity is common in patients with breast cancer. Skeletal metastasis may cause more problems, such as pathologic fractures, in the overweight person.

Some evidence suggests that the cancer recurrence rate may be adversely affected by the patient being overweight.[32,33] Therefore, obesity should be treated by gradual weight reduction through moderate caloric control.

Nutrition and Its Role in Cancer Protection

Epidemiologic and animal studies over a period of years indicate that patterns of food consumption and some dietary components may increase the risk of cancer. The idea that types of diets and individual food components offer protection against cancer risk is unproven. However, the National Cancer Institute and the American Cancer Society have established prudent dietary guidelines for food selection. The reader is referred to the section on *American Cancer Society: Diet and Cancer Protection* (page 38) for this information.

REFERENCES

1. Costa G, Donaldson S. The nutritional effects of cancer and its therapy. Nutr Cancer 1980;2:22–29.
2. Buzby GP, Steinberg JJ. Nutrition in cancer patients. Surg Clin North Am 1981; 61:691–700.
3. Balducci L, Hardy C. Cancer and malnutrition—a critical interaction: a review. Am J Hematol 1985;18:91–103.
4. DeWys WD. Management of cancer cachexia. Semin Oncol 1985;12:452–460.
5. DeWys WD, Begg C, Lavin PT, et al. Prognostic effect of weight loss prior to chemotherapy in cancer patients. Am J Med 1980;69:491–497.
6. Theologides A. Nutritional management of the patient with advanced cancer. Postgrad Med J 1977;61:97–101.
7. DeWys WD. Anorexia in cancer patients. Cancer Res 1977;37:2354–2358.
8. DeWys WD. Anorexia as a general effect of cancer. Cancer 1979;43:2013–2019.
9. Theologides A. Pathogenesis of anorexia and cachexia in cancer. Cancer Bull 1982;34:140–149.
10. Theologides A. Anorexins, asthenins and cachectins in cancer. Editorial, Am J Med 1986;31:696–698.
11. Vickers ZM, Nielsen SS, Theologides A. Food preferences of patients with cancer. J Am Diet Assoc 1981;79:441–445.
12. Nielsen SS, Theologides A, Vickers ZM. Influence of food odors on food aversions and preferences in patients with cancer. Am J Clin Nutr 1980;33:2253–2261.
13. Holland JCB, Rowland J, Plumb M. Psychological aspects of anorexia in cancer patients. Cancer Res 1977;37:2425–2428.
14. Bernstein I. Physiological and psychological mechanisms of cancer anorexia. Cancer Res 1982;42:715s–720s.
15. vanEyes J. Nutrition and cancer: Physiological interrelationships. Ann Rev Nutr 1985;5:435–461.
16. DeWys WD. Pathophysiology of cancer cachexia: current understanding and areas for future research. Cancer Res 1982;42:721s–726s.
17. Shils ME. Nutrition and neoplasia. In: Goodbart RS, Shils ME, eds. Modern nutrition in health and disease. 6th ed. Philadelphia: Lea and Febiger, 1980:1153–1192.
18. Lawrence W. Effects of cancer and nutrition. Impaired organ system effects. Cancer 1979;43:2020–2029.
19. Lawrence W. Nutritional consequences of surgical resection of the gastrointestinal tract for cancer. Cancer Res 1977;37:2379–2386.
20. Kokal WA. The impact of antitumor therapy on nutrition. Cancer 1985;55:273–278.

21. Donaldson SS, Lenon RA. Alterations of nutritional status. Impact of chemotherapy and radiotherapy. Cancer 1979;43:2036–2052.
22. Zook DJ, Yasho JM. Psychologic factors: their effect on nausea and vomiting experienced by clients receiving chemotherapy. Onc Nurs Forum 1983;10:76–81.
23. Hernandez BM, Bonomi P, Hoeltgen T, Roseman DL, Slayton RE, Walter J, Foltz A. Weight gain during adjuvant therapy for stage II breast cancer. Proc Am Soc Clin Oncol 1983;2:108.
24. Heasman KZ, Sutherland HJ, Campbell JA, Elhakim T, Boyd NF. Weight gain during adjuvant chemotherapy for breast cancer. Breast Cancer Res Treat 1985;5:195–200.
25. Donaldson SS. Nutritional consequences of radiotherapy. Cancer Res 1977;37:2407–2413.
26. Dwyer JT. Dietetic assessment of ambulatory cancer patients with special attention to problems of patients suffering from head-neck cancers undergoing radiation therapy. Cancer 1979;43:2077–2086.
27. Young VR. Energy metabolism and requirements in the cancer patient. Cancer Res 1977;37:2336–2347.
28. Cimprich B. Symptom management: constipation. Cancer Nursing 1985;8(Supplement 1):39–43.
29. Schnippr IM. Symptom management: anorexia. Cancer Nursing 1985;8(Supplement 1):33–35.
30. Flaherty AM. Symptom management: nausea and vomiting. Cancer Nursing 1985;8(Supplement 1):36–38.
31. Margie JD, Block AS. Nutrition and the cancer patient. Radner PA: Chilton Book, 1983.
32. Ahmann DL, O'Fallon JR, Scanlon PW, Payne WS, Bisel HF, Edmonson JH. A preliminary assessment of factors associated with recurrent disease in a surgical adjuvant clinical trial for patients with breast cancer with special emphasis on the aggressiveness of therapy. Am J Clin Oncol (CCT) 1982;5:371–381.
33. Boyd NF, Campbell JE, Germanson T, Thompson DB, Sutherland DJ, Meakin JW. Body weight and prognosis in breast cancer. JNCI 1981;67:785–789.

BONE MARROW TRANSPLANT

General Description

An "as tolerated" general diet that omits fresh fruits and vegetables is indicated unless complications arise that require further diet modification (i.e., side effects of pre-transplant conditioning, gastrointestinal graft versus host disease [GVHD]).[1] Fresh fruits and vegetables are avoided because of their gram-negative bacteria content.

Nutritional Inadequacy

The diet is similar to the general hospital diet and is not inherently inadequate in nutrients as compared to the Recommended Dietary Allowance (RDA). However, when the intake is 1,200 kilocalories or less, it is difficult to meet the RDA consistently. A daily multiple vitamin supplement that provides nutrients at a level that is equivalent to the RDA is recommended for persons who consume diets of 1,200 kilocalories or less or for those with food aversions or with intolerances that greatly limit the variety of food choices. (Note: during the transition from central parenteral nutrition to oral intake, vitamins at levels that meet the RDA are provided parenterally.)

Indications and Rationale

Bone Marrow Transplantation (BMT) is a form of therapy for certain hematologic disorders such as aplastic anemia, chronic and acute leukemias, and, more recently, some forms of lymphoma. Critical to a successful transplant is a donor with closely matched histocompatible antigens. The closest match is that of a genetically identical twin (syngeneic). The more common match is a human leukocyte antigen (HLA) identical sibling (allogeneic). In some cases, such as certain lymphomas, the patient's own marrow is aspirated when the patient is in remission and infused later (autologous).[2]

Prior to transplantation, the patient is "conditioned" to prevent possible graft rejection and/or relapse. This conditioning regimen generally consists of several days of high-dose chemotherapy and of total body irradiation.

Nutritional consequences of the "conditioning" phase may include nausea, vomiting, mucositis, esophagitis, xerostomia, thick viscous saliva, dysgeusia, anorexia, early satiety, diarrhea, and steatorrhea. The duration and the intensity of these symptoms and the stress of the treatments are such that protein-calorie malnutrition in some degree is almost a certainty. Another consequence of the conditioning is the loss of immune competence and of the ability of the patient's body to deal with infections. The amounts and the kinds of bacteria in fresh fruits and vegetables are ordinarily no hazard to the healthy person, but may provoke a serious infection in the BMT patient. Strategies for dealing with these problems are a major focus of nutritional care in the post-transplant phase. (See section on *Oncologic and Hematologic Disease*, page 196 on methods for dealing with eating problems).

The primary goal is to provide optimal nutrition for the BMT patient. These patients generally experience a decreased ability to maintain an adequate oral intake owing to mucosal ulceration, severe anorexia that is induced by the transplantation conditioning programs, infection, or GVHD. Frequent monitoring of the nutrient intake and the provision for and the encouragement of adequate kilocalorie and protein intake is essential in the care of the BMT patient.

General Recommendations

Pre-transplant. Patients undergoing a bone marrow transplant should be seen by a dietitian on the day of admission to the hospital to complete a thorough nutritional assessment. A detailed diet history that includes food preferences and dislikes is needed for reference in the post-transplant phase when oral feeding is resumed. Because the hospital stay for the BMT patient is lengthy, a description of the food and the nutrition services is provided to the patient and the family prior to the transplant. The need to avoid fresh fruits and vegetables because of bacterial content, the likely side effects of the "conditioning," and the use of central parenteral nutrition (CPN) to provide nutrients when the oral intake is inadequate are also explained. An understanding of the need for and the cooperation of the patient and the family in the provision of adequate nutrition by mouth in the post-transplant phase is critical to the success of the transplant process.

Post-transplant. Severe oral lesions and anorexia that results from the conditioning regimen is common for the BMT patient for several weeks. Because of a significantly decreased oral intake, CPN is instituted to meet nutritional needs. A daily nutrient (kilocalories, protein, fat) intake from oral and parenteral routes is monitored closely.

An oral intake is encouraged as soon as possible. The patient and the family are made aware of protein and kilocalorie intake goals. Cooperation and encourgement from family members to assist the patient in meeting nutrient intake goals is an important part of the recovery process. When oral feeding is possible, a general diet as tolerated, with the avoidance of fresh fruits and vegetables, is resumed. No other dietary restrictions are needed unless gastrointestinal symptoms occur. Standard CPN monitoring practices are followed (see page 277) as long as CPN therapy continues. In addition, nitrogen balance, prealbumin measures, and daily weights are obtained and evaluated as indicators of nutritional status.

Upon dismissal, the patient should be able to maintain weight on oral intake alone. The patient is counseled regarding nutritional needs and how to meet them in a home or an outpatient setting. Patients are required to maintain food intake records after dismissal from the hospital for a period of 2 weeks. The records are reviewed and evaluated by the dietitian and discussed with the physician who consults with the patient on an out-patient basis. Patients are counseled as needed to assure an adequate oral intake and weight maintenance.

Graft Versus Host Disease (GVHD)

A major complication of bone marrow transplant may be GVHD, which can present as an acute or a chronic state. It is thought that the newly grafted bone marrow recognizes the host's cells as foreign. GVHD is a reaction that involves the body's immune system. GVHD usually causes multiple organ damage, but especially involves the skin, the entire gastrointestinal tract, and the liver.

Gastrointestinal GVHD is a potential major nutritional complication after transplantation. Its symptoms can include abdominal pain, nausea, vomiting, diarrhea, bloody stools, malabsorption, altered intestinal motility, and ileus.

The dietary protocol for the management of gastrointestinal GVHD is:[3]

Step 1. Bowel rest and no food by mouth until the stool volume is less than 500 ml per day for 2 days or more. Nutrition is provided by CPN.

Step 2. The introduction of low residue, low lactose (preferably isosmotic) beverages in small frequent feedings. When symptoms improve advance to the next step. CPN support is provided to meet nutrient and kilocalorie goals.

Step 3. The introduction of solid foods that are of low residue, low lactose, and low fat (approximately 30 g), and that have no gastric irritants (see section on *Peptic Ulcer Disease*). These foods should be taken as tolerated. The slow introduction of foods is necessary, one at a time in frequent small meals. CPN support continues as needed as a nutrient supplement.

Step 4. Gradually liberalize the previous dietary restrictions until a normal diet is tolerated asymptomatically. Discontinue CPN support when the oral intake adequately meets the nutrient needs.

Physicians: How to Order Diet

The diet order should indicate a general diet with no fresh fruits or vegetables. The diet is to begin upon admission at the start of the conditioning process. It is may be maintained up to 6 months post-transplant or as long as determined necessary by the physician. If gastrointestinal GVHD occurs, the diet order should indicate *GVHD diet protocol.*

REFERENCES

1. Aker SN, Cheney CL. The use of sterile and low microbial diets in ultraisolation environments. JPEN 1983;7:390–397.
2. Petz LD, Scott EP. Management of nutritional requirements. In: Blume KG, Lawrence MD, eds. Clinical bone marrow transplantation. New York: Churchill-Livingston, 1983:199–206.
3. Lenssen P, Aker SN. Nutritional assessment and management during marrow transplantation. A resource manual. Seattle: Fred Hutchinson Cancer Center, 1985.

OSTEOPOROSIS

General Description

For persons who have osteoporosis or who are at risk of developing osteoporosis, dietary recommendations emphasize the maintenance of a nutritionally adequate diet, which includes an adequate calcium intake from foods or supplements.

Nutritional Inadequacy

The diet recommended for osteoporosis is not inherently inadequate as compared to the Recommended Dietary Allowance (RDA).

Indications and Rationale

Osteoporosis is a common and potentially disabling disorder that afflicts primarily Caucasian women who are beyond the age of menopause.[1] Osteoporosis is a condition in which bone mass decreases, causing bones to become more susceptible to fracture. The loss of bone mass is most severe in the spine, but involves all of the skeleton. Compression fractures of the spine and fractures of the hip and forearm are serious consequences of osteoporosis.

The pathogenesis of osteoporosis has not been clearly elucidated. Hormonal changes, particularly a reduction in estrogen with natural or with induced menopause, accelerate the rate of bone loss. In addition, women are at a greater risk because they have less bone mass than men.[2] An inadequate calcium intake has frequently been cited as a cause of osteoporosis. Suboptimal consumption of calcium-containing foods in growth and young adult years may reduce the maximal bone mass development and contribute to the later development of osteoporosis.[3] Several research studies suggest that, in adults, a low calcium intake speeds up bone loss and that an increased calcium intake slows the process.[4,5] However, other research has not demonstrated a preventive role for calcium.[6] For persons with osteoporosis, a reduced rate of bone loss and fracture risk has been achieved through the use of calcium in combination with vitamin D, fluoride, and/or estrogen.[7]

Calcium insufficiency may be the result of inadequate calcium intake or decreased availability of calcium. The Second National Health and Nutrition Survey 1976 to 1980 (HANES II) indicates the average daily calcium intake for females does not exceed 85 percent of the RDA of 1,200 mg after the age of 12 years.[8] During the years of peak bone mass development (years 18 to 30), more than 66 percent of all U.S. women fail to consume the RDA of 800 mg of calcium on any given day; after age 35, this percentage increases to over 75 percent.[8,9] A decreased availability of calcium may be attributable to decreased absorptive capacity or to drug interference.[10]

Other dietary constituents, particularly an excess intake of alcohol and caffeine, have been implicated in the development of osteoporosis.[1,11] A stringent restriction of alcohol and of caffeine for the treatment or the prevention of osteoporosis is not warranted, although moderate use may be advisable for other health reasons.

Life-style habits, particularly smoking and inactivity, are associated with osteoporosis.[1] A causal role for smoking is unclear; however, its effect may be through reducing estrogen levels. Exercise, involving weight bearing reduces bone loss and increases bone mass. Exercise that is sufficient to induce amenorrhea in young women may lead to decreased bone mass.[1] Immobilization and prolonged bed rest produce rapid bone loss.

Women who are underweight have osteoporosis more often than women who are overweight.[1] This may be related to numerous factors, which include nutrient intake, smoking, increased stress on bone, or increased estrogen levels with obesity. However, those who have osteoporosis and are overweight may be advised to lose weight, especially if excess weight further limits mobility.

Osteoporosis should be distinguished from osteomalacia. Osteoporosis and osteomalacia are types of osteopenia, a general term that means reduced bone mass. In osteomalacia, there is a defect in the mineralization of protein bone matrix. Osteomalacia is characterized by a low serum calcium and phosphorus and an elevated serum alkaline phosphatase. Symptoms include diffuse bone pain and tenderness. Celiac sprue, pancreatic insufficiency, and short bowel syndrome may cause osteomalacia. In osteoporosis, mineralization is normal, but there is simply too little bone. Osteoporosis is characterized by normal serum calcium, phosphorus, and alkaline phosphatase levels. However, a bone biopsy is the only definitive means of distinguishing between these two forms of metabolic bone disease.

Goals of Dietary Management

The goal of nutritional intervention in osteoporosis is to prevent or to slow further bone loss in order to reduce the possibility of more fractures.

Dietary Recommendations

Persons who have or who are at risk for developing osteoporosis should be advised to maintain a nutritionally adequate diet. Although there are still unanswered questions regarding the role of calcium intake in the development of osteoporosis, current information suggests that it is rational for women to ingest the 1980 RDA[12] for calcium or slightly more (800 to 1,000 mg). It may be reasonable for women at increased risk for osteoporosis to ingest 1,000 to 1,500 mg of calcium. Those at risk for osteoporosis may include peri- and postmenopausal women, women who have had a premature loss of ovarian function, and women who have small bones, have fair skin, are underweight, have had a long-term low calcium intake, or have a strong family history of osteoporosis. Women who have osteoporosis may be advised to consume 1,000 to 1,500 mg of calcium or even slightly greater amounts on the advice of a physician.

Food Sources of Calcium. Obtaining adequate calcium from food sources is preferred (Table 6–42). The approximate calcium content of a diet without milk or other high calcium foods is 200 mg of calcium per 1,000 kilocalories. Diets of 1,500 to 2,500 kilocalories that do not contain milk or other good sources of calcium usually contain 300 to 600 mg of calcium. It is difficult to obtain an adequate amount of absorbable calcium from food sources on a daily basis unless milk or milk products are consumed. Although dark green leafy vegetables contain a moderate to high level of calcium, the calcium is partially bound to phytates and to oxalate, which reduces the amount of calcium that is available for absorption. Tofu, processed with calcium sulfate, and fish with bones are good sources of calcium, but are generally consumed too infrequently or in too small portions to be considered a major source of calcium.

TABLE 6–42   Calcium Content of High Calcium Foods

The following foods contain approximately 300 mg of calcium[13]

1 cup milk (skim, 2%, whole, or chocolate)
$1\frac{1}{2}$ oz cheddar type cheese
2 cups cottage cheese
$1\frac{3}{4}$ cup ice cream or ice milk
1 cup pudding
6 oz low fat yogurt
1/3 cup dry milk powder
3/4 cup collard greens, cooked
1 cup turnip greens, cooked
$1\frac{1}{2}$ cup other greens, cooked
8 oz tofu (processed with calcium sulfate)
3 oz sardines, with bones
5 oz salmon, with bones

Persons who have lactose intolerance and who experience bloating, abdominal cramps, flatulence, or diarrhea with the ingestion of milk may have fewer symptoms if milk and milk products are consumed in small amounts at a time and with meals. Lactase enzyme replacement can also be used. (See *Lactose Intolerance,* page 165, for additional information.)

Calcium Supplements. The use of calcium supplements (Table 6–43) is not advocated in preference to food sources; however, they may be necessary to achieve an adequate calcium intake. Persons who require calcium supplements should be made aware of the various calcium salts, their appropriate use, and the ways of minimizing side effects, such as constipation. More serious side effects from the long-term ingestion of calcium salt supplements are uncommon, but do occur.[14] These side effects include hypercalcemia, hypercalciuria, urolithiasis, and gastric acid rebound. Also, the chronic ingestion of large amounts of calcium and of absorbable alkali, such as calcium carbonate, can induce milk-alkali syndrome (subacute or chronic hypercalcemia with fully or partially reversible renal failure). It is unlikely that milk-alkali syndrome will occur with the ingestion of 1 or 2 g of calcium per day. However, the over zealous person who decides "more is better" may be at greater risk.

TABLE 6–43   Calcium Content of Some Commercial Calcium Carbonate Supplements

Brand	mg of calcium per tablet
Oyster shell calcium (generic, 650 mg size)	260 mg
Tums[R] antacid	200 mg
Os-Cal[R] 500	500 mg
Caltrate[R] 600	600 mg
Ca-Plus[R]	280 mg
Titralac (liquid, 1 teaspoon)	400 mg

Calcium supplementation is generally not encouraged for individuals with hypercalcemia, hypercalciuria, or a history of calcium-containing urolithiasis. Medical consultation is necessary in this case.

If the dietitian makes a recommendation for calcium supplementation, the amount should be documented in the patient's medical record. Several different forms of supplements are available. Usually, calcium carbonate is recommended because it contains the highest percentage of calcium (40 percent). Calcium lactate is 13 percent calcium, and calcium gluconate is only 9 percent calcium. For example, a 650 mg tablet of calcium carbonate contains approximately 260 mg of elemental calcium, whereas an equivalent amount of calcium lactate or calcium gluconate contains 85 and 59 mg of elemental calcium, respectively.

Absorption and utilization of calcium supplements appear to be better when supplements are taken with meals and taken throughout the day rather than in a single dose.[15] Calcium carbonate may cause constipation for some people. (See page 141 for guidelines for preventing constipation.) Calcium-containing antacids are a good source of calcium and have the advantage of being chewable, which may be important for those persons who have difficulty swallowing calcium tablets.

Bone meal and dolomite are not recommended because they may be contaminated with toxic substances, such as lead, mercury, and arsenic. Chelated calcium tablets are not recommended. They are expensive and have no advantage over other types of calcium. Supplemental magnesium is generally not necessary since magnesium is available in adequate amounts from foods in the diet.

An adequate amount of vitamin D is necessary for bone mineralization. If the patient has regular exposure to sunlight or uses vitamin D fortified milk, vitamin D intake is probably adequate. Additional vitamin D, which is present in some calcium supplements, should generally not exceed the RDA of 400 IU per day. Larger amounts of vitamin D should not be taken except under supervision of a physician.

Physicians: How to Order Diet

The diet order should indicate *high calcium diet* or a specific level of dietary calcium intake.

REFERENCES

1. National Institutes of Health Consensus Conference. Osteoporosis. J Am Med Assoc 1984;252:799–802.
2. Riggs BL, Melton LJ III. Involutional osteoporosis. N Engl J Med 1986;314:1676–1686.
3. Sandler RB, Slemenda CW, La Porte RE, Cauley JA, Schramm MM, Barresi ML, Kriska AM. Postmenopausal bone density and milk consumption in childhood and adolescence. Am J Clin Nutr 1985;42:270–274.
4. Recker RR, Saville PD, Heany RP. Effects of estrogens and calcium carbonate on bone loss in postmenopausal women. Ann Intern Med 1977;87:649–655.
5. Recker RR, Heany RP. The effect of milk supplements on calcium metabolism and calcium balance. Am J Clin Nutr 1985;41:254–263.
6. Nilas L, Christiansen C, Rodbro P. Calcium supplementation and postmenopausal bone loss. Br Med J 1984;289:1103–1106.
7. Riggs BL, Seeman E, Hodgson SF, Taves DR, O'Fallon WM. Effect of the fluoride/ calcium regimen on vertebral fracture occurrence in postmenopausal osteoporosis. N Engl J Med 1982;306:422–450.
8. Carroll MD, Abraham S, Dresser CM. Dietary intake source data: United States, 1976–80. Washington D.C., U.S. Govt Printing Office, National Center for Health Statistics, Public Health Service 1983 (Vital and health statistics. Series 11:No 231). (DDHS publication no. (PHS)83–1681).
9. Heany RP, Gallagher JC, Johnston CC, Neer R, Parfitt AM, Whedon GD. Calcium nutrition and bone health in the elderly. Am J Clin Nutr 1982;36(Suppl):986–1013.
10. Allen LH. Calcium bioavailability and absorption: a review. Am J Clin Nutr 1982;35:783–808.
11. Heany RP, Recker RR. Effects of nitrogen, phosphorous, and caffeine on calcium balance in women. J Lab Clin Med 1982;99:46–55.
12. Food and Nutrition Board, National Research Council. Recommended Dietary Allowances. 9th ed. Washington, D.C., National Research Council, 1980.
13. Pennington JAT, Church HN. Bowes and Church's food values of portions commonly used. 14th ed. Philadelphia: J.B. Lippincott, 1985.
14. Health H III, Callaway CW. Calcium tablets for hypertension? A consideration of risks and benefits (editorial). Ann Intern Med 1985;103:946–947.
15. Recker RR. Calcium absorption and achlorhydria. N Engl J Med 1985;313:70–73.

RENAL DISEASE

The kidneys function as excretory, regulatory, and endocrine organs. They excrete waste products, regulate water and electrolyte content of the body, and are the site of the formation of renin, an enzyme involved in the regulation of electrolyte metabolism. Also formed in the kidneys are 1, 25 dihydroxyvitamin D_3 and erythropoetin.[1]

Nephrons are the minute structural units of the kidney that carry out these functions. The number of functioning nephrons is decreased in the diseased kidney. As the disease progresses, the waste products (e.g., urea, creatinine, uric acid, sulfate, and organic acids) increase in the blood, and the capacity of the kidney to excrete and to conserve both water and electrolytes is impaired.

Dietary fats and carbohydrates are metabolized to carbon dioxide and water and thus leave no residue. However, breakdown products of protein, including urea, creatinine, and other nitrogenous substances, must be excreted by the kidneys. The amount of a substance that must be excreted daily to prevent accumulation in the body is called the load. The load of creatinine is fairly constant from day to day and depends on the mass of muscle and similar tissues. In contrast, the load of urea depends on the dietary intake of protein and on tissue catabolism.[2] Thus, if the ability of the kidney to excrete nitrogenous substances deteriorates, measurements of urea or urea nitrogen levels in the blood can be used as an indication of the effectiveness of a protein restricted diet, and the creatinine levels can be used as an indication of the degree of underlying kidney injury.[2]

The normal kidney conserves water in states of water lack by producing only a small volume of concentrated urine, but disposes of an excessive amount of water by producing a large volume of dilute urine. In instances of advanced kidney failure there is a diminished capacity to excrete dilute or concentrated urine, but this usually is not a significant clinical problem.

The kidneys regulate the amount of an electrolyte in the body by excreting larger or smaller amounts of that substance as required. With a diet of ordinary composition, the amount of potassium, phosphate, and hydrogen ion that must be excreted requires that the concentrations in the urine be many times greater than those in the plasma. Catabolism, even to a rather minor degree, increases the acidity of the urine. Thus, with impaired kidney function, there is a tendency toward increased levels of potassium and of phosphorus and toward acidosis.[1]

Increased amounts of sodium and chloride in the body tend to be associated with higher than usual blood pressure and with edema. Excess dietary sodium increases the possibility of edema, weight gain, hypertension, and thirst. Insufficient dietary sodium may result in weight loss, depletion of extracellular fluid volume, orthostatic hypotension, and a further decrease in glomerular filtration rate.[1]

A number of disorders can cause a gradual deterioration of all functions of the nephron. The degree of failure is estimated by measuring creatinine clearance, the milliliters of plasma "cleared" of creatinine during each minute.[3] Compensation for variations in body size is accomplished by expressing the clearance in terms of an average sized person with a surface area of 1.73 m^2. There is a wide range of normal, but the mean normal creatinine clearance is 90 ml per minute per 1.73 m^2 for young men and 84 ml per minute per 1.73 m^2 for young women. There is a 6 ml per minute per 1.73 m^2 per decade decrease with aging. Iothalamate clearance is considered a better measure of renal function status than creatinine clearance. The normal iothalamate clearance, for both men and women, is 110 ml per minute per 1.73 m^2 with a 4 ml per minute per 1.73 m^2 per decade decrease with aging.

Fortunately, kidneys have a great reserve capacity. Kidneys can maintain their functional capacity, usually without symptomatic complications to the individual, even if 60 percent of the nephrons have been destroyed. The patient usually does not become aware of symptoms until the residual kidney function is less than 30 percent. This is reflected clinically by a creatinine clearance of less than 30 to 40 ml per minute per 1.73 m^2. At this level of renal function, serum concentrations of urea and creatinine are elevated. It is important to recognize that the upper limits of serum creatinine concentrations are lower for infants, small children, and adults with reduced muscle mass than for normal-sized adults.[3] Accumulation of protein waste products may contribute to tiredness, nausea, vomiting, anorexia, a general deterioration of health, and weight loss, perhaps both from loss of protein tissue and from decreased fat stores.

Treatment choices consist of (1) limiting dietary protein intake and instituting other modalities to reduce the waste product concentration and to return the electrolyte composition of the body to normal; (2) using a hemodialysis machine to remove the waste products; (3) continuous ambulatory peritoneal dialysis (CAPD), a self-dialysis technique that does not require a machine; (4) continuous cycling peritoneal dialysis (CCPD), using an automated machine to pass the dialysate in and out of the peritoneal cavity at night; and (5) renal transplantation. Dietary management in each treatment modality is discussed in subsequent sections.

REFERENCES

1. Liddle VR. Nutrition for the patient with end-stage renal disease. In: Lancaster LE, ed. The patient with end-stage renal disease. New York, New York: John Wiley & Sons, 1984:92.
2. Burton BT, Hirschman GH. Current concepts of nutritional therapy in renal failure: an update. J Am Diet Assoc 1983;82(4):359–363.
3. Sargent J, Gotch F. Urea kinetics: a guide to nutritional management of renal failure. Am J Clin Nutr 1978;31:1696–1702.

ACUTE RENAL FAILURE

General Description

The diet emphasizes control of protein, sodium, potassium, fluid, and kilocalories according to the use of dialysis and the needs of the individual.

Nutritional Inadequacy

Potential nutritional inadequacies depend on the treatment modality. If a low protein diet is used, nutritional inadequacies are related to the degree of restriction (see Table 6–45). If repetitive dialysis is necessary to treat acute renal failure, nutritional risks exist as with dialysis for chronic renal failure (see page 220).

Indications and Rationale

Acute renal failure is characterized by a sudden decrease in glomerular filtration rate and/or tubular damage. It may be ischemic, hypersensitivity related, or nephrotoxic. Ischemic acute renal failure can result from hemorrhage, shock, or septicemia. Acute renal failure that results from hypersensitivity occurs with systemic or local renal reactions to certain drugs and to contrast dyes. The nephrotoxic type of acute renal failure is caused most often by aminoglycoside antibiotics.[1] Sepsis and trauma often occur along with acute renal failure and are usually the cause of the high morbidity and mortality that are associated with acute renal failure. One-third of the patients with acute renal failure are non-oliguric; the other two-thirds of the patients go through an oliguric and then a diuretic phase. The oliguric phase is marked by azotemia, acidosis, high serum potassium, high serum phosphorous, hypertension, anorexia, edema, and risk of water intoxication (characterized by low serum sodium levels.) In the past, the oliguric phase was thought to occur for 2 to 4 weeks. However, it is not uncommon for it to persist for approximately 6 weeks.[2]

Acute renal failure often occurs in the setting of impaired gastrointestinal tract function owing to surgery or trauma. Nutritional considerations depend on the function of the gastrointestinal tract, the daily urine volume, and whether or not repetitive dialysis is being used.

The amount of protein recommended depends on whether dialysis is used. Thirty to 40 g of protein per day is usually appropriate if dialysis is not being used and if the patient is not highly catabolic. It may be advisable to start dialysis earlier and to use central parenteral nutrition (CPN) to supplement suboptimal oral intake if plasma urea levels rise rapidly as a result of a highly catabolic state. Give 1.0 to 1.5 g of essential and non-essential amino acids per kilogram per day. Lipids may be used in the CPN solution as an additional kilocalorie source.[2]

Kilocalorie requirements can be determined following the guidelines in *Nutritional Assessment* (see page 3). The amount of fluid allowed in acute renal failure generally equals the urine volume plus 500 ml. The amount of dietary sodium used is usually 40 to 90 mEq. If hyperkalemia exists, dietary potassium is restricted to less than 60 mEq per day.[3] Table 6–44 summarizes the dietary restrictions for acute renal failure.

Common Nutritional Problems

A common nutritional concern is poor appetite. High caloric enteral supplements are frequently used to maintain adequate nutrition. Protein supplements may be necessary if the patient is on dialysis and, therefore, requires a higher protein intake.

Goals of Dietary Management

The goals of nutrition therapy in acute renal failure are to maintain the chemical composition of the body as close to normal as possible and to preserve body protein stores until renal function returns. Although these goals are similar to those established for chronic renal failure, they are more difficult to achieve because of the acute nature of the loss of renal function and because of the presence of other life-threatening diseases.

Dietary Recommendations

The food exchange list for protein, sodium, and potassium control can be used for meal planning.

TABLE 6–44 Dietary Restrictions in Acute Renal Failure

Component	Comments
Protein	If not on dialysis, 0.4 to 0.6 g/kg or 30–40 g If on dialysis, 1–1.5 g/kg from dietary and parenteral sources
Kilocalories	Sufficient for weight maintenance Encourage non-protein kilocalories from fats, oils, and simple carbohydrate
Sodium	40 to 90 mEq
Fluid	Limit beverages and foods that are liquid at room temperature to an amount equal to urine volume plus 500 ml
Potassium	If hyperkalemia exists, restrict to ≤60 mEq

Physicians: How to Order Diet

The diet order should indicate the *specific level of protein* (the most common levels are 30 and 40 g), the *specific level of sodium* (the most common levels are 40, 60, and 90 mEq) and the *specific amount of fluid.*

The dietitian calculates caloric needs. Restriction of potassium (usually ≤60 mEq) should be indicated if needed.

REFERENCES

1. Schrier RW. Acute renal failure. JAMA 1982;247:2518–2525.
2. Lazarus JM, Brenner BM. Acute renal failure. Philadelphia: WB Saunders, 1983:797.
3. Anderson CF, Nelson R, Margie J, Johnson J, Hunt J. Nutritional therapy for adults with renal disease. JAMA 1973;223:68–72.

CHRONIC RENAL FAILURE

General Description

The diet emphasizes a controlled intake of protein, sodium, and kilocalories.

Nutritional Inadequacy

Potential amino acid deficiencies exist in diets that provide less total protein than the Recommended Dietary Allowances (RDA) of 0.8 g protein per kilogram of body weight. To counter this risk, approximately 75 percent of the total protein intake should be high biologic value protein.[1]

Diets of 50 g of protein or less per day provide inadequate calcium, iron, phosphorous, thiamine, riboflavin, niacin, and folic acid by the RDA criteria.[2] Therefore, a daily multivitamin that includes folic acid is recommended. Natabec Rx is the currently preferred vitamin preparation because it provides 1 mg folic acid and all other recommended vitamins in one tablet. It also contains vitamin A, which could potentially promote vitamin A toxicity in the future. Other vitamin preparations are being investigated that do not contain vitamin A.

Diets that provide more than 50 g of protein, but less than the RDA, may provide inadequate calcium and iron.[1]

Indications and Rationale

Protein. Preliminary animal research, and even more preliminary human research, suggest that early intervention with protein restriction not only prevents the symptoms of chronic renal failure (CRF), but *may* preserve kidney function.[3–5] The current practice at the Mayo Clinic is to treat CRF with a low protein diet. However, it is uncertain whether the low protein diet retards deterioration of kidney function.

The patient's symptoms, as well as the degree of impairment of renal function, should be considered when the level of protein restriction is determined. Table 6–45 shows the initial suggested intake of protein per kilogram of actual body weight for the corresponding level of renal function in the adult patient.[5] It should be noted that the suggested protein intake is based on actual body weight (corrected for edema), not ideal or desired weight.

TABLE 6–45 Suggested Protein Intake in Chronic Renal Failure

Creatinine Clearance ml/min/1.73 m²	Daily Protein Intake*	
	g/kg	g/70 kg
30 to 20	0.60	42
19 to 5	0.45	32
5	0.40	28

*Plus an amount of protein equal to the 24-hour urinary protein loss.

If proteinuria is present, an amount of protein equal to that lost in the urine, as determined by a 24-hour urine collection, should be added to the calculated daily protein allowance (see *Nephrotic Syndrome* page 232). Approximately 75 percent of the total protein should be of high biologic value (eggs, milk, and meat) to assure an adequate intake of essential amino acids.[3] Diets providing less than 50 g of protein should include egg daily because of the high biologic value of eggs. To minimize the use of dietary protein as a calorie source, it is recommended that high protein foods be distributed throughout the day and not be "saved" for consumption in a single meal.

Close follow-up of patients by the use of 7-day food records is advised so that protein intake can be modified according to the patient's course.

Kilocalories. Utilization of dietary protein is directly influenced by total caloric intake. Therefore, adequate caloric intake is of vital importance to the patient with renal disease (1) to prevent catabolism of body protein, (2) to ensure that dietary protein is not used as an energy source, (3) to maintain a constant body weight, and (4) to favor the preservation of normal vigor and of feelings of well-being.[3,4,6] Patients need to be reminded to maintain an adequate caloric intake, since they often adhere more closely to the protein restriction and neglect their caloric needs. Patients should be encouraged to consume adequate kilocalories from the intake of fats and carbohydrates. Consumption of these non-protein kilocalories, along with the dietary protein, may spare endogenous tissue protein from use as an energy source. Caloric needs can be determined according to the guidelines described in *Nutritional Assessment,* page 3.

Weight reduction should be approached cautiously because of the risk of catabolism of lean body tissue, in addition to fat catabolism. Unless immediate weight loss is compelling, stringent caloric restriction is not recommended since it may be hazardous, especially if renal function is less than 15 percent of normal. A moderate caloric deficit, no more than 250 to 500 Kcal, is recommended.

Sodium. The level of sodium intake should be specific to the patient's needs. Maximal renal function is achieved when sodium intake is adjusted to just below a level that causes edema or hypertension (or both).[4] If edema or hypertension are present, a sodium intake of 60 to 90 mEq per day is often indicated.[1] In the extremely edematous patient, more strict control (less than 60 mEq of sodium per day) and diuretics may be needed initially. The diet should be planned to provide the prescribed level of sodium ± 10 percent.* For example, if a diet of 90 mEq of sodium is requested, the diet should be calculated to provide between 81 and 99 mEq of sodium. A measured amount of added salt is necessary only in rare instances. Most renal patients can conserve sodium reasonably well.

---

*In other situations, such as management of hypertension, the diet prescription is interpreted to mean "less than or equal to" the desired sodium level. The diet may actually provide considerably less than the prescribed level. However, in renal disease, the diet should be planned to provide the prescribed level ± 10 percent.

Potassium. The serum potassium level usually remains within the normal range when urinary volume is normal. Dietary potassium control becomes more important when urine volume decreases to below normal.[6] However, as a precaution, patients should be advised to avoid potassium chloride (salt substitute) unless the physician prescribes it as a medication to correct hypokalemia. With normal urine output, hypokalemia usually does not occur unless excess sodium intake necessitates increased use of diuretics, thereby resulting in a corresponding loss of potassium.

Calcium and Phosphorous. As the glomerular filtration rate declines to 30 percent of normal or less, the dietary phosphate load is greater than the kidney can excrete.[3] Consequently, the serum phosphorous concentration rises and may, in turn, cause the serum calcium level to decrease. The impaired production by diseased kidneys of 1, 25 dihydroxyvitamin D_3 decreases the intestinal absorption of dietary calcium. These factors lead to a lowered serum calcium concentration, which stimulates increased secretion of parathyroid hormone. Renal osteodystrophy and metastatic calcification are two of the demonstrable complications that may result from the body's adjustments to normalize serum calcium and phosphorous levels.

Some degree of restriction of phosphorous and calcium is inherent in a low protein diet.[3,4] On a low protein diet the daily phosphorous intake is already well below the usual American intake (1,500 mg per day). The phosphorous intake can be decreased further if dairy products and whole-grain breads and cereals are eliminated from the diet (see *Appendix 12* for the phosphorous content of foods). However, the use of phosphate binders (aluminum hydroxide or aluminum carbonate) usually is necessary to sufficiently decrease serum phosphorous. Unfortunately, aluminum toxicity is a potential problem, especially in children.[1]

Calcium intake is generally low on a protein controlled diet. Increased calcium needs often are best met by calcium supplements.[4] Calcium carbonate is a weak phosphate binding agent. Dietary phosphorous restriction, in conjunction with calcium carbonate supplementation, may be used to control serum calcium and phosphorous without using aluminum phosphate binders. Table 6–46 summarizes the dietary restrictions in chronic renal failure.

TABLE 6–46 Dietary Restrictions in Chronic Renal Failure

Component	Comments
Sodium	Generally 60 to 90 mEq Calculate sodium level ± 10 percent of diet order
Kilocalories	Sufficient for weight maintenance, weight gain, or slow weight loss (0.2 to 0.4 kg or 1/2 to 1 lb/wk) Encourage non-protein calories (fat, carbohydrate)
Protein	0.4 to 0.6 g/kg body weight + 24-hour urinary protein loss Approximately 75% of protein from high biologic value sources (meat, poultry, fish, egg, milk); use of egg should be encouraged because of high protein quality; high protein foods should be distributed throughout the day
Potassium	Generally no restriction of food sources Avoid potassium chloride (salt substitutes)
Phosphorous	Reduced intake is inherent in low protein diet Further restriction only if serum phosphorous level elevated
Calcium	Calcium carbonate supplements if ordered by physician

Goals of Dietary Management

The goals of dietary management are (1) to control sodium intake, thereby maximizing renal function, preventing edema, and controlling blood pressure; (2) to provide adequate non-protein calories, thereby preventing muscle catabolism, and (3) to limit protein intake, thereby preventing excessive accumulation of nitrogenous waste products and preventing uremic toxicity.

Dietary Recommendations

The food exchange list for protein, sodium, and potassium control is used for meal planning. For most persons, the potassium subgroupings can be ignored at this point.

Chronic Renal Failure and Diabetes

Some compromises must be made in the usual diabetic diet when diabetes mellitus is complicated by renal failure. The requirements of the protein controlled diet generally take priority, especially at extremely low levels of protein intake.[1]

The decrease in protein intake requires a corresponding increase in intake of fat and carbohydrate. Low protein products can be used as a source of kilocalories. To assure adequate kilocalories, one also may have to include simple carbohydrates, such as sugar, jellies, and sugar-sweetened fruit. If simple carbohydrates are consumed, they should be measured carefully and distributed evenly throughout the day to minimize fluctuation in blood sugar levels. Patients often are reluctant to eat simple sugars; thus, the rationale behind their incorporation must be clearly stated to ensure compliance.

The food exchange list for protein, sodium, and potassium control, rather than the diabetic exchange list, is used for meal planning. Consistency in timing and in composition of meals and the use of additional food for increased exercise and to prevent hypoglycemic reactions are still appropriate.

Physicians: How to Order Diet

The diet order should indicate the *specific level of protein* (the most common levels are 30, 40, and 50 g), and the *specific level of sodium* (the most common levels are 60 and 90 mEq).

The dietitian will calculate caloric needs. The diet order should indicate if weight loss is desired. Restriction of potassium, other than to caution against use of potassium chloride, is not included unless specifically requested. Restriction of phosphorous beyond that inherent in the diet, is not included unless specifically requested.

REFERENCES

1. Sargent J, Gotch F. Urea kinetics: a guide to nutritional management of renal failure. Am J Clin Nutr 1978;31:1696–1702.
2. Carron D. A review of vitamin supplements for adults undergoing hemodialysis. CRN Quarterly 1985;9:7–8.
3. Liddle VR. Nutrition for the patient with end-stage renal disease. In: Lancaster LE,

ed. The patient with end-stage renal disease. New York, New York: John Wiley & Sons, 1984:92.

4. Kopple JD. Nutrition management of chronic renal failure. Postgrad Med 1978; 64(5):135–144.

5. Bergstrom J. Discovery and rediscovery of low protein diet. Clin Nephro 1984;21(1):29–35.

6. Burton BT, Hirschman GH. Current concepts of nutritional therapy in renal failure: an update. J Am Diet Assoc 1983;82(4):359–363.

HEMODIALYSIS

General Description

The diet emphasizes controlled intake of kilocalories, protein, fluid, sodium, potassium, and phosphorous. Recommended levels are dependent on the frequency of dialysis and on the individual medical situation.

Nutritional Inadequacy

The dialysis patient is at risk for deficiencies of water-soluble vitamins and minerals, particularly vitamin B_6, folic acid, vitamin C, and iron, because of the loss of these nutrients in the dialysate.[1] A daily multivitamin that includes folic acid and iron is recommended. Natabec Rx is currently the preferred vitamin preparation, but other vitamin preparations not containing vitamin A are under investigation.

Trace minerals also may be lost in the dialysate, but the extent of the losses is unknown. There is not currently an acceptable means of supplementation beyond those provided in Natabec Rx.

The risk of nutrient deficiencies is greater when the patient has poor dietary intake. Poor intake may be the result of poor appetite, of nausea and vomiting, or of limitations on food choices imposed by restriction of potassium or phosphorous.

Indications and Rationale

Although the dialysis machine is capable of duplicating much of the kidney's function, it does not have the flexibility of the normal kidney. Without nutritional intervention, dangerous levels of waste products can accumulate between dialyses.[2] Protein-calorie malnutrition also may occur. Dietary recommendations should be based upon the frequency of dialysis, the level of residual intrinsic renal function, and the size of the patient.

Protein. The protein intake of the patient must be sufficient to maintain nitrogen balance and to replace amino acids and nitrogen lost during dialysis. However, the protein intake must be low enough to prevent excessive interdialytic accumulation of waste products.

At the Mayo Clinic, dietary protein prescription and dialysis therapy are individually tailored according to the patient's actual body weight ("dry weight"), the residual kidney function, and the urea kinetic modelling.[3]

The overall goals of urea kinetic modelling are (1) to individualize the length of dialysis necessary to maintain blood urea nitrogen or urea within a target range and (2) to provide a means for early intervention in patients with poor nutritional status or with excessive protein intake.

Urea kinetic modelling is based on work done by Sargent and Gotch.[3] It is a computerized clinical tool for assessing protein metabolism and for monitoring the efficacy of diet and of the patient's compliance. Urea kinetic modelling utilizes the net protein catabolic rate (PCR). The PCR is a reflection of the amount of protein that is catabolized per kilogram of body weight per 24 hours. It provides useful information for the determination of nitrogen balance. Urea kinetic analysis uses the patient's PCR, the residual renal function, and the dialyzer characteristics to forecast the length of treatment time necessary to maintain a midweek plasma urea or blood urea nitrogen (BUN) within a designated target range. (Plasma or blood urea $\times$ 0.47 = BUN).

Catabolized protein can be either endogenous (muscle catabolism) or exogenous (dietary) in origin. To determine the source of catabolized protein, the patient's reported protein intake from 3- to 5-day food records is compared to the PCR. This comparison indicates if the patient's protein intake is inadequate or excessive. Nutritionally stable patients have a PCR equivalent to the reported dietary protein intake. Correlation of dietary protein intake, the PCR, changes in weight, and changes in serum albumin can assist in the identification and the prevention of catabolism and in the maintenance of optimum nutritional status.

As a general rule of thumb, the protein need for the average adult with minimal residual renal function who requires dialysis three times a week usually can be supplied by a diet that provides 1 g of protein per kilogram of body weight.[4] Approximately 75 percent of the total protein intake should be of high biologic value (eggs, meats, and milk). Some researchers suggest that 1.2 g of dietary protein per kilogram of body weight is desirable and that this amount can be used as a general guide if PCR determinations are not available.[4]

Kilocalories. Adequate caloric intake is necessary to prevent catabolism of lean body tissue. Caloric needs generally remain the same as they were prior to dialysis and can be determined according to the guidelines described in *Nutritional Assessment,* page 3.

Adequate intake of non-protein kilocalories is encouraged to prevent the use of dietary protein for energy. The primary sources of non-protein kilocalories are fats, oils, simple carbohydrates, and low protein products.[2]

Weight reduction should be approached cautiously because of the risk of catabolism of lean body tissue in addition to fat catabolism. Only slow weight loss, no more than 0.2 to 0.4 kg per week (1/2 to 1 pound per week), should be attempted. Correspondingly, the recommended caloric deficit should be no more than 250 to 500 kcal per day.

Sodium. Sodium intake control of 40 to 120 mEq per day is usually necessary to control hypertension and edema. Restriction of sodium is extremely helpful in blunting thirst, and thus prevents excessive fluid intake and weight gain.[2] A higher sodium intake may be encouraged 7 to 9 hours before dialysis in attempt to prevent hypotension or muscle cramps during dialysis. A high sodium intake during dialysis is not encouraged since it contributes to excessive thirst that may persist beyond the dialysis and that may result in excessive weight gain due to edema.

Potassium. Potassium restriction is essential. Hyperkalemia can result in cardiac dysrhythmia and even cardiac arrest.[2] The potassium level of the diet is largely determined by the potassium concentration of the dialysate. With a dialysate concentration of 1 mEq or more of potassium per liter, dietary potassium must be limited to 60 mEq or less per day. With a dialysate concentration of less than 1 mEq of potassium per liter, dietary potassium may be more liberal (up to 100 mEq).

Fluid. Limitation of fluid is often the most difficult aspect of the diet for the dialysis patient. If the body retains excess water, but sodium intake is restricted, a state of hyponatremia and "water intoxication" may occur. This state is characterized by tremulousness and disorientation, but not necessarily edema.

Fluid sources are (1) beverages and foods that are liquid at room temperature, such as ice cream and gelatin; (2) water content of non-liquid foods; and (3) water formed from the oxidation of food. For practical purposes, the water content of non-liquid foods and the water formed from oxidation of food can be disregarded since they are approximately equal to insensible water loss (respiration, perspiration, and fecal losses) in the stable dialysis patient.[4] Insensible loss may be elevated in states of fever, with extensive burns, or in a warm dry environment. Water of metabolism may be substantially increased in catabolic states or with a large oral or parenteral intake of calories. It is reasonable to consider as dietary fluid sources only beverages and foods that melt at room temperature. To achieve the optimal interdialytic weight gain of 1 pound or less per day, the total dietary fluid allowance can be calculated by adding urine volume and 500 ml.

Calcium and Phosphorous. Hypocalcemia and hyperphosphatemia must be controlled in the uremic state to avoid hyperparathyroidism and to minimize skeletal changes and soft-tissue calcification. Serum calcium and phosphorous levels are difficult to alter by dietary means.[2] Phosphorous and calcium are best controlled by the use of phosphate binders and calcium supplements. Limiting dietary protein generally decreases both calcium and phosphorous intake.

Methods for controlling phosphorous have been modified because of the potential for aluminum toxicity with prolonged use of aluminum-containing phosphorous binders. Currently, the first step is to recommend strict dietary phosphorous limitation in conjunction with calcium carbonate supplementation (taken with meals).[5] Usual phosphorous intake can be determined from 3- or 4-day food records. A specific level of phosphorous is not recommended. Rather, particularly high phosphorous foods are proscribed, and lower phosphorous alternatives are recommended. (See *Appendix 12* for phosphorous content of foods and page 242 for high phosphorous foods.) Calcium carbonate is a much weaker and less efficient phosphorous binder than aluminum-containing antacids. Hypercalcemia and an increase in phosphorous sometimes occur on this program. Therefore, calcium and phosphorous must be closely monitored. Persistent elevations in phosphorous may necessitate use of aluminum-containing phosphate binders, which are currently the most effective means of reducing serum phosphorous. Table 6–47 summarizes dietary restrictions with hemodialysis.

Other Nutrition Problems

Patients on chronic maintenance dialysis commonly develop hypertriglyceridemia and/or hypercholesterolemia.[6] Dietary efforts to regulate hypertriglyceridemia consist of weight control and avoidance of alcohol. Simple carbohydrates are an important calorie source, and it is often not feasible to restrict them. Usual recommendations for hypercholesterolemia often are not practical. Total fat intake is generally high since fat is a major non-protein calorie source. However, the use of polyunsaturated fat is recommended. In actual practice, high cholesterol foods, such as eggs and cheese, are not limited because of their

TABLE 6–47 Dietary Restrictions with Hemodialysis

Component	Comments
Protein	1 g/kg body weight, adjusted according to individual dialysis characteristics
Kilocalories	Sufficient for weight maintenance, weight gain, or slow weight loss (0.2 to 0.4 kg or 1/2 to 1 lb/wk) Encourage non-protein kilocalories from fats, oils, and simple carbohydrate
Sodium	40 to 120 mEq, generally 90 mEq Calculate the sodium level ± 10 percent of the diet order
Potassium	If dialysate contains ≥1 mEq potassium/liter, limit to ≤60 mEq potassium If dialysate <1 mEq potassium/liter, limit to ≤100 mEq potassium
Fluid	Limit beverages and foods that are liquid at room temperature to an amount equal to urine volume plus 500 ml
Phosphorous	Restrict dietary phosphorous
Calcium	Calcium carbonate supplements if ordered by the physician

importance as protein sources. Exercise is encouraged to control weight and to promote an increase in high density lipoprotein.

Another common nutrition concern is poor appetite, partly owing to changes in taste acuity and in food preferences, especially for red meat and sweets. Changes in gut motility may also effect appetite.[2] Enteral supplements of high protein and/or high caloric content are frequently needed by the dialysis patient to maintain adequate nutrition. In an attempt to increase protein intake, increased use of dairy products may be encouraged and the serum phosphorous may be allowed to rise slightly above 5.5 mg per deciliter, provided the product of calcium level multiplied by phosphorous level is less than 60.

Goals of Dietary Management

The goals of dietary management are (1) to provide sufficient protein to compensate for essential amino acids and nitrogen lost in the dialysate, to maintain nitrogen balance, and yet to prevent excessive accumulation of waste products; (2) to provide adequate kilocalories to prevent catabolism of lean body tissue; (3) to limit sodium intake to control blood pressure and thirst and prevent edema; (4) to control potassium to prevent hyperkalemia and cardiac arrhythmia; (5) to control fluid intake to prevent hyponatremia and excess interdialytic weight gain; and (6) to limit phosphorous to control hyperphosphatemia and renal osteodystrophy.

Dietary Recommendations

The food exchange list for protein, sodium, and potassium control is used for meal planning. Additional modifications of the list may be necessary for restriction of phosphorous (see *Appendix 12*) and saturated fat.

Physicians: How to Order Diet

The diet order should indicate the *specific level of protein* (generally, the initial order is 1 g protein per kilogram body weight), the *specific level of sodium* (generally, the initial order is 90 mEq sodium. The usual range is 40 to 120 mEq sodium), the *specific level of potassium* (the most common levels are 60 mEq or less daily and 100 mEq or less daily), and the *specific amount of fluid.*

The dietitian will calculate caloric needs. The diet order should indicate if weight loss is desired. Restriction of phosphorous is routinely included. Dietary modifications for hyperlipidemia are included if the patient has hyperlipidemia.

REFERENCES

1. Liddle VR. Nutrition for the patient with end-stage renal disease. In: Lancaster LE, ed. The patient with end-stage renal disease. New York: John Wiley & Sons, 1984:92–105.
2. Harum P. Renal nutrition for the renal nurse. ANNA J 1984;11(5)38–43.
3. Sargent J, Gotch F. Urea kinetics: a guide to nutritional management of renal failure. Am J Clin Nutr 1978;31:1696–1702.
4. Kluthe R, Lüttgen FM, Capetianu T, Heinze V, Katz N, Sudhöff A. Protein requirements in maintenance hemodialysis. Am J Clin Nutr 1978;31:1812–1820.
5. Slatopolsky E, Weerts C, Lopez-Hilker S, Norwood K, Zink M, Windus D, Delmez J. Calcium carbonate as a phosphate binder in patients with chronic renal failure undergoing dialysis. N Engl J Med 1986;315:157–161.
6. Lindner A, Charra B, Sherrard DJ, Scribner BH. Accelerated atherosclerosis in prolonged maintenance hemodialysis. N Engl J Med 1974;290:697–701.

CONTINUOUS AMBULATORY PERITONEAL DIALYSIS

General Description

The diet emphasizes a high protein intake to offset the loss of protein in the dialysate, adequate calories to maintain a desirable weight, and moderate sodium restriction.

Nutritional Inadequacy

As in hemodialysis, the patient undergoing continuous ambulatory peritoneal dialysis is at risk for deficiencies of water-soluble vitamins and minerals. The extent of losses are unknown. A daily multivitamin that includes water-soluble vitamins, particularly folic acid and iron, is recommended. Natabec Rx is currently the preferred vitamin preparation, although, as stated before, it may be discontinued owing to its content of vitamin A.

Indications and Rationale

Continuous ambulatory peritoneal dialysis (CAPD) is a self-dialysis technique that does not require a machine, unlike other dialysis techniques. Perceived benefits of CAPD by the patient include freedom from in-center dialysis, liberalization of diet, and an increased sense of well-being. The major disadvantage of CAPD is the risk of peritonitis with the potential need for hospitalization.

This self-dialysis technique is accomplished by having the patient perform exchanges of dialysate into the peritoneal cavity four to five times daily. Since dialysis is continuous, a steady state of metabolic end products, electrolytes, and fluid can be achieved.[1] Dialysis exchanges vary in volume and in concentration. Currently, each exchange is a volume of 1.0, 1.5, 2.0, or 3.0 liters with a dextrose concentration of 1.5, 2.5, or 4.25 percent. The percent is defined in grams of dextrose per deciliter.

Diabetic patients are frequently placed on CAPD in the hope of better blood glucose control and lower morbidity.[2] Insulin is added to the dialysate, rather than being injected subcutaneously, which results in less fluctuation of plasma glucose levels. In general, the dose of insulin delivered in this manner is usually three to four times that required subcutaneously.

Higher protein intake to offset the loss of protein in the dialysate is critical. Other nutritional goals include adequate calories for achievement and maintenance of desirable body weight and adequate intake of vitamins, minerals, and fluid. Dietary recommendations are individualized according to the number of dialysis exchanges, the volume of each exchange, and dextrose concentration of each exchange. The size of the patient, his or her residual kidney function, and his or her individual needs must also be considered.

Protein. As in hemodialysis, CAPD removes needed nutrients as well as unwanted waste products. Protein losses, primarily albumin, may be 9 g or more per day.[3] A protein intake of 1.2 to 1.5 g per kilogram per day is recommended to replace protein losses. Hemoglobin, serum albumin, urea, and total serum protein are used as the key indicators of adequacy of protein intake. Sudden decreases in these values are seen in patients with inadequate oral intake or with excessive losses accompanying peritonitis.

Much of the literature[1,3] suggests that appetite improves in CAPD patients so that increasing protein intake is easier. However, experience at the Mayo Clinic does not support this observation. Many patients are unable to achieve the 1.2 to 1.5 g protein range.[4] Central parenteral nutrition and maintenance hemodialysis may become necessary in patients who cannot maintain an adequate protein intake.

Calories. Dietary caloric needs of the CAPD patient are generally lower than those for the hemodialysis patient because of the significant calorie contribution from the CAPD exchanges. The literature[1] frequently cites the kilocalorie contribution of the dialysate as 400 to 800 kilocalories. However, the volumes of the exchanges vary greatly and thus affect this rough estimate. Dietary caloric needs can be calculated by determining total caloric needs (see *Nutritional Assessment,* page 3) and subtracting the kilocalories provided by the dialysate.

Generally, it is assumed that 80 percent of the glucose in the dialysate is absorbed. The kilocalories contributed by the dialysate can be estimated by multiplying the grams of glucose (expressed as the monohydrate) by 3.4 Kcal per gram and 80 percent.[5] To calculate kilocalories from the dialysate, the following equation can be used:

Kilocalories from dialysate = glucose concentration (g per liter) × 3.4 (kilocalories per gram) × 0.8 × volume (liters). For example, 2,000 ml of 4.25 percent glucose would provide approximately 231 Kcal (42.5 g/liter × 3.4 Kcal/gram × 0.8 × 2 liters).

Sodium. Restriction of sodium is generally more liberal than for other treatment modalities for CRF. Current practice is to recommend 90 to 150 mEq sodium. Sodium restriction helps prevent fluid retention. If fluid retention were to occur, higher concentrations of dextrose in dialysis exchanges would be required to remove edema fluid. Unfortunately, chronic use of high dextrose concentrations in the dialysate promotes adipose tissue weight gain because of the added caloric intake. More rigorous sodium restriction may therefore be necessary for patients with diabetes mellitus so that lower dextrose concentrations can be used in dialysis. Patients with hypertension, excess fluid weight gain, or congestive heart failure may also benefit from further reduction of sodium intake.

Potassium. Serum potassium is usually kept within normal limits because of the frequency of dialysis, so a potassium restriction is not always needed. However, hypokalemia can occur in patients on five exchanges per day.[3] Hyperkalemia can also occur owing to the higher protein and the corresponding higher potassium content of the diet. Dietary potassium should be limited to approximately 60 mEq to 70 mEq if the serum potassium is elevated. Otherwise, high potassium foods may be used in moderation.

Fluid. Restriction of fluid intake is usually not necessary. Up to 2 liters per day may be tolerated and removed by using higher concentrations of dextrose in the dialysate. Restriction of both fluid and sodium may be necessary to control edema in some patients.

Phosphorous. The experience at the Mayo Clinic is that the need for phosphorous control with CAPD is similar to that in hemodialysis patients. There is no evidence that the need for phosphate binders is reduced.[4] Dietary control of phosphorous is difficult. Food records can be used to assess current intake of phosphorous. (See Appendix 12 for phosphorous content of foods.) The higher meat intake, which is necessary to obtain adequate protein, also increases phosphorous intake. High phosphorous foods (see page 242) should be restricted where possible and substituted with lower phosphorous foods.

Calcium. Increased calcium intake is desirable. However, dairy products are generally limited in an effort to control serum phosphorous. Milk intake is limited to 1/2 cup per day, unless the patient has difficulty consuming adequate protein. Milk may be an alternative for those who cannot obtain sufficient protein from meat. Acceptance of milk is often better than for meat. An increase in the serum phosphorous level slightly above 5 mg per deciliter may be accepted in an attempt to achieve adequate protein intake. Milk intake is limited for the patient who is able to consume adequate protein from meat. Calcium supplements may be used in an effort to maintain serum calcium levels. Table 6–48 summarizes the dietary restrictions for CAPD.

Other Nutrition Problems

The experience at the Mayo Clinic suggests that serum cholesterol and triglycerides increase with the length of CAPD. Kurtz et al[4] reported an increase in the very low-density lipoproteins and a low, but stable, high-density lipoprotein cholesterol fraction. Low-density lipoprotein remained normal throughout therapy.

The reasons for the lipid changes are not known. It has been theorized that triglycerides become elevated because of the higher protein intake and from possible glucose absorption from the dialysate. The increase in triglycerides also may be related to an increase in weight, to changes in fatty acid oxidation, or to a decrease in lipoprotein lipase activity, which results in reduced peripheral triglyceride clearing.[6-8]

Weight control measures and restriction of cholesterol, saturated fat, simple carbohydrate, and alcohol are recommended to manage hyperlipidemia. These

TABLE 6–48 Dietary Restrictions for CAPD

Component	Comments
Protein	1.2 to 1.5 g/kg body weight
Kilocalories	Dietary kilocalorie(s) = total kilocalorie(s) requirement − kilocalorie(s) from dialysate Kcal from dialysate = glucose concentration (g/liter) × 3.4 (Kcal/g) × 0.8 × volume (liters)
Sodium	90 to 150 mEq
Potassium	Use high potassium foods in moderation If serum potassium is elevated, restrict to 60 to 70 mEq
Fluid	Generally not restricted
Phosphorous	Avoid very high phosphorous foods, except meat; limit milk to 1/2 cup per day
Calcium	Calcium carbonate supplements as ordered by the physician
Simple carbohydrates	If hypertriglyceridemia exists, or if above desired weight, limit intake
Alcohol	If hypertriglyceridemia exists, avoid unless prescribed by physician to increase appetite
Saturated fat	If hypercholesterolemia exists, use polyunsaturated fats rather than saturated fats
Cholesterol	If hypercholesterolemia exists, restrict only if able to consume adequate protein from low cholesterol sources

dietary modifications are recommended only to the degree that they are possible without compromising adequacy of protein and non-protein caloric intake. Cholesterol intake usually can not be greatly decreased because of the need for adequate protein. In fact, patients who have nausea or taste acuity changes are often advised to consume eggs in an attempt to meet their protein needs. Generally, polyunsaturated fats can be substituted for saturated fats, and it may be possible to reduce total fat intake slightly. However, since high protein foods are often sources of fat, it may not be possible to greatly reduce fat intake. Simple carbohydrates and alcohol are restricted as a means of controlling hypertriglyceridemia, but also to control weight gain, which may have a greater effect on the hyperlipidemia.

Weight gain is commonly seen in CAPD.[9] The dialysate contributes a significant caloric load. It appears that the weight gain is the result of fat deposition and of correction of protein deficits with an associated increase in the mass of muscle, since hypertension and edema are generally not seen with such weight gains. Avoidance of excessive weight gain is an important aspect of the nutritional care of the CAPD patient, especially for those patients who use higher concentrations of dextrose.

Dehydration may occur with CAPD and should be anticipated when a change is made from hemodialysis to CAPD. Dehydration also may occur in people who are extremely weight conscious and who restrict their caloric and/or sodium intake excessively. A lower concentration of dextrose in the dialysate may be effective in correcting dehydration.

Another common nutrition problem is early satiety. The intra-abdominal volume of the dialysate may cause the patient to feel full and to have difficulty consuming adequate nutrients, particularly protein. It may be helpful for the patient to drain the dialysate prior to meal time and to reinfuse with the fresh exchange at the end of the meal. Small frequent meals also may help to relieve the sense of fullness.

Goals of Dietary Management

The goals of dietary management are (1) to provide sufficient protein to compensate for large losses of nitrogen and essential amino acids in the dialysate and to maintain nitrogen balance; (2) to limit sodium intake to control blood pressure and thirst and to prevent excess edema; (3) to prevent excessive weight gain; (4) to limit phosphorous to control hyperphosphatemia and renal osteodystrophy; and (5) to control hyperlipidemia.

Dietary Recommendations

The food exchange list for protein, sodium, and potassium control can be used for meal planning. Modifications can be made to liberalize sodium and potassium restrictions. Additional modifications may be necessary for restriction of saturated fat or phosphorous (see *Appendix 12*).

Physicians: How to Order Diet

The diet order should indicate *diet for CAPD.*

The dietitian will calculate caloric needs based on the concentration of the dialysate and on the number of exchanges made each day. The diet order should also indicate if weight loss is desired and if a potassium restriction is necessary. The dietitian will follow the preceding guidelines for modification of other dietary constituents.

REFERENCES

1. Bouma S, Dwyer JT. Glucose absorption and weight change in 18 months of CAPD. J Am Diet Assoc 1984;84:194–197.
2. Senekjian H, Koerpel BJ. CAPD in the diabetic patient. Dialysis and Transplantation 1984;13:780–783, 812.
3. Moncrief JW. Continuous ambulatory peritoneal dialysis—impact on management of patients with end-stage renal disease. Nephron 1981;27:226–268.
4. Kurtz SB, Wong VH, Anderson CF, Vogel JP, McCarthy JT, Mitchell JC, Kumar R, Johnson WJ. Continuous ambulatory peritoneal dialysis three-years' experience at the Mayo Clinic. Mayo Clin Proc 1983;54:633–639.
5. Jackson A. Nutritional considerations for adults on CAPD: a literature review. CRN Quarterly 1982;6:12.
6. Pierides AM, Weightman D, Goldfinch M, Alyama P, Kerr D. Hyperlipidemia of regular hemodialysis and successful renal transplantation. Cardiovasc Med 1978;3:185–206.
7. Wochos DN, Anderson CF, Mitchell JC. Serum lipids in chronic renal failure. Mayo Clin Proc 1976;51:660–664.
8. Kark RM, Oyama JH. Nutrition, hypertension and kidney diseases. In: Goodhart RS, Shils ME, eds. Nutrition in the prevention and treatment of disease. Modern Nutrition in Health and Disease, 6th ed. Philadelphia: Lea and Febiger, 1980:1005, 1030.
9. Baig F, Brubaker KA, Ali AS. Nutritional implications in CAPD. Contemp Dial 1982;Mar:37–41.

CONTINUOUS CYCLIC PERITONEAL DIALYSIS

General Description

The diet emphasizes high protein intake to offset loss of protein in the dialysate and adequate caloric intake to maintain a desirable weight.

Nutritional Inadequacy

As in other forms of dialysis, the patient undergoing continuous cyclic peritoneal dialysis is at risk for deficiencies of water-soluble vitamins and of minerals. The extent of losses are unknown. A daily multiple vitamin that includes water-soluble vitamins, particularly folic acid and iron, is recommended. Natabec Rx is currently the preferred vitamin preparation (see previous sections regarding Natabec Rx).

Indications and Rationale

Continuous cyclic peritoneal dialysis (CCPD) is a home dialysis technique that utilizes an automated device to provide nocturnal exchanges.[1] During each night there are three to five exchanges of 2 liters each and of 1 1/2 to 3 hour's duration. During each day there is a single 15-hour exchange. There appears to be less risk of peritonitis with CCPD than with CAPD.

In many regards, the nutritional considerations for CCPD are similar to those for CAPD. As in CAPD, substantial loss of protein in the dialysate means that the patient must maintain a high protein intake. Determination of caloric needs in CAPD and CCPD are similar, including calculations of the kilocalorie contribution of the dialysate. However, restriction of sodium, potassium, and fluid is less often necessary with CCPD than with CAPD because of greater absorption of these nutrients in the 15-hour exchange. Restriction of sodium and fluid are necessary if hypertension or fluid overload is present. Table 6–49 summarizes the dietary restrictions for CCPD.

Goals of Dietary Management

The goals of dietary management are (1) to provide sufficient protein to compensate for large losses of nitrogen and essential amino acids in the dialysate and to maintain nitrogen balance; (2) to prevent excessive weight gain; (3) to limit phosphorous to control hyperphosphatemia and renal osteodystrophy; and (4) to control hyperlipidemia.

Dietary Recommendations

The food exchange list for protein, sodium, and potassium control can be used for planning the diet. Modifications can be made to liberalize sodium and potassium restrictions. Additional modifications may be necessary for restriction of saturated fat and phosphorous (see *Appendix 12*).

Physicians: How to Order Diet

The diet order should indicate the *diet for CCPD*.
The dietitian will calculate calorie needs based on the concentration of the

TABLE 6–49   Dietary Restrictions for CCPD

Component	Comments
Protein	1.2 to 1.5 g/kg body weight
Kilocalories	Dietary kilocalorie(s) = total kilocalorie(s) requirement − kilocalorie(s) from dialysate Kcal from dialysate = glucose concentration (g/liter) × 3.4 (Kcal/g) × 0.8 × volume (liters)
Sodium	Generally not restricted
Potassium	Generally not restricted
Fluid	Generally not restricted
Phosphorous	Avoid very high phosphorous foods except meat; limit milk to 1/2 cup per day
Calcium	Calcium carbonate supplements as ordered by the physician
Simple carbohydrates	If hypertriglyceridemia exists or if above desired weight, limit intake
Alcohol	If hypertriglyceridemia exists, avoid unless prescribed by physician to increase appetite
Saturated fat	If hypercholesterolemia exists, use polyunsaturated rather than saturated fats
Cholesterol	If hypercholesterolemia exists, restrict only if able to consume adequate protein from low cholesterol sources.

dialysate and the number of exchanges each day. The diet order should indicate if weight loss is desired. The dietitian will follow the preceding guidelines for modification of other dietary constituents.

REFERENCE

1. Diaz-Buxo JA, Walker PJ, Chandler JT, Farmer CD, Holt KL. Advances in peritoneal dialysis, continuous cyclic peritoneal dialysis. Contemp Dial 1981;54:23–26.

RENAL TRANSPLANT

General Description

Dietary management following renal transplantation emphasizes control of hyperlipidemia with cholesterol and fat restriction, control of hypertension and/or water retention with mild sodium restriction, and control of weight.

Indications and Rationale

Hypercholesterolemia and hypertriglyceridemia are common in the stable post-transplant patient and place the patient at increased risk for development of occlusive atherosclerosis.[1,2,3] Glucocorticoids (usually Prednisone) contribute to the development of hyperlipidemia. Dietary measures are similar to those for other persons with hypercholesterolemia and hypertriglyceridemia (see page 80). Dietary cholesterol is limited to 300 mg per day. Total fat is limited to 30 to 35 percent of total caloric intake with 10 to 12 percent of these kilocalories to come from polyunsaturated fat and 10 to 12 percent from saturated fat. Alcohol consumption is discouraged,[1,3] and simple carbohydrate intake is limited.

A mild sodium restriction (90 to 150 mEq) is recommended initially following transplantation. High doses of steroids often result in sodium and water retention,[4] and hypertension is common in this population. The sodium restriction may be liberalized if the patient is normotensive and continues to show no signs of edema.

Carbohydrate metabolism is affected by high-dose steroids.[4,5,6] Decreased glucose tolerance, hyperglycemia, glucosuria, and relative resistance to insulin are commonly seen. Therefore, simple carbohydrate is limited in the diet. In practice, some restriction of simple carbohydrate is recommended in order to control weight and hypertriglyceridemia after the patient is stable and no longer shows signs of glucose intolerance.

Increased appetite is another effect of steroid therapy, along with the patient's new-found sense of well-being. A significant weight gain is common. Weight control is important to minimize glucose intolerance and to control hypertriglyceridemia. Medically approved regular exercise is a major adjunct to dietary control of weight and may help lower blood lipid levels.[1]

Fiber is encouraged in moderate amounts for relief of constipation, for possible serum lipid lowering, and for improved glucose tolerance effects.

Protein is not restricted, but amounts exceeding 1.5 g protein per kilogram are not encouraged. A proponent of a higher protein diet (2 g protein per kilogram) bases this recommendation on data from nitrogen balance studies done on patients with chronic Cushing's syndrome.[4,5] A study of transplant recipients showed a protein catabolic rate (PCR) of 1.6 g per kilogram per day at 5 to 20 days post-transplant.[6] The increased PCR was attributable to the administration of steroids (60 mg per day of Prednisone). The rationale for a more "normal" protein intake (1.2 to 1.5 g per kilogram per day), with consideration for some protein catabolism, is to preserve the function of the transplanted kidney.

Recommendations regarding potassium and calcium should be considered and individualized for each patient. Potassium is usually unrestricted. Supplementation with calcium may be necessary. Patients may be calcium depleted if they have been receiving chronic dialysis.[4] In addition, glucocorticoids contribute to osteopenia, i.e., loss of bone minerals.[4,5,6] Supplementation is not initiated until hyperparathyroidism is well regulated. Serum calcium levels need to be closely monitored.

The renal transplant diet should be presented to the patient as a healthy, "normal" diet aimed at contributing to the patient's well-being (Table 6–50).

Goals of Dietary Management

After successful renal transplantation, dietary recommendations are aimed at prevention of side effects from immunosuppressive drugs and at promotion of a nutritionally adequate diet.

Dietary Recommendations

The guide for meal planning for hyperlipidemia (see page 80) can be used. Additional modifications may be necessary to promote high fiber foods (see page 140) and to restrict sodium (see page 77).

TABLE 6–50 Dietary Restrictions Following Renal Transplant

Component	Comments
Kilocalories	Control to avoid excessive weight gain
Protein	Encourage more normal intake; however, not more than 1.2 to 1.5 g/kg is recommended
Cholesterol and fat	Limit cholesterol to ≤300 mg Limit total fat to 30 to 35 percent of kilocalories
Alcohol	Avoid
Simple carbohydrates	Limit
Fiber	Encourage use of high fiber foods
Sodium	90 to 150 mEq

Physicians: How to Order Diet

This diet may be ordered as *renal transplant diet* (*renal Tx diet*). The dietitian will follow the preceding guidelines.

REFERENCES

1. Disler PB, Goldberg RB, Kahn L, Mayers AM, Joffe BI, Seftel HC. The role of diet in the pathogenesis and control of hyperlipidemia after renal transplantation. Clin Nephrol 1981;16:29–34.
2. Ibels LS, Alfrey AC, Weil R III. Hyperlipidemia in adult, pediatric, and diabetic, renal transplant patients. Am J Med 1978;64:634–642.
3. Shen YS, Lukens CW, Alongi SV, Sfeir KE, Dagher FJ, Sadler JH. Patient profile and effect of dietary therapy on post-transplant hyperlipidemia. Kidney Int 1983;24(Suppl):147–152.
4. Liddle VR, Walker PJ, Johnson HK, Ginn HE. Diet in transplantation. Dialysis and Transplantation 1977;6:9–11.
5. Liddle VR, Johnson HK. Dietary therapy in renal transplantation. Proc Clin Dial Transplant Forum 1979;9:219–220.
6. Hoy WE, Sargent JA, Hall D, McKenna BA, Pabico RC, Freeman RB, Yarger JM, Byer BM. Protein catabolism during the postoperative course after renal transplantation. Am J Kidney Dis 1985;5:186–190.

NEPHROTIC SYNDROME

General Description

The diet emphasizes controlled intake of sodium, protein, and kilocalories.

Nutritional Inadequacy

The diet is not inherently inadequate as compared to the Recommended Dietary Allowances (RDA).

Indications and Rationale

Nephrotic syndrome arises from the abnormal passage of plasma proteins into the urine as a result of an increased glomerular membrane permeability.

Such urinary losses of protein result in hypoalbuminemia, hyperlipidemia, and edema. Twenty-four-hour urinary protein excretion greater than 3.5 g is indicative of nephrotic range proteinuria. Nephrotic syndrome may be the result of a wide variety of systemic disease states, or may occur as part of a primary glomerular disease.

A sodium intake range of 60 to 90 mEq sodium usually controls hypertension (often in conjunction with blood pressure medications) and edema after the initial diuresis.

The influence of protein intake on the course of nephrotic syndrome is controversial. An early study recommended a high protein intake of over 3 g protein per kilogram per day to promote positive nitrogen balance and to improve symptoms.[1] More recently, 1.5 g protein per kilogram per day has been recommended.[2,3,4] This recommendation is being reconsidered in light of the work by Hostetter et al that demonstrates that high protein diets may accelerate the course of some renal diseases by enhancing glomerular injury through hyperperfusion.[5] Preliminary work indicates no untoward effects from protein restriction in nephrotic rats[6] and in nephrotic humans (0.8 g protein per kilogram per day in humans).[7] Increased dietary protein intake is shown to have the paradoxical effect of increasing albuminuria without a beneficial effect on body albumin economy.[6] Long-term studies have yet to be reported.

In view of the recent studies, a dietary protein intake of 0.8 to 1 g per kilogram per day is generally recommended for patients without renal failure. However, if a patient with reasonably good renal function has obvious protein calorie malnutrition, has massive proteinuria (greater than 15 g protein per day), is receiving high-dose corticosteroid therapy, or has other conditions that may require a high protein intake to avoid malnutrition, it may be necessary to increase protein to about 1.5 g per kilogram per day.[3] In cases where the glomerular filtration rate is decreased, the amount of protein allowed should be determined in the same way as for other patients with chronic renal failure, with an additional amount of protein equivalent to the 24-hour urinary protein loss.

Caloric intake for patients with nephrotic syndrome should be calculated according to individual needs. (See *Nutritional Assessment* page 3.) Care should be taken to avoid insufficient caloric intake, since this results in catabolism of lean body tissue. Weight reduction should be approached cautiously because of the risk of catabolism of lean body tissue in addition to fat. Stringent caloric restriction is not recommended unless immediate weight loss is compelling. A slow to moderate weight loss of no more than 0.2 to 0.4 kg per week (1/2 to 1 lb per week) and a corresponding caloric deficit of 250 to 500 kilocalories is recommended. Table 6–51 summarizes the dietary restrictions for nephrotic syndrome.

Other Nutrition Problems

Hyperlipidemia is a common manifestation of nephrotic syndrome. The mechanisms that cause increased levels of triglycerides and cholesterol probably involve increased hepatic synthesis and defective peripheral utilization. Hypercholesterolemia occurs in association with modest hypoalbuminemia. Hypertriglyceridemia is associated with greater degrees of hypoalbuminemia.[2] The impact of a low fat, low cholesterol diet on the hyperlipidemia of nephrotic syndrome is probably insignificant. Since the lipid abnormalities are secondary effects, drug therapy (such as use of clofibrate or gemfibrozil) or stringent dietary restrictions are ineffective in influencing a significant change.[4]

Goals of Dietary Management

The primary goals of dietary management are to control hypertension, minimize edema, decrease urinary albumin loss, offset protein malnutrition, slow progression of renal disease, prevent muscle catabolism, and supply adequate energy. Control of hyperlipidemia, which is a common manifestation, is not a primary dietary concern.

Dietary Recommendations

The food exchange list for protein, sodium, and potassium control can be used for meal planning.

TABLE 6–51 Dietary Restrictions in the Nephrotic Syndrome

Components	Comments
Kilocalories	Sufficient for weight maintenance, weight gain, or slow weight loss ($\leq$ 0.2 to 0.4 kg/wk or 1/2 to 1 lb/wk)
Protein	Generally 0.8 to 1.0 g/kg body weight If protein needs are high because of malnutrition and if renal function is good, up to 1.5 g/kg body weight If the glomerular filtration rate is reduced, 0.4 to 0.6 g/kg body weight plus 24-hour urinary protein loss
Sodium	60 to 90 mEq sodium Calculate the sodium level to $\pm$ 10 percent of the diet order
Cholesterol and fat	Stringent dietary restrictions not necessary

Physicians: How to Order Diet

The diet order should indicate the *specific level of protein* (see preceding guidelines) and the *specific level of sodium* (the usual range is 60 to 90 mEq sodium). The dietitian will calculate caloric needs.

REFERENCES

1. Blainey JD. High protein diets in the treatment of the nephrotic syndrome. Clin Sci 1954;13:567–581.
2. Glassock RJ. Principles of management of the nephrotic syndrome. In: Glassock RJ, ed. Current therapy in nephrology and hypertension. Philadelphia: BC Decker, 1984:219.
3. Kaufman CE. Fluid and electrolyte abnormalities in nephrotic syndrome. Postgrad Med 1984;76:135–143.
4. Wagoner RD. Long-term management. In: Wagoner RD, ed. The nephrotic syndrome. New York: Medical Examination Publishing, 1981:33–39.
5. Hostetter TH, Olson JL, Rennke HG, Venkatachalam MA, Brenner BM. Hyperfiltration in remnant nephrons: A potentially adverse response to renal ablation. Am J Physiol 1981;241(1)F85–F93.

6. Kaysen GA, Kirkpatrick WG, Couser WG. Albumin homeostasis in the nephrotic rat: Nutritional considerations. Am J Phsiol 1984;247(1 pt 2):F192–F202.

7. Hutchison FN, Gambertoglio J, Jiminez I, Jones H Jr, Kaysen GA. Effect of reduced dietary protein intake on albumin homeostatis and albuminuria in man (Abstract). Kidney Int 1985;27:141.

Food Exchange Lists for Protein, Sodium, and Potassium Control

Meat and Meat Substitutes

Each exchange contains approximately 7 g protein and 2.5 mEq potassium. The sodium content varies. Portion sizes refer to cooked weights.

Unsalted: 1 mEq sodium

1 oz	Beef, lamb, pork, or veal
1 oz	Poultry
1 oz	Fish: any fresh or frozen
1/4 cup	Salmon or tuna, fresh or unsalted, waterpacked
1 oz	Unsalted cheese
2 Tbsp	Unsalted peanut butter* (limit to 1 serving daily)

Salted: 3 mEq sodium

1	Egg (no salt added)
1/4 cup	Egg substitute (no salt added)
1 oz	Lightly salted meat, fish, poultry (1/4 tsp salt per pound)
1 oz	Liver, heart, kidneys
2 oz (1/3 cup)	Clams, crab, lobster
3 oz (6 medium)	Oysters
2 oz (5 medium)	Shrimp
1 oz	Swiss cheese[†]

High sodium: 8 mEq sodium

1/4 cup	Cottage cheese[†]
1 oz	Cheese[†]: brick, cheddar, colby, mozzarella
2 Tbsp	Regular peanut butter* (limit to 1 serving per day)

*contains 6 mEq potassium and is low biologic value protein
[†] contains 1 mEq potassium

Milk and Milk Products

Each exchange contains approximately 4 g protein, 2.5 mEq sodium, and 4 mEq potassium.

1/2 cup	Skim, 2%, or whole milk
1/2 cup	Half and half
1/4 cup	Evaporated milk
2 Tbsp	Nonfat dry milk (before adding liquid)
2/3 cup	Whipping cream, light
3/4 cup	Whipping cream, heavy
1/2 cup	Yogurt (plain)

Desserts (made with milk)

The following milk products contain additional carbohydrate. Omit one-half serving of carbohydrate supplement in addition to one serving of milk for diabetic patients.

1/3 cup	Custard
1/2 cup	Pudding
1/4 cup	Bread pudding
3/4 cup	Ice cream*
2/3 cup	Ice milk*
1/2 cup	Frozen yogurt dessert*
1/2 cup	Yogurt (flavored)
1/2 cup	Chocolate milk*

*These foods to be included in fluid allowance

Starch

Each exchange contains approximately 3 g of protein and 1.5 mEq of potassium unless otherwise specified. Sodium content is indicated.

Unsalted: less than 1 mEq sodium (average 0.5 mEq)

Bread

1 slice	Unsalted bread
1	Tortilla, 6-in diameter

Cereal

3/4 cup	Corn flakes, unsalted
$1\frac{1}{2}$ cups	Puffed wheat or rice, unsalted, unsweetened
1 biscuit	Shredded wheat, unsalted
1/2 cup	Cooked cereal, no salt
1/2 cup	Grits (cooked, no salt)
1/2 cup	Barley
1 Tbsp	Wheat germ (2 mEq potassium)

Rice and Pasta

1/3 cup	Rice (brown or white), cooked (no salt)
1/2 cup	Pasta, spaghetti, noodles, macaroni (cooked, no salt)

Other Bread Products

$2\frac{1}{2}$ Tbsp	Cornmeal, dry
3 Tbsp	Flour
$1\frac{1}{2}$ cups	Popcorn (popped, no salt)

Crackers

6	Saltines, unsalted, $2\frac{1}{2}$-in square

Salted: 5 to 10 mEq sodium (average 8 mEq)

Bread: 1.5 mEq potassium

1/2	Bagel or English muffin
1 slice	Bread: white (including French or Italian), whole wheat, rye, raisin
4	Breadsticks (unsalted tops)
1/2	Hamburger bun
1	Plain roll

Bread: 3 to 5 mEq potassium

1/2	English muffin
1 slice	Pumpernickel bread

Cereal: 1.5 mEq potassium

3/4 cup	Cereals, ready to eat, unsweetened
1/2 cup	Cereals, cooked (with 1/8 tsp of salt)
1/2 cup	Barley, cooked (with 1/8 tsp of salt)
3 Tbsp	Grapenuts
1/2 cup	Grits, cooked (with 1/8 tsp of salt)
1/2 cup	Barley, cooked (with 1/8 tsp of salt)

Cereal: 5 to 10 mEq potassium

1/2 cup	Bran cereals, flakes, chex, etc.
1/3 cup	Bran cereals, All Bran, Bran Buds

Crackers: 1.5 mEq potassium

10	Animal crackers
3	Arrowroot
3	Graham crackers, $2\frac{1}{2}$-in square
3/4	Matzo, 4 in by 6 in
5	Melba toast, 2 in by $3\frac{3}{4}$ in
3	Rye wafers, 2 in by $3\frac{1}{2}$ in
6	Round butter or whole wheat crackers (low sodium)
6	Saltines, unsalted tops, $2\frac{1}{2}$-in square

Rice and Pasta

1/3 cup	Rice (brown or white), cooked (with 1/8 tsp of salt)
1/2 cup	Pasta, spaghetti, noodles, macaroni (cooked with 1/8 tsp of salt)

Other Bread Products

1 square	Cornbread, 2 in by 2 in by 1 in*
1 small	Croissant†
1/2 cup	Chow mein noodles*
1/2 cup	Croutons
1/4 cup (4 Tbsp)	Dried bread crumbs
2	Pancakes from mix, 4-in diameter*
1	Pita bread, 6-in diameter
1 small	Plain muffin, biscuit, 2-in diameter*
3/4 oz (25 sticks)	Pretzels, unsalted
2	Taco shells, 6-in diameter*
1	Tortilla, 6-in diameter
1	Waffle, 5-in diameter*

*These foods contain one additional fat exchange.
†These foods contain two additional fat exchanges.

Starchy Vegetables

Unsalted: Prepared without salt (less than 1 mEq sodium)

Salted: Prepared with 1/8 tsp of salt per serving. (Approximately 8 mEq sodium)

3 to 5 mEq potassium

1/3 cup	Corn
1 small ear	Corn on the cob, $3\frac{1}{2}$ in
1/4 cup	Sweet potato or yam, canned
1/2 small	Sweet potato, baked
1/3 cup	Lima beans
10 ($1\frac{1}{2}$ oz)	French fried potatoes, 2 to $3\frac{1}{2}$ in long

5 to 10 mEq potassium

1/2 cup	Mashed potato
1 small	Potato, peeled and boiled

10 to 15 mEq potassium

2/3 cup	Parsnips
1 small	Potato, baked
3/4 cup	Squash, acorn, butternut, or winter
1 cup	Pumpkin

Vegetables

Each exchange equals approximately 2 g protein. Unsalted vegetables are prepared without salt (less than 1 mEq sodium). Salted vegetables are canned with added salt or prepared with 1/8 tsp salt per serving (approximately 12 mEq sodium).

One serving of vegetable equals 1/2 cup cooked or 1 cup raw vegetables unless otherwise specified. There are no "free" vegetables.

Moderate Potassium—3 to 5 mEq potassium (average 4 mEq)

Alfalfa sprouts	Escarole	Radishes
Asparagus	Green pepper	Rhubarb
Bamboo shoots	Green string beans	Rutabaga
Bean sprouts	Kale	Summer squash
Beets	Lettuce	Turnip
Cauliflower	Mustard greens	Water chestnuts
Chicory	Okra	Watercress
Chinese cabbage	Onion	Yellow string beans
Eggplant	Peas, green (1/4 cup)	Zucchini
Endive	Pea pods or snow peas	

Higher Potassium—5 to 10 mEq potassium (average 7 mEq)

Artichokes	Chard	Spinach
Beet greens	Collards	Tomatoes
Broccoli	Cucumber	Tomato juice, unsalted
Brussel sprouts	Dandelion greens	Turnip greens
Cabbage	Kohlrabi	Vegetable juice cocktail,
Carrots	Mushrooms	unsalted
Celery	Parsley	

Fruit

Each exchange contains 0.5 to 1 g protein, trace of sodium, and averages of 2, 4, or 7 mEq potassium.

Low potassium–less than 3 mEq potassium (average 2 mEq)

1 small	Apple, fresh, 2-in diameter	1/3 cup	Cranberry juice cocktail
1/2 cup	Apple juice or cider	$1\frac{1}{4}$ cup	Cranberry juice cocktail (low calorie)
1/2 cup	Applesauce		
3/4 cup	Blueberries		
$1\frac{1}{4}$ cup	Cranberries		

Moderate Potassium–3 to 5 mEq potassium (average 4 mEq)

1 cup	Raspberries	1/2 cup	Canned peaches
12	Cherries, fresh	2 halves	Dried peaches
1/2 cup	Canned cherries	1/2 cup	Peach nectar
2 large	Dates	1 small	Pear, fresh
2 medium	Fig, fresh	1 half	Pear, dried
1 medium	Fig, dried	1/2 cup	Pear, canned
$1\frac{1}{2}$	Canned figs	1/2 cup	Pear, nectar
1/2 cup	Fruit cocktail	2 medium	Persimmon, native
1/2 medium	Grapefruit, fresh	3/4 cup	Pineapple, fresh
1/2 cup	Grapefruit juice	1/3 cup	Pineapple, canned
3/4 cup	Grapefruit sections	1/2 cup	Pineapple juice
15 small	Grapes, fresh	2	Plum, fresh, 2 in
1/3 cup	Grape juice	3 or 1/2 cup	Plums, canned
5 medium	Kumquats	2 Tbsp	Raisins
1/2 small	Mango	1 cup	Rhubarb
1 medium	Peach, fresh		

High potassium–5 to 10 mEq potassium (average 7 mEq)

4 medium	Apricots, fresh	$1\frac{1}{4}$ cup	Watermelon
1/2 cup or 4 halves	Canned apricots	1/2	Nectarine, 3 in
7 halves	Dried apricots	1 small	Orange, fresh, $2\frac{1}{2}$
1/2 cup	Apricot nectar	3/4 cup	Orange sections
1/2	Banana, 9 in	1/2 cup	Orange juice
3/4 cup	Blackberries	1 cup	Papaya
$1\frac{1}{4}$ cup	Strawberries	3 medium	Passion fruit
1 medium	Guava	1/2 medium	Pomegranate
1 large	Kiwi fruit	1 medium	Prickly pear
1 cup	Lemon juice*	3 medium	Prunes
1/4 small or 1 cup	Cantaloupe, 6 in	1/3 cup	Prune juice
		1 medium	Tangelo
1/8 medium or 1 cup	Honeydew	2 medium	Tangerine, fresh
		1/2 cup	Tangerine juice

---

*Up to 2 Tbsp of lemon juice may be used per day without considering this as part of the fruit group.

Low Protein Products

Each exchange contains 0.2 g protein, 0.5 mEq sodium, trace potassium, and 100 kilocalories.

1 slice ($1\frac{1}{2}$ oz)	Low protein bread
2 slices	Low protein rusks
1/2 cup, cooked (1/4 cup dry)	Low protein macaroni, ring macaroni, or noodles
1/2 cup, prepared	Low protein gelatin (negligible protein, 1 mEq sodium, 2 mEq potassium, 85 kilocalories)
2	Low protein cookies (0.2 g protein, 2 mEq sodium, 1 mEq potassium, 1 fat serving, and 140 kilocalories)

Fats and Oils

Each exchange contains negligible amounts of protein and a trace of potassium. Sodium varies.

Unsalted: trace of sodium

1 tsp	Margarine, unsalted
1 tsp	Butter, unsalted
1 tsp	Mayonnaise, low sodium
1 tsp	Oil
1 tsp	Shortening
2 Tbsp	Gravy (meat drippings with fat thickened with cornstarch), unsalted

Salted: 2 mEq sodium

1 tsp	Margarine
1 tsp	Butter
1 tsp	Mayonnaise
2 Tbsp	Nondairy creamer
2 Tbsp	Sour cream (limit to one serving per day)

Carbohydrate Supplements

Each exchange contains negligible amounts of protein, sodium, and potassium and 100 kilocalories.

Sugar and syrups

2 Tbsp	Sugar
2 Tbsp	Honey
2 Tbsp	Jelly or jam
2 Tbsp	Syrup

Candy

3 large	Fondant or sugar mints
3 large	Gumdrops
6 pieces	Hard candy, unfilled
20	Jelly beans
1 medium	Lollipop, unfilled

Fruit desserts

1/4 cup	Cranberry sauce or relish
1/2 cup	Fruit ice (sherbert made without milk) (contains 80 ml fluid)
1 twin bar	Popsicle ($2\frac{1}{2}$ oz bar contains 75 ml fluid)

Flavored beverages

1 cup (8 oz)	Carbonated, fruit flavored Kool Aid, artificially flavored lemonade

Flour products

1/4 cup	Cornstarch or tapioca (may be used to thicken sauces and gravies)

Other carbohydrate supplements

1/4 cup	Polycose powder or liquid (contains 2 mEq sodium, use as suggested)

Beverages

One cup (8 oz) of the following beverages contains only a trace of protein and sodium.

Trace potassium	*1 mEq potassium*	*2 mEq potassium*	*4 mEq potassium*
Cola	Limeade	Coffee, instant	Coffee, brewed
Ginger ale		Coffee, decaffeinated, instant, and freeze dried	
Kool Aid			
Root beer		Lemonade, from frozen concentrate	
Seven-up		Tea	

12 oz of beer contain 1.5 mEq sodium and 3 mEq potassium.
4 oz of wine contain a trace of sodium and 3 mEq potassium.

Common Foods High in Phosphorus[1]

	Milligrams of Phosphorus Per Exchange*
Milk Group	
Yogurt (plain)	165
Pudding	130
Milk (including chocolate and evaporated)	125
Half and Half	115
Ice cream	100
Custard	100
Meat and Meat Substitutes	
Cheese (processed)	215
Cheese (Swiss)	175
Cheese (cheddar, mozzarella)	145
Liver	130
Fish (salmon, bass, mackerel)	120
Lentils	120
Egg	90
Cottage cheese	70
Starch	
Cereal (100 percent bran)	400
Cereal (All Bran, Bran Buds, granola-type)	265
Cereal (Bran Chex, bran flakes)	150
Waffle (frozen)	135
Cooked cereal (instant)	135
Biscuit (from mix)	130
Cake, white (from mix)	115
Wheat germ	80
Bread (whole wheat)	70
Lima Beans	60
Vegetables	
Mushrooms	80
Peas	50
Fats and Oils	
Nondairy creamer	50
Carbohydrate Supplements	
Cola beverage	30

*As listed in the *Food Exchange Lists for Protein, Sodium, and Potassium Control* (see page 235)

REFERENCE

1. Pennington JAT, Church HN. Bowes and Church's food values of portions commonly used. 14th ed. Philadelphia: JB Lippincott, 1985.

General Description

Potassium is widely distributed in foods, but is highest in fruits and vegetables. General guidelines are given for increasing or decreasing potassium intake.

Indications and Rationale

Hypokalemia. Hypokalemia is associated most often with the use of diuretics, but also may be induced by other drugs (such as corticosteroids), gastrointestinal disturbances, (such as diarrhea and vomiting), some renal disturbances, and some endocrine disorders.[1,2] In many instances, parenteral or oral administration of potassium supplements is warranted.

Treatment of hypokalemia that occurs with diuretic therapy for hypertension may consist of (1) restriction of dietary sodium to lessen urinary potassium wastage, (2) substitution of a potassium-sparing diuretic for a potassium-wasting one, (3) use of potassium chloride supplements or potassium chloride salt substitutes, (4) use of foods high in potassium, or (5) reduction of the dosage of potassium-wasting medications, if adequate blood pressure control can be maintained at a lower dosage.[1,2]

Many potassium chloride supplements are poorly accepted because of their unpleasant taste. Supplements of potassium citrate and potassium bicarbonate are better tolerated, but less effective, than potassium chloride.

Salt substitutes that contain potassium chloride may be a reasonable alternative, since they generally cost less and are more palatable than prescription potassium chloride supplements.[3] Some patients develop a tolerance over time to the bitter, metallic taste of salt substitutes.[1] Although there is some variation among brands of potassium chloride salt substitutes, the usual potassium content is 10 to 13 mEq of potassium per gram.* Five grams (1 teaspoon) of these salt substitutes would provide 50 to 65 mEq of potassium. If a potassium chloride salt substitute is recommended to the patient, a specific dose should be indicated. Many dietetic "low sodium" products use potassium chloride instead of sodium chloride, a substitution that substantially increases the potassium content of these foods.

The usual American diet provides 50 to 150 mEq of potassium daily.[4] It is difficult for most patients consistently and reliably to increase dietary intake of potassium beyond this level. A range of 40 to 60 mEq of potassium from potassium chloride supplements is a frequently prescribed dose. When a similar increase in potassium is attempted with food, the total intake of calories or sodium (or both) often is appreciably increased also. Attempts to increase dietary potassium may be successful if the patient requires only a very low level of potassium supplementation to prevent hypokalemia, if the patient's usual diet is extremely low in potassium, or if therapy adjunctive to potassium supplements is required.

Hyperkalemia. A decrease in urinary output of potassium and an increase in serum potassium levels occur in advanced renal failure, hypoaldosteronism,

---

*Potassium chloride provides 13.4 mEq of potassium per gram.

and adrenal insufficiency. Excessive use of potassium-sparing diuretics also may result in hyperkalemia.[5] Treatment includes dietary restriction of potassium and reduction of the dosage or discontinuation of the use of the potassium-sparing diuretics.[5]

Both endogenous and exogenous sources can increase input of potassium into the serum.[6] Typically, the exogenous sources include a high dietary intake and excess intake of salt substitutes that contain potassium chloride. Treatment includes dietary restriction and discontinuation of salt substitutes or other dietetic foods containing potassium chloride. The low protein diet used for the predialysis patient is inherently restricted in potassium. In the usual diet, high protein foods contribute significant amounts of potassium. Restricting protein generally reduces dietary potassium intake as well.

The primary endogenous source of potassium is muscle and tissue catabolism.[6] One of the primary objectives in the dietary management of chronic renal failure is the prevention of muscle catabolism.

Food Sources of Potassium[7]

Low Potassium (<3 mEq potassium per serving)

Meats, meat substitutes (such as eggs), breads, pasta, and cereals generally are low in potassium.

Fruits

Apple	
fresh	1 small
sauce	1/2 cup
Blueberries	3/4 cup
Cranberries	$1\frac{1}{4}$ cups
Cranberry juice cocktail	$\frac{1}{3}$ cup
Cranberry juice cocktail	
(low calorie)	$1\frac{1}{4}$ cup

Nuts

Almonds	6 whole
Brazil nuts	2 medium
Cashews, roasted	4 large
Filberts or hazelnuts	5
Mixed nuts	8–12 nuts
Pumpkin seeds	2 tsp
Pecans	5 halves
Walnuts	4 halves
Sunflower seeds	1 Tbsp without shell

Dairy Foods

Cheese	1 oz
Cottage cheese	$\frac{1}{4}$ cup

Beverages

Coffee (decaffeinated and regular, instant or freeze dried)	1 cup
Postum	1 cup
Tea	1 cup
Lemonade	1 cup

Miscellaneous
>   Olives
>> black   5 medium
>> green   9–10 medium
>   Sweet chocolate   1 oz
>   Tofu   4 oz
>   Wheat germ   1 Tbsp

Moderate Potassium (3–5 mEq potassium per serving)

In general, dietary products and most fruits and vegetables contain moderate amounts of potassium.

Fruits

Apple juice	1/2 cup	canned	1/2 cup
Cherries, canned	1/2 cup	dried	2 halves
Cherries, fresh	12 large	Pears	
Dates	$2\frac{1}{2}$ medium	fresh	1 small
Figs, canned	1/2 cup	nectar	1/2 cup
Figs, fresh or dried	2 medium	canned	1/2 cup
Fruit cocktail	1/2 cup	dried	1 half
Grapes		Persimmon	2 medium
fresh	15 small	Pineapple	
canned	1/3 cup	fresh	3/4 cup
juice	1/3 cup	canned	1/3 cup
Grapefruit		juice	1/2 cup
fresh	1/2 medium	Plums	
canned	3/4 cup	fresh	2 small
juice	1/2 cup	canned	1/2 cup or 3
Mango	1/2 small	Raisins	2 Tbsp
Peaches		Raspberries	1 cup
fresh	1 medium	Rhubarb	1 cup
nectar	1/2 cup		

Vegetables—all portions are 1/2 cup cooked or 1 cup raw unless otherwise indicated.

Alfalfa Sprouts	Okra
Asparagus	Onion
Bamboo shoots	Peas
Bean sprouts	Peapods or Snow peas
Beets	Radishes
Cauliflower	Rutabaga
Chicory	Summer squash
Chinese cabbage	Sweet potato or
Corn, kernel	canned yam
Eggplant	1/3 cup, cooked,
Endive	or 1/2 small
Escarole	Turnip
Green beans	Watercress
Green pepper	Water chestnuts
Kale	Yellow beans
Lettuce	Zucchini
Mustard greens	

Dairy Foods
Milk	1/2 cup
Yogurt	1/2 cup

Miscellaneous
Brewed coffee	1 cup
Canned soup	6 oz
Cocoa powder	2 Tbsp
Peanut butter	2 Tbsp
Peanuts	1 oz or 25

High Potassium (5–10 mEq potassium per serving)

The following foods are high in potassium. Many low sodium dietetic foods, such as low sodium canned soups, also are considered to be high in potassium because the sodium chloride is replaced with potassium chloride.

Fruits
Apricots, fresh	4 medium
canned	1/2 cup or 4 halves
dried	7 halves
nectar	1/2 cup
Banana	1/2 of 9-in length
Berries	
Blackberries	3/4 cup
Strawberries	$1\frac{1}{4}$ cup
Melon	
Cantaloupe	1/4 small or 1 cup
Honeydew	1/8 medium or 1 cup
Watermelon	$1\frac{1}{4}$ cup
Kiwi	1 large
Lemon juice	1 cup
Nectarine	1/2 3-in diameter
Orange, fresh	1 $2\frac{1}{2}$-in diameter
sections	3/4 cup
juice	1/2 cup
Papaya	1/2 medium or 1 cup
Pomegranate	1/2 medium
Prunes	3 medium
Prune juice	1/3 cup
Tangerine, fresh	2 $2\frac{1}{2}$-in diameter
juice	1/2 cup
Tangelo	1 medium

Vegetables—all portions are 1/2 cup cooked or 1 cup raw unless otherwise indicated.

Artichoke	1 large	Celery
Beet greens		Chard
Broccoli		Collards
Brussels sprouts		Cucumbers
Cabbage		Dandelion greens
Carrots		Kohlrabi

Boiled potato	1 small	Tomatoes	
Mashed potato		Tomato juice	
Mushrooms		Turnip greens	
Parsley		Vegetable juice	
Spinach		cocktail	

Miscellaneous

Chocolate, bitter	1 oz
Low sodium baking powder	1 tsp
Sunflower seeds	1/4 cup
Low sodium canned soups	1/2 cup

Very High Potassium (10–15 mEq potassium per serving)

The following foods contain very high amounts of potassium.

Vegetables

Baked potato	1 small, 2-in diameter
Squash, acorn, hubbard, butternut, winter	3/4 cup
Parsnips	2/3 cup
Pumpkin	1 cup

Miscellaneous

Salt substitute	1/4 tsp

REFERENCES

1. Longford HG. Potassium in hypertension: the case for its role in pathogenesis and treatment. Postgrad Med 1983;73:227–233.
2. Fischer RG. Managing diuretic-induced hypokalemia in ambulatory hypertensive patients. J Fam Pract 1982;14:1029–1036.
3. Sopko JA, Freeman RM. Salt substitutes as a source of potassium. JAMA 1977;238:608–610.
4. Food and Nutrition Board Research Council. Recommended Dietary Allowances, 9th ed. Washington, DC: National Academy of Science, 1980:173.
5. Madias NE, Zelman SJ. What are the metabolic complications of diuretic treatment. Geriatrics 1982;37:93–99.
6. Elms JJ. Potassium imbalance—causes and prevention. Postgrad Med 1982;72:165–171.
7. Pennington JAT, Church HN. Bowes and Church's food values of portions commonly used. 14th ed. Philadelphia: JB Lippincott, 1985.

UROLITHIASIS

General Description

Generous fluid intake is recommended in the management of all types of stone disease. Other diet modifications are based on the type of stone disease and are generally directed at reduction of excessive intake of a particular dietary constituent.

Indications and Rationale

The major components of urinary stones are calcium, oxalate, uric acid, phosphate, and cystine. Chemical analysis of stones can determine the predominant components. Recommendations for or contraindications to dietary modification are discussed for each of these constituents and for other nutritional factors affecting urolithiasis.[1,2,3]

Fluid

Dilution of the urine is of primary importance.[4] The goal is to minimize precipitation of the offending substance into urinary stones. Fluid intake should be distributed throughout the day to assure a constantly high urine output. In moderate climates, the patient should be advised to drink 250 to 300 ml (8–10 ounces) of fluid per hour while awake and on each occasion during the night that the person arises to void. The amount of fluid that must be consumed to maintain the recommended urine volume is greater in warm climates and for physically active people.

At Least Half of the Fluid Ingested Should Be Water.　Any other form of fluid is acceptable, except for milk products and tea in certain conditions. Although some fruit juices contain oxalate, the beneficial effect of providing fluid and the resulting urine dilution is more important than the potential increase in oxalate absorption.[5]

REFERENCES

1. Smith LH, Van Den Berg CJ, Wilson DM. Nutrition and urolithiasis. N Engl J Med 1978;298:87.
2. Benson EA, Brannen GE, Bush WH. Urinary tract stones—medical management. Postgrad Med J 1985;77:193–198,201.
3. *National Dairy Council* Diet and Urolithiasis. Dairy Council Digest 1983;54:1–5.
4. Pak CYC, Sakhaee K, Crowther C, Brinkley L. Evidence justifying a high fluid intake in treatment of nephrolithiasis. Ann Intern Med 1980;93:36–38.
5. Pak CYC, Smith LH, Resnick MI, Weinerth JL. Dietary management of idiopathic calcium urolithiasis. J Urol 1984;131:850–852.

CALCIUM RESTRICTION

General Description

Calcium intake can be controlled by restricting milk and foods containing large amounts of milk.

Nutritional Inadequacy

The diet may be inadequate in calcium, depending on the degree of restriction. Calcium supplements are not advised.

Indications and Rationale

In normal persons, urinary calcium excretion has little correlation with calcium consumption, since intestinal absorption of calcium decreases when dietary intake is excessive.

Half of the patients with idiopathic calcium urolithiasis (ICU) have normal urinary calcium levels. The other 50 percent of patients with ICU have elevated urinary calcium, which can be divided into three categories. Ten percent of these patients have renal hypercalciuria due to a renal "leak" of calcium. The remaining 90 percent are equally divided between absorptive hypercalciuria type I, which is elevated irrespective of dietary calcium intake, and absorptive hypercalciuria type II, which has elevated urinary calcium only with high dietary calcium intake. (Fig. 6–3)

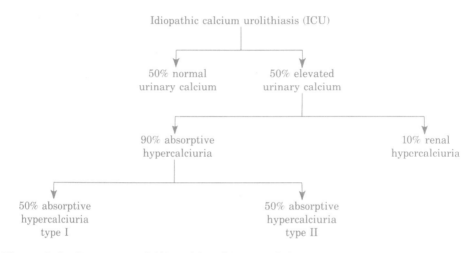

Figure 6–3 Occurrence of idiopathic calcium urolithiasis.

A dietary calcium restriction of 400 to 600 mg per day is recommended to control hypercalciuria in patients with absorptive hypercalciuria type II. (A simultaneous oxalate restriction is required. See *Oxalate Restriction,* page 251.) Restriction of calcium to less than 400 mg daily yields no additional clinical benefit and usually is not recommended, since a calcium intake below this level may result in a negative calcium balance.

An excessive amount of calcium, greater than 1 g per day, should be avoided because it may produce hypercalciuria significant enough to promote stone formation even when intestinal calcium absorption is normal.[1] Patients with absorptive hypercalciuria type I and renal hypercalciuria should limit their calcium intake to approximately 800 mg a day.

Excessive amounts of dietary sodium, animal protein, and sugars can aggravate hypercalciuria. Therefore, excesses of these dietary constituents should be avoided in patients with hypercalciuria. Patients should be encouraged to eat a normal balanced diet.

A moderate sodium restriction (90 to 150 mEq per day) may be beneficial to patients with hypercalciuria by reducing the saturation of calcium salts in the urine.[1,2] When thiazide diuretics are used to reduce the urinary excretion of calcium, high sodium intake can overcome the response. Therefore, a 90-mEq sodium restriction should be followed in conjunction with thiazide medication. (See *Hypertension*, page 71.)

Intake of dietary protein should not exceed 120 g daily,[3,4] since excessive animal protein may increase urinary uric acid from purine load.

A high fiber diet, including unprocessed bran, has been shown to increase fecal calcium excretion by binding calcium and preventing its absorption. The bran provides phytic acid, which, combined with dietary calcium in the intestine to form calcium phytate, is excreted[5] in the stool, thus lessening the excretion of calcium via the kidney.

Hypercalciuria is a common complication of spinal cord injury (SCI) and nonweight-bearing immobilization. Hypercalciuria may lead to negative calcium balance and osteoporosis, thus resulting in fractures of the long bones in the lower extremities. Hypercalciuria is also associated with a high incidence of urolithiasis in SCI patients. However, bladder stones in SCI patients frequently are the consequence of indwelling Foley catheters and of bladder infections.[6]

Calcium is not routinely restricted for SCI patients. Adequate calcium is recommended to prevent negative calcium balance and its long-term consequences.

Goals of Dietary Management

The goals of dietary management are to reduce the level of calcium in the urine and to maintain a dilute urine.

Dietary Recommendations

Sufficient restriction of calcium generally can be accomplished by avoiding or limiting milk and foods containing large amounts of milk. The calcium content of a diet that includes a variety of foods, but no milk products, can be estimated as approximately 200 mg calcium per 1,000 kilocalories per day. For most persons this is equivalent to 300 to 500 mg calcium per day. Limited amounts of milk or milk products can be permitted in order to achieve the desired level of calcium[7] (Table 6–52).

TABLE 6–52 Calcium Restriction

General Recommendations	Disorder	Additional Recommendations
Fluid: 250–300 ml/hour while awake and upon awakening at night; at least 50% as water	Absorptive hypercalciuria, type II	Low calcium diet, 400 to 600 mg/day; Low oxalate diet (see Table 6–54)
Sodium: Moderate restriction, 90–150 mEq/day, or avoidance of excessive sodium intake	Renal hypercalciuria and absorptive hypercalciuria, type II	Moderate calcium diet, 800 mg/day; avoid excessive calcium intake
Avoid dietary excesses and deficiencies	Hypercalciuria resulting from immobilization (SCI)	Encourage adequate calcium intake, 800 to 1,000 mg/day

Low Calcium Diet, 400 to 600 mg

- Limit the following foods to a total of 1/2 cup (or one ounce of cheese) a day: milk, including whole, low fat, chocolate, and butter milk; yogurt; cheese; cottage cheese; ice cream; sherbet; custard; pudding; and cream.*

Moderate Calcium Diet, Less Than 1 g per day

- Limit the preceding foods to a total of 1 to 2 cups (or ounces for cheese).

Physicians: How to Order Diet

The diet order should indicate the *specific level of calcium* desired, such as 400 to 600 mg or 800 to 1,000 mg.

The dietitian will make additional recommendations according to the preceding guidelines.

REFERENCES

1. Pak CYC, Smith LH, Resnick MI, Weinerth JL. Dietary management of idiopathic calcium urolithiasis. J Urol 1984;131:850–852.
2. Muldowney FP, Freaney R, Moloney MF. Importance of dietary sodium in the hypercalciuria syndrome. Kidney Int 1982;22:292–296.
3. Lemann J, Piering WF, Lennon EJ. Possible role of carbohydrate-induced calciuria in calcium oxalate kidney-stone formation. N Engl J Med 1969;280:232–237.
4. Hegsted M, Schuette SA, Zemel MB, Linkswiler HM. Urinary calcium and calcium balance in young men as affected by level of protein and phosphorus intake. J Nutr 1981;111:553–562.
5. Shah PJR, Williams G, Green NA. Idiopathic hypercalciuria: its control with unprocessed bran. Br J Urol 1980;52:426–429.
6. Lamid S, El Ghatit AZ, Melvin JL. Relationship of hypercalciuria to diet and bladder stone formation in spinal cord injury patients. AM J Phys Med 1984;63:182–187.
7. Pennington JAT, Church HN. Bowes and Church's food values of portions commonly used. 14th ed. Philadelphia: JB Lippincott, 1985.

OXALATE RESTRICTION

General Description

Oxalic acid occurs primarily in food of plant origin. The diet excludes foods that are high in oxalates and is intended to provide less than 50 mg of oxalate per day.

Nutritional Inadequacy

There are no nutritional inadequacies inherent in an oxalate-restricted diet.

---

*Some other foods—sardines, fish canned with bones, quick-cooking cereals, quick breads, sweet potato, beet greens, Swiss chard, collards, dandelion greens, kale, mustard greens, okra, spinach, turnip greens, endive, escarole, rhubarb and dried fruits—may contribute a substantial amount of calcium to the diet if used frequently and in large amounts. It is not necessary to restrict these foods unless a diet history reveals a high frequency of use and the situation warrants their exclusion.

Indications and Rationale

Oxalic acid, or oxalate, is the end product of both glyoxylic acid and ascorbic acid metabolism. Normal urinary excretion of oxalate is less than 60 mg per 24 hours, of which approximately 10 percent comes from oxalate in the diet. However, large fluctuations in urinary oxalate may be attributable to variations in diet.[1]

Dietary calcium intake and intestinal oxalate absorption are inversely related. Calcium normally combines with oxalate in the intestinal lumen and makes it less available for absorption. Therefore, a diet extremely low in calcium may increase urinary oxalate excretion.

Urine is commonly supersaturated with calcium oxalate, since this compound is poorly soluble. Small increases in urinary oxalate concentration greatly increase the potential for crystal formation. Control of dietary oxalate may be of benefit to those who are susceptible to urinary oxalate lithiasis, since increased urinary excretion of oxalate is likely after ingestion of high oxalate foods.

Restriction of oxalate, in addition to restriction of calcium, is recommended for absorptive hypercalciuria type II. A low calcium diet tends to increase oxalate absorption from the diet because of decreased availability of calcium to bind oxalate.[2] Once absorbed into the body, the oxalate is not metabolized, but excreted into the urine. An oxalate- and calcium-restricted diet effectively reduces the rate of stone formation. However, many persons find strict, long-term adherence to a low calcium and oxalate diet difficult[3] (Tables 6–53 and 6–54).

Enteric hyperoxaluria is a consequence of intestinal malabsorption.[4] The increase in urinary oxalate excretion is attributable to enhanced absorption of dietary oxalate. Oxalate is normally sequestered by calcium in the intestinal lumen and is poorly absorbed. In malabsorptive states, fatty acids bind with calcium so that oxalate is more available for absorption. The malabsorbed fatty acids and bile salts also increase colonic permeability to oxalate. A low fat diet may be warranted if steatorrhea is significant. Calcium restriction is contraindicated because of the mechanisms of increased oxalate absorption. In fact, calcium supplements up to 1 g a day[9] may be recommended.

Oxalate is an end product of ascorbic acid metabolism; therefore, ascorbic acid supplementation may increase urinary oxalate excretion. If supplementation with ascorbic acid is warranted, limit the level to less than approximately 1 g per day.

TABLE 6–53 Oxalate Restriction

General Recommendations	Disorder	Additional Recommendations
Oxalate: Low oxalate diet.	Idiopathic hyperoxaluria.	Moderate to high calcium intake recommended (2 or more glasses milk/day).
Fluid: 250–300 ml/hour while awake and upon awakening at night; 50% as water.	Absorptive hypercalciuria, type II.	Low calcium diet (see page 251).
Ascorbic Acid: Avoid excessive supplementation.	Enteric hyperoxaluria.	High calcium intake (supplement with 1 g or more calcium—as calcium carbonate) (see page 210). Low fat diet if there is significant steatorrhea.

TABLE 6–54 Approximate Oxalate Content of Selected Foods[5-7]*

Foods	Little or No Oxalate, <2 mg oxalate/serving	Moderate Oxalate, 2–10 mg oxalate/serving	High Oxalate Foods, >10 mg oxalate/serving
Beverages	Beer, bottled Carbonated cola (limit to 12 oz/day) Distilled alcohol Lemonade or limeade without peel Wine: red, rose, white	Coffee (limit to 8 oz/day)	Draft beer Ovaltine and other beverage mixes Tea Cocoa
Milk	Buttermilk Whole, low fat, or skim milk Yogurt with allowed fruit		
Meat and substitutes group	Eggs Cheese Beef, lamb, or pork Poultry Fish and shellfish	Sardines	Baked beans canned in tomato sauce Peanut butter Tofu

Vegetables	Avocado
	Brussels sprouts
	Cauliflower
	Cabbage
	Mushrooms
	Onions
	Peas, green, fresh, or frozen
	Potatoes, white
	Radishes
		Asparagus
		Broccoli
		Carrots
		Corn:
		  sweet, white
		  sweet, yellow
		Cucumber, peeled
		Green peas, canned
		Lettuce
		Lima beans
		Parsnips
		Tomato, 1 small or juice (4 oz)
		Turnips
			Beans: green, wax, dried
			Beets: tops, root, greens
			Celery
			Chives
			Collards
			Dandelion greens
			Eggplant
			Escarole
			Kale
			Leeks
			Mustard greens
			Okra
			Parsley
			Peppers, green
			Pokeweed
			Potatoes, sweet
			Rutabagas
			Spinach
			Summer squash
			Swiss Chard
			Watercress

Fruits/Juices	Apple juice
	Avocado
	Banana
	Cherries, Bing
	Grapefruit, fruit and juice
	Grapes, green
	Mangoes
	Melons:
	  Cantaloupe
	  Casaba
	  Honeydew
	  Watermelon
	Nectarines
	Peaches
	Pineapple juice
	Plums, green or yellow
		Apple
		Apricots
		Black currants
		Cherries, red sour
		Cranberry juice (4 oz)
		Grape juice (4 oz)
		Orange, fruit and juice (4 oz)
		Peaches
		Pears
		Pineapple
		Plums, purple
		Prunes
			Blackberries
			Blueberries
			Currants, red
			Dewberries
			Fruit cocktail
			Grapes, purple
			Gooseberries
			Lemon peel
			Lime peel
			Orange peel
			Raspberries
			Rhubarb
			Strawberries
			Tangerine
			Juices made from the above fruits

TABLE 6-54 Approximate Oxalate Content of Selected Foods[5-7]* *(continued)*

Foods	Little or No Oxalate, <2 mg oxalate/serving	Moderate Oxalate, 2-10 mg oxalate/serving	High Oxalate Foods, >10 mg oxalate/serving
Bread/Starches	Breakfast cereals Macaroni Noodles Rice Spaghetti Bread	Cornbread Sponge cake Spaghetti, canned in tomato sauce	Fruit cake Grits, white corn Soybean crackers Wheat germ
Fats & Oils	Bacon Mayonnaise Salad dressing Vegetable oils Butter, margarine		Nuts: Peanuts, almonds, pecans, cashews, walnuts
Miscellaneous	Coconut Jelly or preserves (made with allowed fruits) Lemon, lime juice Salt, pepper (limit to 1 tsp/day) Soups with ingredients allowed Sugar	Chicken noodle soup-dehydrated	Chocolate, cocoa Vegetable soup Tomato soup Marmalade

*Considerable variation in the oxalate content of a single type of food exists. Factors such as growing conditions, age of the plant, bioavailability, and gastrointestinal abnormalities all affect individual absorption of oxalate.[8] Therefore, the foods have been categorized into low, moderate, and high oxalate groups, rather than giving an exact value. The data available on the oxalate content of foods is limited and variable. Many foods have been analyzed for oxalate content using specific name brands or varieties. Data have been extrapolated to include the broader category of food for which analysis of oxalate content is available.

Goals of Dietary Management

The goals of dietary management are to reduce the level of oxalate in the urine and to maintain a dilute urine.

Dietary Recommendations

The dietary recommendations for an oxalate-reduced diet are given in Table 6-53.

Physicians: How to Order Diet

The diet order should indicate *low oxalate diet*.

The dietitian will make additional recommendations according to the preceding guidelines.

REFERENCES

1. Finch AM, Kasidas GP, Rose GA. Urine composition in normal subjects after oral injestion of oxalate-rich foods. Clin Sci 1981;60:411-418.
2. Jaeger P, Portmann L, Jacquet A, Burckhardt P. Influence of the calcium content of the diet on incidence of mild hyperoxaluria in idiopathic renal stone formers. Am J Nephrol 1985;5:40-44.

3. Hodgkinson A. Comment: Is there a place for a low-oxalate diet? J Hum Nutr 1981;35:136.
4. Stauffer JQ. Hyperoxaluria and calcium oxalate nephrolithiasis after jejunoileal bypass. Am J Clin Nutr 1977;30:64–71.
5. Kasidas GP, Rose GA. Oxalate content of some common foods: determination by an enzymatic method. J Hum Nutr 1980;34:255.
6. Ney DM, Hofmann AF, Fischer C, Stubblefield N. The low oxalate diet book for the prevention of oxalate kidney stones. San Diego: University of California, 1981.
7. Krause M, Mahan L. Food nutrition and diet therapy. 7th ed. Philadelphia: WB Saunders, 1984:944–945.
8. Brinkley L, McGuire J, Gregory J, Pak CYC. Bioavailability of oxalate in foods. Urology 1981;17:534–538.
9. *National Dairy Council* Diet and Urolithiasis. Dairy Council Digest 1983;54:1–5.

ACID-ASH AND ALKALINE-ASH DIETS

General Description

Foods that render the urine acid are spoken of as "acid-ash" foods since the ash remaining after their combustion is acid in reaction. Foods that leave alkaline ash after combustion cause the urine to become alkaline.

Nutritional Inadequacy

There are no nutritional inadequacies inherent in diets that promote changes in the pH of the urine.

Indications and Rationale

Dietary manipulations that alter the pH of the urine may be useful in the management of infection type urinary stones and, together with methenamine mandelate, some urinary tract infections.

Description of foods as either "acid-ash" or "alkaline-ash" is based on the reaction of the ash that remains after the combustion of foods under laboratory conditions. Acid-ash foods tend to promote a more acidic urine. Conversely, alkaline-ash foods tend to promote a more alkaline urine. Tables are available that list amounts of acid or alkali to be derived from the metabolism of various foods, but there are enough uncertainties in the interpretation of these data that diets planned to manipulate the pH of the urine should be regarded as qualitative rather than quantitative.[1]

An acid-ash or alkaline-ash diet is generally considered to be supplemental to acidifying or alkalinizing medications. Therefore, advising the patient simply to avoid excessive use of particular foods may be sufficient in conjunction with medical treatment.

Catabolic states tend to favor an acid urine. Even such a minor process of catabolism as overnight fasting results in an acid urine. In addition, the average diet is somewhat "acid-ash."

The use of cranberry juice has gained popular appeal and may be self-prescribed by some persons. Normal amounts of cranberry juice may be drunk, if desired, since it is a liquid; however, it contains oxalate and provides no apparent benefits.[2]

Alkalinization of the urine may retard formation of uric acid or lysine calculi.

Goals of Dietary Management

The goal of acid- and alkaline-ash diets is to supplement the effect of medications in altering the pH of the urine.

Dietary Recommendations

Both the acid-ash and the alkaline-ash diets tend to become monotonous so that compliance by the patient often is poor. A strict dietary regimen rarely is necessary. Since diet generally is considered an auxiliary measure to acidifying or alkalinizing medications, it may be sufficient to simply avoid excessive use of particular foods. For example, if medical treatment is directed at acidifying the urine, the diet should not contain large amounts of alkaline-ash foods; complete avoidance of all alkaline-ash foods, however, probably would not yield any further benefit and is unwarranted.

Potentially Acid or Acid-Ash Foods

Meat	Meat, fish, fowl, shellfish, eggs, all types of cheese, peanut butter, peanuts
Fat	Bacon, nuts (Brazil nuts, filberts, walnuts)
Starch	All types of bread (especially whole wheat), cereal, crackers, macaroni, spaghetti, noodles, rice
Vegetable	Corn, lentils
Fruit	Cranberries, plums, prunes
Desserts	Plain cakes, cookies

Potentially Basic or Alkaline-Ash Foods

Milk	Milk and milk products, cream, buttermilk
Fat	Nuts (almonds, chestnuts, coconut)
Vegetables	All types (except corn, lentils), especially beets, beet greens, Swiss chard, dandelion greens, kale, mustard greens, spinach, turnip greens
Fruit	All types (except cranberries, prunes, plums)
Sweets	Molasses

Neutral Foods

Fats	Butter, margarine, cooking fats, oils
Sweets	Plain candies, sugar, syrup, honey
Starch	Arrowroot, corn, tapioca
Beverages	Coffee, tea

Physicians: How to Order Diet

The diet order should indicate *acid-ash* or *alkaline-ash diet.*

REFERENCES

1. Dwyer J, Foulkes E, Evans M, Ausman L. Acid/Alkaline ash diets: time for assessment and change. J Am Diet Assoc 1985;85:841–845.
2. Kahn DH, Panariello VA, Saeli J, et al. Effect of cranberry juice on urine. J Am Diet Assoc 1977;58:16–24.

PURINE RESTRICTION

General Description

Specific kinds of meats and meat extracts are high in purines.

Nutritional Inadequacy

There are no nutritional inadequacies inherent in a purine-restricted diet.

Indications and Rationale

Persons with disorders affecting purine metabolism, such as gout and urinary uric acid lithiasis, may be advised to reduce their intake of purine.

Uric acid stones may develop as a result of hyperuricuria, dehydration, or excessive acidity of the urine. Uric acid is the end product of purine metabolism. Foods high in purines generally have a high acid-ash content and tend to acidify the urine and increase urinary excretion of uric acid. Exclusion of foods extremely high in purines may be helpful.

Goals of Dietary Management

The goals of a purine restriction are to supplement the effect of medication by making the urine more acidic and by decreasing urine levels of uric acid.

Dietary Recommendations

Historically, dietary efforts to reduce purine intake have been relatively comprehensive. All meats, fish, and poultry contain moderate to high amounts of purine. Some vegetables contain low to moderate amounts of purine. Efforts to greatly restrict these foods generally are unnecessary because of their relatively insignificant effect compared to that of medications aimed at reducing uric acid excretion. It generally is sufficient to simply avoid an excessive intake of purines since the diet is considered an auxiliary measure to medications.

Specific Dietary Recommendations

Avoid excessive intake of meat, fish, and poultry. Avoid extremely high purine foods, such as organ meats (liver, heart, tongue, kidneys), sweetbreads, brains, anchovies, sardines, meat extracts, gravy, broth, and bouillon. Reduce weight if overweight.

Physicians: How to Order Diet

The diet order should indicate *purine control*.

OTHER DIETARY CONSTITUENTS

Phosphate

Attempts to control the formation of phosphate-containing stones through the use of a low-phosphate diet and phosphate-binding agents have been largely unsuccessful.

Cystine

Cystinuria is an inherited disorder that involves gastrointestinal and renal transport of the amino acids cystine, lysine, arginine, and ornithine. The only major complication in this disorder is the tendency to form cystine stones because of the low urinary solubility of cystine. Cystine is the end product of methionine metabolism. Urinary excretion of cystine can be lowered by reducing the dietary intake of methionine, and this can be accomplished by decreasing the total protein content of the diet. Stringent restriction of protein rarely is recommended; however, excessive dietary protein (greater than 120 g per day) should be avoided.[1,2] Acidification of the urine increases solubility of cystine, and avoidance of alkaline-ash foods increases the effectiveness of acidifying agents such as ammonium chloride.

REFERENCES

1. Pak CYC, Smith LH, Resnick MI, Weinerth JL. Dietary management of idiopathic calcium urolithiasis. J Urol 1984;131:850–852.
2. Mahalko JR, Sandstead HH, Johnson LK, Milne DB. Effect of a moderate increase in dietary protein on the retention and excretion of Ca, Cu, Fe, Mg, P, and Zn by adult males. Am J Clin Nutr 1983;37:8–14.

TYRAMINE CONTROLLED DIET

General Description

The diet restricts foods that contain large amounts of tyramine either naturally or through aging. Aging is a process that increases tyramine content by protein breakdown. Foods that have high levels of other pressor amines and foods that have been implicated in hypertensive reactions during monoamine oxidase therapy are also restricted.

Nutritional Inadequacy

The tyramine-controlled diet is not inherently inadequate in nutrients when compared to the Recommended Dietary Allowance (RDA). However, for those diets in which kilocalories are restricted to 1,200 Kcal or less, it is difficult to meet the RDA consistently. A multiple vitamin supplement that provides nutrients at a level that is equivalent to the RDA is recommended for persons who consume 1,200 Kcal or less. A multiple vitamin supplement may also be warranted for persons who have food aversions or intolerances that greatly limit the variety of food choices.

Indications and Rationale

The diet should be used as a precautionary measure for all patients who take monoamine oxidase inhibitor drugs. These drugs, such as tranylcypromine (Parnate) and phenelzine (Nardil), are utilized in the treatment of depression and of anxiety disorders.

The concomitant ingestion of foods that have a high concentration of tyramine or other pressor amines may precipitate a hypertensive crisis that is characterized by headaches and nausea. Tyramine and other pressor amines are normally degraded in the body by the enzyme monoamine oxidase. Monoamine oxidase inhibitors interfere with this process, and the result is the accumulation of a variety of amine substances in the adrenergic nerve terminals. The ingestion of tyramine may trigger the sudden release of large quantities of these pressor amines from their nerve terminal storage sites. Some of the released catecholamines are strongly active vasopressor materials; therefore, a hypertensive crisis may occur.

Goals of Dietary Management

In patients who take monoamine oxidase inhibitors, it has been reported that as little as 6 mg of tyramine may cause increased blood pressure and that 25 mg may induce a hypertensive crisis. Thus, the intake should be kept below 5 mg per day.[1]

Dietary Recommendations

In general, only fresh foods or freshly prepared frozen or canned foods should be eaten. Avoid any protein food that has been aged, improperly handled, stored, or refrigerated.

1. Cottage cheese, cream cheese, farmer's cheese, and ricotta cheese may be used.
2. Bakery-type products made with yeast are allowed.
3. Check labels of canned and packaged foods carefully.
4. Remember tyramine restriction when selecting foods in a restaurant.
Table 6–55 presents foods that are high in tyramine.

TABLE 6–55   Food Sources of Tyramine[*,1,2]

Food Group	Types of Food
Beverages	Beer, liqueurs, red wines including Chianti, sherry
Meat and Meat Substitutes	Caviar Cheese, aged and processed Herring, pickled or dried Liver Sausage: dry, summer, pepperoni, hard salami, bologna
Vegetables	Chinese pea pods Italian green beans Fava beans
Fruits	Avocado in large amounts
Soups	Soups packaged with yeast products
Miscellaneous	Brewer's yeast Soy sauce in large amounts

*Data available on the content of tyramine and other pressor amines show a great deal of variation. The tyramine content is likely to vary among different brands of a particular food, since several factors related to the preparation, processing, and storing of foods may contribute to their tyramine content. The tyramine content may also vary with the time the food is left unrefrigerated, i.e., the longer the time, the greater the protein degradation. For practical purposes, the diet is intended to prohibit or limit foods that tend to be high in tyramine or other pressor amines and foods that have been implicated in the development of a hypertensive crisis in patients who take monoamine oxidase inhibitors.

In addition to the aforementioned dietary restrictions, certain medications should be avoided while receiving an MAO inhibitor. These include many cold tablets and decongestants, most allergy and asthma medications, some high blood pressure pills, and the pain medication Demerol. Prior to beginning an MAO inhibitor, the physician should evaluate all the medications taken, including over the counter preparations. The patient should be reminded to consult a physician or pharmacist prior to taking any new medication.[3,4]

Physicians: How to Order Diet

The diet order should indicate *tyramine control* or request dietary precautions during the use of monoamine oxidase inhibitors.

REFERENCES

1. McCabe BJ. Dietary tyramine and other pressor amines in MAOI regimens: A review. J Am Diet Assoc 1986;86:1059–1064.
2. Lippmann S. Monoamine oxidase inhibitors. Am Fam Physician 1986;34:113–119.
3. Ziscook SA. A clinical overview of monoamine oxidase inhibitors. Psychosomatics 1985;26:240–251.
4. Adverse reactions to MAOIs. Biol Ther Psychiatry 1985;8:1–4.

CHAPTER 7

SPECIALIZED NUTRITION SUPPORT

ENTERAL NUTRITION SUPPORT
OF ADULTS

General Description

The term "enteral" nutrition includes both the ordinary ingestion of food by mouth and the provision of nutrients via the gastrointestinal tract by means of a tube. Patients unable to take adequate nutrients by mouth require an alternative form of nutritional support. Some patients may need nutritional support via the intravenous route. Many others are capable of digesting and absorbing nutrients delivered through feeding tubes introduced into the alimentary tract at various levels. Tube feeding has been shown to be an effective method for repairing and for preventing nutritional deficiencies.[1]

The approach to enteral tube feeding should be a cooperative team effort and should include the physician, dietitian, nurse, and pharmacist. When the patient is dismissed from the hospital with a plan for continuing tube feeding, social service input should also be available.

Indications and Rationale

Any disease process that adversely affects oral intake may ultimately lead to significant nutritional deprivation and depletion. Patients who cannot eat, will not eat, or should not eat, yet who have some degree of functioning of the gastrointestinal tract, are candidates for enteral tube feeding (Table 7–1).

Enteral feeding has a number of distinct advantages over parenteral feeding for the patient whose gastrointestinal tract is functional. Advantages include maintenance of gastrointestinal structural and functional integrity, enhanced utilization of nutrients delivered enterally versus parenterally, greater ease and safety of administration, lower cost, and better patient acceptance and tolerance.[2]

Enteral tube feeding is contraindicated in patients with peritonitis, intestinal obstruction, and intractable vomiting or severe diarrhea. Enteral feeding is not recommended during the early stages of short bowel syndrome or in the presence of severe malabsorptive states.[3] Parenteral nutrition should be considered when a properly managed trial of tube feeding fails to meet nutritional

TABLE 7–1 Indications for Tube Feeding

Nutritional Disorder	Cause
Oral intake inadequate or contraindicated	Mechanical: stroke, central nervous system disorders, coma, oropharyngeal and esophageal disorders, partial obstruction Poor appetite: chemotherapy, radiation therapy, drug effect, nausea, depression Transitional feeding: advance from parenteral to oral intake
Increased nutritional requirements	Burns, trauma, sepsis, surgical or medical stress
Digestive and absorptive disorders	Inflammatory bowel disease, short bowel syndrome, pancreatitis, irradiated bowel, proximal and distal intestinal fistulae
Metabolic and excretory disorders	Glycogen storage disease Hepatic encephalopathy Renal disease

goals, aggravates the primary condition, or creates secondary problems such as pulmonary aspiration or unmanageable diarrhea.

Determination of Nutrient Needs

Assessment of the nutritional status of every patient is fundamental and includes four key components: nutritional history screen, anthropometric procedures, clinical examination, and biochemical data. Nutritional assessment is a process that documents the presence of malnutrition, identifies nutrient needs, aids the clinician in selecting the best method for providing nutrients, and allows for objective monitoring of nutritional support efforts. For tube-fed patients, nutritional assessment is not necessary only to evaluate nutritional status. The assessment also is needed to estimate requirements in order to select the correct type and amount of formula, and to estimate the need for vitamin, mineral, and fluid modifications. (See *Nutritional Assessment*, page 3, for a more complete discussion of these methods and a review of techniques for nutritional assessment.)

Kilocalories. The patient's caloric requirements determine the quantity of formula required daily. Most tube feeding formulations provide 1.0 kilocalorie per milliliter, although concentrations at 1.5 and 2.0 kilocalories per milliliter are available. Consideration of the patient's sensitivity to volume and the overall fluid requirements may necessitate the selection of a more concentrated or a more dilute formula.

Protein. The amount of protein provided by a formula is dependent on the amount of formula administered daily, as well as on the concentration of protein. The patient's nutritional requirements should be met by adjusting the quantity of formula, by selecting a formula with a different protein density, or by adding a protein module to the formula. Most commercial formulas contain a kilocalorie-to-nitrogen ratio of 150:1 (with a range between 100:1 and 200:1), which is thought to be optimal for seriously ill patients. Nitrogen balance techniques can help in deciding whether the supply of protein is adequate for the individual patient. (See *Nutritional Assessment,* page 3).

Vitamins, Minerals, and Trace Elements. It is important to note at what quantity enteral formulations meet or exceed the Recommended Dietary Allowances (RDA) for vitamins and minerals. Most commercial formulations provide 100 percent or more of the RDA for vitamins and essential minerals in 1,500 to 2,000 ml. Supplemental vitamins and minerals should be provided when the quantity of formula does not assure adequacy. The individual's nutritional status should also be monitored and the amounts of vitamins and minerals adjusted accordingly. Known essential trace elements are present in commercial formulas, and current clinical practice is to supplement with additional trace elements only if a deficiency is detected.

Water. Fluid balance in tube-fed patients requires daily monitoring, since these patients are susceptible to overhydration as well as to dehydration. Water requirement for a healthy adult is 1 ml for each kilocalorie ingested.[4] The amount of water in the tube feeding formulas varies. The amount of additional water needed can be calculated from the composition of the formula, based on the percentage of moisture and on the caloric density of the product. Generally, about 20 percent of the volume of the formula should be given as additional water. Conveniently, the additional water is given to flush the tube following feedings.

Water requirement is also dependent on the renal solute load and on extrarenal losses. Those patients with impaired renal concentrating ability (infants and elderly patients) require extra water to eliminate the solute load. Extrarenal losses due to diarrhea, vomiting, or fistulas should be monitored and replaced accordingly. Insensible water loss increases 13 percent for each degree centigrade above normal body temperature.[5] Insensible losses vary considerably, but likely average 800 to 1,000 ml daily. This happens to be approximately equal to the water derived from metabolism. By virtue of this coincidence, urinary volume is approximately equal to the volume of fluids ingested (i.e., "intake" equals "output").[6]

Nutritional Formulations

A wide variety of commercially prepared formulas currently are available that have variable sources and concentrations of protein, carbohydrate, and fat. Consequently, they differ in caloric density, kilocalorie-to-nitrogen ratio, electrolyte and mineral content, and osmolality. Commercial products offer many distinct advantages over hospital or home-blended mixtures, including a known nutrient composition, controlled osmolality and consistency, ease in preparation and storage, bacteriological safety, and in most instances lower cost.[7,8]

Table 7–2 displays the nutrient content of commercial formulas that have been selected as standard tube feedings at the Mayo Clinic. *Appendix 13* presents other available formulations. Data are derived from manufacturers' analysis and are presented on the basis of nutrients per 1,000 ml. The volumes needed to assure 100 percent of the RDA for vitamins should be noted, and supplements should be provided as needed. These formulas are often categorized as polymeric, monomeric, special formulas, and supplemental nutrient sources. Each category emphasizes the product characteristics that are important for most effective utilization.

Polymeric Formulas. Polymeric formulas are composed of intact proteins, disaccharides and polysaccharides, variable amounts of fat, residue, and lactose. The osmolality of polymeric formulas is usually lower than other more "elemental" diets. In general, these formulas require a functioning gastrointestinal tract for digestion and absorption of nutrients.

TABLE 7-2 Nutrient Content Mayo Medical Center Enteral Nutrition Formulary

Formula	Kcal/ml	Non protein Kcal:gN	Osmolality mOsm	Moisture %	Volume for 100% RDA Vits (ml)	Protein g	Total Fat (MCT fat) g	CHO g	Na/K mEq	Protein	Fat	Carbohydrate
Malabsorption and maldigestion												
Ensure Plus (Ross Laboratories)	1.5	146:1	600	76	1,600	55	53 (0)	200	50/55	Sodium & calcium caseinates, soy protein isolates	Corn oil	Corn syrup sucrose
Ensure (Ross Laboratories)	1.06	153:1	450	83	1,887	37	37 (0)	145	37/40	Sodium & calcium caseinates, soy protein isolates	Corn oil	Corn syrup sucrose
Osmolite (Ross Laboratories)	1.06	153:1	300	83	1,887	37	39 (17)	145	28/26	Sodium & calcium caseinates, soy protein isolates	MCT oil, corn oil, soy oil	Hydrolyzed corn starch
Travasorb MCT (Travenol Laboratories)	1.0 or 2.0	102:1	312	75	2,000	49	33 (26)	123	15/45	Lactalbumin, potassium caseinate	MCT oil, sunflower oil	Cornsyrup solids
		102:1	590	42	1,000	98	66 (53)	246	30/90			
Vital High Nitrogen (Ross Laboratories)	1.0	125:1	460	85	1,500	42	11 (5)	185	20/34	Whey, soy, & meat protein hydrolysates, free essential amino acids	Safflower oil, MCT oil	Hydrolyzed corn starch, sucrose
Special Formulas												
Hepatic Aid II (Kendall McGaw)	1.1	148:1	560	78	0	44	36 (0)	169	$<$15/$<$6	Crystalline amino acids (high branch-chain, low aromatic amino acids)	Soybean oil, lecithin, mono & diglycerides	Maltodextrin, sucrose
Amin-Aid (Kendall McGaw)	2.0	830:1	1,095	87	0	19	46 (0)	366	$<$15/$<$6	Crystalline essential amino acids including histidine	Soybean oil, lecithin, mono & diglycerides	Maltodextrin, sucrose
Supplement												
Polycose (Ross Laboratories)	2.0 (3.8/g)	NA	850	NA	0	0	0	500	25/5	NA	NA	Hydrolysis of corn starch
MCT Oil (Mead Johnson Pharmaceutical)	7.7 (8.3/g)	NA	0	NA	0	0	927 (927)	0	0	NA	Fractionated coconut oil	NA
Citrotein (Sandoz Pharmaceutical)	0.66	76:1	495–515	93	1,350	41	2 (0)	122	31/18	Egg albumin	Soy oil	Sucrose, maltodextrin

NA = not applicable

Polymeric formulas are usually subdivided into blended food products (Complete, Vitaneed), lactose-containing products (Carnation Instant Breakfast, Meritene, Sustacal), lactose-free products that are hypercaloric (TwoCal HN, Ensure Plus), and normocaloric products. Normocaloric formulas can be subdivided into those that are isosmotic (Osmolite, Isocal), those that are hyperosmotic (Ensure, Precision LR), and those that are higher in nitrogen content (Precision HN, Ensure HN).

Monomeric Formulas. Monomeric formulas, or "elemental" diets, are composed of low molecular weight nutrients and require minimal digestive and absorptive capabilities. Protein sources include short-chain peptides and amino acids. Carbohydrates consist of oligosaccharides and sucrose. Fat sources are usually medium-chain triglycerides and small amounts of essential fatty acids. Monomeric diets have minimal residue because nutrients provided in the more "elemental" form are more efficiently absorbed. The products are of greater osmolality than polymeric formulas because of the small molecular weight of the nutrients. Osmotic diarrhea is one of the more common side effects. The lower molecular weight nutrients result in poor palatability. Therefore, these formulas should be administered through a tube.

Special Formulas. Special formulas include products designed for patients who have specific medical conditions that may respond by nutrient modification. In patients with hepatic encephalopathy, which is associated with chronic liver disease, the use of formulas high in branched-chain amino acids (leucine, isoleucine, and valine) and low in aromatic amino acids (phenylalanine, tyrosine, and tryptophan) and methionine may increase the ratio of serum branched-chain amino acids (BCAA) to serum aromatic amino acids (AAA).[9] The efficacy of high BCAA-low AAA formulas in hepatic encephalopathy has not been shown conclusively.[9-11] Newer formulations are now available to meet the nutritional needs of traumatized and septic patients.[9] Recent information on metabolic processes during stress has led to the development of formulas specifically designed with increased branched-chain amino acid content.[12] Patients with chronic renal failure may benefit from the use of formulas containing nitrogen in the form of essential amino acids and histidine.[13] However, conventional protein sources should be given if patients are receiving hemodialysis.

Supplemental Nutrient Sources. These products provide one or more nutrients and are not nutritionally complete. Such products can be added to food or to formulas in order to alter nutrient content and caloric density. By adding carbohydrate, protein, or fat modules to formulas, the patient's nutritional requirements can be met more closely.[14]

Formula Selection. Selection of the appropriate formula is based on the individual patient's medical and nutritional status. Digestive and absorptive capabilities indicate whether a monomeric or a polymeric formula is needed. Individual nutrient requirements further specify the type and the amount of formula necessary to provide adequate nutritional support and whether supplemental sources of nutrients are required. Ongoing assessment of the nutritional status while the patient is receiving tube feeding indicates the effectiveness of the nutritional program.

Tube Feeding Access Routes

The route for tube feeding depends on the anticipated duration of feeding, the condition of the gastrointestinal tract (e.g., esophageal obstruction, prior gastric or small bowel resections), and the potential for aspiration. Access to the gut can be accomplished at the bedside (nasogastric tube, percutaneous endoscopic gastrostomy, percutaneous endoscopic gastrojejunostomy) or in the operating room (gastrostomy, jejunostomy).

Nasal Intubation. Nasal intubation for gastric or transpyloric feeding is the simplest and the most commonly used approach for tube feeding. This technique is preferred for patients in whom eventual resumption of oral feeding is anticipated. Maximum patient comfort and acceptance is possible when a small-diameter, soft feeding tube is used. Access to the duodenum and the jejunum is possible with long weighted tubes for those patients at risk for aspiration.

Tube Enterostomies. Tube enterostomies generally are indicated when long-term tube feeding is anticipated, when obstruction makes nasal intubation impossible, or when there is a risk of aspiration. Conventional gastrostomies require a surgical procedure with the use of a general anesthesia. For high-risk patients the morbidity and mortality rates are high. Percutaneous endoscopic placement of a gastrostomy has advantages, and can be performed at the bedside with minimal or no sedation. Potential complications appear to be relatively minor and infrequent.[15,16] Enthusiasm has been generated for the needle catheter jejunostomy, which is placed at the time of laparotomy.[17] Indications for the placement of a needle catheter jejunostomy include preoperative malnutrition for which postoperative nutritional support is planned, emergency or elective major upper abdominal operations, and the anticipated need for postoperative chemotherapy or radiation therapy. Jejunal access permits early postoperative feeding because, unlike the stomach and the colon, the small bowel is less affected by postoperative ileus. Jejunal feedings also minimize the risk of vomiting and of aspiration from the infusions and do not necessarily interfere with oral intake.

Administration of Tube Feeding

Proper administration of enteral formulas ensures safe delivery of desired nutrients, maximum patient tolerance, and optimum nutritional support. Choice of the specific method for tube feeding (e.g., intermittent or continuous infusion), control of the initial rate and concentration of the formula, and a systematic progression to reach nutrient requirements are all important factors for tube feeding administration.

Methods of Feeding. Tube feeding methods include continuous, intermittent, and bolus infusion. The choice of technique depends mainly on gastrointestinal function, feeding site, and, ultimately, patient response.

Intermittent Infusion. The most common method for the administration of tube feedings is delivery on an intermittent or "meal-type" basis. For intermittent feeding, the total quantity of formula needed for a 24-hour period is divided into equal portions, and the required fractions are administered in six to eight feedings. Each feeding usually is administered by gravity over a 20- to 40-minute period. Rate of intermittent infusion (rather than volume) has been cited as a major reason for symptoms of intolerance.[18]

General clinical practice is to administer intermittent feedings as follows:

Slow	6 ml per minute	240 ml per 40 minutes
Moderate	8 ml per minute	240 ml per 30 minutes
Regular	12 ml per minute	240 ml per 20 minutes

It has been shown that up to 30 ml per minute can be administered without subjective complaint in some patients.[18]

There are limited studies that examine the effects of varying volume while controlling the rate of administration. However, present data suggest that infusion of volumes in excess of 350 ml per meal may be less physiologically tolerated because of delayed gastric emptying.[18] Delivery of larger volumes of total intake, when needed, may require more frequent feedings or continuous infusion.

An advantage of the intermittent feeding method is that it requires only simple equipment. In the absence of infusion pumps, however, feedings must be closely monitored, and the procedure actually may become time consuming. Intermittent infusion may be more physiologic than continuous infusion since it parallels a more normal feeding pattern, and the gastric distention it causes may stimulate gastrointestinal activity.[19]

Continuous Infusion. Continuous infusion is the controlled delivery of a prescribed volume of formula at a constant rate over a period of time (8 to 24 hours). This method is considered to be advantageous since gastric pooling is minimized and fewer gastrointestinal side effects are experienced.[20] Additionally, the length of time required to advance a patient to the desired volume of formula to meet nutritional goals can be minimized with continuous feeding. Controlled, continuous infusion, therefore, may be the most cost effective means of providing specialized nutritional support. Continuous infusion is particularly indicated if the tube location is intestinal, if the patient has taken nothing by mouth for a significant period of time, or if the patient is debilitated or has impaired gastrointestinal function.

A constant infusion rate can be insured by utilizing an infusion pump. Continuous drip by gravity is possible, but accuracy is less easily achieved.

Bolus Feeding. Bolus feeding is the intermittent, rapid administration of large volumes of formula. It usually is given by syringe. This method of feeding is least cumbersome to the patient, but the possibility of aspiration, regurgitation, and gastrointestinal side effects is greatly increased. A rate of 30 ml per minute with a volume less than 350 ml per feeding appears to mark physical tolerance limits.[18]

Initiation of Tube Feeding. Regardless of the choice of feeding technique, a systematic approach to initiating tube feeding is mandatory to assure optimal patient tolerance. Generally, the initial infusion rate should be slow and the concentration should be isosmolar (i.e., approximately 300 mOsm). Table 7–3 outlines suggested guidelines for initiating tube feedings.

Rate. Infusion rates should not exceed the patient's ability to manage the volume provided. Clinical case reports commonly recommend initial administration rates of 25 to 50 ml per hour.[3] The patient should be monitored for symptoms of intolerance. For gastric feedings, aspiration of gastric residual should be done routinely before each feeding. If the volume exceeds that infused during the preceding hour,[21] the rate should be decreased.

Concentration. Initial formula concentration should be isosmotic (i.e., approximately 300 mOsm). Hypertonic formulas adversely affect gastric emptying and lead to either distention or to dumping syndrome. Formulas with a high osmolality pull fluid from surrounding tissues into the intestinal lumen and could lead to intestinal distention and increased motility if the volume is large enough. There is also significant correlation between protein malnutrition

TABLE 7–3 Administration of Tube Feedings

Initial Feeding

Rate: 25–50 ml/hr
Conc: Isosmotic (300 mOsm)

Progression of Feedings

Gastric Feeding		Intestinal Feeding
Intermittent Administration	Continuous Administration	Continuous Administration Only
1. Increase concentration to full strength.* 2. Increase rate: Slow: 6 ml/minute (240 ml/40 min) Moderate: 8 ml/minute (240 ml/30 min) Regular: 12 ml/minute (240 ml/20 min)	1. Increase concentration to full strength.* 2. Increase rate 25–50 ml/hr as tolerated each 8–12 hours until desired daily volume reached.	1. Increase rate 25–50 ml/hr as tolerated every 8–12 hours until desired daily volume reached. 2. Increase concentration to full strength.

Antiaspiration measures:
1. Position: Elevate head of bed 30 to 45° during infusion.
2. Tube placement: Check placement each shift or before each intermittent feeding.
3. Gastric retention: Aspirate residual each shift or before each intermittent feeding.

*Full strength refers to osmolality listed in column 4 of Table 7–2.

(characterized by serum albumin levels less than 3 g per deciliter) and the development of diarrhea at the initiation of tube feedings.[21] The initial diarrhea generally is alleviated by diluting the formula and by slowly increasing the flow rate and the concentration. It is general clinical practice, therefore, that hyperosmolar formulas be diluted to an isosmotic (approximately 300 mOsm) concentration. There usually is no need to dilute isosmotic formulas, and initial delivery can begin at full strength concentration.

Progression of Feeding. The site of feeding (gastric versus intestinal) is important in determining the advancement of rate and of formula concentration. For gastric feeding, it is general practice to increase the concentration of the formula first. Once full strength is achieved, the rate of administration can be increased according to tolerance. For duodenal or jejunal feeding, the rate of administration should be increased by 25 to 50 ml per hour per day until the necessary volume is reached. The concentration is then increased until full strength is achieved.[22]

Rate and concentration should not be altered simultaneously. If the feeding is not tolerated, reduce the rate or the concentration to the level of tolerance, then gradually increase again.

One should realize that with low volumes and dilute formulas, nutritional requirements are not met. Most patients with a normal intestinal tract tolerate advancement to maintenance needs within 48 hours. Patients with shortened or compromised small bowel, severe debilitation, or lack of oral feedings for a week or more may benefit from a less aggressive progression. Prolonged disease of the gastrointestinal tract results in both functional and anatomic atrophy. These changes can be reversed by slow and gradual challenges in the form of small, then progressively larger, feedings.

Complications and Their Prevention

The complications associated with tube feeding fall into three major categories: mechanical, gastrointestinal, and metabolic. The most frequently seen problems are minimized or prevented through proper formula and equipment selection, controlled administration, and careful monitoring.

Mechanical Complications. Mechanical problems are often associated with the tube type and its position. Mucosal erosions are more likely to occur when large diameter tubes are used. Such tubes also may reduce the competency of the lower esophageal sphincter, thereby increasing the risk of gastroesophageal reflux and aspiration.[23] Tubes that are small in diameter (e.g., 8 or 9 F) and more pliable are associated with less irritation and better tolerance. However, small lumen tubes are more likely to become occluded, usually from residual of the feedings or from particulate matter from pulverized medications administered through the tubes. In an attempt to prevent obstruction of the tubes, irrigation with 20 to 50 ml of water or cranberry juice should occur every 8 to 12 hours and whenever the feeding is interrupted.[24] Also, only liquid forms of medications should be administered through small tubes. Pharmacologic activity of medications that are administered with tube feedings may be either enhanced or diminished; care should be taken when drugs are given with the feeding.[19,25] Displacement of nasogastric tubes can be disastrous and can be avoided if care is taken during intubation. Placement of a radiopaque tube can be confirmed by a chest roentgenogram, by auscultation over the left upper quadrant of the abdomen during instillation of air with a syringe, or by aspiration of gastric contents. Displacement of tubes also can occur with altered gastric motility, vomiting, or coughing. Weighted tubes placed transpylorically can help alleviate this problem. Tube position should be checked periodically and before initiation of each feeding. Mechanical complications seen most frequently with enterostomy feedings include leakage of gastrointestinal contents around the stoma site with subsequent skin erosion, wound infection, and tube dislodgement. Proper tube maintenance and routine site care help control such complications.[26]

Gastrointestinal Complications. Gastrointestinal side effects of tube feeding include delayed gastric emptying, nausea, vomiting, cramping abdominal pain, and diarrhea (Table 7–4). Such problems frequently are related to the rate and/or concentration of the formula being administered. A systematic progression in the feeding rate or the concentration and use of a feeding pump may decrease the risk of gastrointestinal side effects.[27]

Vomiting and pulmonary aspiration are more likely to occur when gastric emptying is delayed. This risk can be lessened by elevating the upper part of the patient's body to a 30° angle, by positioning the tube beyond the pylorus, and by checking for gastric residual before each feeding. The residual should not exceed the amount infused during the preceding hour. If the residual is excessive, the feeding should be held and the residual rechecked in 1 hour. If large volume residuals persist, reduction in the formula concentration and/or the rate

TABLE 7–4 Common Tube Feeding Problems and Causes

Vomiting	Diarrhea	Constipation
Improper tube placement Tube too large Rate of feeding too fast Residual volume from previous feeding too great Osmolality of feeding too high Medications given with feeding	Rate of feeding too fast Osmolality of feeding too high Intolerance to formula ingredients (e.g., lactose) Medications (e.g., antibiotics) Severe protein and calorie malnutrition Malabsorption Bacterial overgrowth	Lack of bulk in the diet Inadequate fluid Lack of activity

may alleviate the problem.[22] Pharmacologic intervention with metoclopramide also may be employed.[28]

Diarrhea with enteral feedings can result from lactase deficiency, concomitant antibiotic treatment, infectious diarrhea from contaminated formulas, and excessive osmotic loads.[29] Diarrhea that persists during the administration of formula feedings may lessen with a reduction in the rate or the concentration of solution. Perseverance with small feedings may promote adaptation, with a return to more nearly normal intestinal enzyme production and motility. If formulas are changed while adaptation is taking place, the second formula used is likely to be credited with being less prone to produce diarrhea. Anti-diarrheal agents should be used with the objective of maintaining an optimal delivery of nutrients. Infectious diarrhea can be prevented by paying close attention to technique in the preparation and handling of formulas. Any formula manipulation—either at the time of preparation or administration—should be carried out with clean technique. Most commercial formulas are in ready-to-feed form and are packaged in sterile containers to which feeding sets are attached. Feeding sets or containers should be changed daily. In general, enteral formulas should not be opened and at room temperature for longer than 8 hours, but this may be more limited for specific products. Any remaining formula that is opened and unused should be refrigerated and should be discarded after 24 hours. Tube feeding products also should be labeled with the expiration time and date.

Metabolic Complications. The metabolic complications with tube feeding consist of excesses and deficiencies of almost every nutrient. The onset and severity, however, are generally moderate, and most complications can be treated easily. In one report, 30 to 40 percent of 100 patients experienced at least one metabolic complication.[30] Hyperkalemia (40%), hyponatremia (31%), hypophosphatemia (30%), and hyperglycemia (29%) were the most frequently observed complications. In another series, 43 percent of 83 patients required modification of the enteral formulation in order to meet fluid and electrolyte requirements.[14] Additional reasons cited for formula modifications were organ dysfunction (31%), vitamin deficiencies (12%), electrolyte imbalances (27%), and fatty-acid deficiencies (12%). Thus, administration of formulas with a fixed composition may increase the likelihood of iatrogenic complications. Such metabolic complications usually are managed easily when patients are routinely monitored.

Tube Feeding at Home

Enteral tube feeding has been increasingly offered to patients going home. The demand for this service and the need to coordinate its application have been growing steadily owing to many factors. Primarily, the acknowledgment of nutrition as a strong component of medical care and the recognition that continued nutritional support is frequently needed at the time of dismissal have led to an extension into the outpatient or the home setting. The rapid development of sophisticated enteral formulas and delivery systems have made home tube feeding feasible and practical. Changing health care reimbursement patterns also have increased the emphasis on home care. Industry has responded with the appearance of a multitude of private home nutrition support companies. Each offers to manage home care services on behalf of the medical center with varying intensity and scope.

Patient Education

Education is a joint health care team effort. The dietitian and the nurse provide individualized training of the patient and family members. Instructional responsibilities should be identified, and a time table for implementation should be established. The techniques for instruction include oral instruction, written guidelines, staff demonstration, return demonstration by the patient and family, and assumption of full responsibility for tube feeding prior to dismissal. In our institution a Home Enteral Coordinator reviews and reinforces instruction and certifies that the patient is ready for dismissal.[31]

Supplies such as formula, administration equipment, and site care items are arranged for the patient prior to dismissal. Avenues for financial assistance with the home nutrition program are also identified.[32] Responsibility for the home tube-fed patient continues beyond dismissal. Frequent telephone contact and return appointments are used to follow the progress of nutritional rehabilitation, to assist with solving problems, and to adjust the enteral program according to changes in needs. Follow-up of patients referred into the Mayo Clinic program reveals that, although many problems with tube feeding are experienced, the majority can be resolved at home. Also, most patients report that they can maintain or improve their level of function.[31]

Physicians: How to Order Diet

The diet order should indicate:

1. The *brand name from the hospital formulary* or the *type of feeding*, e.g., polymeric, monomeric, or special formula

2. The *manner of feeding*, e.g., continuous, or number and interval of intermittent feedings

According to the preceding guidelines, the dietitian will determine the amount of formula required to provide an appropriate caloric and protein level, the degree of dilution, if needed, and the amount of supplemental water.

REFERENCES

1. Heymsfield SB, Bethel RA, Ansley JD, Nixon DW, Rudman D. Enteral hyperalimentation: an alternative to central venous hyperalimentation. Ann Intern Med 1979;90:63–71.

2. McArdle AH, Palmason C, Morency I, Brown RA. A rationale for enteral feeding as the preferable route of hyperalimentation. Surgery 1981;90:616–623.

3. Bethel RA, Jansen BS, Heymsfield SB, Ansley JD, Hersh T, Rudman D. Nasogastric hyperalimentation through a polyurethane catheter: an alternative to central venous hyperalimentation. Am J Clin Nutr 1979;32:1112–1120.

4. Food and Nutrition Board, National Research Council. Recommended Dietary Allowances. 9th ed. Washington, D.C.: National Academy of Science, 1980:168.

5. Hayes MA, Williamson RJ, Heidenreich WF. Endocrine mechanisms involved in water and sodium metabolism during operation and convalescence. Surgery 1957;41:353–386.

6. Shils ME, Randall HT. Diet and nutrition in care of the surgical patient. In: Goodhart RS, Shils ME, eds. Modern nutrition in health and disease. 6th ed.: Philadelphia: Lea and Febiger, 1980:1082–1124.

7. Keighley MR, Mogg B, Bentley S, Allan C. "Home brew" compared with commercial preparation for enteral feeding. Br Med J 1982;284:163.

8. Gormican A, Liddy E. Nasogastric tube feedings: practical considerations in prescription and evaluation. Postgrad Med 1975;53:71–76.

9. Skipper A. Specialized formulas for enteral nutrition support. J Am Diet Assoc 1986;86:654–658.

10. McGhee A, Henderson JM, Millikan WJ, Bleier JC, Vogel R, Kassouny M, Rudman D. Comparison of the effects of hepatic-aid and a casein modular diet on encephalopathy, plasma amino acids, and nitrogen balance in cirrhotic patients. Ann Surg 1983;197:288–293.

11. Eriksson LS, Persson A, Wahren J. Branched-chain amino acids in the treatment of chronic hepatic encephalopathy. Gut 1982;23:801–806.

12. Cerra FB, Mazuski J, Teasley K, Nuwer N, Lysne J, Shronts E, Konstantinides N. Nitrogen retention in critically ill patients is proportioned to the branched chain load. Crit Care Med 1983;11:775–778.

13. Steffee WP, Anderson CF. Enteral nutrition and renal disease. In: Rombeau JL, Caldwell MD, eds. Clinical nutrition Vol. I: Enteral and tube feeding. Philadelphia: WB Saunders, 1984:262.

14. Freed BA, Hsia B, Smith JP, Kaminski MV. Enteral nutrition: frequency of formula modification. JPEN 1981;5:40–45.

15. Larson DE, Fleming CR, Ott BJ, Schroeder KW. Percutaneous endoscopic gastrostomy. Mayo Clinic Proc 1983;58:103–107.

16. Ponsky JL, Gauderer MWL, Stellato IA. Percutaneous endoscopic gastrostomy. Review of 150 cases. Arch Surg 1983;118:913–914.

17. Page CP, Carlton PK, Andrassy RJ, Feldtman RW, Shield CF. Safe, cost-effective postoperative nutrition: defined formula diet via needle catheter jejunostomy. Am J Surg 1979;138:939–945.

18. Heitkemper MM, Martin DL, Hansen BC, Hanson R, Vanderberg V. Rate and volume of intermittent enteral feeding. JPEN 1981;5:125–129.

19. Rombeau JL, Jacobs DO. Nasoenteric tube feeding. In: Rombeau JL, Caldwell MD, eds. Clinical nutrition Vol. I: Enteral and tube feeding. Philadelphia: WB Saunders, 1984:261.

20. Woolfson AMJ, Ricketts CR, Hardy SM, Saour JN, Pollard BJ, Allison SP. Prolonged nasogastric tube feeding in the critically ill and surgical patient. Postgrad Med J 1976;52:678–681.

21. Cobb LM, Cartmill AM, Gilsdorf RB. Early postoperative nutritional support using the serosal tunnel jejunostomy. JPEN 1981;5:397–401.

22. Rombeau JL, Barot LR. Enteral nutrition therapy. Surg Clin North Am 1981;61:605–620.

23. Hayhust E, Wyman M. Morbidity associated with prolonged use of polyvinyl feeding tube. Am J Dis Child 1975;129:72–74.

24. Newmark SR, Simpson MS, Beskitt MP, Black J, Sublett D. Home tube feeding for long-term nutritional support. JPEN 1981;5:76–79.
25. Melnik G, Wright K. Pharmacologic aspects of enteral nutrition. In: Rombeau JL, Caldwell MD, eds. Clinical nutrition Vol. I: Enteral and tube feeding. Philadelphia: WB Saunders, 1984:513–541.
26. Torosian MH, Rombeau JL. Feeding by tube enterostomy. Surg Gynecol Obstet 1980;150:918–927.
27. Cataldi-Betcher EL, Seltzer MH, Slocum BA, Jones KW. Complications occurring during enteral nutritional support: a prospective study. JPEN 1983;7:546–552.
28. Lindor KD, Malagelada JR. Symposium on upper gastrointestinal motility disorders: gastric motility disorders: an overview. South Med J 1984;77:943–946.
29. Bernard M, Forlow L. Complications and their prevention. In: Rombeau JL, Caldwell MD, eds. Clinical nutrition Vol. I: Enteral and tube feeding. Philadelphia: WB Saunders, 1984:542–569.
30. Vanlandingham S, Simpson S, Daniel P, Newmark SR. Metabolic abnormalities in patients supported with enteral tube feeding. JPEN 1981;5:322–324.
31. Nelson JK, Palumbo PJ, O'Brien PC. Home enteral nutrition—observations of a newly established program. Nutr Clin Pract 1986;1:193–199.
32. Public and Private Insurance Coverage of Parenteral and Enteral Nutrition Services. A background paper on definitions and standards for specialized nutrition support services. American Society for Parenteral and Enteral Nutrition 1983.

PARENTERAL NUTRITION SUPPORT
OF ADULTS

General Description

Parenteral nutrition (PN) is a form of intravenous therapy that provides the opportunity to replenish or to maintain nutritional status.[1] Nutrients include amino acids (nitrogen), dextrose (carbohydrate), fat, electrolytes, minerals, vitamins, and trace elements that are in an appropriate volume of fluid. Central parenteral nutrition (CPN) is delivered through a large diameter vein, usually the subclavian or the superior vena cava. Peripheral parenteral nutrition (PPN) is delivered through a smaller vein, usually in the forearm.

Indications and Rationale

In general, the dictum "if the gut works, use it" should be heeded whenever possible. Parenteral nutrition should be utilized whenever nutritional support is needed and the enteral route is not available, is inadequate, or is contraindicated. It must be recognized that it is difficult to establish an absolute criteria for the utilization of PN in hospitalized patients. Variations in the nature and in the extent of individual nutritional problems demand the exercise of clinical judgment.

The American Society for Parenteral and Enteral Nutrition recently approved and published their "Guidelines for Use of Total Parenteral Nutrition in the Hospitalized Adult Patient".[2] The recommendations are summarized in Table 7–5.

Central parenteral nutrition (CPN) is indicated when the volume and the concentration of the solution precludes peripheral administration, when the anticipated duration of therapy is greater than 2 weeks, and when substantial depletion of body fat and protein has occurred. Because the central route often is utilized to provide complete patient nutrition, its usage commonly is referred to as "total parenteral nutrition" (TPN). Peripheral parenteral nutrition (PPN) is preferred when the solution concentration is less than 1,000 milliosmoles (mOsm) per liter and duration of therapy can be less than 2 weeks.

PN Component Products

Hospital pharmacies compound PN solutions just prior to their administration because of the relative chemical instability of the formulations. Component

TABLE 7–5 Guidelines for the Use of Parenteral Nutrition in the Hospitalized Adult Patient[2]*

I. Clinical settings where TPN should be a part of routine care.
  A. Patients with the inability to absorb nutrients via the gastrointestinal tract.
    1. Massive small bowel resection.
    2. Diseases of the small intestine.
    3. Radiation enteritis.
    4. Patients with severe diarrhea.
    5. Patients with intractable vomiting.
  B. Patients who are undergoing high-dose chemotherapy, radiation, and bone marrow transplantation.
  C. Patients with moderate to severe pancreatitis.
  D. Patients with severe malnutrition in the face of a nonfunctional gastrointestinal tract.
  E. Severely catabolic patients with or without malnutrition when the gastrointestinal tract is not usable within 5 to 7 days.
II. Clinical settings in which TPN usually would be helpful.
  A. Patients who have major surgery.
  B. Patients with moderate stress.
  C. Patients with enterocutaneous fistulae.
  D. Patients with inflammatory bowel disease.
  E. Patients with hyperemesis gravidarum.
  F. Moderately malnourished patients who require intensive medical or surgical intervention.
  G. Patients in whom adequate enteral nutrition cannot be established within a 7- to 10-day period of hospitalization.
  H. Patients with inflammatory adhesions with small bowel obstruction.
  I. Patients who receive intensive cancer chemotherapy.
III. Clinical settings in which TPN is of limited value.
  A. Minimal stress and trauma in the well-nourished patient when the gastrointestinal tract is usable within a 10-day period.
  B. Immediate postoperative or post-stress period.
  C. Proven or suspected untreatable disease state.
IV. Clinical settings in which TPN should not be used.
  A. Patients who have a functional and usable gastrointestinal tract that is capable of the absorption of adequate nutrients.
  B. When the sole dependence on TPN is anticipated to be less than 5 days.
  C. Patients who are in need of urgent operation should not have that operation delayed solely in favor of TPN.
  D. Whenever aggressive nutritional support is not desired by the patient or legal guardian and when such action is in accordance with hospital policy and existing law.
  E. Patients whose prognosis does not warrant aggressive nutritional support.
  F. When the risks of TPN are judged to exceed the potential benefits.

*With permission from the American Society for Parenteral and Enteral Nutrition.

products of PN formulation typically include water, amino acids, dextrose, electrolytes, vitamins, and trace elements. Fat emulsions are infused through another intravenous site, are infused concurrently with the parenteral nutrition solution by means of a "piggyback" administration system, or are added directly to the PN solution. Tables 7–6, 7–7, 7–8, and 7–9 display the content of standard PN formulas that are available for routine use in the Mayo Medical Center.

TABLE 7–6 Adult Parenteral Nutrition Formulary for the Mayo Medical Center

Standard Formulas	CPN-D*	PPN-A†
Dextrose	10%, 15%, 20% or 25%	5%
Amino Acids	4.25%	4.25%
Sodium	36.5 mEq/L	36.5 mEq/L
Potassium	30.0 mEq/L	30.0 mEq/L
Calcium	4.7 mEq/L	4.7 mEq/L
Magnesium	5.0 mEq/L	5.0 mEq/L
Chloride	35.0 mEq/L	35.0 mEq/L
Phosphorus	15.0 mmol/L	15.0 mmol/L
Acetate	70.5 mEq/L	70.5 mEq/L
Nitrogen	7.15 g/L	7.15 g/L

*Central parenteral nutrition with standard electrolytes
†Peripheral parenteral nutrition with standard electrolytes

TABLE 7–7 Standard Adult Multivitamin Injection

Vitamin	Amount per Dose per Day
A (retinol)	3300 IU
D (ergocalciferol)	200 IU
E (dl-alpha tocopheryl acetate)	10 IU
C (ascorbic acid)	100 mg
B_1 (thiamine)	3.0 mg
B_2 (riboflavin)	3.6 mg
B_6 (pyridoxine)	4.0 mg
B_{12} (cyanocobalamin)	5 μg
Folic Acid	400 μg
Niacinamide	40 mg
Dexpanthenol	15 mg
Biotin	60 μg

TABLE 7–8 Standard Adult Trace Element Injection

Trace Element	Amount per Dose per Day
Zinc	4 mg
Copper	1 mg
Manganese	500 μg
Chromium	10 μg

TABLE 7–9 Fat Emulsions

10% and 20% Fat Emulsion	500 ml

Amino Acids. In the United States, the source of nitrogen that is typically used in parenteral nutrition is a synthetic crystalline amino acid solution(s), which is available with or without added electrolytes and minerals. The products that are available for adults may be categorized by use; such as general use, renal disease, hepatic disease, and use in the traumatized patient. A comparison of amino acid products and their contents may be found in *Appendix 14.*

General amino acid preparations are analogous in quality to the amino acid profile of egg albumin. Although these products differ somewhat in composition, in general, they may be considered to be therapeutically equivalent.

The efficacy of essential amino acid products for use in renal failure patients and the utilization of solution(s) that contain increased concentrations of branched chain amino acids and decreased aromatic amino acids for hepatic encephalopathy and for stress or trauma are controversial.

Dextrose. Solutions of dextrose in concentrations of 10 percent through 70 percent are mixed with the appropriate amount of amino acids to obtain the desired solution. The dextrose that is utilized in formulating intravenous solutions is dextrose monohydrate. Therefore, 3.4 Kcal per gram of dextrose should be used in the calculation of caloric content.

Electrolytes. Electrolytes and minerals are either provided as part of the general amino acid product or they may be added separately as individual salts. *Appendix 14* lists the electrolyte products that are used typically in the compounding of parenteral nutrition solutions.

The requirements for electrolytes vary according to the individual patient needs. For most patients, the electrolytes that are provided with the amino acid products are adequate in maintenance amounts. (Note that calcium is not provided as part of an amino acid product.) In order to minimize the possibility of calcium phosphate precipitation, calcium, as calcium gluconate, is added after the amino acids and the dextrose are mixed. To correct derangements of plasma electrolyte concentrations and to compensate for losses, changes can be made in the amounts of several electrolytes that are provided in the parenteral solution. If deficits are extensive, corrections may be more effectively made by using separate replacement solutions.

Vitamins. The composition of multivitamin products for intravenous use has been formulated according to the recommendations of the American Medical Association, Nutrition Advisory Group (AMA-NAG).[3] One adult and one pediatric multivitamin formulation are available commercially from several manufacturers (See *Appendix 14*). These formulations are used as a daily maintenance dosage for patients who receive PN, and the formulations are also useful in other situations where administration by the intravenous route is required. Patients with multiple vitamin deficiencies or with markedly increased requirements may be given multiples of the daily dosage as indicated by the clinical status. Supplementation of the daily multivitamin dosage with a single vitamin may be necessary for a specific vitamin deficiency.

Trace Elements. Trace elements are those nutrients that make up less than 4.0 g (or 0.01 percent) of the total body content. Trace elements are available commercially as combination products or as single entity injections. The multiple trace element injection that is used currently in the Mayo Medical Center is listed in Table 7–8. Single entity (trace element) products are also available. One ml of the multiple trace element injection contains zinc, copper, manganese, and chromium in amounts that are suggested for the daily administration by the American Medical Association's Nutrition Advisory Group for stable, adult patients.[4] Other trace elements may be supplemented in appropriate daily doses, as the specific patient deficiencies dictate.

Fat Emulsions. Intravenous fat emulsions are isotonic preparations of either 10 percent or 20 percent fat, as soybean oil or a blend of safflower oil and soybean oil. A comparison of fat emulsion products and their contents is found in *Appendix 14*. Although the products differ somewhat in composition, they may be considered therapeutically equivalent. *Appendix 14* provides a more detailed listing of the composition of Intralipid (Kabi Vitrum).

Fat emulsions may be administered by direct addition to the PN solution, by piggyback infusion into the PN solution, or by infusion through a separate vein. Currently available are 3-in-1 systems that provide fat, dextrose, and protein in one intravenous container for PN. In the past, intravenous fat has been used only in the quantities needed to prevent essential fatty acid deficiency. However, recent studies have provided strong evidence that a combination of dextrose and fat is optimal for most patients.[5] The use of fat emulsions is relatively contraindicated in patients with familial hyperlipidemia and with pathologic hyperlipidemia that is associated with nephrotic syndrome or with pancreatitis. Also, caution should be exercised in the administration of fats to patients with an impaired ability to clear fat emulsion. This may include advanced hepatic disease, end-stage renal disease, and severe sepsis. Patients with an egg allergy should be carefully evaluated before being given fat emulsion, since phospholipid from egg yolk is used as an emulsifying agent.[6]

"Missing Nutrients". Although total parenteral nutrition (TPN) is the provision of nutrients totally by the intravenous route, not all nutrients may be or can be provided. In the Mayo Medical Center, iron, iodine, vitamin K, and selenium are not routinely included in standard PN formulas. Patients who receive PN formulas should be monitored for the need of these nutrients.

Patient Monitoring

All patients who receive parenteral nutrition are monitored by the Nutrition Support Team. The assessed nutrient needs are compared with the PN solution that is provided and adjustments are made as needed. Initial height and weight, daily weight, daily intake and output, twice daily temperature, daily urine glucose, and the quantity of food intake during the transition from PN to enteral diet are the criteria that are monitored. These criteria should be documented in the medical record. Table 7–10 summarizes Nutrition Support Team members' roles in monitoring patients receiving central parenteral nutrition.

Serum laboratory tests also are monitored on a routine basis. Form 1 and Table 7–11 lists the tests and the frequencies that are suggested for baseline and routine monitoring. Additional tests at more frequent intervals may be necessary during periods of patient stress or metabolic instability.

Complications

The complications of CPN therapy may be divided into three categories, which are technical, septic, and metabolic. With proper patient monitoring and with scrupulous techniques, most of these complications can be prevented. Table

TABLE 7–10 Nutrition Support Team

The Nutrition Support Team automatically monitors patients on Central Parenteral Nutrition to assure that the documentation is complete, as well as to assess the CPN regimen. The team also serves as a resource to educate medical, nursing, pharmacy, and dietetic staff regarding current parenteral nutrition standards and hospital policies and procedures.

The Nutrition Support Team meets with the Nutrition Consulting Service Consultant to review patients on CPN as well as to participate in care of patients who are referred to the Nutrition Consulting Service.

Each team member recommends consultation with the Nutrition Consulting Service when appropriate.

Nurse Coordinator

1. Coordinates the monitoring of patients on CPN according to stated responsibilities and discusses discrepancies with the appropriate people involved.
2. Collects data that are relevant to CPN therapy.

Dietitian

1. Monitors the nutrition assessment including the estimate of nutrient requirements.
2. Assures the consistency and the application of nutritional support (see also *Appendix 14*).
3. Coordinates nutrition consultations.

Pharmacist

1. Identifies CPN patients for team monitoring.
2. Monitors patient's drug therapy for chemical and for therapeutic drug nutrient interactions and compatibilities.

Physician

1. Meets with the Nutrition Support Team to review the status of patients who are started on CPN and to review problems that have been identified by the Nutrition Support Team's monitoring.
2. Provides formal nutrition consultation as requested by the primary physician.
3. Discusses with the primary physician any issues that are not resolved by the Nutrition Support Team.

7–12 describes the most common complications in each category with the possible etiology, signs and symptoms, recommended treatment, and guidelines for their prevention.[7]

Physicians: How to Order Parenteral Nutrition

Before parenteral nutrition is initiated, several questions should be considered. What are the indications for parenteral nutrition? Can enteral feedings be used? What is the anticipated duration of therapy? Should central or peripheral administration be employed? Has the position of the central catheter been verified by roentgenogram? Baseline laboratory measurements should also be requested and the nutritional needs of the patient estimated.

TABLE 7–11 Adult Parenteral Nutrition Laboratory Monitoring Guidelines*

Test	Base Line[†]	Day 2	3	4	7	14	21	28	35	42
Chemistry Group										
Albumin	X				X	X	X	X	X	X
Alk. Phos.	X				X	X	X	X	X	X
AST	X				X	X	X	X	X	X
Bilirubin	X				X	X	X	X	X	X
Calcium	X				X	X	X	X	X	X
Creatinine	X				X	X	X	X	X	X
Glucose	X	X	X	X	X	X	X	X	X	X
Potassium	X				X	X	X	X	X	X
Sodium	X				X	X	X	X	X	X
Phosphorus	X				X	X	X	X	X	X
Total Protein	X				X	X	X	X	X	X
Uric Acid	X				X	X	X	X	X	X
Electrolyte Panel										
Creatinine	X				X	X	X	X	X	X
Chloride	X				X	X	X	X	X	X
HCO3	X				X	X	X	X	X	X
Potassium	X	X	X	X	X	X	X	X	X	X
Sodium	X	X	X	X	X	X	X	X	X	X
Urea	X				X	X	X	X	X	X
Essential Element Screen										
Copper	X				X	X		X		X
Iron	X				X	X		X		X
Magnesium	X				X	X		X		X
Zinc	X				X	X		X		X
Individual										
ProTime	X				X	X		X		X
Heme Group[‡]	X									
Triglycerides[‡,§]	X									
Selenium								X		

*The laboratory tests and frequencies listed are suggested for the routine monitoring of adult patients who receive parenteral nutrition. Additional laboratory monitoring tests at more frequent intervals may be necessary during periods of patient stress or metabolic instability.

[†]Baseline tests preceding initiation of parenteral nutrition.

[‡]Baseline. Additional test frequency determined by primary service.

[§]Repeat level prior to the start of the second bottle of fat emulsion.

The Physician's Adult Parenteral Nutrition Order Sheet, in use at the Mayo Medical Center, contains the contents and the descriptive information of standard parenteral nutrition formulas that are available for patients with normal metabolic needs (Forms 1 and 2). A central parenteral nutrition formula is intended for administration through a central vein (e.g., subclavian). A peripheral parenteral nutrition formula may be administered through a peripheral (e.g., forearm) vein. In general, the use of peripheral parenteral nutrition should be limited to therapy less than 2 weeks in duration and less than 1,000 mOsm per liter of formula. Patient tolerance of PPN decreases markedly as the duration of the therapy or the concentration of the solution increases.

On initiating parenteral nutrition, the indications for parenteral nutrition should be identified and routine laboratory monitoring initiated (bottom of Form 1). The Order Sheet (Form 1) lists various options for the final dextrose concentration. Most patients can be adequately nourished with dextrose concentrations of 15 or 20 percent in a standard electrolyte formula. Fat should be provided on a daily basis and should contribute between 25 and 50 percent of the

TABLE 7–12 Complications of Parenteral Therapy[7]*

MAJOR TECHNICAL COMPLICATIONS

Complication	Etiology	Signs and Symptoms	Treatment	Prevention
Catheter insertion				
1. Pneumothorax	Subclavian venipuncture Unusual anatomy	Dyspnea Chest pain Cyanosis	Observation if small	Use internal jugular for high risk patients
	Improper training		Chest tube if large or progressive	Trained and approved doctor
	Multiple punctures			Stop after three to four attempts and get help
	Failure to remove respirator			Ambu during procedure except during thrust of needle
	Slow leak			Repeat chest film
2. Malposition	Anatomical	Pain or tingling in the ear or the neck area on the side of insertion or NONE	Reposition with guidewire or fluoroscopy or new puncture	Proper position if possible
	Needle passed through vein	No free reflux of blood	Catheter removal	
3. Subclavian artery puncture	Incorrect insertion	Return of bright red blood under high pressure Hematoma	Remove needle Elevate head of bed Pressure to puncture site Close patient observation	Strict adherence to technique
4. Carotid artery puncture	Internal jugular catheterization	Hematoma untreated may lead to tracheal obstruction	Local application of direct pressure	
5. Catheter embolism	Shearing off section of catheter	Cardiac irritability	Radiologic or surgical removal	Never pull back catheter through needle
6. Air embolism	During catheter threading	Dyspnea Chest pain Tachycardia Tachypnea Cyanosis Paresis Cardiac arrest	Needle aspiration of heart Left side down in steep Trendelenberg position	Trendelenberg position during insertion Keep hub covered at all times Valsalva Maneuver each time catheter open to air

Complication	Cause	Clinical signs	Treatment	Prevention
Catheter maintenance				
1. Air embolism	Tubing disconnection	Dyspnea Chest pain Tachycardia Tachypnea Cyanosis Disorientation Paresis Cardiac arrest	As above Reconnect tubing Contact MD	Tape tubing connections Luer-loks
	Patent tract after removal of catheter			Ointment and/or occlusive dressing for 12–24 hr
2. Catheter obstruction	Mechanical (pump) failure Kink in catheter	Solutions stop running Occlusion alarm	Adjust pump Reset alarm Aspiration of catheter	Hourly monitoring of solution Close observation during dressing change
3. Thrombosis	Mechanical irritation Patient's hypercoagulable state	Distended collateral veins and chest wall Acute unilateral edema of arm, neck, and face Pleuritic chest pain Inability to thread catheter	Catheter removal Intravenous heparin Venogram	Not always possible Heparin in TPN solution Do not cycle TPN if low AT-III

MAJOR SEPTIC COMPLICATIONS

Complication	Cause	Clinical signs	Treatment	Prevention
Catheter-related sepsis	Inadequate asepsis during catheter insertion, inadequate dressing care and solution maintenance or solution preparation Immunosuppression	Glucose intolerance Spiking temperature Elevated white count Hypotension Disorientation Inflammation or drainage from catheter exit site	Removal of catheter Culture of solution Chest film Cultures of urine, sputum, draining wounds Blood culture (central and peripheral) Catheter removal with tip culture (new puncture or guidewire) Antimicrobial therapy when indicated	Rigid adherence to specific policies and procedures Inspection of catheter site for each dressing change procedure
Septic thrombosis	Untreated catheter sepsis Bacteremic seeding from unknown or other source	Same as catheter-related plus unilateral pain and swelling in arm, shoulder, and neck area	Venogram Remove catheter and culture tip Intravenous heparin Antimicrobial therapy	Immediate response to suspected sepsis Periodic changes of catheter (i.e., new puncture or over a guidewire) when other septic source known

TABLE 7–12 Complications of Parenteral Therapy[7]* *(continued)*

MAJOR METABOLIC COMPLICATIONS

Complication	Etiology	Signs and Symptoms	Treatment	Prevention
Hyperglycemia	Diabetes mellitus Too rapid initiation	Elevated blood glucose Glycosuria	Regular insulin subcutaneously or intravenously Slow rate	Coordinate initiation and insulin requirement Start slow with step increments (i.e., day 1—1 liter, day 2—2 liters, day 3—2 or 3 liters)
	Infection or sepsis		Addition of regular insulin Slow rate until blood glucose stable	
	Drug related (i.e., steroids)		(May increase fat source for calories)	Advance more slowly
	Stress from major surgery		Slow rate or stop infusion	Halve infusion rate during surgery Stop hypertonic solution and infuse dextrose solution or Lactated Ringers solution several hours to 24 hr pre- and postoperatively
Hyperglycemic hyperosmolar nonketotic dehydration	Uncontrolled hyperglycemia	Elevated blood glucose level (500–1,000 mg/100 ml or higher) Glycosuria Osmotic diuresis Metabolic imbalances Lethargy Coma Death	Stop hypertonic solution Hydration with free water Judicious doses of IV insulin and potassium Close laboratory and patient monitoring	Immediate and proper control of blood glucose level to <200
Hypoglycemia	Sudden decrease or stop of infusion due to mechanical problem	Blood glucose in range of 40 mg/100 ml Lethargy	Bolus dextrose infusion Monitor serum glucose	Accurate administration with hourly patient monitoring
Hyperkalemia	Inability to utilize administered potassium Decrease in renal function Low cardiac output Systemic sepsis	Cardiac arrhythmias Bounding or diminished pulses	Stop infusion Change to low potassium solution	Close metabolic monitoring

	Causes	Signs/Symptoms	Treatment	Monitoring
Hypokalemia	Increased requirement with anabolism; Excessive GI losses	Cardiac arrhythmias; Muscle weakness; Impaired respiratory function	Increase potassium in solution; Measure and replace losses	Close metabolic monitoring
Hypophosphatemia	Lack of phosphate supplementation; Excessive use of phosphate binders (i.e., antacids); Increased demand during anabolism	Lethargy; Altered speech; Peripheral paresthesias; Increased respirations; Coma	Add phosphate to solution; May require peripheral repletion; Adjust amount per patient	Close metabolic monitoring; Standard solutions
Hypocalcemia	Lack of or insufficient supplementation	Paresthesia twitching positive Chvostek's sign	Add or adjust calcium in solution	Close metabolic monitoring
Hypomagnesemia	Lack of or insufficient amounts of magnesium in solution	Tingling sensation around mouth; Paresthesia; Dizziness; Disorientation	Add or adjust magnesium in solution	Standardized solutions; Close metabolic monitoring
Essential fatty acid deficiency	Lack of fat supplement	Dry, scaly skin; Hair loss	IV administration of 10% or 20% fat emulsion	Routinely include fat emulsion infusion each week (i.e., twice a week)
Vitamin K deficiency	Deficient oral intake, severe diarrhea, obstructive jaundice, prolonged antibiotic therapy	Hematuria, ecchymoses, bleeding, purpura, increased prothrombin time	Weekly administration PO or IM of Vitamin K	Monitoring prothrombin level
Iron deficiency	Excessive blood loss	Pallor, fatigue, listlessness, exertional dyspnea, headache, paresthesia	IM Iron Dextran, or whole blood	Serial determination of hemoglobin and mean cell volume, serum iron
Zinc deficiency	Chronic illness; Diseases that predispose to excessive gastrointestinal loss	Diarrhea, CNS disturbances, skin lesions, poor wound healing, alopecia, anorexia, growth retardation	Refeed and treat illness; Addition of zinc to solution	Serial determination of serum zinc

* Reprinted with permission from the American Society for Parenteral and Enteral Nutrition.

FORM 1 PHYSICIAN'S ADULT PARENTERAL NUTRITION ORDER SHEET
(Use a new sheet for each daily order)

PLEASE WRITE SPECIFIC ORDERS. Unless otherwise specified, these orders
will begin upon completion of any currently existing parenteral nutrition orders.

CLINIC NO.

NAME

ROOM NO.

STANDARD FORMULAS — ORDER ALL VITAMINS AND TRACE ELEMENTS BELOW

☐ **CENTRAL** PARENTERAL NUTRITION (CPN-D)
with Standard Electrolytes

	FINAL CONC.
Dextrose	☐ 10% ☐ 15% ☐ 20% ☐ 25%
Amino Acids	4.25 %
Sodium	36.5 mEq/L
Potassium	30.0 mEq/L
Calcium	4.7 mEq/L
Magnesium	5.0 mEq/L
Chloride	35.0 mEq/L
Phosphorus	15.0 mmol/L
Acetate	70.5 mEq/L

Grams Nitrogen		7.15	g/L	
Total kilocalories	510	680	850	1020 kcal/L
Approx. Osmolarity	1090	1340	1595	1845 mOsm/L
Approx. Volume		1000	mL	

☐ **PERIPHERAL** PARENTERAL NUTRITION (PPN-A)
with Standard Electrolytes

	FINAL CONC.
Dextrose	5%
Amino Acids	4.25%
Sodium	36.5 mEq/L
Potassium	30.0 mEq/L
Calcium	4.7 mEq/L
Magnesium	5.0 mEq/L
Chloride	35.0 mEq/L
Phosphorus	15.0 mmol/L
Acetate	70.5 mEq/L

Grams Nitrogen	7.15 g/L
Total kilocalories	340 kcal/L
Approx. Osmolarity	835 mOsm/L
Approx. Volume	1000 mL

OPTIONAL ADDITIVES TO STANDARD ELECTROLYTES
☐ INCREASE Total Sodium to _____ mEq/liter
  as: (check one) ☐ Chloride ☐ Acetate ☐ Phosphate
☐ INCREASE Total Potassium to _____ mEq/liter
  as: (check one) ☐ Chloride ☐ Acetate ☐ Phosphate
☐ Regular Insulin _____ units/liter
☐ Other _____

Formulas for less than standard electrolyte concentrations must be ordered in Non-Standard Formula section.

FLOW RATE (Specify one)

_____ mL/hour

_____ liters/day

To be completed by Nurse
Time Needed _____

NON-STANDARD FORMULA ☐ **CENTRAL** ☐ **PERIPHERAL**

Dextrose	_____ % (Final Conc.)
Amino Acids	_____ % (Final Conc.)
Other _____	_____ % (Final Conc.)
Sodium	_____ mEq/L
Potassium	_____ mEq/L
Calcium	_____ mEq/L
Magnesium	_____ mEq/L
Chloride	_____ mEq/L
Phosphorus	_____ mmol/L

_____   _____
_____   _____

Unless specified otherwise, Pharmacy will compound such that the Na: Cl ratio
is approximately 1:1; the balance of anions to be provided primarily as acetate.

DAILY VITAMIN AND TRACE ELEMENTS
☐ **Standard Adult Multivitamin**
  Injection to one bottle daily
  (see Hospital Formulary for contents.)
☐ **Standard Adult Trace Element**
  Injection to one bottle daily
  (see Hospital Formulary for contents.)
☐ Other _____

INTRAVENOUS FAT EMULSION
☐ 10% Fat Emulsion (1.1 kcal/mL)
☐ 20% Fat Emulsion (2.0 kcal/mL)
Volume _____ ☐ Central
Flow Rate _____ ☐ Peripheral

COMPLETE THIS SECTION WHEN <u>INITIATING</u> PARENTERAL NUTRITION AND CHECK EACH APPLICABLE BOX BELOW

Indication for Parenteral Nutrition

	NO	YES

☐ Bowel obstruction due to: _____
☐ Ileus
☐ Malabsorption/Maldigestion due to: _____
☐ Fistula/Abscess
☐ Pancreatitis
☐ Inflammatory Bowel Disease
☐ Short Bowel
☐ Bone Marrow Transplant
☐ Other: _____

NO ☐   YES ☐ Initiate Laboratory Monitoring-see back of form
      ☐ Enteral feeding was considered before
         parenteral nutrition initiated.
      ☐ Anticipated duration of therapy greater
         than 7 days
      ☐ X-ray verification of central catheter
         position completed.
      ☐ Order Nutrition Consult

SPECIAL INSTRUCTIONS _____

Date _____ Time _____ Dr. _____

See reverse for Guidelines for Ordering Adult Parenteral Nutrition Solutions and Laboratory Monitoring Guidelines

Form 2. Guidelines for Ordering Adult Parenteral Nutrition Solutions
(These guidelines may not be applicable to some patients)

Kilocalories

Several methods exist for estimating energy requirements. The most widely used formulas are those of Harris and Benedict:

$$\text{For Males,} \quad BEE = 66.4 + 13.7(W) + 5(H) - 6.8(A);$$

$$\text{For Females,} \quad BEE = 655 + 9.6(W) + 1.8(H) - 4.7(A);$$

where BEE is basal energy expenditure, A is age in years, W is weight in kilograms, and H is height in centimeters. Adjustments to the calculated BEE for various forms of stress, fever, surgery, sepsis, or burns often overestimate the actual BEE when measured by indirect calorimetry. Therefore, for patients suspected of having greatly increased energy requirements, measurement of oxygen consumption is recommended.

For unstressed patients, measured energy expenditures range between 20 and 25 kilocalories per kilogram. Thus, caloric intakes between 25 and 35 kilocalories per kilogram of actual body weight should be adequate for nearly all hospitalized patients. At the other extreme, there appears to be no advantage to regimens providing less than 20 kilocalories per kilogram even in obese patients. Weight reduction is a long-term process. Patients sick enough to require central parenteral nutrition for less than 20 kilocalories per kilogram or greater than 35 kilocalories per kilogram are discussed with the primary service, to determine whether or not such levels of caloric intake are actually indicated.

Amino acids provide 4 kcal per gram and dextrose monohydrate 3.4 kcal per gram. Fat emulsions provide 1.1 kcal per milliliter (10%) or 2.0 kcal per milliliter (20%).

Protein

The recommended dietary allowance (RDA) for protein for normal healthy adults is 0.8 g per kilogram. The minimum requirement for the maintenance of nitrogen balance in otherwise healthy adults is between 0.4 and 0.5 g per kilogram. Fever, sepsis, surgery, trauma, and burns increase the protein catabolism and, therefore, the amount of amino acids and/or of protein that must be supplied in order to achieve nitrogen balance. The most direct way for assessing nitrogen requirements in acutely ill patients is to measure 24-hour urinary nitrogen. If one multiplies urinary nitrogen (plus an allowance of 1 to 2 g for fecal and other losses) times 6.25, an estimate of the grams of protein catabolized can be obtained.

Most hospitalized patients can be adequately maintained on protein intakes between 1.0 and 1.5 g per kilogram of actual body weight. Intakes greater than 2 g per kilogram should not be ordered in the absence of documentation of the rate of protein catabolism by 24-hour urinary nitrogen. When such orders are received, they are discussed with the primary service. In some rare instances (e.g., graft-versus-host reactions), it may be necessary to give as much as 3 to 4 g of amino acids per kilogram in order to meet nitrogen requirements. However, such patients require close monitoring to assure that they do not receive excess nitrogen loads.

Vitamins

A standard adult multiple vitamin supplement can be ordered from the existing Physician's Adult Parenteral Nutrition Order Sheet. In nearly all circumstances, this supplementation is adequate to prevent the development of vitamin deficiency. If, however, vitamin deficiency has already occurred, it may be necessary to supplement individual vitamins as indicated.

Trace Elements

The standard adult trace element package is described in the Parenteral Nutrition Order Sheet. Patients who are severely malnourished may need additional zinc supplementation. The decision regarding trace element supplementation should be made after the initial measurement of zinc, as indicated in the Laboratory Monitoring Guidelines.

Concentration of Solutions

The Physician's Adult Parenteral Nutrition Order Sheet contains various options for dextrose concentrations. Most patients can be adequately nourished with dextrose concentrations of 15 or 20 percent. In many circumstances, dextrose concentrations of 25 percent provide an excess of kilocalories as glucose. The complications of caloric excess are beginning to be recognized and include hyperglycemia, excessive fluid retention, electrolyte disturbances (especially hypokalemia and hypophosphatemia), and perhaps an increased susceptibility to fatty liver. In addition, provision of glucose in excessive amounts increases the production of carbon dioxide and, therefore, may be contraindicated in patients with pulmonary insufficiency.

Uses of Intravenous Fat

In the past, intravenous fat has been used to prevent essential fatty acid deficiency. However, recent studies have provided strong evidence that a combination of glucose and fat is optimal in most patients. Current recommendations are that fat be provided on a daily basis to provide between 25 and 50 percent of the total kilocalories. CPN orders that provide no fat on a daily basis or that provide fat at a concentration of greater than 60 percent of the total calories are discussed with the primary service. As noted in the Laboratory Monitoring Guidelines, serum triglycerides should be checked prior to initiating fat infusion and, again, immediately prior to the second day's infusion of intravenous fat. Infusion rates should be no faster than 500 ml of 10 percent fat per 4 hours or 500 ml of 20 percent fat per 8 hours, but can be given on a continuous 24-hour infusion if so desired.

Special Formulations

The Physician's Adult Parenteral Nutrition Order Sheet lists standard solutions that are available through the pharmacy. Special solutions can be mixed when indicated, e.g., in patients who require fluid restriction and in patients who require alterations in amino acid mixtures (e.g., patients in hepatic and/or renal failure). Questions regarding special preparations should be referred to the pharmacy or Nutrition Consulting Service.

total kilocalories. The standard multivitamin and trace element injections should be provided on a daily basis.

Additional electrolytes may be added to the standard formulas in the space provided. Formulas with less than standard electrolyte concentrations or alterations in dextrose or in amino acids must be ordered in the non-standard formula section. Medications may be added to PN formulas only when chemically stable and when their continuous intravenous dosing is appropriate and consistent with the continuous infusion of PN. Nutrient requirement guidelines for adult patients with normal metabolic needs are indicated on the Order Sheet (Form 2). PN should be ordered daily. Questions on the ordering of PN should be referred to the hospital pharmacies.

REFERENCES

1. Fleming CR, McGill DB, Hoffman HN, Nelson RA. Total parenteral nutrition. Mayo Clin Proc 1976;51:187–199.
2. A.S.P.E.N. Board of Directors. Guidelines for use of total parenteral nutrition in the hospitalized adult patient. JPEN 1986;10:441–445.
3. AMA Department of Foods and Nutrition. Multivitamin preparations for parenteral use. A statement by the nutrition advisory group. JPEN 1979;3:258–262.
4. AMA Department of Foods and Nutrition. Guidelines for essential trace element preparations for parenteral use. A statement by an expert panel. JAMA 1979;241:2051–2054.
5. Jeejeebhoy KN. Carbohydrate-lipid utilization: mixed fuel delivery for total parenteral nutrition. In: Deitel M, ed. Nutrition in clinical surgery. Baltimore: Williams & Wilkins, 1985:121.
6. Dickerson RN. Clinical utility of intravenous lipid emulsion. Hosp Pharm 1986;21:564–569.
7. Griggs BA, Ingalls M, Ayers N, Champagne C. A basic nursing guide to providing TPN for the adult patient. Washington, DC: American Society for Parenteral and Enteral Nutrition, 1984.

CHAPTER 8

NORMAL NUTRITION AND THERAPEUTIC DIETS IN INFANTS, CHILDREN, AND ADOLESCENTS

PEDIATRIC NUTRITIONAL ASSESSMENT

A nutritional assessment program can increase the quality of care given to pediatric patients by identifying patients at risk for development of nutritional deficiencies and by promoting earlier nutritional intervention. Nutritional assessment provides an objective basis for dietary recommendations and for evaluation of nutritional support. This information provides data to evaluate the nutrition of the individual at a given moment in time. Serial assessments are essential for facilitating optimal intervention and for monitoring growth and nutritional status over longer periods of time.

Nutritional assessment includes clinical assessment, anthropometrics, dietary evaluation, and biochemical data. Selection of parameters, techniques, and standards relevant to a specific population is important to maximize cost and to benefit effectiveness. Table 8–1 presents guidelines for three levels of nutritional assessment.

Clinical Assessment

In general, clinical assessment of nutritional status in children is similar to that for adults (see *Nutritional Assessment* page 3). Clinical signs of nutritional deficiencies are usually the last to appear, are nonspecific, and should lead to further laboratory assessment.

Anthropometric Evaluation

Accurately determined anthropometric measurements are one of the best indicators of nutritional status in children. These measurements include height, weight, skinfolds, mid-arm circumference, and head circumference. Height (or length if the child is less than 2 years old) and weight are generally considered to be the most important measures of normal growth and nutritional status in

TABLE 8–1 Guidelines for Selection of Nutritional Assessment Techniques

	Indications	Anthropometrics	Clinical	Laboratory Data	Dietary
Screening	All children	Height Weight Weight for height Head circumference in children less than 2 yr	Health history and general physical appearance	Hemoglobin Hematocrit (at least once in first 15 months)	Dietary history of usual intake, feeding skills, and behaviors Use of supplements
Intermediate (add)*	Child at risk identified from screening or with disease known to affect nutritional status	Body composition including triceps skinfold (TSF) and arm muscle circumference measurements, if indicated	Physical exam for evidence of nutritional deficiency or excess	Serum albumin Mean corpuscular volume (MCV)	3–7 day food record
In-depth (add)*	Identification of specific nutrient deficiency or excess Child with severe nutritional deficiencies Evaluation of response to nutritional therapy	Growth velocity, if indicated (see section on "Failure to Thrive")		Specific vitamin and mineral levels; prealbumin	

*Add indicates that the techniques recommended at a given level should be in addition to those recommended at the previous level.

children because the standards available are based on large groups of healthy growing children and have been used successfully for a number of years. Skinfold and mid-arm circumference measurements require reliable equipment, considerable skill, and practice for accuracy. In addition, interpretation of the results can be complex, and the norms currently available are not universally accepted.[1-3]

Measurements of Height and Length. Growth graphs from the National Center for Health Statistics (NCHS) (see *Pediatric Appendix 5*, page 494) are used to assess a child's growth progress over time. The graphs are based on a cross-sectional sample of healthy children from the United States from 1963 to 1975.[4] Proper technique in obtaining the measurements and exact age are essential for valid use of the graphs.

Measurement Technique; Birth to 36 Months. Record the weight of the nude child. Recumbent length, without shoes, should be measured using a length board with a fixed headboard and a movable right angle footboard. This requires two people—one to position the child and the other to obtain the measurement. Values on the birth- to 36-month graph are based on recumbent length. Therefore, standing height should not be recorded on this graph.

Measurement Technique; 2 to 18 years. Weight should be taken in light clothing without shoes. Height should be measured without shoes with the child standing against a fixed scale on a rigid surface wide enough to provide back and heel support. A right angle moveable headboard should be lowered until it touches the head. Values on the 2- to 18-year graph are based on standing height. Therefore, recumbent length should not be recorded on this graph.

Interpretation. Measurements that consistently fall on a percentile between the 5th and 95th percentiles generally indicate normal growth. Crossing percentiles within the 25th and 75th percentiles is not unusual and likely represents normal growth. However, crossing percentiles in a progressively upward or downward direction, or measurements near the upper or lower end of the normal percentiles, may indicate nutritional or health problems.

Measurements below the 5th and above the 95th percentiles may indicate a need for further evaluation and follow-up. Weight for length or height greater than the 95th percentile is suggestive of obesity.[5] Follow-up measurements should be done every 1 to 3 months for infants and young children and every 3 to 6 months for older children.

Decreased weight-for-height may suggest a state of acute malnutrition, whereas decreased height-for-age may suggest chronic undernutrition. Weight-for-height has replaced weight-for-age as the criterion by which acute protein-calorie malnutrition (PCM) is determined because the latter failed to account for the effect of height differences. Weight-for-height or length is independent of age and is useful mainly before the onset of puberty. Standard growth charts after the age of 10 years in girls and 11.5 years in boys should be used cautiously since the pubescent growth spurt occurs at different ages and may result in deviations from the norm in heights and weights.

Measurements of Head Circumference. Head circumference is closely related to growth in body length up to 2 years of age. After this age, slower head circumference growth makes it an ineffective measurement of nutritional status. It is primarily a screening measurement for micro- and macrocephaly owing to non-nutritional abnormalities. However, a small head circumference in infants or in older children with failure-to-grow may indicate severe and long-term caloric deficit during the first 2 years of life.[6]

Growth Graphs and Evaluation for Special Groups; Developmental Disabilities. For children with genetic abnormalities that result in growth retardation and developmental delay, weight-for-height or length may be more useful in assessing growth adequacy and nutritional needs than height- or weight-for-age. The Baldwin-Wood Tables (see *Pediatric Appendix 6*, page 500) can be used to assess weight-for-height among these children.[7]

"Height-age" can be useful in estimating advisable weight. Height-age is the age at which the child's height would be at the 50th percentile. Advisable weight would be the 50th percentile weight for that age with a range of 25 to 75th percentile.

Cronk has developed growth graphs of the first 6 years of life for children with Down's syndrome. These graphs correct for the slower growth rate of children with Down's syndrome (see *Pediatric Appendix 7*, page 502, and *Developmental Disability*, page 318, for further discussion).[8,9]

Growth Graphs and Evaluation for Special Groups; Premature Infant. Growth progress of the premature infant (less than 38 weeks of gestation) can be followed either by the child's "adjusted age" or on a growth graph for premature infants developed by Babson.[10] Adjusted age is the infant's birth age minus the number of weeks of prematurity. This age should be used for approximately the first 18 months of life or until catch-up growth is completed. The use of Babson's growth chart allows growth progress to be monitored prior to 40 weeks from conception and can be used for 12 months post-term (see *Pediatric Appendix 8*, page 510, and section on *Low Birth Weight Infant*, page 327, for further discussion).

Growth Graphs and Evaluation for Special Groups; Southeastern Asian Children. Growth graphs based on Thai children can be useful in monitoring growth in children with Southeastern Asian ancestry.[13,14]

Estimation of Body Fat and Protein Status. Children with decreased weight-for-height (less than 5th percentile) have increased morbidity and longer hospitalizations.[11] Further nutritional assessment may be beneficial in identifying how decreased body weight has altered total body composition and how body composition is changed by nutritional therapy. Measurements of total body fat and body protein may indicate the area(s) and the severity of compromise.

Body Fat. Since approximately 50 percent of body fat is subcutaneous fat, a simple and fairly reliable measurement of body fat, and thus of caloric reserves, is triceps skinfold. Measurement techniques, which have been published by Frisancho, should be followed.[12] The average of three triceps skinfold measurements should be compared to the triceps skinfold percentile tables published by Frisancho (see *Pediatric Appendix 9*, page 511).

Edema may falsely increase the skinfold measurement. Measurements of infants can be quite difficult and require frequent practice and much patience.

Values below the 5th percentile are considered abnormally low, and nutritional intervention should be considered. Measurements greater than the 90th percentile for age indicate a need for close medical supervision and for dietary counseling. Those greater than the 95th percentile may need to be treated.[12]

Body Protein. Upper arm circumference and triceps skinfold are necessary for estimating arm muscle circumference and arm muscle area.[12] The nomogram (see *Pediatric Appendix 10*, page 512) can be used for making these calculations.[15] These values can then be compared with arm muscle circumference and arm muscle area percentile tables (see *Pediatric Appendix 9*, page 511) to estimate body muscle mass relative to other children of the same age and sex.[12]

Height-age standards, instead of those for chronological age, should be used for children with decreased height-for-age, since these measurements are, to a certain extent, height-dependent.

Values below the 5th percentile are considered abnormal. Further evaluation or intervention is recommended.[11]

Dietary Assessment

Dietary assessment may include a retrospective or prospective estimate of the child's intake. Information regarding the child's development, socioeconomic status, eating attitudes and behavior, and those of his family is useful. Assessment of parent-child interaction and the psychosocial environment of the family are also valuable components in the overall evaluation.

Qualitative information of dietary intake from food frequency and usual meal and snack patterns is generally adequate for screening purposes. The diet should be evaluated for adequacy of food sources of key nutrients.

For infants on formula and solids, an accurate estimate of retrospective dietary intake is usually obtainable from the parents. Kilocalories, protein, and other key nutrients can be calculated. The diet history should include formulas and/or breast milk used, age at introduction of solids, the variety of solids used, vitamin and mineral supplements given, and problems such as vomiting, diarrhea, constipation, and colic.

Retrospective quantitative information about the older child's past intake is extremely difficult to get from the child or from his parents. Children of school age and older may or may not be able to give accurate nutritional histories and should be evaluated individually as to maturity and level of dietary awareness. Frequently, it is helpful to interview the parents and child separately. A prospective food intake record should be initiated under the supervision of a dietitian if quantitative information is warranted by other indices of the nutritional assessment.

Evaluation of Nutritional Adequacy. Key nutrients for growing children include kilocalories, protein, iron, calcium, and vitamins A, D, and C. The diet also should be evaluated for the content of foods with low nutrient density, for the interference of these foods with intake of other more nutritious foods, and for adverse affects of these foods on dental health. The dietary history also should include information about past diets, including a vegetarian diet, diets for chronic disease, and for weight reduction. Food aversions, sensitivities, vitamin and mineral or food supplements, and medications also need to be evaluated because these factors can potentially enhance or pose a risk to nutritional and health status.

Assessment of Feeding Skills and Attitudes. Feeding skills and attitudes are an integral part of normal physical and psychosocial development. An initial assessment of the child's ability to feed himself and the appropriateness of the texture of food eaten for the age of the child should be made. A more detailed discussion of the assessment of feeding skills is included in the sections of *Developmental Disability* (page 316) and *Healthy Infants, Children, and Adolescents* (page 293).

Knowledge of child and adolescent behavior, especially as it relates to food and eating habits, is essential. Periods of increased or decreased appetite, food jags, binges, disinterest, willingness to try new foods, or lack of it are common at various stages throughout childhood and adolescence. Dietary assessment should include the appropriateness of the child's attitudes and behaviors for his age.

Biochemical Data

Biochemical data may either confirm nutrient excesses or deficiencies suspected from other nutritional assessment parameters or identify clinically unapparent nutritional abnormalities. There is not a simple set of tests that can give an estimate of overall or individual nutrient stores, nor are the tests uniformly precise and accurate. Laboratory studies should be selected on the basis of the patient, level of assessment, evaluation of other nutritional assessment parameters, and risk factors determined from the family history. *Pediatric Appendix 13*, page 515, presents selected references for pediatric laboratory values.

Iron Deficiency Anemia. Screening for iron deficiency is a reasonable part of all routine nutritional assessment, since it is one of the most common nutritional problems of children in our society. Hemoglobin and hematocrit can be used to screen for iron deficiency anemia, and mean corpuscular volume (MCV) should be added whenever possible. All three parameters require the use of age-specific norms. Of the three, hematocrit, which measures the percent of packed red cells in whole blood, is the least sensitive indicator for identifying children with iron deficiency anemia, and MCV is the most sensitive.[5] In addition, it must be recognized that anemia is a late manifestation of iron deficiency, but also may be attributable to other nutritional or non-nutritional factors. When hemoglobin, hematocrit, and/or MCV are below normal for age, a treatment trial with an iron supplement should be initiated with follow-up laboratory studies for a response. Differential diagnosis of iron deficiency anemia, however, would require measurement of ferritin or serum iron, total iron binding capacity, percent saturation, and transferrin. In iron deficiency anemia, ferritin, which is a measure of body reserves, is low, serum iron and transferrin may be low-to low-normal, total iron binding capacity is above normal, and percent saturation is low.

Protein Status. Serum albumin is an appropriate screening test to measure visceral protein status in the hospitalized patient. Because it has a half-life of approximately 20 days, it is considered a good indicator of long-term body protein nutriture. Liver secretory proteins with shorter half-lives, such as prealbumin (about 2 days) and creatinine height index,[16] can be useful in assessing treatment progress for those patients where protein-calorie nutrition intervention was initiated.

Other Studies. Other biochemical studies can be used to further identify the extent and severity of malnutrition. Assessment of the vitamin and mineral status of a malnourished child is essential in the rehabilitation process. When biochemical data is outside the normal range, the studies may need to be repeated for confirmation before additional studies are ordered or treatment is initiated. The type of studies and/or treatment are dependent on the biochemical abnormalities.

REFERENCES

1. Owen GM. Measurement, recording and assessment of skinfold thickness in childhood and adolescence: report of a small meeting. Am J Clin Nutr 1982;35:629–638.

2. Bishop CM, Bowen PE, Ritchey SJ. Comparison of two newly developed sets of upper arm anthropometric norms for American adults (letter). Am J Clin Nutr 1982;36:554–557.
3. Frisancho AR. Reply to letter by Bishop et al. Am J Clin Nutr 1982;36:557–560.
4. Hamill PVV, Drizd TA, Johnson CL, Reed RB, Roche AF, Moor WM. Physical growth: national center for health statistics percentiles. Am J Clin Nutr 1979;32:607–629.
5. Hubbard VS, Hubbard LR. Clinical assessment of nutritional status. In: Walker WA, Watkins JB, eds. Nutrition in pediatrics. Boston: Little, Brown, and Company, 1985:121.
6. Fomon SJ. Nutritional status. In: Fomon SJ, ed. Infant nutrition. 2nd ed. Philadelphia: WB Saunders, 1974:459.
7. Jelliffe DB. The assessment of the nutritional status of the community. Monograph No. 53. Geneva: World Health Organization, 1966.
8. Cronk CE. Growth of children with Down's syndrome: birth to age three years. Pediatrics 1978;61:564–568.
9. Personal communication: CE Cronk, Sc D Associate Professor of Nutrition and Food Sciences, Drexel University, Philadelphia, PA.
10. Babson SG, Benda GI. Growth graphs for the clinical assessment of infants of varying gestational age. J Pediatr 1976;89:814–820.
11. Merritt RJ, Blackburn GL. Nutritional assessment and metabolic response to illness of the hospitalized child. In: Suskind RM, ed. Textbook of pediatric nutrition. New York: Raven Press, 1981:285.
12. Frisancho A. New norms of upper limb fat and muscle areas for assessment of nutritional status. Am J Clin Nutr 1981;34:2540–2545.
13. Chavalittamrong B, Vathakanon R. Height and weight of Bangkok children. Standards of height and weight of Bangkok children. Journal of the Medical Association of Thailand 1977;61(Suppl 2):1–28.
14. Khanjanasthiti P. The anthropometric nutritional classification in Thai infants and preschool children. Journal of the Medical Association of Thailand 1977;60(Suppl 1):1–19.
15. Gurney JM, Jelliffe DB. Arm anthropometry in nutritional assessment: nomogram for rapid calculation of muscle circumference and cross-sectional muscle and fat areas. Am J Clin Nutr 1973;26:912–915.
16. Viteri FE, Jorge A. The creatinine height index: its use in the estimation of the degree of protein depletion and repletion in protein/calorie malnourished children. Pediatrics 1970;46:696–706.

NORMAL NUTRITION

HEALTHY INFANTS, CHILDREN, AND ADOLESCENTS

General Description

The Recommended Dietary Allowances (RDA) (page 39) for normal infants are based on estimations of intake of breast-fed infants with satisfactory growth. There are few data on the nutritional requirements for preschoolers, school age children, and adolescents. The recommended allowances for these groups are only estimates based on extrapolations of infant and adult data with estimations for growth.

Nutritional Requirements for Infants

Energy. The average intake of healthy, growing infants (see *RDA* page 39) is one of the best measures of caloric need. The higher caloric demand of infants, as compared with adults, is related to the relatively greater body surface heat loss and to the larger percentage of metabolically active tissue. During the first year, approximately 85 to 90 percent of the estimated energy intake is used for body maintenance and growth. By 9 to 12 months of age, an average of 15 percent of the total energy intake is used for increasing physical activity.[1]

Protein. The RDA for protein at birth is 2.2 g per kilogram per day. This decreases to 2 g per kilogram per day during the latter half of the first year as growth decelerates. The requirements for carbohydrates and fats have not been specifically determined. The usual caloric distribution of the diet of infants drinking human milk or infant formulas is approximately 40 to 50 percent from fat and 40 to 45 percent from carbohydrate. However, of the total caloric intake, a maximum of 60 percent from carbohydrates and a minimum of 30 percent from fat is recommended in order to ensure adequate caloric intake and satiety.[2] The recommended intake for essential fatty acids is 3 percent of total kilocalories.[3]

Fluid. In neonates, the daily turnover of water is approximately 15 percent of body weight. Since the immature kidneys of young infants are less able to concentrate urine, more fluid is required, particularly in warm climates. A fluid intake of 120 to 150 ml per kilogram per day is recommended.[3] This recommendation is ordinarily met by human milk and by commercial formulas.

Minerals. Estimations of the minerals needed for infants, except for iron and fluoride, are based on averages from breast milk. Breast milk may provide inadequate iron and fluoride in some situations. Iron-fortified commercially prepared formula contains adequate amounts of all minerals except fluoride.

Supplemental iron is recommended after 6 months of age for breast-fed term infants and after 4 months of age for infants fed non-iron-containing formulas. An intake of 1 mg per kilogram per day maintains hemoglobin levels in term infants.[4] The recommended allowances of 10 and 15 mg per day for the first and second half of the first year, respectively, are based on 1.5 mg per kilogram per day.

A fluoride supplement of 0.25 mg per day is recommended for all breast-fed infants who are not living in an area where the water is adequately fluoridated and for infants fed commercial ready-to-feed formulas. The amount of fluoride in human milk varies only slightly with the amount in the mother's diet. However, unsupplemented breast-fed infants of mothers drinking fluoridated water have been shown to have a rate of dental caries comparable to formula-fed infants with adequate fluoride intake.[4] When powdered or concentrated formulas are used, the requirement for fluoride depends on the fluoride content of local water. If the water and fluoride concentration is less than 0.3 parts per million, 0.25 mg per day of fluoride should be supplemented. Formulas mixed with fluorinated water do not need further supplementation. Excessive fluoride ingestion, 0.1 to 0.3 mg per kilogram of body weight, causes dental fluorosis.[5]

Vitamins. Human milk provides adequate levels of all vitamins when the mother's diet is nutritionally balanced. However, there have been reports of rickets in breast-fed black infants, in infants who consumed or whose nursing mothers consumed vegan diets, and in infants who had minimal sunlight exposure.[6,7] In addition, unsupplemented breast-fed infants have been shown to have decreased bone mineral concentrations by 12 weeks of age compared to babies receiving 400 international units (IU) of vitamin D per day.[7,8] Therefore, a daily supplement of 400 IU is recommended for breast-fed infants who are not exposed regularly to sunlight.[4,9] Commercial infant formulas are supplemented with all the necessary vitamins.

Table 8–2 provides information on types of feeding and the recommended vitamin and mineral supplementation.

TABLE 8–2 Vitamin and Mineral Supplementation for Infants

Type of Feeding	Iron	Vitamin D	Fluoride	Other
Breast	Additional iron from a supplement or an iron-fortified infant cereal is needed after 6 months of age	Vitamin D supplementation may be recommended if the infant has little exposure to sunlight	Fluoride supplementation may be recommended	None
Formula	Supplementation is needed by 4 months of age if the formula does not contain iron	No supplementation needed	Fluoride supplementation may be recommended, based on the fluoride content of the water supply	None
Cow's milk plus solid food (after 6 months of age)	Additional iron from a supplement or from an iron-fortified infant cereal is needed	No supplementation needed	Fluoride supplementation may be recommended	None

Human Milk. Breast feeding provides numerous benefits to both the infant and the mother. These include the nutritional and immunologic benefits of human milk for the infant and the psychological, physiologic, social, and hygenic benefits of the breast feeding process for the mother and infant.[10] Human milk is ideally suited for the infant.[10] Its composition averages 7 percent protein, 55 percent fat (4 percent as essential fatty acids), and 38 percent carbohydrate. The composition varies with the stage of the feeding (i.e., there is a higher proportion of fat at the end of the feeding), with the time of day, and with the length of nursing. Human milk supplies approximately 20 kilocalories per ounce, or 67 kilocalories per 100 ml.

The advantages of human milk are numerous. Human milk has a solute concentration compatible with the infant's immature kidneys. The fat in human milk is better absorbed because of its higher concentration of bile salt-stimulated lipase. Human milk contains antibodies and other immune factors that may reduce the incidence of certain infections and conditions in the infant. The incidence of gastroenteritis, otitis media, and asthma has been shown to be less frequent among breast-fed infants, even in industrialized countries, than among formula-fed infants. The incidence of upper respiratory infections and eczema appears to be equally common in breast-fed and formula-fed infants.[11,12]

Most drugs are excreted into breast milk at concentrations that are not harmful to the infant. Breast feeding is contraindicated only when the medications or chemicals that are taken by the mother and transmitted to the infant via breast milk are harmful to the infant. This includes anticoagulants, some antibiotics, anticancer drugs, tranquilizers, and sedations. Nursing mothers should contact their physicians before taking any medications. Nicotine from heavy cigarette smoking and "street drugs," including alcohol and marijuana, are also harmful to the nursing infant (Table 8–3).

TABLE 8–3 Acceptability of Drugs in Nursing Mothers[3]*

Contraindicated	Adverse Effect ("Infant" indicates actual observation)
Chloramphenicol	Infant: bone marrow depression
Metronidazole (Flagyl)	Blood dyscrasia, neurologic effects, possibly carcinogenic
Tetracycline	Infant: enamel hypoplasia, discoloration
Reserpine	Infant: lethargy, nasal congestion, diarrhea
Quinine	Infant: thrombocytopenia
Pyrimethamine	Bone marrow depression, convulsions
Meprobamate	Concentration to four times higher in milk than plasma
Lithium	Plasma concentration in infant is up to half that of mother
Primidone (Mysoline)	Contraindicated on manufacturer's advice
Ergot alkaloids	Infant: ergotism
Cascara and most laxatives	Infant: diarrhea
Propylthiouracil	Concentration up to 12 times higher in milk than plasma
Tetrahydrocannabinol	Infant: drowsiness
Phenytoin, Trimethadione Iodides	Infant: goiter

Allowed Judiciously	Adverse Effect
Valium	Infant: sedation with high doses
Theophyllin	Infant: thrombocytopenia, 1 case
Sulfonamide	Hemolytic anemia in G-6PD-deficiency
Nalidixic acid	Hemolytic anemia and kernicterus possible
Nicotine	Infant: nicotine intoxication
Isoniazid	Hepatitis, neuropathy
Phenobarbital and Morphine	Infant: sedation with hypnotic doses
Atropine	
Alcohol	Infant: sedation, congenital anomalies

Unknown Effects
Large doses of Salicylate, Caffeine, Methyldopa, Imipramine, Phenothiazine, Thorazine, Prochlorperazine, Trifluoperazine, Phenolphthalein (Ex-Lax)

Acceptable
Dicumarol, Warfarin, Guanethidine, Propranolol, Penicillins, Chloral hydrate, Antihistamines, occasional use of Aspirin, Acetaminophen

*With permission: Krieger I. Pediatric disorders of feeding, nutrition and metabolism. New York: John Wiley & Sons, 1982: 1, 31.

Breast feeding may not be possible if the mother is chronically ill. Furthermore, a special formula or feeding device may be necessary if the infant needs a modified infant formula (see *Infant Formulas and Feedings, Appendix 1*, page 464) or if the infant is unable to nurse. Concern has been raised about the transmission of environmental contaminants, especially pesticide residues, in breast milk. Thus far, no harmful effects have been shown, although investigations are being continued and extended to include contamination of cow's milk and other infant foods.[13]

Formulas. Commercially prepared formulas are patterned after human milk and are adjusted to meet the recommended allowances. The protein is slightly higher than human milk and has been treated to produce a fine, easily digested curd. Vegetable oils are used instead of butterfat as the fat source. Subsequently, the cholesterol content is extremely low, less than 3 mg per 100 ml. (Cow's milk has about 20 mg of cholesterol per 100 ml, and human milk has about 30 mg per 100 ml.) Studies of infants who received either breast or bottle feedings have not shown differences in plasma cholesterol concentration or in the incidence of arteriosclerosis.[3] The major disadvantage of commercial formulas is the absence of immunologic properties in human milk.

The use of soy-based formulas for infants has grown to approximately 20 percent of the total formula sold. However, the use of soy formulas in the prevention of allergic disease in infancy is controversial, and various studies show conflicting results. Soy protein formulas can be recommended for vegetarian families, for the management of children with galactosemia, and for infants with a family history of infantile eczema.[9]

Cow's Milk. Cow's milk contains higher levels of most nutrients than breast milk. Exceptions are lactose, ascorbic acid, niacin, and vitamin A. The protein in cow's milk is three times greater than in human milk. The higher protein and mineral content of cow's milk causes a higher renal solute load, which increases obligatory water loss. Supplementary water may lessen the effects of the increased solute load, but adequate water consumption is difficult for the infant to achieve. Newborn infants are at risk for development of hypernatremia and of irreversible central nervous system damage because of their small free water surplus and their limited capacity for renal solute excretion. In addition, the protein in cow's milk is not well utilized, and the fat is not absorbed as efficiently as the fat in human milk. Furthermore, only about 1 percent of the total kilocalories is in the form of essential fatty acids.[3] Another disadvantage of cow's milk is a curd that is larger, tougher, and more slowly digested. This can result in gastrointestinal blood loss and a higher incidence of allergic reactions (allergies). In addition, heating cow's milk concentrates the protein and the electrolytes because of water evaporation and therefore further potentiates dehydration and hypernatremia. When an infant over 6 months of age is eating approximately 200 g of solid foods each day (1.5 jars of commercially strained baby food), there is no objection to feeding homogenized, vitamin D-fortified whole milk.[14] Milk reduced in fat, such as 2% or skimmed milk, is not recommended during the first year of life. Infants fed skim milk receive insufficient energy to support maintenance requirements. Growth is achieved, but at a reduced rate. Energy is obtained by the mobilization of body fat and is clinically evidenced by a substantial reduction in triceps and subscapular skinfold thicknesses. A further consideration may be whether an infant who is required to mobilize stores of body fat in order to supply energy requirements is able simultaneously to synthesize the lipids essential for myelination of the nervous system.[15] Therefore, whole cow's milk is not recommended for infants during the first 6 months of life. The following chart provides a comparison of RDA for normal infants with composition of human milk, cow's milk, and commercial formula (Table 8–4).

Introduction of Solid Foods. The newborn infant has a number of primitive adaptive reflexes, such as suckling, swallowing, and rooting, that probably develop as survival mechanisms and that help to promote the acquisition of liq-

TABLE 8–4 Comparison of Recommended Dietary Allowances for Normal Infants with Composition of Human Milk, Cow's Milk, and Milk-based (Commercial) Formula[16]**

Nutrient	Dietary Allowances 0–6 Months	Dietary Allowances 6–12 Months	Human Milk per 1,000 ml*	Cow's Milk (Whole) per 1,000 ml	Commercial Milk-based Formula per 1,000 ml
Weight, kg	6	9			
lb	13	20			
Height, cm	60	71			
in	24	28			
Water, ml			897	894	875
Energy, Kcal	kg × 115	kg × 105	718	620	670
Protein, g	kg × 2.2	kg × 2.0	10.6	33.4	15–16
Fat, g			44.9	33.9	36–37
Carbohydrate, g			70.6	47.3	70–72
Vitamin A, RE	420	400	656	315	340–500
IU	1,400	2,000	2,470	1,279	1,700–2,500
Vitamin D, μg	10	10	1.3–3.3	10[†]	10
Vitamin E, mg TE	3	4		5.7	5.7–8.5
Ascorbic acid, mg	35	35	51	10	55
Thiamin, mg	0.3	0.5	0.14	0.39	0.4–0.7
Riboflavin, mg	0.4	0.6	0.37	1.65	0.6–1.0
Niacin, mg NE	6	8	2.0	0.85	7–9
Vitamin B₆, mg	0.3	0.6	0.11	0.43	0.3–0.4
Vitamin B₁₂, μg	0.5	1.5	0.46	3.63	1.5–2.0
Folacin, μg	30	45	51	51	50–100
Calcium, mg	360	540	328	1,208	550–600
Phosphorus, mg	240	360	144	945	440–460
Sodium, mg	115–350[‡]	250–750[‡]	141	498	250–390
Potassium, mg	350–925[‡]	425–1,275[‡]	523	1,544	620–1,000
Magnesium, mg	50	70	31	132	40–50
Iodine, μg	40	50	30–100		40–70
Iron, mg	10	15	0.3	0.5	1.4–12.5[§]
Zinc, mg	3	5	1.8	3.9	2.0–4.0

*One liter of human milk = 1.025 g; 1 liter of cow's milk = 1.017 g.
[†]Assumes fortification of cow's milk with 10 μg vitamin D.
[‡]Allowances for sodium and potassium are ranges considered to be safe and adequate.
[§]Values for formula not fortified and fortified with iron.
**From Food and Nutrition Board. Recommended Daily Allowances. 9th Ed. National Research Council—National Academy of Sciences, Washington, D.C., 1980.

uid foods. Most primitive reflexes disappear by 3 to 4 months of life. Table 8–5 correlates the infant's digestive and neuromuscular development with nutritional requirements and implications for feeding during the first year of life.

The age to introduce solids cannot be definitely determined since each infant matures at a different rate. However, by 4 to 6 months most infants are physiologically ready for semisolid foods. Feeding solids before this may lead to poor eating habits and overfeeding, since infants are unable to communicate when they are full. In addition, when solid foods are introduced earlier, the infant may be fed a diet that varies from the recommended caloric distribution of 7 to 16 percent of kilocalories from protein, 35 to 55 percent from fat, and the rest from carbohydrates.[2]

A reasonable schedule for the introduction of solid foods is presented in Table 8–6.

Starting with iron-fortified cereal, 1 to 2 teaspoons of a single ingredient baby food are introduced at 4- to 5-day intervals so that food sensitivities can be readily determined. Semisolids and solids should both be given at a feeding.

As foods other than milk or formula are introduced, the composition of the total diet should be considered (Table 8–7). For example, the infant may receive fewer kilocalories and other nutrients required for growth and development when certain strained foods, like fruit or vegetables, are substituted for human milk or formula.[2] The infant's acceptance of specific foods should be considered when planning a nutritionally-balanced diet.

By the end of the first year of age, the infant consumes about 300 to 450 g (10 to 15 ounces) of solid food each day, and thus the amount of human milk or formula decreases to about 750 ml each day.[1] Total milk intake should not exceed 1 L per day.[3] Most children can be weaned from the breast or bottle to a cup by this time, although they may need assistance with drinking from the cup for several months beyond the first year.

Nutritional Needs of Preschool and School-Age Children

Energy.   Energy needs vary widely, depending on the stage of growth and the level of activity of the child. As growth decelerates during the first 3 years, the caloric needs decrease from 115 to 100 kilocalories per kilogram. Caloric requirements are fairly stable from the fourth year until puberty and are similar for boys and girls, at an average of 85 kilocalories per kilogram (see *RDA* on page 39). However, several studies have shown that the energy intake per kilogram of body weight is different between the sexes and decreases with age. Median intakes of boys decreased from 87 to 71 kilocalories per kilogram per day and of girls from 78 to 61 kilocalories per kilogram per day.[13]

Protein.   The current RDA for protein is based on the maintenance requirement for adults (0.8 g per kilogram) plus an additional amount for growth and for adjustment of protein utilization efficiency. The protein allowance decreases from 1.8 g per kilogram at 1 to 3 years to 1.5 g per kilogram by 4 to 6 years of age. Normally, the preschool and school-age child consumes approximately 10 to 15 percent of the total kilocalories from protein sources. Generally, this results in a protein intake of almost twice the recommended amount.[16] The protein allowance for school-age children is 1.2 g per kilogram of body weight, or 5.7 percent of the caloric recommendation.[13]

Other Nutrients.   There are no allowances established for carbohydrates or fats. However, it has been recommended that 1 to 2 percent of the total kilocalories be from linoleic acid to assure an adequate essential fatty acid intake.[13]

The recommendations for minerals and vitamins have been determined by interpolation with arbitrary allowances for growth (see *RDA,* page 39). Several dietary surveys have shown low intakes of iron, vitamin A, and ascorbic acid in certain population groups, but clinical symptoms of deficiency are rare or are not a major nutritional problem.[17,18]

Meeting Nutritional Requirements.   The 1-year-old begins to show an increasing curiosity in his expanding world while he exhibits a decreasing interest in food at mealtimes. The child is beginning to discern flavors and textures and so may suddenly decide to dislike foods that were liked before. The child also likes to feel and explore foods with his fingers and to feed himself.

By 2 to 3 years of age, the child begins to show signs of independence, and as a result, food jags may limit the variety of foods selected. Parents report a high degree of dissatisfaction with appetite and interest in food shown by this age group.

TABLE 8–5 Development Patterns, Nutritional Needs, and Implications for Feeding*

	Birth	1 Mo	2 Mo	3 Mo	4 Mo	5 Mo	6 Mo	7 Mo	8 Mo	9 Mo	10 Mo	11 Mo	12 Mo
NUTRITIONAL RE-QUIREMENTS	Rapid growth requires greater quantity of protein, energy, and other essential nutrients.												
					Iron stores depleted.		Begin fluoride if necessary.						
	Human milk meets nutritional requirements for term infants. Commercially prepared formulas are the approved alternative.									Amount of milk needed is diminished. Meats are an important source of protein and iron.			
DIGESTION	Enzymes present to digest milk.												
		Little saliva.											
			Starches poorly digested, utilized.										
		Butterfat poorly utilized.											
										Stomach acid volume increases.			
DEVELOPMENTAL ABILITIES		Rhythmic suck.		Drooling.									
		Infant will stick out tongue when spoon introduced (tongue protrusion reflex).											
					Starts to chew.								
						Can use tongue to put food in back of mouth.							
							Opens mouth to spoon.						
							Feeds self cracker.						
									Will turn face away when full.				
												Easily chews soft table foods.	

Infant will turn his head to the same side, open mouth, and may begin to suck when cheek is stroked (rooting reflex).

Sleeps 5 to 8 hours at night.

Sleeps 8 to 12 hours at night.

Lifts head.

Hands to mouth constantly.

Reaches for objects.

Reaches for objects out of reach.

Transfers objects hand-to-hand.

Sits with support.

Sits alone.

Child will use thumb and fingers to pick up objects (thumb-finger grasp).

Child will use thumb and fore-finger to pick up objects (pincer grasp).

Drinks from cup.

IMPLICATIONS FOR FEEDINGS

Breast milk or commercially pre-pared formula only. No solids necessary.

May begin iron-fortified cereals.

Can sit in high chair.

Begin to use cup.

Begin fruits, vegetables.

Finger foods. Gradually add and increase foods from all food groups.

Regular mealtimes. Adjust quantity of intake.

Offer juices, milk from cup.

Allow weening from the bottle; wean from breast if desired.

*Every child is an individual. This chart is meant as a guideline.

TABLE 8–6 Food Introduction by Age

Age	Food to Introduce
4 to 6 months	Infant cereal
5 to 7 months	Vegetables, fruits, and their juices
6 to 8 months	Protein foods*—cheese, yogurt, cooked beans, meat, fish, chicken, turkey, egg*

*Emphasize lean meat with more frequent use of fish and poultry and less frequent use of egg yolks.

TABLE 8–7 Dietary Recommendations for the First Year of Life*

Basic Four Food Groups	Major Nutrients Supplied	Number of Servings Recommended Per Day
Milk Whole milk, cheese, cottage cheese, yogurt, ice cream, creamed soups	Protein, calcium, riboflavin, B_{12}	By 4 to 6 months: 30 to 32 ounces breast milk or formula By 9 months: 24 ounces 9 to 12 months: 16 to 24 ounces breast milk, formula, or whole milk 1 ounce cheese = 3/4 cup milk 1/2 cup cottage cheese = 1/4 cup milk 1/2 cup ice cream = 1/4 cup milk 1/4 cup pudding = 1/4 cup milk
Meat Beef, lamb, veal, fish, poultry, eggs, dry beans, peanut butter	Protein, niacin, iron, thiamin	4 to 6 months: none 6 to 8 months: 1 to 2 servings 9 to 12 months: 2 servings 1 serving = 1 ounce lean meat, poultry, fish; 1 egg; 1/4 cup cooked dried beans, peas, or lentils; 2 tablespoons peanut butter
Grain Whole-grain enriched or fortified breads, cereal, crackers, rice, spaghetti, noodles, rolled oats or tortillas	Carbohydrates, thiamin, iron, niacin	4 to 6 months: 1 to 2 servings cereal 6 to 12 months: 2 to 3 servings 12 months: 4 servings 1 serving = 1/2 slice bread; 1/4 cup cooked cereal
Fruits and Vegetables Should include vitamin C every day, vitamin A every other day Sources of vitamin C; citrus fruit, strawberries, fortified juices, tomato, broccoli Sources of vitamin A: carrots, spinach, sweet potato, apricots, winter squash	Carbohydrates, vitamins A and C	4 to 6 months: 1 serving fruit 6 to 8 months: 2 servings fruit, 1 to 2 servings vegetable 9 to 12 months: 4 servings; 1 or more from each vitamin group 1 serving = 1/4 cup juice, 1/2 piece of fruit, 1/4 cup cooked vegetables

*These are general guidelines for the average child.

TABLE 8–8 Guide to Food Intake and Average Serving Sizes for Children and Teens

Food Group	Servings Per Day	Average Size of Serving				
		1 Year	2 to 3 Years	4 to 6 Years	7 to 10 Years	11 to Teen
Milk	4					
Milk, (whole, skim, dry, evaporated, butter-milk, yogurt, or pudding)		1/2 cup	1/2 to 3/4 cup	3/4 cup	3/4 to 1 cup	1 cup
Meat	3 or more					
Egg		1	1	1	1	1
Lean meat, fish, poultry		1/2 oz (2 Tbsp)	1/2 oz (2 Tbsp)	3/4 oz (3 Tbsp)	$1\frac{1}{2}$ to 2 oz	2 to 3 oz
Peanut butter		none	1 Tbsp	2 Tbsp	2 to 3 Tbsp	2 to 3 Tbsp
Legumes (dried peas and beans)		none	1/2 cup	1/2 to 3/4 cup	1/2 to 3/4 cup	
Fruits and Vegetables	4 or more					
Vegetables		3 Tbsp	3 Tbsp	1/4 cup	1/3 cup	1/2 cup
Fruits		3 Tbsp	3 Tbsp	1/4 cup	1/3 cup	1/2 cup
Breads and Cereals	4 or more					
Whole grain bread		1/2 slice	1 slice	$1\frac{1}{2}$ slices	1 to 2 slices	1 to 2 slices
Ready-to-eat cereals		1/2 oz	3/4 oz	1 oz	1 oz	1 oz
Cooked cereals		1/4 cup	1/3 cup	1/2 cup	1/2 cup	1/2 cup
Spaghetti, macaroni, noodles, rice		1/4 cup	1/3 cup	1/2 cup	1/2 cup	1/2 cup
Crackers		1 to 2	1 to 2	2 to 3	3 to 4	3 to 4

Amounts of foods such as fats, oils, desserts, and sweets should be determined by individual caloric needs.

The 4- to 5-year-old child's appetite may vary greatly from meal to meal and from day to day. The child is a great imitator and may quickly follow the example set by a parent or by an older brother or sister. The use of food refusal as a bargaining device or to obtain attention also is common and should not be condoned. These changes are considered "normal" for these age groups and should be expected. Preschool children tend to dawdle during mealtime due to limited interest in food and to their developing feeding skills. Consequently, time and patience are required by parents during meals.

The school-age child needs guidance in the selection of foods that are good sources of minerals and vitamins and that provide adequate protein and kilocalories so that growth can continue. Normal weight children are able to balance their energy intake with their energy requirement via appetite regulation.

A child's nutrient requirements, in relation to body size, are greater than adults. Therefore, care givers need to be creative when planning eating times in order to provide an interesting, nutritionally balanced diet. The serving guidelines for children that help to ensure a nutritionally adequate diet are listed in Table 8–8.

Establishing Good Eating Habits. Eating habits and attitudes about food learned during childhood are likely to become lifelong practices. As the child gains more independence and as the peer group exerts increasing influence, healthy eating habits and a positive attitude toward food can provide the basis for proper food selection when the decision is theirs alone. Optimal eating habits can be developed by considering the following suggestions:

1. Parental and sibling attitudes have an impact on the child's request for and attitude toward food. Parents need to establish regular mealtimes, encourage breakfast, and provide nutritious snacks in a pleasant atmosphere. New foods should be introduced at the beginning of the meal when the child is hungry and in a form easily handled.

2. Growth rate, mastery of fine and gross motor skills, and personality development affect what and how much the child eats. Utensils needed and portion sizes must be consistent with the child's developmental level. Undernutrition or skipping meals negatively affects the quality of physical and mental effort necessary to participate in normal learning experiences.

3. Emotional stresses or involvement with other activities that conflict with mealtimes may influence food and nutrient intake. These situations should be minimized or eliminated whenever possible.

4. Negative eating behaviors should be ignored, positive behaviors should be encouraged and praised, and favorite foods should not be used as a reward.

5. If the child does not eat at mealtime, wait for the next regularly scheduled snack or meal.

6. It is important to recognize symptoms of obesity during childhood (see *Obesity*, page 184).

The American Heart Association has made general dietary recommendations for healthy American children above 2 years old and for adolescents. They include fat control, limitation of cholesterol, and decreased salt intake. (See page 37 for these guidelines.)

Nutritional Requirements of the Adolescent

Traditionally, adolescents are thought to be a "vulnerable group" because of increased nutritional requirements and because of their reputation for having the poorest nutritional intake. However, little data are available either to describe the quantitative nutritional requirements of this group or to verify that nutritional status is poor.[19]

The greatest demand for energy and nutrients occurs during the peak in the growth spurt, which varies according to gender and with each individual. Limitations of either kilocalories or protein during this stage has been demonstrated to inhibit growth.[13] Each adolescent, especially those with early maturation, must be evaluated according to his or her unique maturation stage and biologic age. Tanner's stages of maturity (see *Obesity,* page 184) can be helpful for estimating the caloric needs of the child. The use of a standard table of nutrient requirements based on chronologic age is not recommended when applied to the individual adolescent because of the wide variation in both timing and magnitude of growth. For practical purposes, however, the Recommended Dietary Allowances are convenient and generally are satisfactory when applied to the general population.[3] Individual needs can be verified through dietary interview and follow-up.

Caloric and protein requirements are summarized in Table 8–9.

TABLE 8–9 Adolescent Caloric and Protein Requirements

	Age	Kilocalories per kilogram per day	Protein g per kilogram per day
Males	11–14	60	1.00
	15–18	42	0.85
	19–22	41	0.80
Females	11–14	48	1.00
	15–18	38	0.84
	19–22	38	0.80

Information concerning the vitamin requirements of adolescents is scarce. However, one would expect that vitamin needs would increase as a result of increased caloric needs, tissue synthesis, and skeletal growth. The data on mineral requirements are slightly more extensive than vitamins, but still are controversial.

Meeting Nutritional Requirements. Generally, adolescents' nutritional health is quite good. However, marginal or subclinical deficiencies of some vitamins and minerals were observed in adolescents of low socioeconomic status, adolescents of certain ethnic groups, and adolescent females. Nutrients most often consumed in insufficient amounts were iron, calcium, riboflavin, and vitamin A.[13,18] Adolescents' need for iron increases as the result of expanding blood volume and of increased muscle mass. In addition to increased needs, females must replace iron lost through menstruation. Many weight-conscious adolescent females consume low kilocalorie diets, which makes it even more difficult to achieve iron requirements. Insufficient intakes of calcium and riboflavin have been associated with decreased dairy food and increased soft drink consumption. This trend affects calcium absorption by altering the calcium-to-phosphorus ratio of 1:1 at a time when increased calcium is needed for bone mineralization. Although low intakes or low plasma levels of vitamin A are often cited, evidence of a clinical deficiency is rare.[20,21]

Nutrient needs can best be met when the diet contains a wide variety of foods. The recommended allowances of all nutrients (with the possible exception of iron) can be met by following the basic four food guidelines, as indicated in Table 8–8.

Eating Habits. The many healthy food habits developed in childhood should be encouraged throughout adolescence. By respecting the adolescent's ideas about food, it is easier to emphasize the positive aspects of their practices and to build on them.

Adolescence is a period of alteration in life-style and self-concept, as well as a time of physical growth and of increased nutritional needs. The average adolescent is involved in an extremely busy schedule of school, extracurricular activities, and perhaps part-time employment. Time schedules may lead to the omission of some meals, especially breakfast, or to an increased frequency of eating (two to six times per day). A greater number of meals are eaten away from home, especially "fast" foods and vending machine "snacks." Frequent intake of sugar-containing snacks is associated with a greater incidence of dental caries.[22,23] Emotional instability and altered body image may cause intermittent stress and may therefore lead to abnormal eating habits, such as overeating, weight reduction, anorexia nervosa, or bulimia. Greater independence from the family and the desire to be accepted by peers often influence altered eating practices, such as vegetarianism, changing the diet in hopes of improving athletic performance, fad dieting, and indulging in alcohol. In addition, chronic chemical abuse can alter the nutritional status of the teenager. For example, the adolescent who has increased needs for growth and development may be susceptible to nutritional deficiencies as a result of chronic alcohol abuse and subsequent changes in the quality, quantity, and frequency of foods consumed.

All of these factors put certain groups of adolescents at greater risk for suboptimal nutrition. Many factors are considered important enough to be described in greater detail in their own specific section of this manual. The following information and suggestions for the chemically dependent teen may be beneficial in the establishment of an educational program.

Nutrition Education for the Chemically Dependent Teen

Instructing the chemically dependent teen is extremely educational for both patient and nutrition educator. An understanding of the teen's world and the use of a variety of nutrition-related topics and teaching techniques contributes greatly toward a positive experience.

It is important to understand the teenager's general concept of self and to know about the specific audience before attempting to share nutritional information. Teaching sessions can be facilitated by asking staff members who are familiar with the group about behaviors, the teaching techniques they have found to be beneficial for this specific group, the age range and educational limitations of the group, and the number of participants. Groups and sessions can vary significantly; therefore, the speaker must be flexible with the information presented and with the teaching techniques utilized.

The nutrition-related topics can be general or specific. General topics include wellness, normal growth, nutritional needs, common deficiencies, meeting nutritional needs for this age group, and eating habits and effects of alcohol on nutrition and/or disease. Specific topics include fad diets, health foods, caffeine, fiber, vegetarianism, anorexia, and bulimia. Many times a combination of general and specific topics best meet the needs of the audience. A few key areas may be incorporated into each session and the other topics presented according to the interest of the group. Whenever possible, surveying the group prior to a session and identifying areas of interest is helpful.

A variety of teaching techniques contribute toward presentation flexibility. A 20- to 30-minute presentation is optimal, unless group activities or audio-visual materials are used. Active audience involvement is essential. Many times the question (by the speaker) and answer (by the group) type of session can be effective in stimulating group participation. Having a group member write responses on a board may help to facilitate group interaction and to reinforce the learning of key issues. Another way to obtain group involvement is to establish small group tasks that require group presentation on completion. However, this may be unsuccessful if the task is too difficult for the group, if not enough guidance is given, or if groups are large and supervision is limited. A post-test may be useful for the speaker to get feedback on what the group has learned and to summarize key points. This can be given for written response by the individual or by small groups or for oral response with the entire group. The method used depends upon the time available and the number of participants in the group. A beneficial way to end each session is to summarize the nutritional information and to point out its relationship to the underlying disorder and its treatment.

REFERENCES

1. Kien CL. Energy metabolism and requirements in disease. In: Walker WA. Nutrition in pediatrics: basic science in clinical application. Boston: Little, Brown, 1985:87.
2. Fomon SJ. Infant nutrition. Philadelphia: WB Saunders, 1974:152, 182.
3. Krieger I. Pediatric disorders of feeding, nutrition and metabolism. New York: John Wiley and Sons, 1982:1, 31.
4. Committee on Nutrition. Fluoride supplementation. Pediatrics 1986;78:758–760.
5. Fomon SJ, Filer LJ, Anderson TA, Ziegler EE. Recommendations for feeding normal infants. Pediatrics 1979;63:52–59.
6. Bachrach SB, Fisher J, Parks JS. An outbreak of vitamin D deficiency rickets in a susceptable population. Pediatrics 1979;63:871–877.
7. Edidin DV, Levitsky LL, Schey W, Dumbovic N, Campos A. Resurgence of nutritional rickets associated with breast feeding and special dietary practices. Pediatrics 1980;65:232–235.
8. Greer FR, Scarey JE, Levin RS, Steechen JJ, Asch PS, Tsang RC. Bone mineral content and 25-hydroxyvitamin D concentration in breast-fed infants with and without supplemental vitamin D. J Pediatr 1981;98:696–701.
9. American Acadamy of Pediatrics. Pediatric nutrition handbook. 2nd ed. Elk Grove Village, Illinois: Am Acad Peds, 1985:1.
10. American Dietetic Association. Position paper of the American Dietetic Association: promotion of breast feeding. J Am Diet Assoc 1986;86:1580–1585.
11. Pipes PT. Nutrition in infancy and children. 3rd ed. St. Louis: Time Mirror, Mosby College Publishing, 1985:57,175,229.
12. Kovar MG, Serdula MK, Marks JS, Fraser DW. Review of the epidemiologic evidence for an association between infant feeding and infant health. Pediatrics (suppl) 1984;74:615–638.
13. Beal VA. Nutrition in the life span. New York: John Wiley & Sons, 1980:171,321.
14. Committee on Nutrition. The use of whole cow's milk in infancy. Pediatrics 1983;72:253–255.
15. Fomon SJ, Filer LJ, Ziegler E, Bergmann K, Bergmann RL. Skim milk in infant feeding. Acta Paediatr Scand 1977;66:17–30.
16. Robinson CH. Nutrition during infancy. In: Robinson CH, Lawler MR, Chenoweth

WL, Garwick AE. Normal and therapeutic nutrition. 17th ed. New York: MacMillan, 1986:280.

17. Ad Hoc Committee to Review the Ten-State Nutrition Survey: Nutrition, growth, development and maturation: Findings from the ten-state nutrition survey of 1968–1970. Pediatrics 1973;51:1095–1099.

18. Abraham S, Carroll MD, Dresser CM, Johnson CL. Dietary intake findings, United States 1971–1974. DHEW Publ. No. (HRA) 77-1647. Washington, D.C., U.S. Government Printing Office, 1977.

19. Heald FP. New reference points for defining adolescent requirements. In: McKigney JI, Munro HN, eds. Nutrient requirements in adolescence. Massachusetts: MIT Press, 1978:295.

20. Heald FP. The adolescent. In: Jelliffe DD, Jelliffe EFP, eds. Nutrition and growth. New York: Plenum Press, 1979:239.

21. Greenwood CT, Richardson DP. Nutrition during adolescence. World Rev Nutr Diet 1979;33:1–41.

22. Bibby BG. The cariogenicity of snack foods and confections. J Am Dent Assoc 1975;90:121–132.

23. Garn SM, Cole PE, Solomon MA, Schaefer AE. Relationships between sugar foods and the decayed, missing, filled, teeth in 1968–1970. Ecol Food Nutr 1980;9:135–138.

YOUNG ATHLETES

Consideration of the nutritional needs of the young athlete must emphasize not only the increased requirements for exercise, but also the requirements to support normal growth. Nutritional assessment for this population involves evaluation of the following: kilocalorie, protein, vitamin, mineral, and fluid needs.

Energy

Determination of the caloric requirements for the young athlete involves consideration of a number of variables, including body size, age, and level of activity. To date, there are no universal guidelines for calculating energy costs of activities for this group. The average daily energy requirement during adolescence is 40 to 60 kilocalories per kilogram per day.[1] Depending on the level of activity, the growing athlete may require an additional 600 to 1,200 kilocalories per day.[2]

In general, physical activity increases caloric expenditure and automatically increases the appetite, with the result that more food is ingested. In most instances, sufficient kilocalories are consumed to maintain appropriate body weight and to support growth. Although it is unlikely that a teen in heavy physical training will gain too much weight, caloric intake greater than the daily expenditure is not recommended because it results in unnecessary fat deposition. The increased caloric requirements are best met by increasing food servings from each of the major food groups (see *Appendix 6*) without significantly altering the proportions of the micro- or macronutrients of the diet.[3] The distribution of the total kilocalories should be approximately 55 percent carbohydrate, 30 percent fat, and 15 percent protein.

Protein

For many years it has been generally believed that physical activity does not significantly increase the need for dietary protein. However, recent data suggests that protein metabolism may change somewhat during endurance exercise or rigorous weight training.[3,4] A substantial decrease in the rate of protein synthesis during exercise has been reported,[5] and it is estimated that protein can provide up to 5.5 percent of the total caloric cost of exercise. It is premature, however, to use this data as justification for increased protein intake for the physically active teen.

The Recommended Dietary Allowance (RDA) for protein for teens is 45 to 56 g per day for males and 44 to 46 g per day for females.[6] The observation that this population's diet usually exceeds the RDA suggests that supplementation of a diet with extra protein is unnecessary.

Vitamins and Minerals

Vitamin supplements are generally not recommended for the young athlete for several reasons. First, excess water-soluble vitamins cannot be stored in the body effectively and, thus, are rapidly excreted in the urine when tissue saturation occurs. Second, fat-soluable vitamins are retained and stored in the body, and daily high-potency supplements of vitamins A and D are known to be toxic and sometimes fatal. Third, a nutritionally balanced diet that contains approximately 1,800 kilocalories each day usually provides satisfactory levels of all vitamins.[3]

The most significant effect of exercise on mineral nutrition is loss of the electrolytes, sodium, potassium, and magnesium through sweat.

Sodium requirements for the young athlete have not been determined. Deficits can be replaced on a regular basis by salting foods to a satisfying taste. Salt tablets are rarely needed and, if ingested, may cause gastrointestinal disturbances that result from fluid movement into the gut.

The amount of potassium and magnesium lost through sweat is negligible when the environmental temperature is mild and the exercise level is moderate. However, potassium losses may occur under conditions of moderate to extreme heat with profuse sweating. Usually, normal food intake is sufficient to replace losses.

Electrolyte replacement beverages may be provided to replenish minerals lost in sweat, but generally are not recommended because of their glucose content. With intense exercise, even a small amount of carbohydrates can block fluid movement from the stomach into the intestinal tract, thus delaying gastric emptying.[7] The sugar content of sport drinks should not exceed 2.5 g per 100 ml (1/2 teaspoon sugar per 1/2 cup). Most have two to three times that amount. Therefore, if used, the sport drinks should be diluted by 50 percent: 1/2 cup drink with 1/2 cup water.[4]

Iron is a mineral of major importance for maintenance of optimal athletic condition. Iron is an essential component of hemoglobin, which is necessary for oxygen transport; therefore, adequacy of the iron status significantly affects endurance and physical performance. A condition known as sports anemia, runners anemia, or pseudoanemia has been reported in some athletes, especially those involved in long-distance running or swimming or those subjected to recurrent trauma.[8] Suggested causes of sports anemia include inadequate iron intake, decreased intestinal absorption of iron, blood loss, expansion of blood volume, intravascular hemodialysis caused by onset of heavy training, and trauma that results in hemoglobinuria and inadequate dietary protein intake.[3]

The iron deficient teen should be identified and provided with iron supplements and dietary counseling regarding food sources of iron. There are no documented daily recommended iron requirements for the growing teen. However, the RDA of 10 mg for preadolescents (7 to 10 years of age) and 18 mg for adolescents (11 to 15 years of age) appear to be reasonable goals.

Fluids

The young athlete has a significantly greater water requirement per proportional weight than does the adult. A useful formula for daily maintenance water requirements for this age group is 100 ml per kilogram for the first 10 kg of body weight, 50 ml per kg for the next 10 kg of body weight, and 25 ml per kg of additional water for the next 10 kg of body weight (i.e., a 25 kg child would need approximately 1,625 ml per day). Above 30 kg of body weight, the requirements approximate normal adult values (see *Nutritional Needs for Physical Performance,* page 21).[5]

Hydration during sports events and strenuous training should be monitored. Since thirst is not a reliable indication of hydration, the athlete should drink 5 to 6 ounces of fluid every 10 to 15 minutes during prolonged exercise. A weight loss of 1 kg indicates a need for 1 L of water replacement.[9] Under no circumstances should fluid restriction be used as a way to control body weight.

Carbohydrate Loading

Carbohydrate loading or glycogen packing of the muscles is not advised, since long-term effects of it on young athletes are not known.[4,7] Diarrhea can result if the loading is done with simple and refined sugars. No definite research has been published to support individual cases of cardiac arrythmias, elevated serum triglycerides, and destruction of muscle fibers by excessive storage of glycogen.

Achieving Competing Weight

A young athlete who wants to reduce body fat to a level desired for competition needs a well-planned program of exercise and a prescribed diet that is sufficient to support the needs of training while protecting muscle tissue from being used as a source of energy. The amount of fat to be lost is estimated by assessing the existing level of body fat and projecting the optimal level of fatness desired for the specific sport. These assessments can be made by hydrostatic weighing or by use of a skin fold caliper. For the average teen athlete, a desired rate of fat reduction to achieve an appropriate level of fatness is approximately 2 pounds per week.[10] This fat reduction can be accomplished by creating a negative energy balance of approximately 1,000 kilocalories daily.[10] Energy expenditure is increased in training activities, so the desired negative energy balance can occur while the athlete has a food intake of no less than 2,000 kilocalories daily.[10] This restricted caloric intake is maintained for the few weeks that are required to reduce fatness to the desired level. Once the desired level of fatness has been achieved, caloric intake is increased to maintain a desired competing weight and to satisfy the energy needs of athletic training and normal growth. Weight and level of fatness should be monitored and should remain stable during the competing season.

Athletes attempting to gain weight should increase weight as muscle mass, not fat. Muscle mass is increased only through muscle work supported by an appropriate increase in food intake. No food, vitamin, drug, or hormone increases muscle mass. It is recommended that the high kilocalorie diet required to support muscle growth from increased work be low in animal fats and cholesterol.[11]

In summary, as physical training increases, more energy is needed for the young athlete. Therefore, food intake must be adjusted and consideration given to appropriate balance of fats (30 percent), carbohydrates (50 to 55 percent), and proteins (15 percent). Supplements of vitamins and minerals are not needed, since the athlete usually meets these needs by increasing kilocalories and by eating a variety of foods. Hydration during sports events and strenuous training should be monitored. A weight loss of 1 kg indicates a need for intake of 1 L of water. Carbohydrate loading is not recommended. Weight loss and weight gain for the young athlete should be done under the supervision of a qualified health professional.

REFERENCES

1. Consotazio C. Physical activity and performance of the adolescent. In: McKigney JI, Munro HN. Nutrient requirements in adolescence. Massachusetts: MIT Press, 1978:203.
2. Nutrition Committee, Canadian Pediatric Society. Adolescent nutrition: sports and diet. Can Med Assoc J 1983;129:552–553.
3. Worthington-Roberts R. Nutritional considerations for children in sports. In: Pipes P. Nutrition in infancy and childhood. St. Louis: Times Mirror/Mosby College Publishing, 1985:312–346.
4. National Dairy Council. Food power: a coach's guide to improving performance. 1983.
5. Ziegler M. Nutritional care of the pediatric athlete. Clin Sports Med 1982;1:371–378.
6. Committee on Dietary Allowances, Food and Nutrition Board. Recommended dietary allowances. Washington, D.C.: National Academy of Science, 1980.
7. Katch F, McArdle W. Nutrition, weight control, and exercise. In: Katch F, McArdle W, eds. Optimal nutrition for exercise and sport. Philadelphia: Lea & Febiger, 1933:33.
8. Pate RR. Sports anemia: a review of the current research literature. Phys Sports Med 1983;11:115–126.
9. Narins D, Belkengren R, Sapala S. Nutrition and the growing athlete. Pediatric Nursing 1983;May/June:163–168.
10. Smith N. Nutrition and the adolescent athlete. Curr Concepts Nutr 1982;11:63–70.
11. Smith N. Gaining and losing weight in athletics. JAMA 1976;236:149–151.

VEGETARIAN DIET

General Description

The reasons for adopting a vegetarian diet are many and include religion, ethics, and economics. Vegetarianism is a term that embraces a variety of dietary practices. The diet is classified according to the extent by which animal foods are excluded (see *Vegetarian Diet* on page 29).

Infants, children, and adolescents who follow vegetarian dietary practices are at high risk for the development of nutritional deficiencies because of their rapid growth rates and the need for kilocalories and nutrients to support growth.[1]

Nutritional Adequacy

The American Dietetic Association recognizes that well-planned vegetarian diets are consistent with good nutrition status.[1] The extent to which food selection and feeding patterns meet the dietary recommendations for infants, children, and adolescents is dependent on the type of vegetarian diet chosen and on the degree of careful meal planning by the parent(s).

The primary indicator of nutritional adequacy is normal growth and development. Evidence shows that children with a reasonable amount of animal protein in the diet will likely grow normally (i.e., lacto- or lacto-ovovegetarians). To date, all published data imply that the more limited vegetarian diets are inadequate to support the maximum growth potential of infants and children.[2] However, there may be an association between more strict forms of vegetarianism and a variety of life-styles and attitudes that may adversely affect growth independent of food intake.[3]

Energy. Adequate caloric intake for vegetarian infants and children is seldom a problem when some animal protein is used. However, if the restrictions of total vegetarianism are imposed, the infant or child may have difficulty consuming adequate kilocalories as the result of the limited capacity of the stomach to tolerate sufficient volume of low energy density foods and because of the lower fat content.[3]

Protein. The quantity and quality of protein consumed in a vegetarian diet is important, since protein requirements are higher throughout periods of growth. When caloric needs are met with a good variety of foods, the quantity of protein should be adequate.

The quality of protein, or the amino acid composition of a food, is rarely a concern when some animal foods are consumed. In a vegetarian regimen, it is necessary to combine vegetable proteins that complement each other, since all vegetable proteins contain relatively limited quantities of one or more essential amino acids. See *Vegetarian Diet,* Table 3–5 (page 31) for a scheme for combining complementary proteins.

Vitamins and minerals. The most successful way to meet vitamin and mineral needs is through dietary diversity. The possibility of deficiency states is a concern only when all foods of animal origin are excluded. The most common deficiencies include the vitamins B_{12}, D, and riboflavin and the minerals calcium, iron, and zinc.[4] Mineral deficiency can occur for two reasons: inadequate intake and low bioavailability.

Low vitamin B_{12} intakes during pregnancy and lactation by vegan mothers may produce a B_{12} deficiency in the infant. Both fetal stores and breast milk supply limited amounts of B_{12} and must be supplemented by additional B_{12}.[5] A B_{12} supplement, or the consumption of B_{12}-fortified foods, is considered essential for all vegans (Table 8–10). Sea plants, such as seaweeds and algae, may contain some B_{12}, but this source is too variable to be considered a reliable source of B_{12}.

TABLE 8–10 Vitamin and Mineral Sources of Plant Foods

Food group	B_{12}	D	Riboflavin	Calcium	Iron*	Zinc
Cereals, whole grains, breads	Fortified cereal or yeast		Brewer's yeast, wheat germ, grains		Fortified cereals, white or brown rice	Whole grains, brown rice
Legumes, meat analogs, soy products	Fortified soy milk, meat analogs	Fortified soy milk	Beans, soybeans	Fortified soy milk, great northern & navy beans	All legumes	All legumes
Nuts, seeds			Almonds	Almonds, filberts, sunflower & un-hulled sesame seeds	Almonds, pecans	Almonds, pecans
Fruits					Dates, prunes, raisins	
Vegetables			Avocados, broccoli, leafy greens, mushrooms	Leafy greens†	Greens, spinach, broccoli	Spinach
Oils		Fortified margarine, cod liver oil				

* Iron absorption may be enhanced by consumption of ascorbic acid-rich foods at the same meal. Ascorbic acid sources are citrus fruits and juices, tomatoes, broccoli, strawberries, green or red sweet peppers, dark green leafy vegetables, and potatoes with the skins.
† Avoid oxalic acid sources: spinach, chard, parsley, and beet greens.

Newborn infants of vegan mothers are predisposed to vitamin D deficiency. A vitamin D supplement or the consumption of fortified foods is imperative (see Table 8–10) for pregnant women, infants, and children who consume no foods of animal origin. (There have been no reported cases of riboflavin deficiencies in vegans. However, when milk products are not used, other food sources of riboflavin must be consumed [see Table 8–10]).

Since calcium is necessary for normal growth, an inadequate calcium intake compounded with insufficient vitamin D jeopardizes growth potential. Therefore, the vegan diet must include plant foods with high calcium content (see Table 8–10). It is important to remember that calcium bioavailability may be decreased by oxalic acid, dietary fiber, and phytates.[6]

Iron from foods is absorbed as either heme (animal sources) or nonheme (plant sources) iron. Heme iron is absorbed much better than nonheme iron. Nonheme iron absorption is significantly improved when some heme iron or a source of ascorbic acid is consumed at the same meal.[1] Phytic acid, oxalic acid, large amounts of plant fiber, phosvitin in egg yolks, and tannic acid in tea decrease absorption.[6] It is important to emphasize the consumption of at least one food high in iron and one high in ascorbic acid for each meal (see Table 8–10).

Little is known about zinc and its bioavailability in relation to the vegan diet.[1] High levels of phytic acid and of dietary fiber may decrease the absorption of zinc. Yeast fermentation (leavened bread) often decreases phytate levels in whole wheat flour, thereby improving zinc availability. Plasma zinc levels appear to be inversely related to fiber intake, rather than dietary zinc content per se.[3] Refer to Table 8–10 for food sources.

Goals of Dietary Management

The nutritional goal in vegetarian diets for infants, children, and adolescents is to achieve an intake that meets all known nutrient needs and that supports normal growth and development.

With proper meal planning, consumption of a vegetarian diet can support normal growth and development. The use of food groups may be beneficial when devising meal patterns. The major nutrients contributed by standard food groups are listed in Table 8–11.[6]

In addition, the following dietary practices and meal plan (Table 8–12) should be encouraged for vegan infants and children:

1. Breast feed infants for at least 6 months and preferably longer (one must pay careful attention to the mother's diet).

2. Toddlers should use fortified soy formulas or milk whenever possible.

3. Supplemental vitamins and minerals may be necessary in the older child or adolescent when soy milk is not used.

4. B_{12} must be supplemented.

5. Certain foods may be considered unsafe for infants and toddlers: honey; home canned fruits and vegetables owing to the potential for food-born illness; vegetable juices, such as carrot or spinach, which have high nitrate content; whole nuts (nut butters may be used); and granolas because of the potential for choking.[3]

Physicians: How to order diet

The diet order should indicate *vegetarian diet*. The dietitian determines food preferences and establishes a nutritionally adequate diet.

TABLE 8–11 Food Guide for Lacto-ovovegetarian Diets[6]

Food Group	1 to 3 yr Both Sexes	4 to 6 yr Both Sexes	7 to 9 yr Both Sexes	10 to 12 yr Both Sexes	13 to 17 yr M	13 to 17 yr F	18 to 19 yr M	18 to 19 yr F	20+ yr M	20+ yr F	Standard serving
Cereals, whole grains, breads	3	3 to 4	4	5	7	5	9	5	8	6	1 slice whole grain or enriched bread or 3/4 cup cooked cereal or 1 oz dry cereal
Legumes, meat analogs, textured vegetable protein (TVP)	1/8	1/4	1/2	1/2	3/4	1/2	$1\frac{1}{2}$	1	1	3/4	1 cup cooked legume or 2 to 3 ounce meat analog or 20 to 30 g textured vegetable protein
Nuts, seeds	1/8	1/4	1/2	3/4	1	3/4	2	1	1	1	$1\frac{1}{2}$ oz or 3 Tbsp
Milk, milk products	2 to 3	2 to 3	3	4	4	4	2 to 3	2 to 3	$1\frac{1}{2}$	$1\frac{1}{2}$	1 cup milk*
Eggs	1	1	1	$1\frac{1}{2}$	$1\frac{1}{2}$	$1\frac{1}{2}$	$1\frac{1}{2}$	$1\frac{1}{2}$	$1\frac{1}{2}$	$1\frac{1}{2}$	1 medium egg
Fruits, vegetables	2 to 3	3 to 4	4	5	5	5	6	5	6	5	1/2 cup juice or 1 medium piece or 1 cup raw or 1/2 cup cooked
Oils	1/3 to 1	2/3 to 1	2/3 to 1	1	1	1	1	1	1	1	1 Tbsp

Minimum Number of Servings Daily

*Common portions of dairy foods and their milk equivalents in calcium content:
1 inch cube cheddar-type cheese = 1/2 cup milk
2 Tbsp cream cheese = 1 Tbsp milk
1/2 cup yogurt = 1/2 cup milk
1/2 cup ice cream or ice milk = 1/3 cup milk
1/2 cup cottage cheese = 1/4 cup milk

TABLE 8–12 Diet Plan for the Vegan Child[*][4]

Food Group	Standard Serving Size	Daily Servings		
		6 mo to 1 yr	1 to 4 yrs	4 to 6 yrs
Enriched cereals or grains	1 to 5 Tbsp	1/2 (1/2 to $2\frac{1}{2}$ Tbsp) finely ground	1	2
Breads	1 slice	1	3	4
Legumes, meat analogs, soy products, nuts, seeds (grind for toddlers)	1 to 6 Tbsp	2 cooked and sieved	3 chopped	3
Fortified soy milk (Isomil, Nursoy, ProSobee, Soy-alac, etc.)	1 cup	3	3	3
Fruits (include two servings of citrus fruit or juice each day)	1/4 to 1/2 cup	3 pureed	4 juice or chopped	5
Vegetables green leafy or deep yellow	1/4 to 1/3 cup	1/4 (1 to $1\frac{1}{2}$ Tbsp)	1/2 (2 to $2\frac{1}{2}$ Tbsp)	1
other		1/2 (2 to $2\frac{1}{2}$ Tbsp) cooked and pureed	1 chopped	1
Oils	1 tsp	0	3	4
Miscellaneous				
Brewer's yeast	1 Tbsp	0	1	1
Molasses	1 Tbsp	0	1	1
Wheat germ	1 Tbsp	0	optional	optional

*Truesdell DD, Acosta PB. Feeding the vegan infant and child. Copyright, The American Dietetic Association. Reprinted by permission from JOURNAL OF THE AMERICAN DIETETIC ASSOCIATION 1985;85:837.

REFERENCES

1. Position paper on the vegetarian approach to eating. J Am Diet Assoc 1980;77:61–69.
2. Dietz WH, Dwyer JT. Nutritional implications of vegetarianism for children. In: Suskind RM, ed. Textbook of pediatric nutrition. New York: Raven Press, 1981:179.
3. MacLean WC, Graham GG. Vegetarianism in children. Am J Dis Child 1980;134:513–519.
4. Truesdell DD, Acosta PB. Feeding the vegan infant and child. J Am Diet Assoc 1985;85:837–840.
5. Johnston PK. Getting enough to grow on. Am J Nurs 1984;84:336–339.
6. Fanelli MT, Kuczmarski RJ. Food selection for vegetarians. Dietetic Currents 1983;10:1–4.

OTHER NUTRITIONAL CONSIDERATIONS

DEVELOPMENTAL DISABILITY

Children with developmental disabilities require the same nutrients as normal healthy children; however, the amounts needed may vary. These children are at risk for stunted growth, poor weight gain or obesity, anemia, food allergies, adverse food and drug interactions, constipation, and poor dental health. In addition, they have many feeding problems, both physical and psychosocial in origin, that may affect nutritional intake and status.[1] The goals of nutritional care are to assure adequate nutritional intake to promote maximum growth potential and feeding skills. Developmental disability includes a wide variety of conditions, each of which has a different impact on nutritional needs, feeding skills, and problems. Therefore, the dietitian in charge of their care should have knowledge of normal development and behaviors and of how the condition or its treatment affects nutritional status.

Nutritional Assessment

Lack of standards, particularly for growth, make nutritional assessment of the developmentally delayed child difficult.[2] It is important, therefore, that nutritional assessment be done frequently so that full growth potential and nutritional health are realized. Nutritional assessment should include feeding assessment, in addition to the more traditional parameters discussed in the section *Pediatric Nutritional Assessment,* page 287.

Anthropometrics. Growth is difficult to evaluate. There are few standards for developmentally delayed children, and obtaining accurate measurements is difficult due to the spasticity or the uncooperativeness of the child. Recumbent length may be necessary rather than height. Appropriate adjustment should be made before the measurement is plotted on a height graph. In some conditions, growth retardation and abnormal body composition are attributable to genetic or to biologic defect.[1] Syndromes in which growth retardation is frequently seen are presented in Table 8–13.

TABLE 8–13   Syndromes Associated with Growth Retardation

Cerebral Palsy
de Lange's syndrome
Down syndrome
Hurler's syndrome
Prader-Willi syndrome
Silver's syndrome
Trisomy 13 and 18
Turner's syndrome
William's syndrome

Height-age (see *Pediatric Nutritional Assessment,* page 287) can be used to estimate a child's ideal weight range and caloric need. However, it is important to assure that malnutrition is not contributing to the growth deficit. Weight-for-height ratio is also helpful in the evaluation of weight control for those children below normal height for age.[3] The Baldwin-Wood Tables (*Pediatric Appendix 6,* page 500) are useful for evaluating weight-for-height in the older child. Cronk's growth graphs for children with Down syndrome for ages 1 to 6 years (*Pediatric Appendix 7,* page 502) can be used for the young child with Down syndrome. The graphs reflect the relatively slower growth of these children that begins at about 6 months of age, and can aid in early detection of failure-to-thrive or tendency to be overweight among Down syndrome children.[4,5]

Dietary Assessment. Dietary assessment should include an evaluation of caloric and nutrient intake for growth stage, consistency and texture of the diet for the child's feeding skill level, and medications being used. For children on anticonvulsant medication, attention should be given to adequacy of folic acid, calcium, phosphorus, ascorbic acid, vitamins B_6, B_{12}, and D, zinc, and magnesium.[6] Diets of children with reduced caloric requirements should be assessed carefully for nutrient adequacy because these diets need to be more nutrient dense than normal. Children with severe mental retardation who cannot feed themselves are at risk for inadequate caloric and nutrient intake. Care should be taken to estimate the amount and type of food actually consumed, as opposed to the amount offered, since a significant portion of the food may be refused or spilled.[6] Children who receive the majority of their kilocalories from milk or milk-based supplements may be at risk for iron deficiency anemia. Dietary adequacy also may be affected by bizarre eating habits such as pica, poor appetite and early satiety, food allergies, and rumination. Rumination is the chronic regurgitation of ingested food, which may or may not be re-swallowed, and frequently results in chronic undernutrition.

Food is often used for behavior modification. The impact of the amount, frequency, and type of food on nutritional and dental status should be evaluated.[7] Caretakers should be encouraged to use things other than food for behavior modification.

Feeding Assessment. Feeding assessment involves evaluation of feeding skills and behaviors that may influence nutritional status.[6] Occupational, physical, and speech therapists can aid in assessing feeding skills, problems, and capabilities.[8]

The development of feeding skills in developmentally delayed children usually proceeds in the same sequence as that of normal children. However, the chronologic age at which the developmental stages occur is unpredictable.[1] Physical malformations, neuromotor dysfunction, and psychosocial factors can interfere with the development of feeding skills.[9] Some developmentally delayed children are hypersensitive in the oral area and may require a densensitization program before more textured food or spoon feeding can be introduced. Factors influencing the development of feeding skills are presented in Table 8–14.

TABLE 8–14 Factors Influencing Development of Feeding Skills

Sitting balance
Head and neck control
Jaw, lip, and tongue control
Sucking, swallowing, chewing, and drinking abilities
Persistence of primitive reflexes
Arm, eye, and hand control
Grasp

The degree of motor dysfunction that involves the mouth area and the degree of the developmental disability that interferes with self-feeding has been found to correlate with inadequate dietary intake and growth. Pneumonia, due to repeated aspiration of food, is a problem for some of those children that may necessitate a feeding gastrostomy. (See *Enteral Nutrition Support of Adults,* page 261.) Table 8–15 describes appropriate textures and foods for various feeding skills.[3]

Developmentally delayed children can present with many of the same food-related behaviors as normal children, though perhaps at a different age. They

TABLE 8–15 Guidelines for Selection of Food for Feeding Skill Level*

Feeding Skill Level	Type of Food Indicated	Examples
Sucking	Use fluids	Milk/Formula
Elevation of tongue: moves food to back of mouth	Continue using fluids	Milk/Formula
Swallowing (with head forward and no gagging; elevation of back and tongue)	Introduce blended diet	Baby food; thick purees; mashed potatoes; applesauce; custard; ice cream; yogurt; mashed banana
Up-and-down chewing with jaw control and minimal drooling	Start finely ground foods	Oatmeal: cottage cheese; finely ground meat; scrambled egg; well-mashed cooked vegetables; egg salad; peanut butter if no tongue thrust
Lateral tongue movement	Begin coarsely ground foods	Ground meats in gravy; tuna fish; chopped fruits and vegetables; fine coleslaw; cheese; rice; liverwurst; banana slices; flavored yogurt
Rotary chewing	Use chopped foods	Crackers; finely chopped meats; fruits and vegetables; salad greens; coleslaw; macaroni; dry cereal
Reaches for and grasps objects; brings hands to mouth	Begin finger feeding with large pieces	Crackers; teething biscuit; oven-dried toast; cheese sticks
Voluntary release	Finger feeding with small pieces	Dry cereal; small pieces of meat; cottage cheese
Puts lips on cup rim	Begin cup feeding	
Reaches for spoon; ulnar deviation of wrist	Self-feeding	Foods that adhere to spoon; cooked cereal; mashed potato; applesauce; cottage cheese
Increased rotary movement of jaw	Increase texture and variety	Chopped meats; raw vegetables and fruits

*Adapted from Zeman FJ. Nutrition in handicapping condititons. In: Zeman FJ, ed. Clinical nutrition and dietetics. New York: Macmillan, 1983:595.

can be expected to have periods of reduced food intake, food jags, and attempts to control their parents by the acceptance or the rejection of food.[1] In addition, some feeding problems can develop as a result of feeding being associated with unpleasant circumstances in children who must be fed frequently or in whom feeding is time-consuming due to chewing and swallowing dysfunction.[3] Feeding assessment should evaluate what are normal and abnormal behaviors and how these behaviors interfere with the development of feeding capabilities and adequate nutrient intake.

Dietary Recommendations

Energy. Children with developmental disabilities have varied kilocalorie needs. Children with Down syndrome, spastic cerebral palsy, Prader-Willi syndrome, myelomeningocele, and other disorders that limit activity usually have decreased energy needs, and obesity is a common problem. Children with hyperactivity, hypertonia, and athetoid cerebral palsy frequently have greatly increased requirements for kilocalories. Generally, caloric recommendations based on height or height-age are more appropriate than those based on age or weight alone.[1] In addition, the stage of sexual maturation of the older child should be considered because some of these children undergo early pubescence and others undergo delayed puberty. Tanner's stages of maturity and their effect on caloric requirements are discussed in *Obesity,* page 184. The guidelines in Table 8–16 are useful for making an initial estimate of caloric need. Any estimate of caloric need must be individualized, however, and must have periodic follow-up to assess growth progress and possible need for dietary change.

TABLE 8–16 Guidelines for Estimating Caloric Requirements in Children with Developmental Disabilities

Condition	Caloric Recommendation
Ambulatory, ages 5 to 12 years	13.9 Kcal/cm height
Nonambulatory, ages 5 to 12 years	11.1 Kcal/cm height[11]
Cerebral palsy with decreased levels of activity	10 Kcal/cm height
Cerebral palsy with normal or increased levels of activity	15 Kcal/cm height
Athetoid cerebral palsy, adolescence	Up to 6,000 Kcal[1,12]
Down syndrome, boys ages 5 to 12 years	16.1 Kcal/cm height
Down syndrome, girls ages 5 to 12 years	14.3 Kcal/cm height[13]
Myelomeningocele	Approximately 50% of RDA for age after infancy. May need as little as 7 Kcal/cm height[14]

Protein. Protein requirements are thought to be the same as for normal children of the same height-age.

Fluids. The developmentally delayed child may not be able to respond to thirst or to express a need to drink. Some children may not be able to adequately close their lips to hold and swallow liquids easily. These children are at risk for dehydration and constipation. Thickened fluids, such as milkshakes, sherbet, gelatin, and soups, may be helpful to assure adequate fluid intake.

Fiber. Many developmentally delayed children cannot chew raw or fibrous foods. Lack of fiber in the diet, coupled with low fluid intake and immobility, frequently results in constipation. In addition, diets that consist primarily of dairy-based supplements, rather than a well-balanced diet, may result in constipation. Unprocessed bran, which can be soaked or cooked in a liquid, whole grain cereals, and prunes or prune juice may help prevent constipation.[8] (See *Constipation and Encopresis,* page 345, for further discussion of dietary recommendations.)

Nutrient-Drug Interactions. Drug therapy is frequently used in the treatment of children with developmental or behavioral problems or seizures and may affect nutritional requirements. Anticonvulsants may increase the requirements for folic acid, vitamin B_{12}, and D and may affect bone and dental health. Supplementation, however, should not be given routinely, but rather individualized based on biochemical and/or radiologic data with frequent review and adjustments. Central nervous system stimulants can result in appetite suppression and decreased growth. Growth rate of children on these drugs should be monitored frequently. Steroids can cause increased appetite and obesity.[10]

Nutrition Education. Nutrition education of parents, caretakers, and the child, if possible, should be anticipatory and preventive in focus. The diet should be palatable and as close to normal as possible in terms of texture, taste, and variety. Eating is frequently one of the few pleasures in the life of a severely disabled child. In addition, it is easier to teach proper feeding behaviors than to try to change bad habits. Education should include feeding methods, food preparation, nutritional needs, and special diets when appropriate. It requires a team effort that includes the dietitian, physician, nurse, and occupational, speech, and physical therapists. Due to the prevalence of psychosocial feeding problems among handicapped children, parents and caretakers need to be educated about normal feeding behaviors and appropriate strategies to prevent or to resolve feeding problems.[10] Inability to recognize developmental readiness to acquire new skills can result in failure to provide the child with appropriate stimuli.[1,3,15] For example, failure to progress from pureed foods to a more textured diet at the appropriate time may result in the child refusing lumpy foods at a later date. In addition, limited expectations for the developmentally delayed child can affect how the caretaker interacts with the child during feeding and can therefore hinder development of full capabilities. Whenever possible, the child should be taught adequate food selection by good role modeling, particularly if the child is to be largely responsible for his or her own food selection.

Obesity prevention should be discussed with caretakers or parents of children. Ideally, this education should begin, for parents of a child with myelomeningocele, during the first hospitalization to close the spinal cord defect. When the infant's weight-for-height exceeds the 75th percentile, parents should be advised to limit high kilocalorie, low nutrient-dense foods in order to slow the rate of weight gain.[10] Children with Down syndrome are also at risk for obesity, and parents or caretakers should be educated regarding obesity prevention at the first signs of inappropriate weight gain.

REFERENCES

1. Pipes PL, Pritkin R. Nutrition and feeding of children with developmental delays and related problems. In: Pipes PL, ed. Nutrition in infancy and childhood. St Louis: Times/Mirror/Mosby College Publishing, 1985:347.
2. Garn SM, Weir HF. Assessing the nutritional status of the mentally retarded. Am J Clin Nutr 1971;24:853–854.
3. Zeman FJ. Nutrition in handicapping conditions. In: Zeman FJ, ed. Clinical nutrition and dietetics. New York: Macmillan, 1983:595.
4. Cronk CE. Growth of children with Down's syndrome: birth to age 3 years. Pediatrics 1978;61:564–568.
5. Cronk CE. Personal communication.
6. Ekvall S. Assessment of nutritional status. In: Palmer S, Ekvall S, eds. Pediatric nutrition in developmental disorders. Springfield, IL: Charles C. Thomas, 1978:502.
7. Rast J, Ellinge-Allen JA, Johnston JM. Dietary management of rumination: four case studies. Am J Clin Nutr 1985;42:95–101.
8. Smith MAH. Guides for nutritional assessment of the mentally retarded and the developmentally disabled. Memphis: The Child Development Center, University of Tennessee Center for Health Science, 1976.

9. Howard RB. Nutritional support of the developmentally delayed child. In: Suskind RM, ed. Textbook of pediatric nutrition. New York: Raven Press, 1981:577.

10. Krick J, VanDuyn MS. The relationship between oral-motor involvement and growth: a pilot study in a pediatric population with cerebral palsy. J Am Diet Assoc 1984;84:555–559.

11. American Dietetic Association. Infant and child nutrition: concerns regarding the developmentally disabled. J Am Diet Assoc 1981;78:443–449.

12. Culley W, Middleton T. Caloric requirements of mentally retarded children with and without motor dysfunction. J Pediatr 1969;75:380–384.

13. Palmer S. Cerebral palsy. In: Palmer S, Ekvall S, eds. Pediatric nutrition in developmental disorders. Springfield, IL: Charles C. Thomas, 1978:42.

14. Culley WJ, Goyak K, Jolly DH, Mertz ET. The caloric intake of children with Down's syndrome (mongalism). J Pediatr 1965;66:772–776.

15. Llenado M, Grogan C. Myelomeningocele. In: Palmer S, Ekvall S, eds. Pediatric nutrition in developmental disorders. Springfield IL: Charles C. Thomas, 1978:55.

16. Rice BL. Nutritional problems of developmentally disabled children. Pediatr Nurs 1981; (Sept/Oct):15–18.

FAILURE TO THRIVE

Failure-to-thrive is a term used to describe physical growth failure in infants and young children that may be accompanied by retarded motor and social development. The etiology may be attributable to an identifiable disease process commonly called "organic," it may be psychosocial in origin and referred to as "non-organic," or multiple etiologies may be present.

Numerous guidelines have been proposed to define failure-to-thrive. Fomon defines it as a rate of gain in length and/or weight less than two standard deviations below the mean for at least 56 days in infants under 5 months of age or for at least 3 months in older infants.[1] Other criteria used to define failure-to-thrive utilize the NCHS Growth Curves (see *Pediatric Appendices 4 and 5*, pages 480 to 494) and include the following:

1. Weight less than 80 percent of the 50th percentile for age[2]
2. Weight less than the 3rd percentile of the NCHS growth curve[2]
3. A drop of two or more percentile ranks in weight/height[2]
4. Weight/height less than 80 percent on a calculation of:[3]

$$\%\text{wt/ht} = \frac{\text{actual weight}}{\text{median wt for ht-age}} \times 100$$

5. $\dfrac{\text{Height-age}^4}{\text{Chronologic age}}$ of less than 0.8

Growth deficits are usually manifested in weight first, then height, and, finally, head circumference.

Common organic etiologies that either increase nutritional requirements or result in diminished intake or excessive losses of kilocalories include congenital heart disease,[5] gastrointestinal disorders,[6] cystic fibrosis, central nervous system disturbances, and, rarely, endocrine disorders.[7] Children with renal disease[8] or with constitutional short stature also may present as failure-to-thrive. A detailed patient, family, and growth history, physical examination, and nutritional history frequently can rule out obvious organic causes. Children with non-organic failure-to-thrive may exhibit physical symptoms associated with feeding, such as vomiting, foul-smelling stools, diarrhea, poor appetite, falling asleep during feeding, and rumination.

In cases without obvious organic etiology, a feeding trial that provides adequate kilocalories is usually initiated either on an outpatient or inpatient basis. Organic etiologies may be investigated after failure of the feeding trial or simultaneously, provided the diagnostic procedures do not interfere with the feeding trial.

Dietary Recommendations

Nutrition Assessment. A detailed nutrition history taken from the child's parents or caretakers should include a recent or prospective dietary food intake record and a history of food intake that includes whether the child was breast or bottle fed, types of formulas given, when solids were introduced, and age at weaning. The nutrition history should also include eating patterns and habits, food allergies, excessive losses of food via vomiting or diarrhea, food likes and dislikes, family eating patterns, and how the family views the feeding behaviors and problems. The food intake record should be evaluated for adequacy of kilocalories, protein, and other key nutrients for which suspected deficiencies might exist. In cases of suspected inadequate or inappropriate offering of feedings, the diet history may not be reliable, and hospitalization is usually warranted. The practitioner should unobtrusively observe the parents while they are feeding the child.

Anthropometric procedures performed with care are essential and include, at a minimum, height or length, weight, and head circumference (in infants). Measurements should be plotted over time on the NCHS growth curve.

Feeding Trial. A feeding trial of adequate kilocalories is initiated to determine the etiology of the failure-to-thrive when there are no obvious organic causes. On an outpatient basis, the parents are instructed in the amount, type, and frequency of feedings to be given and on how to keep a food diary. Close follow-up to evaluate growth progress and dietary intake is conducted by the physician and the dietitian. In the hospital, daily kilocalories and protein intake, weight, feeding frequency and duration, special techniques required to feed, and losses from vomiting or diarrhea are recorded. The diet offered should be appropriate for the child's developmental age and should be as close to his home diet, in terms of types of food, as possible. The patient is initially fed amounts as desired on a regular schedule. If the intake is not adequate, further steps are taken to increase intake, such as increasing the caloric density of the feedings and more frequent feedings.

There are many differences of opinion in the literature as to what constitutes an adequate caloric intake for the child recovering from failure-to-thrive. Recommendations range from caloric levels that are adequate to promote normal rates of growth in most healthy infants of similar age[1] to caloric levels that are 50 percent higher than normal for age.[9] An initial caloric goal that is based on the Recommended Dietary Allowances for the patient's height-age (age at which the child's height is at the 50th percentile of the NCHS growth curve) and weight is usually adequate to produce weight gain in the child who does not have increased energy requirements or excessive losses. Weight gain can be expected to begin in 2 to 17 days in infants less than 6 months. The lag time is greater for older infants and children.[3,10]

Evaluation of feeding trials result in three classifications.

1. *Adequate intake with weight gain.* Many factors affect weight gain in relation to energy intake, even in the normal healthy infant. However, some

guidelines are available to evaluate whether the weight gain is appropriate for the energy intake. In the first 6 months of life, the average weight gain per unit of energy intake is estimated to be 3.6 g per 100 Kcal. It is about 1.4 g per 100 Kcal in the second 6 months.[3]

This classification suggests psychosocial and/or environmental problems. The parents are then instructed in how to provide adequate nutrition for their child and are encouraged to come to the hospital or the clinic to feed the child under supervision of the nursing staff. Parent and child interactions are recorded and used to further educate the parents.

2. *Adequate intake with no weight gain.* Increase caloric intake to that estimated for catch-up growth, and/or investigate for non-organic etiologies of the failure-to-thrive.

3. *Inadequate intake with no weight gain.* Investigate whether the poor intake is attributable to poor feeding techniques, to the use of inappropriate foods, or to specific mechanical or neuromotor dysfunction.

Catch-up Growth. The diet should be increased to provide for catch-up growth once weight gain is established. Catch-up growth requires kilocalories and protein far in excess of those normal for age. Peterson et al[2] have formulated the following method of estimating caloric and protein requirements for catch-up growth.

1. Plot height and weight on NCHS growth curves. (See *Pediatric Appendices* pages 480–494).

2. Determine weight-age (age at which present weight is at the 50th percentile).

3. Determine ideal weight (50th percentile for present age).

4. Calculate:

$$\frac{\text{Predicted Kcal/kg}}{\text{for catch-up growth}} = \frac{(\text{RDA Kcal/kg for wt-age}) \times (\text{ideal wt in kg})}{\text{actual wt in kg}}$$

5. Repeat the process to determine protein catch-up requirements.

Ellerstein and Ostrov[10] have developed the concept of "growth quotient" (GQ) to evaluate the patient's rate of growth. The GQ can be used to determine if catch-up growth is occurring.

$$GQ = \frac{\text{mean daily wt gain (over a specified time)}}{\text{normal daily wt gain for age}}$$

NCHS growth charts (see *Pediatric Appendices* pages 480 to 494) or incremental growth normal tables[11] can be used to determine normal weight increments for age. A GQ of 1.00 represents average growth rate. This expression of growth rate is especially helpful in the evaluation of catch-up growth in older children recovering from failure-to-thrive whose actual weight gains appear small.[10]

Patient Education and Follow-up. In the outpatient setting, parent education should begin as soon as the diagnosis is made. Appropriate community resources should be contacted, and close follow-up should be arranged. For the hospitalized child, parent education should be initiated by the health care team while the patient is in the hospital. The dietitian educates the parents as to what the child's nutritional needs are and how to provide them. The parents need to be advised that their child's appearance will change dramatically with catch-up growth. The child may even appear fat at first, but the child's weight for height should normalize with time. Frequently, the caloric density of the food needs to be increased because most children have a limited capacity for volume of food. Specific instructions should be given to the parents. A nutrition care referral should be sent to the public health nutritionist or the outpatient dietitian.

REFERENCES

1. Fomon SJ. Infant nutrition. 2nd ed. Philadelphia: WB Saunders, 1974:81.
2. Peterson KE, Washington J, Rathbun J. Team management of failure-to-thrive. J Am Diet Assoc 1984;84:810–815.
3. Kien CL. Failure-to-thrive. In: Walker WA, Watkins JB, eds. Nutrition in pediatrics: basic science and clinical application. Boston: Little, Brown and Company, 1985:757.
4. Fiser RH, Meredith PD, Elders MJ. The child who fails to grow. Am Family Phys 1975;11:108–119.
5. Ehlers KH. Growth failure in association with congenital heart disease. Pediatr Ann 1978;7:35–57.
6. Lavy U, Bauer CH. Pathophysiology of failure-to-thrive in gastrointestinal disorders. Pediatr Ann 1978;7:20–33.
7. Abrams CA. Endocrinologic aspects of failure-to-thrive. Pediatr Ann 1978;7:58–72.
8. Friedman J, Lewy JE. Failure-to-thrive associated with renal disease. Pediatr Ann 1978;7:73–82.
9. Whitten CF, Pettit MG, Fischhoff J. Evidence that growth failure from maternal deprivation is secondary to undereating. JAMA 1969;209:1675–1682.
10. Ellerstein NS, Ostrov BE. Growth patterns in children hospitalized because of caloric-deprivation failure to thrive. Am J Dis Child 1985;139:164–166.
11. Baumgartner RN, Roche AF, Himes JH. Incremental growth tables: supplementary to previously published chart. Am J Clin Nutr 1986;43:711–722.

LOW BIRTH WEIGHT INFANT

General Description

All infants of low birth weight (less than 2,500 g) are not alike. Infants who are normally grown, but premature, differ from infants who are malnourished in utero and gestationally more mature. Generally, the smaller and/or more malnourished the infant at birth, the greater the nutritional requirements in the early months of life. The nutritional requirements of similar size infants in the two groups are usually considered to be similar, except for perhaps kilocalories, but their ability to feed and their feeding tolerance may vary considerably. More mature infants who are small may be able to suck and to swallow feedings on their own, whereas premature infants who are less than 34 weeks of gestation usually cannot. Small-for-date infants are at greater risk for hypoglycemia in the early days after birth since they have virtually no glycogen stores, and they usually require more kilocalories for growth than their age-matched counterparts.[1] Very-low-birth-weight (VLBW) infants of less than 1,200 g and sick larger infants may need special nutritional support that combines parenteral and enteral nutrition, regardless of their gestational age.

Nutritional Considerations

Much remains unknown about the nutritional requirements of premature infants. A useful, though arbitrary, goal of nutritional care is the maintenance of in-utero growth rates and body composition while maintaining homeostasis. This goal is rarely achievable in practice due to the preterm infant's immature organ systems, but it remains a standard against which to measure the nutritional care of the infant. Babson[2] has published growth curves based on the growth of healthy premature infants from birth to 12 months from term (see *Pediatric Nutritional Assessment* page 287 and Appendix 8, page 504). The growth curves can be used to evaluate the premature infant's progress in terms of both rate of increments in height, weight, and head circumference and rate of growth in a parameter compared to other parameters. The nutritional goal for small-for-date infants is to provide for catch-up growth to reach their growth potential as quickly as possible.[3]

Nutritional requirements are believed to be higher for the low-birth-weight infant than for the healthy term infant for many reasons, including fewer nutrient reserves, less efficient absorption and utilization of nutrients, greater losses of nutrients, and their rapid growth rate.[1] Actual requirements for most nutrients remain unknown, but useful estimates have been proposed from the research data available.

Goals of Dietary Management

Kilocalories. Estimates of caloric requirements are approximately 50 kilocalories per kilogram per day for basal expenditures plus 70 to 75 kilocalories per kilogram per day for activity, specific dynamic action, fecal loss, cold stress, and growth.[4] We have generally found that healthy low-birth-weight infants gain an average of 20 to 30 g per day on intakes of 120 to 130 kilocalories per kilogram per day. Chronic bronchopulmonary dysplasia, congenital heart defects, frequent seizure activity, and intrauterine growth retardation may greatly increase caloric requirements.

Enteral Nutrition Requirements. Estimates of requirements and advisable intakes for protein and major minerals and electrolytes calculated by a factorial method based on the composition of fetal weight gain in the third trimester with adjustments for dermal and urinary losses, intestinal absorption, and growth have been published by Ziegler et al.[5] and are summarized in Table 8–17.

TABLE 8–17 Advisable Enteral Intakes

Nutrient	800–1,200 g Infant (per kg/day)	1,200–1,800 g Infant (per kg/day)
Protein (g)	4	3.5
Sodium (mEq)	3.5	3
Potassium (mEq)	2.5	2.3
Chloride (mEq)	3.1	2.5
Calcium (mg)	210	185
Phosphorus (mg)	140	123
Magnesium (mg)	10	8.5

Protein. Protein quality, as well as quantity, requires consideration when feedings for the premature infant are planned. In addition to the eight amino acids known to be essential to adults, histidine, tyrosine, cystine, and taurine may be essential to premature infants because of the infants' immature enzyme systems.[5] Whey predominant protein appears to result in fewer serum amino acid disturbances,[6] less risk of late metabolic acidosis,[4] and greater efficiency of nitrogen retention.[7] Whey protein eliminates the risk of lactobezoar formation when compared to casein predominant milk protein.[8]

Fat. The premature infant is at risk for the development of essential fatty acid deficiency as soon as 5 to 8 days after birth due to low endogenous reserves at birth.[9] As early as possible after birth at least 3 percent of the caloric intake should be provided by linoleic acid. However, large amounts of polyunsaturated fats should be avoided because they cause an increase in Vitamin E requirement. Long chain saturated fats are not well absorbed by the premature infant's gut. Medium chain triglycerides are better absorbed, presumably because they are not dependent on duodenal intraluminal bile salts, which are inadequate in the premature infant. Human milk fat, though mainly saturated, is well absorbed due to its unique triglyceride configuration and to the presence of bile salt-activated lipase in the milk.[4] Fat usually comprises approximately 50 percent of the energy intake for the premature infant.[4]

Carbohydrate. Lactose may not be efficiently absorbed in the early days of postnatal life since lactase activity does not mature until near term. Glycosidases, which facilitate the absorption of glucose polymers, are active in even the very premature infant's gut. Thus, glucose polymers are absorbed well and offer an additional advantage of adding less osmotic load to the feeding than lactose or monosaccharides.[4]

Minerals. Two thirds of fetal bone mineralization takes place in the last trimester of pregnancy. Bone mineral content is low in both premature and small-for-date infants, even at term.[10] The fetal accretion rates and the advisable intakes (see Table 8–17) to achieve those rates for calcium and phosphorus are approximately four and five times higher, respectively, than is provided by human milk. Adequate vitamin D is also necessary for good bone mineralization and growth after birth. Deficiencies of vitamin D, calcium, and phosphorus have been associated with osteopenia, rickets, and decreased bone mineral content in these infants.[6] In order to assure adequate bone growth and mineralization in these infants, close attention should be given to the provision of the levels of calcium and phosphorus that are estimated to achieve fetal accretion rates and to the provision of adequate vitamin D, as suggested by Ziegler.[5]

Vitamins and Trace Elements. Nutritional requirements for vitamins and for trace elements remain largely undefined for premature infants. Advisable intakes based on current data have been published by Ziegler,[5] by the American Academy of Pediatrics Committee on Nutrition (AAP),[4] and by Tsang et al.[11] For most nutrients, the levels recommended are the same as those for term infants, except for greater amounts for vitamins D, E, C, folic acid, zinc, copper, and iron. Recommendations for those nutrients are compared in Table 8–18.

The requirement for vitamin E increases with the amount of polyunsaturated fatty acid and iron in the diet. The premature infant is born relatively deficient in vitamin E and is at risk for subsequent hemolytic anemia. While the need for vitamin E supplementation is generally agreed upon, the amount recommended varies from 5 to 30 International Units (IU) or more per day.[4–6,11–14] A vitamin E to polyunsaturated fatty acid ratio of at least 1 should be maintained to prevent hemolytic anemia in the premature infant.[4] In addition, the use of pharmacologic doses of vitamin E to reduce the severity of retrolental fibroplasia and of bronchopulmonary dysplasia is the subject of much controversy and research.[15,16] While the data are yet inconclusive, it seems de-

TABLE 8–18 Advisable Daily Intakes for Selected Vitamins and Trace Elements for Low-birth-weight Infants

Nutrient	Ziegler[5]	AAP[4]	Tsang[11]
Vitamin D (IU)	600	500	400
Vitamin E (IU)	30	5 to 25 0.7/100 Kcal 1 E/g linoleic acid	25 for 2 to 4 wk, then 5
Vitamin C (mg)	60	35	35
Folic Acid (μg)	60	50	65
Copper (μg)	60/100 Kcal	90/100 Kcal	100 to 200/kg
Zinc (mg)	0.5/100 Kcal	0.5/100 Kcal	0.8 to 1.2/kg
Iron (mg)	2 to 3/kg (begin at 2 wk)	2 to 3/kg (begin at 1 to 2 mo)	2/kg (begin when birth weight doubled)

sirable to provide sufficient vitamin E from birth to raise the infant's serum level to normal as quickly as possible and to maintain that level.

Negative balances of zinc and copper among premature infants in the early weeks of life[4] and reports of late deficiencies of these two trace elements have raised concern over what the requirements for these nutrients are in these infants.[16] Current recommendations range from approximately 0.6 to 1.2 mg per kilogram per day for zinc and 70 to 200 μg per kilogram per day for copper.[4,5,11]

The low-birth-weight infant is at risk for the development of iron deficiency anemia due to relatively low iron stores at birth, rapid growth rate, and diagnostic phlebotomies. However, iron is not utilized for hemoglobin synthesis in the early weeks of life and the administration of iron may predispose the infant to vitamin E deficient hemolytic anemia.[4,8] Provision of 2 to 3 mg per kilogram per day of ferrous iron, beginning at approximately 1 month of age and continuing until 1 year of age, appears safe and aids in establishing adequate iron reserves in the premature infant.[4]

Provision of adequate nutrition for the low-birth-weight infant requires careful selection of the type of feeding to be given and monitoring for adequacy of nutrient intake. Supplements of 400 IU of vitamin D and 25 IU of vitamin E are usually given until the infant reaches 2 kg. Other nutrients may need to be supplemented as well, depending on the nutrient content of the feeding given. The nutritional requirements of premature infants is just beginning to be understood. Thus, nutrition feeding programs and protocols need to be frequently updated and revised.

Enteral Feedings

Human Milk. Whenever possible, mothers of low-birth-weight infants should be encouraged to breast feed. The advantages of human milk include its anti-infection factors, the improved absorption of fat, a more desirable protein composition, a low renal solute load, the presence of epidermal growth factor, and the psychological benefit to the mother and infant.[6]

There is, however, controversy about whether human milk alone is adequate for premature infants, particularly those less than 1,500 g at birth. Protein levels in human milk generally have been considered too low to support adequate growth. Recent studies have shown that the milk of mothers of preterm infants is slightly higher in protein than that of mothers of term infants,[6] but it falls rapidly during the first weeks of lactation. The greater concentration of protein in the milk of mothers of preterm infants may only be a function of the smaller volume of milk produced by these mothers.[17] Studies comparing sodium, chloride, magnesium, and caloric content of milk of mothers of term and of preterm infants have produced variable results.[6] Calcium and phosphorus levels are the same in milk of mothers of preterm and of term infants and are not considered adequate for the preterm infant. Bone fractures, rickets, and decreased bone mineral content have been seen in premature infants fed breast milk exclusively.[4,6,16] Supplementation with calcium, phosphorus, and vitamin D is warranted, particularly for the breast fed very-low-birth-weight infant.

Whether or not human milk can result in adequate growth in the premature infant is also a topic of controversy. Most researchers agree that pooled milk of mothers of term infants is not adequate for the preterm infant and should not be used. Studies by Gross[18] and others[6] have shown that adequate growth can be achieved by using the milk from the infant's own mother. However, many preterm infants cannot tolerate sufficient volumes of human milk for growth and require caloric supplementation of the milk. Considering all the possible inadequacies of human milk, even from the preterm infant's own mother, we choose to supplement the milk with one of two commercially available human milk supplements until the infant reaches 2 kg (see *Infant Formulas and Feedings,* page 458).

Formulas. Special formulas designed to meet the expected nutritional needs of low-birth-weight infants have been developed. These formulas provide greater concentrations of certain nutrients in more readily absorbable forms than standard formulas for term infants. In these formulas, the protein is predominantly whey, fat content is part long chain fatty acids and part medium chain triglycerides, and carbohydrate is part lactose and part glucose polymers. Calcium and phosphorus content is designed to achieve bone intrauterine accretion rates in the infant. The exact composition of the formulas varies and should be supplemented with nutrients as needed. (See *Infant Formulas and Feedings,* page 458, or manufacturers information). Higher caloric concentrations are available to enable the infant to consume adequate calories in limited fluid volumes. We have found that most infants who weigh less than 2,000 g need formula concentrations of at least 24 kilocalories per ounce for adequate growth without excess fluid intake.

The use of soy-protein formulas in feeding premature infants has been associated with lower nitrogen retention, lower phosphorus levels, osteoporosis, and rickets. These formulas are not advisable, except for specific therapeutic indications, and then should not be used for more than 3 to 4 weeks.[19]

Feeding Process. The immaturity of the gastrointestinal tract and the limited ability of other organ systems to metabolize and excrete nutrients and waste products present many challenges to the provision of adequate nutrition for the low-birth-weight infant. Establishment of adequate enteral nutrition is hindered by the small stomach capacity, slow gastrointestinal motility, immature enzyme systems of the gastrointestinal tract, as well as risk of development of necrotizing enterocolitis.

As discussed, small-for-date infants are different from premature infants with regard to feeding. The more mature infant who is small for gestational age usually feeds more vigorously and more actively than the gestationally immature infant and requires less special support, particularly at weights above 1,800 g. Small and/or immature infants usually do not suck and swallow well enough to meet their nutritional needs and require continuous or intermittent orogastric or oroduodenal tube feedings. If the low-birth-weight infant is well and free of respiratory distress, the first feedings are begun within 4 to 6 hours of birth. Enteral feedings should be introduced slowly, according to tolerance. Feedings should begin with sterile water or, if available, maternal colostrum, then advance to half strength formula or human milk, and, finally, to full strength. Volume of the feedings is increased gradually over 7 to 10 days to achieve approximately 120 to 130 kilocalories per kilogram per day. After 1 week of well-tolerated enteral feedings, the infant who weighs less than 2,000 g is advanced to premature infant formulas that are concentrated to 24 kilocalories per ounce, or one of the commercially available human milk supplements is added to the breast milk from the premature infant's mother. Bottle or breast feeding is introduced gradually as tolerated by the infant.

A 2 kg infant is usually able to ingest and to tolerate sufficient quantities of human milk or regular infant formula for growth. A multivitamin supplement that provides the equivalent of the Recommended Dietary Allowances for term infants is advisable, at least until the infant is consuming 300 kilocalories per day.[20]

Parenteral Nutrition

Parenteral nutrition that supplies all or part of the nutritional needs may be necessary to nourish the very-low-birth-weight or the sick infant. The solutions and nutrient levels chosen should be designed to meet, as nearly as possible, the special needs of the premature infant. The references on page 335 (in the chapter *Sick Infants, Children, and Adolescents*) may be helpful.

REFERENCES

1. Rickard K, Gresham E. Nutritional considerations for the newborn requiring intensive care. J Am Diet Assoc 1985;66:592–599.
2. Babson G, Benda GI. Growth graphs for the clinical assessment of infants of varying gestational age. J Pediatr 1976;89:814–820.
3. Georgieff MK, Hoffman JS, Pereira GR, Bernbaum J, Hoffman-Williamson M. Effect of neonatal caloric deprivation of head growth and one-year developmental status in preterm infants. J Pediatr 1985;107:581–587.
4. Committee on Nutrition, American Academy of Pediatrics. Nutritional needs of low-birth-weight infants. Pediatrics 1985;75:976–986.
5. Ziegler EE, Biga RL, Fomon SJ. Nutritional requirements of the premature infant. In: Suskind RM, ed. Textbook of pediatric nutrition. New York: Raven Press, 1981:29.
6. Reynolds JW. Nutrition of the low-birth-weight infant. In: Walker WA, Watkins JB, eds. Nutrition pediatrics. Boston: Little, Brown and Company, 1985:649.
7. Darling P, Lepage G, Tremblay P, Collet S, Kien LC, Roy CC. Protein quality and quantity in preterm infants receiving the same energy intake. Am J Dis Child 1985;139:186–190.
8. Brady MS, Rickard KA, Ernest JA, Schreiner RL, Lemons JA. Formulas and human milk for premature infants: a review and update. J Am Diet Assoc 1982;81:547–555.
9. Development of essential fatty acid deficiency in the premature infant given fat-free TPN. Nutr Rev 1985;43:14–15.
10. Minton SD, Steichen JJ, Tsang RC. Decreased bone mineral content in small-for-gestational-age infants compared with appropriate-for-gestational-age infants: normal serum 25-hydroxyvitamin D and decreasing parathyroid hormone. Pediatrics 1983;71:383–388.

11. Tsang RC, ed. Vitamin and mineral requirements in preterm infants. New York: Marcel Dekker, 1985.
12. Ehrenkranz RA. Vitamin E and the neonate. Am J Dis Child 1980;134:1157–1165.
13. Bell EF, Filer LJ. The role of vitamin E in the nutrition of premature infants. Am J Clin Nutr 1981;34:414–422.
14. Committee on Fetus and Newborn. Vitamin E and prevention of retinopathy of prematurity. Pediatrics 1985;76:315–316.
15. Hittner HM, Godio LB, Rudolph AJ, et al. Retrolental fibroplasia efficacy of vitamin E in a double blind chemical study of preterm infants. N Engl J Med 1981;305:1365–1371.
16. Ziegler EE. Infants of low birth weight: special needs and problems. Am J Clin Nutr 1985;41:440–446.
17. Anderson DM, Williams FH, Merkatz RB, Schulman PK, Kerr DS, Pittard WB. Length of gestation and nutritional composition of human milk. Am J Clin Nutr 1983;37:810–814.
18. Gross SJ. Growth and biochemical response of preterm infants fed human milk or modified infant formula. N Engl J Med 1983;308:237–241.
19. Committee on Nutrition. Soy-protein formulas: recommendations for use in infant feeding. Pediatrics 1983;72:359–363.
20. American Academy of Pediatrics, Committee on Nutrition. Vitamin and mineral supplement needs in normal children in the United States. Pediatrics 1980;66:1015–1021.

SICK INFANTS, CHILDREN, AND ADOLESCENTS

General Description

The impact of illness on the nutritional requirements of children is extremely variable and also varies during the course of an illness. In pediatric patients, the special nutritional requirements of the disease are superimposed on relatively high requirements for growth and limited endogenous reserves.[1] The nutritional goals for short-term acute illnesses include the prevention of significant losses of nutrients and the facilitation of recovery of body mass from losses caused by illness or trauma. Catch-up growth occurs in the days following the acute illness, provided adequate nutrition is available. The goal of nutritional care with chronic disease is to provide adequate kilocalories and nutrients for growth in addition to the kilocalories and nutrients needed to replace losses or to meet increased requirements due to the disease.

In addition to the parameters discussed in the section *Pediatric Nutritional Assessment* (pages 287 to 293), consideration should be given to the nature and severity of the illness or trauma and to the ability of the child to take in adequate nutrition by oral, enteral, parenteral, or any combination of these methods. In addition, there must be ongoing frequent re-evaluation of the nutritional status of the patient and the care plan. The following discussion is limited to general nutritional considerations that are not discussed elsewhere under specific disease states.

Malnutrition can develop rapidly in a seriously ill infant or child and can affect the rate of recovery from illness or injury.[2] The initial goal of nutrition for the acutely ill pediatric patient is to minimize protein losses and to meet the metabolic requirements of the brain for glucose by the provision of protein-sparing carbohydrate, either enterally or parenterally. How soon such therapy is instituted depends on the size of the child and on whether protein-sharing carbohydrate has been given from the onset of the illness or trauma (Table 8–19).

TABLE 8–19 Maximum Number of Days to Start Full Nutritional Support* (Assuming carbohydrate has been administered from the start of the illness or trauma)

Size of Child	Days
Term Infant	4
10 kg child	5
30 kg child	8
50 kg child	15

* Adapted from: Seashore JH. Nutritional support of children in the intensive care unit. Yale J Biol 1984;57:111–134.

Full nutritional support should be started promptly for children who have lost weight prior to the illness or whose metabolic requirements are increased by the disease.[3]

Nutritional Considerations

Energy Needs. The energy recommendations of the National Research Council for children are designed for normal healthy growing children and include a substantial allowance for activity. Activity is decreased with illness, but increased energy needs are imposed by the illness. Trauma (operative or accidental), thermal injury, sepsis with or without fever, and congenital heart disease all result in various degrees of hypermetabolism.[4] Increased requirements may be offset by decreases in needs in some cases, so that the recommended dietary allowance for energy for age may be appropriate. Guidelines to meet the maintenance energy needs of the ill child are presented in Table 8–20.[5] Other formulas for estimating energy needs during illness, which may be more accurate, have been proposed. However, it is important to remember that there is a paucity of data regarding the metabolic response of the child to illness or trauma, and that much of the information is extrapolated from adult research data.

TABLE 8–20 Maintenance or Hospital Energy Requirements for Children

Weight	Energy Requirements
3–10 kg	100 Kcal/kg
11–20 kg	1,000 Kcal + 100 kcal/2kg > 10 kg
>20 kg	1,500 Kcal + 100 kcal/5 kg > 20 kg

Seashore has published guidelines to estimate energy requirements based on a formula for basal metabolic rate that does not rely on calculation of body surface area and includes adjustments for activity, illness, and growth.[3] The formula for basal metabolic rate (BMR) is:

$$BMR (Kcal/day) = (55 - 2 \times age\ in\ years) \times weight\ in\ kg$$

This formula can be used for children who are between the 10th and 90th percentiles for weight. For under- or overweight children, weight-age should be used (see *Pediatric Nutritional Assessment*, page 287), rather than chronologic age. Table 8–21 presents guidelines for the estimation of total daily energy needs.

Another method for estimating the energy needs of the sick child uses the *Nomogram for Estimation of Basal Caloric Requirements (Appendix 6)* and Wilmore's Scale for Estimating Energy Requirements for Illness (Fig. 8–1).[6]

TABLE 8–21 Estimation of Energy Requirements*

	Add
BMR: (55 − 2 × age) × kg =	_____
Maintenance: 20% × basal = (Includes specific dynamic action and amount of energy needed for equilibrium in the resting but awake state with minimal muscular movements).	_____
Activity: 0 to 25% × basal = (0% for comatose state, 25% for hospitalized child who ambulates 2 to 3 times a day, 50% for active non-hospitalized child).	_____
Sepsis: 13% for each 1°C above normal × basal =	_____
Simple Trauma: 20% × basal =	_____
Multiple Injuries: 40% × basal =	_____
Burns: 50 to 100% × basal =	_____
Growth and Anabolism: 50 to 100% × basal = (100% for growth in infancy and adolescence; 50% for the years in between)	_____
	TOTAL _____

*With Permission From: Seashore JH. Nutritional support of children in the intensive care unit. Yale J Biol Med 1984;57:111–134.

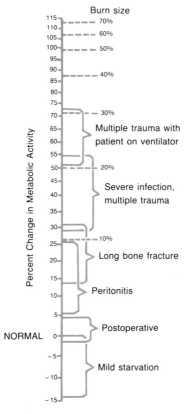

Figure 8–1 Scale for Estimating Energy Requirements for Illness[*][6]

*With Permission From: Wilmore DW. Energy and Energy Balance. In: Wilmore DW, ed. The metabolic management of the critically ill. New York: Plenum, 1977:36.

1. Determine basal metabolic energy needs from the nomogram (Columns I to V using the patient's height, weight, age, and sex).

2. Add an allowance for activity. Generally 20 to 25 percent is needed for the hospitalized child.

3. Add an allowance for illness. Determine the impact of the disease state on the basal metabolism from the scale in Figure 8–1. (Percent change in metabolic activity × BMR.)

Assessment of basal energy requirements by indirect calorimetry is warranted in situations of more long-term critical illness when a more precise estimate of energy expenditure is needed. The Harris and Benedict formula for resting energy expenditure is not appropriate for children; however, it can be used for adolescents.

Protein Needs. Protein requirements are increased by severe trauma or illness. The initial response of the body to illness or to stress is the mobilization of protein for the synthesis of proteins associated with the immune response. In addition, there is an increased metabolism of amino acids in the liver for gluconeogenesis, which results in a negative nitrogen balance.[7] Protein requirements are related to (1) the previous nutritional state of the infant or child, (2) the length and severity of the catabolic state, and (3) the amount of the extrarenal losses that may be occurring. (See *Burn* and *Inflammatory Bowel Diseases* sections, pages 338 and 421).

Protein requirements during the recovery may nearly double to 11 percent or more of the total calories.[2] Nitrogen balance can be affected by changes in either caloric or nitrogen intake.[8] A kilocalorie-to-nitrogen ratio of 150 to 250:1 (24 to 40 kilocalories per g of protein) is recommended to promote nitrogen retention in ill children.[9]

Vitamins and Mineral Needs. Provision of levels of vitamins and of minerals to meet the recommended dietary allowance for age is generally considered adequate, except when there are large losses related to specific disease states, such as burns, renal disease, and malabsorption states. Additional supplementation of the nutrients involved is discussed in those sections.

Nutritional Support

Nutritional care planning for the sick child includes determination of the child's nutritional requirements, selection of the most appropriate avenue for the delivery of the kilocalories and nutrients that are necessary to prevent nutritional depletion, and selection of the most appropriate feeding or formula.[2]

Oral Feeding. The gastrointestinal tract should be used whenever possible, preferrably by oral ingestion. High protein and/or high kilocalorie supplements added to the diet may be useful, since children are rather limited in their ability and their willingness to increase their volume of dietary intake. Small frequent feedings of familiar foods, rather than three large meals, may result in greater intake. Close follow-up of intake is necessary to evaluate the success of the nutritional care plan and to make adjustments to ensure adequate nutritional intake.

Enteral Feeding. Tube feeding, either alone or in conjunction with other avenues, may be necessary to achieve adequate intake when oral intake is inadequate. Commercially prepared formulas are preferred because of better sanitation and reliability of nutritional content. Generally, however, the nutrient contents of the enteral products available today are formulated for adults and do not fit the nutritional needs of the growing child very well. The product chosen should be evaluated for nutritional adequacy (see page 264 for nutritional content of enteral products) and appropriate supplements should be provided. Supplements of calcium and of vitamin D are frequently needed to meet the recommended dietary allowances for children. See also the section of pediatric *Enteral Nutrition,* page 450.

Parenteral Nutrition. Parenteral nutrition is appropriate only when the gastrointestinal tract cannot be used. In younger children, a parenteral nutrition solution designed for children, rather than adults, should be used. (See section on pediatric *Parenteral Nutrition,* page 458).

REFERENCES

1. Panel report on nutritional support of pediatric patients. Am J Clin Nutr 1981;34:1223–1234.
2. Merritt RJ, Blackburn GL. Nutritional assessment and metabolic response to illness of the hospitalized child. In: Suskind RM, ed. Textbook of pediatric nutrition. New York: Raven Press, 1981:285.
3. Seashore JH. Nutritional support of children in the intensive care unit. Yale J Biol Med 1984;57:111–134.
4. Kien CL. Energy metabolism and requirements in disease. In: Walker WA, Watkins JP, eds. Nutrition in pediatrics: basic science and clinical application. Boston: Little, Brown and Company, 1985;87.
5. Holliday MA, Segar WE. The maintenance need for water in parenteral fluid therapy. Pediatrics 1957;19:823–832.
6. Wilmore DW. Energy and energy balance. In: Wilmore DW, ed. The metabolic management of the critically ill. New York: Plenum, 1977:36.
7. Scrimshaw NS. Significance of the interactions of nutrition and infection in children. In: Suskind RM, ed. Textbook of pediatric nutrition. New York: Raven Press, 1981:229.
8. LeLeiko NS, Murray C, Munro HN. Enteral support of the hospitalized child. In: Suskind RM, ed. Textbook of pediatric nutrition. New York: Raven Press, 1981:357.
9. Reimer SL, Michener WM, Steiger E. Nutritional support of the critically ill child. Pediatr Clin North Am 1980;27:647–660.

NUTRITIONAL MANAGEMENT OF DISEASES AND DISORDERS

ALLERGY

General Description

Symptoms of food allergy vary among individual children. Treatment involves elimination of the offending food(s) from the diet. Nutrient deficiencies may result from this reduced variety of foods in the child's diet. Therefore, the energy and nutrient intake of the child with food allergies should be carefully monitored.

Nutritional Inadequacy

Vitamin or mineral supplements may be indicated, depending on the specific foods or groups of foods that must be eliminated from the diet. An assessment of the diet for nutritional adequacy should be done for each individual child.

Indications and Rationale

Despite the strides made in many areas of health care, much confusion still exists in the area of food allergy. This confusion may be explained first by the fact that the term "food allergy" is used indiscriminately to describe many types of adverse reactions to foods. Secondly, the problem of food allergy is complex. Finally, the diagnostic procedures and laboratory tests presently available are inadequate to account for the many clinical observations made with regard to reactions to foods.

Adverse reactions to foods and to food additives may be broadly classified into two types: immunologic reactions (food allergy) and non-immunologic reactions (food intolerance). Non-immunologic reactions may be attributable to a pharmacologic or a toxic action of the food or the result of an enzyme deficiency. Examples of food or food additive "intolerances" are lactose intolerance and reactions to tartrazine or to sulfite compounds. The exact incidence of all adverse

TABLE 8-22 Food Families and Related Food Items

Food Family	Related Foods
Apple	Apple, pear, quince
Aster	Lettuce, chicory, endive, escarole, artichoke, dandelion, sunflower seeds, tarragon
Beef	Cow's milk
Beet	Beet, spinach, chard, lamb's quarters
Bird	All fowl and game birds, including chicken, turkey, duck, goose, guinea fowl, pigeon, quail, and pheasant; eggs
Blueberry	Blueberry, huckleberry, cranberry
Buckwheat	Buckwheat, rhubarb, garden sorrel
Cashew	Cashew, pistachio, mango
Chocolate	Both white and regular chocolate, cocoa, and cola
Citrus	Orange, lemon, grapefruit, lime, tangerine, kumquat, citron
Crustacean	Crab, lobster, shrimp
Fish	All true fish, either freshwater or saltwater, including tuna, sardine, catfish, trout, and crappie
Fungus	Mushroom, yeast, molds, antibiotics
Ginger	Ginger, cardamom, turmeric
Gooseberry	Currant, gooseberry
Grape	Raisin
Grass	Wheat, corn, rice, oats, barley, rye, wild rice, cane, millet, sorghum, bamboo sprouts
Laurel	Avocado, cinnamon, bay leaves, sassafras
Mallow	Cottonseed, okra
Melon (gourd)	Watermelon, cucumber, cantaloupe, pumpkin, squash, other melons
Mollusk	Oyster, clam, abalone, mussel
Mustard	Mustard, turnip, radish, horseradish, watercress, cabbage, kraut, Chinese cabbage, broccoli, cauliflower, Brussels sprouts, collards, kale, kohlrabi, rutabaga
Myrtle	Allspice, guava, clove, pimento
Onion	Onion, garlic, asparagus, chives, leeks, sarsaparilla
Palm	Coconut, date
Parsley	Carrot, parsnip, celery, parsley, celeriac, anise, dill, fennel, angelica, celery seed, cumin, coriander, caraway
Pea	Peanuts, peas (green, field, black-eyed), beans (navy, lima, pinto, string, soybeans, etc.), licorice, acacia, tragacanth
Plum	Plum, cherry, peach, apricot, nectarine, wild cherry, almond
Potato	Potato, tomato, eggplant, peppers (including green pepper, red pepper, chili pepper, paprika, cayenne, and capsicum, but not black and white peppers)
Reptile	Turtle, rattlesnake, frog
Rose	Strawberry, raspberry, blackberry, dewberry, loganberry, youngberry, boysenberry
Walnut	English walnut, black walnut, pecan, hickory nut, butternut

reactions to foods is unknown. However, food intolerances outnumber immunologic or food allergy reactions.

Food allergy may appear at any age, but true allergic reactions to foods are most common in infants and in young children and decrease in frequency with age.[1] Allergic reactions are most commonly caused by relatively few foods, including milk, eggs, nuts, soy, wheat, and peanuts.[2-4] The causative food is called an allergen. The allergic reaction may be immediate or delayed and may affect the skin (hives, itching, eczema), the respiratory system (swelling of the throat, sneezing, coughing, wheezing, nasal stuffiness), the gastrointestinal tract (vomiting, diarrhea, cramping) and the cardiovascular system (anaphylactic shock, irregular heart beat). Symptoms of food allergy are not uniform and may change with the same food for an individual child. A child who is allergic to one food is usually allergic to food in related food families. Peanuts, for example, belong to the pea family; persons who cannot eat peanuts may not be able to eat beans or peas. They usually are able to tolerate nuts because true nuts are in a different food family. The food family list[5] is shown in Table 8–22.

Food allergies are difficult to diagnose. The diagnosis usually is made by history, by response to elimination diets, and by reintroduction of foods into the diet. Verification by allergic skin testing or by radioallergosorbent testing (RAST) may be helpful in identifying a true allergic reaction.

Goals of Dietary Management

The goal of management is to design a diet that does not include the offending food(s), but ensures the child's nutritional needs.

Dietary Recommendations

Table 8–23 summarizes the guidelines for the dietary management of food allergies. There is no standard procedure for identifying suspected food allergies in children. Offending foods can often be identified by the patient and by taking a diet history. Having the patient or parent keep a 7-day food record is helpful. This record should include not only foods eaten and avoided, but also any adverse reactions that occur each day. A diet can be devised that does not include suspected foods. To determine which of the suspected foods produces an adverse reaction, foods can be added back to the diet one at a time at 4- to 5-day intervals until an adverse reaction occurs or tolerance is shown. Food records also should be completed by the patient and monitored by the dietitian while food challenges are being done.

TABLE 8–23 Guidelines for Dietary Management of Food Allergy

Treatment Guidelines	Recommendations
Identification of allergen	Use diet history and food-symptom record
	Add suspected food(s) back to the diet at 4- to 5-day intervals to verify adverse reaction or tolerance
	Use monomeric formula followed by challenge tests in a closely supervised hospital setting when an extremely limited number of foods appear to be tolerated
Diet design	Omit offending food(s) and foods in same food families
	Suggest substitutions for foods omitted to maintain nutrient adequacy of diet

Children with multiple suspected food allergies or intolerances who appear to tolerate an extremely limited number of foods or who have food allergies or intolerances that are difficult to identify by the method already described may need to have all food eliminated. These children are given a monomeric (elemental) formula (see page 564) exclusively while they are hospitalized for a period of 7 to 10 days. Monomeric formula is used because it is hypo-allergenic. All other foods are avoided during this trial, and the child's allergy symptoms are monitored. If the symptoms resolve, suspected foods are added back to the diet in a double-blind fashion to reproduce the clinical exacerbation of allergy. Results of challenge feeding may be correlated with results of skin testing and of specific IgE antibodies. In this method, specific food allergies or intolerances usually can be identified.

Periodically, challenges with foods that are known to cause an allergic reaction should be done, since a significant number of children can tolerate the food as they grow older. Challenge with foods believed to cause anaphylactic reactions should not be done.[4]

Physicians: How to Order Diet

The diet order should indicate *elimination diet to identify food allergy(ies) and/or intolerances*. The dietitian designs and monitors the diet using the procedure described.

REFERENCES

1. Foucard T. Developmental aspects of food sensitivity in childhood. Nutr Rev 1984;42:98–104.
2. May CD. Food allergy: perspective, principles, practical management. Nutr Today 1980;Nov–Dec:28–31.
3. Sampson HA, Jolie PL. Increased plasma histamine concentrations after food challenges in children with atopic dermatitis. N Engl J Med 1984;311:372–376.
4. Forbes GB, Woodruff CW. Hypersensitivity to food. In: Forbes GB, Woodruff CW, eds. Pediatric nutrition handbook. Elk Grove, IL: American Academy of Pediatrics, 1985:257–266.
5. Rapaport HG, Linde SM. The complete allergy guide. New York: Simon & Schuster, 1970.

BURN

General Description

Adequate nutrition in the severely burned child is one of the major factors that contributes to the recovery from the burn injury. Nutritional status often determines the morbidity and the mortality of the injury. Besides the need to replace losses from the burn and to meet increased metabolic demands, the child's needs for growth and development must be met. This is particularly important for the infant, who has high nutrient needs relative to size. Infants are at risk for delay in cerebral growth and function if nutrition is inadequate for a length of time. Resistance to infection, immune response, and healing are often determined more by the nutritional status of the child than by any other factor.

Indications and Rationale

The burned child has greater caloric and protein requirements per kilogram than the burned adult. Quantitatively, hypermetabolism, the accelerated rate of tissue breakdown, and the exhaustion of body reserves that is experienced after a severe burn is greater than after any other form of injury. Negative nitrogen and caloric balance is seen with a lower percentage of body surface area burned in children than in adults. Early provision of adequate nutritional intake is essential. Failure to supply sufficient kilocalories, protein, and other nutrients to meet metabolic demands results in rapid consumption of endogenous fuel reserves with weight loss, delayed wound healing, and increased risk of septic complications. In general, energy expenditure and nitrogen loss are functions of burn injury extent, immobilization, nutritional status prior to burn injury, and ambient temperature.

Goals of Dietary Management

The goals of dietary management are to replace nutrient losses that are associated with the burn in order to correct body deficits, to provide sufficient nutrients to promote energy, nitrogen balance, and healing, and to assure normal growth.

Dietary Recommendations

Energy. During the immediate post-burn period, or "ebb phase", the metabolic rate and energy demands are decreased for a few hours to a few days. This early response is followed by the longer "flow phase," which is characterized by increased oxygen consumption, heat production, negative nitrogen balance, and weight loss. Caloric requirements after the ebb phase can be estimated:[1]

$$[(RDA \text{ for kilocalories for age}) \times (\text{kg pre-burn body weight})]$$
$$+ [(40 \text{ Kcal} \times (\% \text{ total body surface area of burn})]$$

Nutritional intervention should be initiated before the fourth day post-burn. Ideally, by the end of the first post-burn week daily caloric intake should reach appropriate levels to satisfy nutritional requirements.[2]

Limiting metabolic demands is as important as providing the child with an adequate caloric intake. A child who is upset and distressed consumes more energy, since pain, anxiety, and fear stimulate the release of catecholamines.[2] In addition, a child who is treated in a warm, dry environment requires less energy than one treated in a room that has a lower temperature and a higher humidity.

Protein. Protein needs for the burned child are higher than the protein needs of a healthy child. Nitrogen losses from the wound increase protein needs and vary with the size of the wound. Gluconeogenesis, if not readily suppressed by exogenous glucose, leads to reduced efficiency of amino acid utilization for maintenance of body protein synthesis.[3] There is evidence that high protein diets, with the emphasis on high quality protein intake, lead to improved survival in children, largely because infection is more easily controlled.[4]

Nitrogen utilization is highly dependent on adequate caloric intake. A kilocalorie-to-nitrogen ratio of 130 to 150 kilocalories to 1 g of nitrogen (21 to 24 kilocalories per gram of protein) should be provided.[2,3,5]

Few studies have been conducted to quantify the protein needs of burned children. Sutherland has reported only a small weight loss and a negative nitrogen balance of short duration when the protein intake of children whose burns were less than 50 percent of their total body surface area equaled (3 g protein per kilogram per day) + (1 g protein × percent of total body surface area of burn). Results from a Boston Shriners Burn Institute study indicate that the requirements for protein are approximately three times the recommended dietary allowance for healthy children.[3]

Vitamins and Minerals. Protein and caloric sources cannot be utilized efficiently if the intake of vitamins and minerals is inadequate. The exact requirements of burned children are not known, but levels of intake have been suggested at five times the RDA for the B vitamins, 10 times the RDA for vitamin C, and two times the RDA for fat-soluble vitamins. These levels are somewhat arbitrary, and the utilization of and the requirement for many of the essential nutrients need further investigation.[3]

In children, zinc and copper deficiencies are likely if more than 20 percent of the total body surface has been burned. Clinical trials of zinc and copper supplementation have not conclusively demonstrated acceleration of wound healing, alteration in the type of infection, or decline in the rate of infection. However, the length of hospitalization, adjusted for percentage of body surface burned, decreases slightly with supplementary zinc and copper. This decrease occurs even though the average serum levels of zinc and copper do not reach normal levels. Optimal levels of supplementation are approximately 10 to 30 mg zinc sulphate and 0.08 mg per kilogram copper sulphate per day, if given in addition to a diet. Zinc administration by itself decreases serum copper levels and may lead to anemia. Therefore, zinc administration alone may not be appropriate and, if done, necessitates careful monitoring of serum zinc and copper levels.[6]

Monitoring. Frequent re-evaluation and revision of the nutrition program during the burn patient's treatment is important. Metabolic requirements decrease as the burn wound heals, or after surgical closure. Septic complication, on the other hand, further increases hypermetabolism and may dictate more aggressive therapy. Closure of the wound with a graft, in the absence of infection, returns metabolic demands to normal; but this effect of wound closure is at least partially countered by autografting itself because of increased caloric needs and increased protein losses from the donor site.[5]

The child should be weighed on admission and daily, if possible. Weight is the easiest and the most constant parameter with which to monitor nutritional status,[5] although early post-burn fluid retention and later diuresis can lead to inaccuracies. Ideally, weight should slowly rise over the weeks of hospitalization in accordance with the normal growth curve of the child. (This is often difficult to achieve, however; the goal is for the child to gain weight or at least to maintain pre-burn weight.)

Other conventional assessment tools for evaluation of nutritional status are not always reliable for use with burn victims. Anthropometry of the arm is invalid if the tissue is distorted from the burn. Serum values are not always reliable indicators of nutritional status in patients who are receiving multiple blood transfusions.[7]

Enteral and Parenteral Alimentation. Whenever possible, the oral or the enteral route should be used to supply the patient's nutritional needs. Nasogastric tube feeding may be necessary if the seriously burned child cannot meet his or her caloric needs by oral intake. Tube feeding can be given with a feeding pump during the night to supplement nutrition taken orally during the day. Since no abnormalities of digestion caused by burns have been described, commercial liquid isotonic tube feedings, rather than elemental diets, can be administered.[1] (See *Enteral Nutrition Support of Adults*, page 261, and *Enteral Nutrition Formulas, Appendix 13.*)

Children with severe burns over 60 percent of the body surface or more may not be able to tolerate the large enteral volume that is required for adequate nutrition.[5] Few children consume more food during than before hospitalization. Septic complications often are associated with paralytic ileus, thus preventing oral or enteral feeding. In these cases, nutritional requirements may be met through parenteral nutrition.

Motivation and Goal Setting. The child should participate with the dietitian in the planning of meals that are acceptable and that meet the child's nutritional needs. Intake should be monitored daily. The child should be told why eating is important for recovery. Motivation is often enhanced by informing the child and the child's parents about the goals for caloric and protein intake and about the daily progress toward attaining these goals.

Food should be provided in frequent feedings, rather than in three large meals, to encourage adequate intake. Unpleasant or painful procedures should not be scheduled immediately before meal times. Meals should not be interrupted for laboratory tests, physicians visits, or nursing treatments.

Physicians: How to Order Diet

The diet order should indicate a *diet for a child with burns*. The dietitian plans the diet based upon the preceding guidelines.

REFERENCES

1. Luterman A, Adams M, Curreri PW. Nutritional management of the burn patient. Critical Care Quarterly 1984;7:34–43.
2. Curreri PW, Luterman A. Nutritional support of the burned patient. Surg Clin North Am 1978;58:1151–1156.
3. Young VR, Motil KJ, Burke JF. Energy and protein metabolism in relation to requirements of the burned pediatric patient. In: Suskind RM, ed. Textbook of pediatrics. New York: Raven Press, 1981:309–340.
4. Alexander JW, Macmillan BG, Stinnett JD, Ogle CK, Bozian RC, Fisher JE, Oakes JB, Morris MJ, Krummel R. Beneficial effections of aggressive protein feeding in severely burned children. Ann Surg 1980;192:505–517.
5. Solomon JR. Nutrition in the severely burned child. Prog Pediatr Surg 1981;14:63–79.
6. Pochon JP. Zinc and copper-replacement therapy—a must in burns and scalds in children? Prog Pediatr Surg 1981;14:151–172.
7. Bell SJ, Molnar JA, Krasker WS, Burke JF. Dietary compliance for pediatric burned patients. J Am Diet Assoc 1984;84:1329–1333.

CANCER

Children with cancer are more likely to be malnourished than other hospitalized children.[1] These children are at risk for developing malnutrition, both from the tumor itself and from chemotherapy, radiation therapy, and surgery administered as treatment. Overt malnutrition is seen in as many as 17 percent of the children with newly diagnosed localized tumors and in 37 percent of those with metastatic disease.*[2] These children sometimes enter aggressive treatment programs with little or no nutritional reserve.

Children must receive optimal nutritional support so they can grow and develop to their full potential. A good nutritional status also makes more aggressive cancer treatment possible. Malnutrition in cancer patients has the associated risks of an increased morbidity and mortality, a decreased capacity to withstand aggressive treatment, and an increased susceptibility to infections.[3] Donaldson et al related poor nutritional status to shorter survival in cases of localized disease in an early state. However, this may reflect disease that is more difficult to control, rather than a factor that causes the disease to be more difficult to control.[4] Recognition of lowered nutritional status as a possible risk factor in the subsequent relapse of disease or in ultimate death can lead to these children being followed more closely, thereby prompting earlier detection of recurrence or relapse.[4]

Etiology of Malnutrition

Malnutrition is commonly seen in children with active disease, in those who have suffered a relapse, and in those undergoing aggressive treatment for their disease.[4] Malnutrition results when the child's intake is less than the required needs. Inadequate intake can result from a variety of reasons. Anorexia and early satiety are frequently seen at diagnosis and following treatment. Taste changes have been reported in the literature when chemotherapy treatment results in gastrointestinal side effects.[5] Children may also learn taste aversions to foods eaten just prior to the treatment. Malabsorption may result from radiation therapy or from chemotherapy, such as methotrexate. There may be excess nutrient loss owing to steroid induced diabetes, to severe renal protein loss, or to persistent nausea and vomiting.[6] Malnutrition itself can also cause malabsorption.

Location of the tumor can affect nutritional status. There is a higher incidence of malnutrition among children with leukemia,[7] metastatic Ewing's sarcoma, retinoblastoma, glioma, and neuroblastoma who have relapses.[8] Children with hypothalamic tumors may experience hyperphagia or aphagia, depending upon the location of the tumor.[2] Head and neck surgery may result in severe problems with chewing and with swallowing. Gastrectomy can result in vitamin B_{12} malabsorption and in dumping syndrome. Massive intestinal resection may result in malabsorption of vitamin B_{12} or of bile acids.

Acute effects of radiation of the head and neck areas include nausea, anorexia, mucositis, esophagitis, decreased smell and taste sensation, damage to developing teeth, and decreased salivation. Thoracic radiation may result in inflammation and in cell damage in the pharynx and the esophagus. Stomach radiation may be associated with nausea, vomiting, and ulcer formation. Colitis may result from radiation of the colon.[1]

Cancer chemotherapeutic agents are used in the treatment of nearly all

*Malnutrition is defined as inadequate growth with weight to height ratio below the 20th percentile of the national standard and/or a serum albumin of 3.0 g/dl.

childhood neoplasms. Most agents are associated with nausea and vomiting. Mucositis of the oral cavity and of the upper gastrointestinal tract painfully interferes with the ingestion of nutrients. Continual mucosal toxicity can manifest as diarrhea, proctitis, and mucosal ulceration and bleeding. Vincristine and vinblastine may cause constipation and even adynamic ileus.[2]

Corticosteroid hormones have known nutritional consequences, particularly after long-term administration. These hormones exert an endocrine effect that results in polyphagia, hyperglycemia, and glycosuria, as well as obesity. Fluid and electrolyte disturbances, including edema and hypokalemic alkalosis, may occur.[2]

Nutritional Assessment

Weight–height percentile is believed to be the most reliable anthropometric indicator of nutritional status in the child with cancer. This parameter is easily obtained and should be checked frequently while the child is hospitalized and at every follow-up visit as an outpatient. Height–weight percentile can be used to reliably predict nutritional status because of its high direct correlation with triceps, skinfold, and mid-arm muscle circumference measurements. A low weight–height percentile alerts physicians and dietitians to patients who need immediate nutritional support.[8]

Laboratory data used for nutritional assessment may be affected by the patient's disease or its treatment. Hemoglobin and hematocrit values in children with leukemia, lymphoma, and Hodgkin's disease reflect the disease state, rather than nutritional status. Chemotherapeutic agents that cause bone marrow suppression decrease total lymphocyte count. The complete blood count must be used cautiously with patients who have solid tumors because, once treatment begins, complete blood count reflects treatment effects, rather than nutritional status. Furthermore, serum albumin does not clearly reflect weight–height percentiles, caloric intake, or dietary protein intake in the pediatric cancer patient. Serum magnesium has been shown to decrease with use of the chemotherapeutic agent cisplatinum. Other serum alterations may be found with the introduction of new chemotherapeutic agents.[8]

A careful dietary history that determines the adequacy of caloric and protein intakes and that determines changes in weight–height percentiles may be the most reliable indicator of nutritional status.[8]

Nutritional counseling by the dietitian should provide the patient and the patient's parents with practical suggestions that can help improve the intake, in spite of the side effects of cancer treatment (see *Cancer,* page 196, for specific examples). Prime emphasis should be placed on caloric intake. Patients who reportedly have intakes that are approximately 80 percent of the RDA for kilocalories, but greater than 155 percent of the RDA for protein, have done better. In follow-up, these children's intake remained greater than 125 percent of the RDA for protein.[8] Parents may express interest in special diets, megavitamin therapy, and health food supplements, and this should be discussed during nutritional education.[9]

Parents should be encouraged to be with their children at mealtimes when a child is hospitalized for cancer treatment. An effort should be made to avoid interrupting mealtime with tests, with treatments, or with discussion of upsetting topics. If nausea is present after a treatment, meals should be planned to avoid this time. A calm, positive attitude can help a child increase his or her intake more effectively than trying to force the child to eat. Some children eat better in a room other than their hospital room where treatment has taken place. A pleasant distraction during mealtime, such as watching a favorite television program or the promise of a small reward, may be helpful. Small quantities of food should be encouraged at frequent intervals, and nutritious snacks can be small meals in themselves. Nutritional supplements, such as Instant Breakfast, Ensure, or Polycose, are well-tolerated. Children should be able to take part in the planning of their diets. New foods can be offered if the child's sense of taste has been altered and if old favorite foods no longer have appeal.

Nutritional support should be considered when the weight of the child with cancer falls to 10 percent below his ideal,[10] or pre-illness,[11] weight. The child's intake can be supplemented by night-time tube feedings (see *Enteral Nutrition Support of Adults,* page 261) if he or she is not able to consume adequate kilocalories. Peripheral parenteral nutrition can supplement enteral intake if the child can tolerate a limited amount of food, but cannot be used as the sole access for nutritional support because of the limited tolerance of small veins for hypertonic solutions. Total parenteral nutrition (TPN) is necessitated if the child is unable to tolerate enteral feedings owing to severe gastrointestinal disturbances, such as obstructions, fistulas, ileus, malabsorption, or protracted vomiting.[11] When total parenteral nutrition was used with Wilm's patients, it was not sufficient in itself to restore lost weight. TPN needed to be continued until the end of the intense treatment period in order to reverse and to prevent recurrence of the protein energy malnutrition associated with treatment.[3]

Data on long-term nutritional status of children who have had cancer are limited. A survey of the effects of treatment in children with acute lymphocytic leukemia revealed that growth was slower than normal during the 2.3- to 3-year period of treatment. However, 5 years after diagnosis 19 of 22 children had weights within one standard deviation of normal average children. All but two of 22 resumed normal growth after cessation of therapy.[2]

REFERENCES

1. Kein CL. Nutrition in cancer. In: Walker WA, Watkins JB, eds. Nutrition in pediatrics. Boston: Little, Brown and Company, 1985:497–515.
2. Donaldson SS. Effects of therapy on nutritional status of the pediatric cancer patient. Cancer Res 1982;42:729s–736s.
3. Rickard KA, Kirksey A, Baehner RL, Grosfeld JL, Provisor A, Weetman RM, Boxer LA, Ballantine TVN. Effectiveness of enteral and parenteral nutrition in the nutritional management of children with Wilms' tumors. Am J Clin Nutr 1980;33:2622–2629.
4. Donaldson SS, Wesley MN, DeWys WD, Suskind RM, Jaffe N, van Eys J. A study of the nutritional status of pediatric cancer patients. Am J Dis Child 1981;135:1107–1112.
5. Bernstien IL. Learned taste aversions in children receiving chemotherapy. Science 1978;200:1302–1303.
6. van Eys J. Malnutrition in children with cancer. Cancer 1979;43:2030–2035.
7. Smithson WA. Personal communication. Mayo Clinic.
8. Carter P, Carr D, van Eys J, Coody D. Nutritional parameters in children with cancer. J Am Diet Assoc 1983;82:616–622.
9. Carter P, Carr D, van Eys J, Ramirez I, Coody D, Taylor G. Energy and nutrient intake of children with cancer. J Am Diet Assoc 1983;82:610–615.
10. Filler RM, Dietz W, Suskind RM, Jaffe N, Cassady JR. Parenteral feeding in the management of children with cancer. Cancer 1979;43:2117–2120.

11. Lukens JJ. Supportive care for children with cancer . . . the use of nutritional therapy. Am J Pediatr Hematol Oncol 1984;6:261–265.

CONSTIPATION AND ENCOPRESIS

General Description

Dietary recommendations include a varied and nutritionally balanced diet with adequate fiber and fluid.

Nutritional Inadequacy

The diet is adequate in nutrients when compared to the Recommended Dietary Allowances (RDA). However, the diet for each child should be assessed for nutritional adequacy. On the basis of this assessment, vitamin supplementation may be necessary.

Indications and Rationale

Constipation is a common problem in infants and children, yet it is often ignored or incorrectly treated. Constipation is not a disease, but it can have many unpleasant consequences, such as abdominal pain, distention, flatulence, diarrhea by overflow, and nausea. This variety of symptoms can disrupt childhood activities and can create parental anxiety. The spectrum of problems of fecal elimination ranges from simple constipation to chronic retention and may be either functional or organic in origin. Constipation can be associated with anal lesions, such as fissures and ulcers, and may also be a manifestation of more serious disorders, such as Hirschsprung's disease or even malabsorption. Table 8–24 lists the most common causes of constipation-encopresis.[1]

TABLE 8–24 Causes of Constipation-Encopresis*

Constipation Without Encopresis	Encopresis Without Constipation	Constipation With Encopresis
Lack of fecal bulk	Neurogenic	Anatomic obstruction
Unusually firm stools	Psychogenic	Spinal cord lesion
Interference with contraction of the voluntary muscles of defecation		Psychogenic
Anatomic obstruction		
Psychogenic		

*With Permission From: Fitzgerald JF. Encopresis, soiling, constipation: what's to be done? Pediatrics 1975;56:348–349.

Constipation is defined as the passage of excessively dry stools, stools of insignificant size, or infrequent stools (less often than every other day).[2] In practice, parents may perceive constipation in a variety of ways, and inappropriate perceptions should be clarified. Encopresis is defined as fecal soiling of clothing that persists regularly beyond the usual age of completion of toilet training (between ages 4 to 5 years).[3]

One of the most common causes of simple constipation in infants is a change in feeding practices. These alterations can be as minor as a change from breast milk to formula, a change from one formula to another, or the introduction of new foods into the diet. Inappropriately chosen diets also cause constipation in children. Such diets are limited in variety and usually include only a few favorite foods. Fruits and vegetables are typically missing in most of these children's diets. Frequently, these children do not eat regular, well-balanced meals.

There is evidence that fiber intake in children is low. In a 1975 survey of 2,000 households, 75 percent of the children ate less than four servings per day of fruits and vegetables, and 62 percent ate less than four servings of breads and cereals.[4] The Health and Nutrition Examination Survey (HANES) data also revealed that a substantial number of children have low intakes of fiber-containing foods.[4]

Goals of Dietary Management

The goal of dietary management is to help the child establish a varied and nutritionally well-balanced diet, with high-fiber meals and adequate fluid intake.

Dietary Recommendations

Recommendations for the child include the regular use of a wide variety of foods, ample fiber, and adequate fluid. Management initially involves an assessment of food and fluid intake. This assessment helps the dietitian identify current problems and formulate the dietary recommendations and consider growth, and development and activity needs (see *Pediatric Nutritional Assessment,* page 287, and *Normal Nutrition,* page 293). Dietary modification is indicated if an inappropriate diet is a major cause of the patient's constipation.

Fiber. The American Academy of Pediatrics' Committee on Nutrition states that, although no firm recommendations can be made at this time, a "substantial amount" of fiber probably should be eaten by all children (except those less than 1 year old) to ensure normal laxation. Solid foods, when introduced, should include whole-grain breads and cereals, fruits, and vegetables. A diet for children that emphasizes high-fiber foods (many of which are of low-caloric density) to the exclusion of other common foods should not be advised.[4]

The diet should include enough fiber (vegetables, fruits, and whole-grain breads and cereals) so that the bulk left in the bowel after digestion encourages the movement of intestinal contents and stimulates periodic evacuation. In general, foods can be classified in order of increasing fecal bulk as follows: protein, fat, milk, digestible carbohydrate, and carbohydrate with nondigestible material. The fiber content of food is listed on page 143. Quantitative recommendations for fiber intake for children have not been established.

Two major areas of concern exist when the fiber intake of children is increased. The first concern is the small stomach capacity of children. Fiber-rich foods are bulky, filling, and have a low-caloric density. Therefore, many children may be unable to consume sufficient kilocalories on a high-fiber diet. The second area of concern is the influence that fiber can have on the absorption of essential minerals, such as calcium, iron, phosphorus, zinc, and magnesium.

Bran, the most concentrated source of food fiber, should be used in moderation. Large amounts may cause flatulence, abdominal pain, and discomfort. Commercially available bran preparations have been recommended in amounts ranging from 15 to 45 g per day for infants and 30 to 60 g per day for children.

It is usually recommended that these preparations be added to foods and be given in at least three divided doses a day. Bran preparations usually are not well accepted by children. It often is possible to achieve an adequate fiber intake in the diet without bran supplements.

Fluid. Many children do not regularly take an adequate amount of fluid. Fluid intake, essential to bowel function, is especially important with a higher fiber diet. There are several formulas for estimating water requirements. The minimum requirement of water approximates 60 ml per kilogram of body weight per day. An intake greater than this may be necessary. However, an excessive fluid intake is considered to be two and a half times this amount.[5] Guidelines for maintenance water requirements are shown in Table 8–25.

TABLE 8–25 General Guidelines for Daily Maintenance Water Requirements*[6]

Patient Weight (kg)	Water Requirement (ml)
10–20	1,000 plus 50 (weight minus ten)
>20	1,500 plus 20 (weight minus twenty)

*From Robbins S, Thorp JN, Wadsworth C. Tube feeding of infants and children (monograph). Silver Spring, MD: American Society for Parenteral and Enteral Nutrition, 1981:4.

Other Considerations. Certain foods have been cited as causing constipation or as being inappropriate for treatment. However, there is no conclusive documented evidence. These foods include milk and cheese, apples in any form, and carrots. If the child's diet is limited in variety and predominately includes these foods, one would expect that the child would be constipated, but the cause would be more related to the limited diet than to these specific foods.

Other components of the constipation-encopresis treatment program may include regular exercise; use of bulk agents, stool softeners, and lubricants; and the encouragement of elimination on a regular basis.

Follow-up is essential. The patient or parent should keep a 3- to 5-day food record at least monthly so that recommended changes can be monitored and modifications made, if needed.

Physicians: How to Order Diet

The diet order should indicate *constipation-encopresis.*

REFERENCES

1. Fitzgerald JF. Encopresis, soiling, constipation: what's to be done? Pediatrics 1975;56:348–349.
2. Almy TP. Constipation. In: MH Sleisenger, ed. Gastrointestinal disease. Philadelphia: WB Saunders, 1973:320–325.
3. Johns C. Encopresis. Am J Nurs 1985;85:153–156.
4. American Academy of Pediatrics. Plant fiber intake in the pediatric diet. Pediatrics 1981;67:572–575.
5. Greene HL, Ghishan FK. Excessive fluid intake as a cause of chronic diarrhea in young children. J Pediatr 1983;102:836–840.
6. Robbins S, Thorp JN, Wadsworth C. Tube feeding of infants and children (monograph). Silver Spring, MD: American Society for Parenteral and Enteral Nutrition, 1981.

CYSTIC FIBROSIS

General Description

The diet for cystic fibrosis should meet the patient's nutritional needs with an emphasis on increased kilocaloric and protein intake. Some patients may experience an intolerance to fat and may be more comfortable with a limited fat intake. High kilocalorie, high protein nutritional supplements may be needed in addition to regular meals when the patient cannot maintain an adequate intake. Infants with cystic fibrosis are given a predigested, medium chain triglyceride-containing formula. Solid foods are usually added in less than recommended amounts to the infant's diet for age, because solids are a less desirable source of kilocalories and of protein than is formula.

Nutritional Inadequacy

The diet for patients with cystic fibrosis is planned to meet the Recommended Dietary Allowance (RDA) for kilocalories and for all other nutrients. Nutritional deficiencies in cystic fibrosis are most likely to occur in the first years of life, when growth rates are greatest. However, many variables influence the nutritional status of cystic fibrosis patients. Nutritional deficiencies may occur at any time and with a varying degree of severity, depending on the degree of steatorrhea, the degree of azotorrhea, the growth rate, the presence and severity of chronic respiratory disease and infection, and the quantity and quality of the foods consumed.

Supplemental vitamins should be prescribed for all cystic fibrosis patients. Multivitamin capsules, tablets, or drops that contain C and B complex should be given daily to meet the RDA. In addition, water-soluble forms of vitamins A, D, E, and K are required (Table 8–26). If needed, iron should also be given.

TABLE 8–26   Vitamin Preparations

Vitamin	Brand Name	Manufacturer	How Supplied	Recommended Daily Doses
Multivitamin supplement containing A, B complex, C, D, and E	Poly-Vi-Sol	Mead Johnson & Company	Drops Tablets	Recommended Dietary Allowance for age
A (water-soluble)	Aquasol A	USV Armour Pharmaceutical Company	Drops Capsules	Recommended Dietary Allowance for age
E (water-soluble)	Aquasol E	USV Armour Pharmaceutical Company	Drops Capsules	Infants, 25 to 50 IU Children, 100 to 200 IU
D (water-soluble)	Drisdol	Winthrop Laboratories	Drops Capsules	400 IU
K (water-soluble)	Synkayvite	Roche Laboratories	Tablets	Advisable intake, 15 μg

Caloric supplements, such as medium chained triglyceride oil and commercial formulas, are generally not well accepted by the patient. In our experience, a beverage such as an instant breakfast can be used to increase calories and protein without the patient experiencing aversion or flavor fatigue.

Indications and Rationale

Cystic fibrosis is an hereditary disorder that affects infants, children, adolescents, and adults. This disorder is found predominately in Caucasians and occurs in about 1 of every 2,000 live births.[1] People with cystic fibrosis are now commonly living to adulthood, with the current median age of survival approaching 20 years.[2] A number of physical signs, such as growth retardation, failure to gain weight, abdominal protuberance, lack of subcutaneous fat, and poor muscle tone, are seen in individuals with the disease.

The basic defect that causes the disease is as yet unknown. Cystic fibrosis is characterized by excessively viscid exocrine gland secretions that may obstruct the pancreatic and bile ducts, the intestine, and the bronchi. The major criteria for diagnosing cystic fibrosis include elevated concentration of electrolytes in the sweat of the patient, pulmonary involvement, pancreatic insufficiency, and a family history for the disorder.[2] Pancreatic insufficiency, gastrointestinal malabsorption, and frequent pulmonary infections predispose individuals with cystic fibrosis to undernutrition. Inadequate lipase activity accounts for the most profound clinical effects, although all three pancreatic enzymes (amylase, protease, and lipase) are either insufficient or missing. The resulting steatorrhea leads to significant energy loss and to malabsorption of fat-soluble vitamins, essential fatty acids, some minerals, and bile salts.

Specific therapy for cystic fibrosis is not possible since the basic defect remains unknown. Treatment is aimed toward control of the pulmonary obstructive process, prevention of pulmonary infection, and correction of pancreatic and nutritional deficiencies. Treatment consists of chest physical therapy, aerosal inhalation, antibiotics, pancreatic enzyme replacement, vitamin and mineral supplementation, and a high kilocalorie, high protein diet. Nutrition is of prime importance in the treatment of individuals with cystic fibrosis. Undernutrition contributes to pulmonary complications, to susceptibility to infection, to poor growth, and to decreased energy and motivation. Nutritional support is needed to offset (1) nutrient losses that are secondary to pancreatic insufficiency and malabsorption, (2) a general increase in metabolic rate, and (3) an increased expenditure of energy during chest therapy, labored respiration, and periods of infection and fever.

Goals of Dietary Management

The primary goal of nutritional therapy for the cystic fibrosis patient is to encourage caloric, protein, vitamin, and mineral intakes in sufficient quantities to achieve consistent growth and weight gain. When this goal is achieved, catch-up growth needs should be identified and encouraged.

Normal ranges on the growth curves are used as guidelines for determining energy and nutrient needs for the infant and the young child, whereas ideal weights for height are the guidelines used for the older child. Children with cystic fibrosis are often remarkably underweight for height and age. Although the lack of weight gain is attributed largely to pancreatic insufficiency, the severity of pulmonary disease correlates better with the growth curve (the more severe the pulmonary disease, the less the slope of the growth curve) than does the degree of malabsorption.[3]

Dietary Recommendations

Nutritional recommendations for infants and children with cystic fibrosis have been outlined by the Cystic Fibrosis Foundation[5] and appear in Table 8–27.

Infants. The infant is unique because milk is the prime nutrient source of the kilocalories, protein, and other nutrients that are necessary for satisfactory growth and development. The milk may be ingested as breast milk or as commercial formula. Breast milk is not as good a choice for feeding as a pre-digested medium chained triglyceride commercial formula, such as Pregestimil or Portagen, since the energy requirement for infants with cystic fibrosis is 150 to 200 percent of the Recommended Daily Allowances (RDA) and the protein intake requirement is 200 percent of the RDA. These formulas have the advantage of reducing, but not eliminating, the need for enzyme supplements. In order to meet caloric and protein needs, it may be necessary to concentrate the formula or to add a glucose polymer supplement.

Generally, formulas alone become inadequate to meet needs at 5 to 6 months of age. Infants should begin solid foods at that time and increases made as tolerated. The infant's ability to chew is dependent on his or her stage of development and varies among infants of the same age. Strained foods, particularly for the young infant with respiratory difficulty, are preferred because of their soft consistency. Pureed or chopped table foods are begun as soon as tolerated. Strained or pureed foods may be needed for a longer time for the infant with cystic fibrosis. Certain infant foods that have a laxative effect, such as strained plums or prunes, should be avoided.

Children and Adolescents. Individual tolerances among patients vary greatly. Foods that usually are not tolerated include high fat foods, such as gravy, salad dressing, rich desserts, and fried foods. Condiments, such as catsup, chili sauce, horseradish, pepper, and pickles, may be irritants to the gastrointestinal tract and may therefore cause discomfort, even though they contain little or no fat. Abdominal distress occurs in many cystic fibrosis patients following the

TABLE 8–27 Nutrient Guidelines for Infants and Children with Cystic Fibrosis*[5,6]

Age	Kilocalories per kilogram per day	Protein grams per kilogram per day	Fat grams per day
Infants (to 1 yr old)	150 to 200	4	Infants Normal 30 to 60 Moderate 30 to 50 Low-fat 30 to 40
Children (1 to 9 yr old)	130 to 180	3	Other children Normal 50 to 120 Moderate 50 to 70 Low-fat 30 to 50
Males (9 to 18 yr old)	100 to 130	2.5 to 3	
Females (9 to 18 yr old)	80 to 110	2.5 to 3	

*With permission from: Schwachman H. Nutritional considerations in the treatment of children with cystic fibrosis. In: Suskind RM, ed. Textbook of pediatric nutrition. New York: Raven Press, 1981:511.

ingestion of dried beans and peas, cabbage, broccoli, sauerkraut, and strong-flavored greens. Although these foods contain little or no fat or spices, any food that persistently causes distress should be omitted from the diet.

Five to six feedings a day are often needed to meet nutrient needs for those individuals with lack of appetite.

Energy. The total energy requirement is generally increased owing to malabsorption and to chronic infections. The voracious appetite seen in the child who is malabsorbing nutrients is not seen in the child with cystic fibrosis. For the most part, these children have poor appetites and generally eat, at most, 80 percent of the recommended daily amount of kilocalories, in spite of increased caloric requirements that are created by cystic fibrosis and its complications.[4] An increase of 50 percent to 100 percent of the RDA for caloric intake is recommended for the cystic fibrosis child and adolescent (see Table 8–27). In practice, however, the initial goal should be to reach the RDA.

Protein. A child or adolescent with cystic fibrosis requires 150 percent of the RDA for protein.

Fat. Some restriction of fat intake has often been recommended in an attempt to reduce the abdominal symptoms of malabsorption. However, dietary fat, as a high density source of kilocalories, improves the palatability of food and provides essential fatty acids.

In our experience, it is useful to plan the initial diet with fat controlled to 30 percent of kilocalories and with foods that are well-tolerated. The diet and its fat content can be liberalized, as tolerated, by gradually introducing new foods and noting any signs of distress caused by these foods. Any food that persistently causes distress should be omitted from the diet. The patient learns how much fat and what combination of foods causes gastrointestinal distress. These patients, especially adolescents, should be free to adjust their diets, instead of being bound to a strict regimen. Some patients would rather experience some discomfort and occasionally enjoy foods they might not eat routinely. Others prefer to be more restrictive with their diets in order to avoid discomfort and inconvenience. The patient should be permitted to make these decisions.

Sodium. Most, if not all, children with cystic fibrosis lose excessive amounts of sodium and chloride in their sweat; therefore, additional salt is needed in the diet. The child needs more salt during periods of extremely hot weather, febrile illness, and strenuous physical exertion than during times of sedentary activity. This salt can be provided by liberal use of table salt.

Assessment of the Diet. A food record of at least 3 days should be completed for the initial nutritional consultation. This food record helps the dietitian formulate initial dietary recommendations. Re-evaluation is needed at regular intervals to determine whether the original recommendations were adequate to support growth and to evaluate the foods that are being added back to the diet. Re-evaluation is also needed because growth and the disease process change the child's nutritional needs.

Weight gain and linear growth must be assessed when the adequacy of nutritional intake is evaluated.

Physicians: How to Order Diet

The diet order should indicate *diet for cystic fibrosis*. The dietitian determines the content and the caloric level according to the principles stated herein.

REFERENCES

1. Barry MM. Cystic fibrosis. J Am Diet Assoc 1979;75:446–449.
2. Hubbard VS, Mangrum PJ. Energy intake and nutrition counseling in cystic fibrosis. J Am Diet Assoc 1982;80:127–131.
3. Sproul A, Huang N. Growth patterns of children with cystic fibrosis. J Pediatr 1964;65:664–676.
4. Chase HP, Long MA, Lavin MH. Cystic fibrosis and malnutrition. J Pediatr 1979;95:337–347.
5. Ad Hoc Nutrition Committee, Cystic Fibrosis Foundation. Present status of nutrition in cystic fibrosis. Atlanta, Georgia, March 1978.
6. Shwachman H. Nutritional considerations in the treatment of children with cystic fibrosis. In: Suskind RM, ed. Textbook of pediatric nutrition. New York: Raven Press, 1981:511.

DIABETES MELLITUS

General Description

The diet for children with diabetes is planned to be adequate in essential nutrients to ensure normal growth and maturation. The kilocalorie content of the diet must meet changing energy needs for growth and activity levels, yet must prevent obesity. Total fat, saturated fat, and cholesterol are controlled in the diet for diabetes in an effort to minimize vascular complications. The prevention, the delay of development, or the progression of other complications associated with diabetes should also be considered in the diet design.

The diet for diabetes is planned with five or six feedings a day in an effort to distribute caloric intake in a way that minimizes fluctuations in blood glucose concentrations, and to provide nutrients at the time of maximal insulin action in order to ensure efficient energy utilization. The meal plan must be individualized to reflect the child's likes and dislikes and to be consistent with the personal, cultural, and/or racial food choices of the child and the family.

Nutritional Inadequacy

The diet for diabetes is planned to meet the Recommended Dietary Allowances (RDA) for kilocalories and all nutrients. The diet must be assessed and adjusted periodically to maintain a normal rate of growth and maturation.

Indications and Rationale*

The nutrient needs of the child with diabetes are the same as those of the child who does not have diabetes (see *Healthy Infants, Children, and Adolescents,* page 293). However, greater attention must be given to the timing of meals and snacks and the consistency of intake from day to day. Regular and intermediate insulins are administered at specific times each day, and meal and snack times are planned to correlate with the peak action times of these insulins. Therefore, it is important that meals are eaten at regular times each day, with day-to-day variation not to exceed more or less than 15 minutes. A consistent distribution of kilocalories, carbohydrate, and protein among meals and snacks

---

*See *Diabetes Mellitus,* page 100, for a more complete description and discussion of diabetes.

is recommended to stabilize changes in blood glucose and to allow more predictable results following changes in insulin dose. The carbohydrate in the diet is distributed so that 25 to 30 percent is provided at each meal and 8 to 10 percent at each snack. The diet for the infant and the young child is planned with mid-morning, mid-afternoon, and bedtime snacks. Diets for older children are planned with mid-afternoon and bedtime snacks; if needed, a mid-morning snack can also be included. Protein foods from the meat and/or milk exchange lists are included with each meal and snack. However, if breakfast and lunch or lunch and dinner are closely spaced, it may be appropriate to plan just a fruit or a starch exchange for the snack between these meals. The use of simple carbohydrates is not recommended for the child with diabetes in order to minimize plasma glucose fluctuations. Judicious use of noncaloric artificial sweeteners is suggested because there are inadequate data on the safety of the use of these products by children (see *Diabetes Mellitus*, page 100, and *Appendix 10* for *Nutritive and Non-nutritive Sweeteners*).

The young child who has diabetes needs the help of a family member to plan and prepare the diet. As the child gets older, the child needs to be encouraged to make decisions at meal times, with parents available for support. This assists the child in becoming more independent with meal selections, both at home and away from home.

The diet for diabetes is based on the food exchange lists (see *Diabetes Mellitus, Food Exchange Lists,* page 114, and *Infant Formulas and Feedings* in *Pediatric Appendices,* page 458).

Goals of Dietary Management

The goals of dietary management for children with diabetes are to provide nutrients and kilocalories to achieve normal growth and development, to maintain or attain an appropriate body weight for height and age, and to prevent hyperglycemia and hypoglycemia. The diet prescription should be individualized in the meal plan design, the educational component, and the follow-up program.

Nutritional management is an integral part of overall diabetes therapy, which also includes insulin administration, regular participation in physical activity, and emotional support and guidance (see *Diabetes Mellitus,* Community Support Program, page 113).

Determining Energy and Protein Needs. Kilocalorie needs of the child are determined primarily from the present dietary intake, which is obtained by a thorough diet history. Supportive data for energy needs include the RDA for age and sex of the child, as determined by the *Nomogram for Estimating Caloric Requirements* (see *Appendix 6*), and the estimated level of activity. The protein level of the diet should meet the RDA for the child's age and weight and should represent about 15 to 20 percent of the total kilocalories of the diet.

Determining Dietary Fat and Sodium Needs. The American Heart Association has made general dietary recommendations for healthy American children above 2 years old and for adolescents. These recommendations are relevant to the child with diabetes, since such persons are at greater risk for atherosclerosis than are nondiabetics. The recommendations include (1) the control of fat intake to 30 percent of total kilocalories (10 percent saturated, 10 percent polyunsaturated, 10 percent monounsaturated), (2) the limitation of cholesterol to 100 mg per 1,000 calories (not to exceed 300 mg per day), and (3) the elimination of salt at the table and the limitation of intake of high salt-containing foods.[1]

When designing the diabetic meal plan, these recommendations should be considered as a means of slowing the disease process and of establishing eating habits that, in adulthood, may help to deter atherosclerosis. For children with elevated serum lipids, a diet should be used with the total fat controlled to 20 to 25 percent of total calories (equal amounts of the three types of fatty acids) and the cholesterol controlled to 150 to 200 mg per day.[2]

Fiber. Few studies have been reported of children with diabetes who have achieved improved blood sugar control from use of fiber-supplemented diets; the studies that have been reported have contradictory results.[3] However, as a general health measure, increased use of whole grain breads and cereals, fresh fruits, and uncooked vegetables is appropriate for the child. (See *Diabetes Mellitus, Fiber,* page 106.)

Changing Preferences and Needs. The diet history aids in planning the distribution of nutrients among meals and snacks by the consideration of likes and dislikes, school and activity schedules, use of fast food and restaurant meals, use of convenience foods, and family eating patterns. The diet is planned to modify existing food practices as realistically as possible and to ensure optimal nutrition for activity and normal growth and development. The diet should be re-evaluated periodically to accommodate the child's changing nutritional needs and preferences.

School Lunch. The child with diabetes may choose to eat a school lunch or a lunch brought from home. If a school lunch is chosen, the child can learn to select foods from the school cafeteria menu. The school lunch menu is often published in local newspapers, or it can be obtained from the school. The child and the parents can plan the child's lunch by reviewing the menu and deciding which items should be eaten and which should be avoided. The school food service can usually be contacted to get serving sizes of casseroles, pizza, and other menu items. A school lunch may have to be supplemented with foods from home to meet the needs of the diet.

The United States Department of Agriculture (USDA) has established a meal pattern for five age or grade groups that reduces the minimum portion size for children age 8 and under and offers more food to children age 12 and over.[4] The school lunch pattern established for ages 9 to 12 years is shown in Table 8–28. This pattern is used if portions are not adjusted for age or grade groups.

TABLE 8–28 USDA School Lunch Pattern

Components	Minimum Daily Quantities
Meat or meat alternate	2 ounces
Vegetable and/or fruit	3/4 cup
Bread or bread alternate	8 servings per week
Milk	1/2 pint

To include school lunch in the meal plan, the following lunch meal plan usually works well:

> 2 meat exchanges
> 2 to 3 fat exchanges
> 3 starch exchanges
> 1 milk exchange
> 1 to 2 vegetable and/or fruit exchanges

Skim milk is increasingly more available in school lunch programs. If skim milk is not available, the meal plan should allow for the type of milk the school serves. If the school offers only one type of milk, USDA regulations state that it must serve low fat milk (either skim or 2%).

Eating For Extra Activity. The diet probably needs to be adjusted when the child with diabetes engages in activities more strenuous than those in the normal daily routine. Because of individual tolerances and needs, the child may have to try different amounts of food for a given amount of exercise; too much may result in excessive elevation in blood glucose, too little may result in hypoglycemia.

TABLE 8–29 Diet and Exercise

Types of Exercise and Examples	If Blood Sugar Is:	Increase Food Intake By:	Suggestions of Food To Use
Exercise of short duration or of moderate intensity	80 mg or above	May not be necessary	
Examples: walking a half mile or leisurely biking for duration of one-half hour or less	less than 80 mg	10–15 g of carbohydrate per one-half hour	1 fruit or 1 starch exchange
Exercise of moderate intensity	80–180 mg	10–15 g of carbohydrate per hour of exercise	1 fruit or 1 starch exchange
Examples: tennis, swimming, jogging, leisure cycling, gardening, golfing, vacuuming for a one-hour duration	less than 80 mg	25–50 g of carbohydrate prior to exercise, then 10–15 g per hour of exercise	½ meat sandwich with a milk or a fruit exchange
	180–300 mg	Not necessary to increase food	
	400 mg or greater*		
Strenuous activity or exercise	80–180 mg	25–50 mg of carbohydrate, depending on intensity and duration	½ meat sandwich with a milk or fruit exchange
Examples: football, hockey, raquetball, basketball games, or tennis (singles); strenuous cycling or swimming, shovelling heavy snow for one-hour duration	less than 80 mg	50 g of carbohydrate, monitor blood sugars carefully	1 meat sandwich (2 slices of bread) with a milk and a fruit exchange
	180–300 mg	10–15 g of carbohydrate per hour of exercise	1 fruit or 1 starch exchange

*High blood sugar may reflect inadequate insulin therapy, and exercise may cause the blood sugar to increase further.

The guidelines in Table 8-29 may be helpful in planning additional snacks for activity.

The added carbohydrate is taken as a snack before starting the activity and is taken in addition to the normal meal plan. Use of these guidelines and observation of blood glucose patterns before and after activity periods should allow the child to identify more closely how much extra food is needed for specific types and durations of exercise.

Physical education and recess periods ideally should be scheduled early in the morning or after lunch. If this is not possible, changes in the composition and/or the timing of meals and snacks may be necessary.

The child with diabetes should be instructed to carry a readily available source of carbohydrate (sugar cubes, pure sugar candy) to be used in the event of an insulin reaction.

Diet During Illness. The stress of illness, whether attributable to infection or to any other cause, can raise the blood sugar and thus cause diabetes to go out of control.[5] Even when a child is unable to eat, the stress of illness can bring on hormonal changes that may raise the blood sugar and thereby change insulin requirements. Many diabetics feel that, because they are unable to eat, they do not need to take insulin. Diabetics should take at least the usual amount of insulin when ill, especially if the blood glucose is normal or elevated. If the blood glucose is decreased, the amount of insulin may be decreased to 2/3 of the usual dose. Changes in appetite and in the ability to tolerate the usual meal plan may require that the child's diet be modified during times of illness. Insulin and carbohydrate are needed during these times to prevent ketoacidosis.

Eating and drinking are extremely important for the diabetic when he or she is ill. If eating is difficult, it may be helpful to modify food choices to those

TABLE 8–30 Carbohydrate Content of Foods That May be Used During Illness

Fruit and Milk (15 g carbohydrate per exchange)

The following foods may be substituted for either one fruit or one milk exchange:
$\frac{1}{2}$ cup orange juice
$\frac{1}{3}$ cup grape juice
5 ounces *regular* carbonated beverage
1 twinbar popsicle (3 ounces)
3 pieces of hard candy
1 tablespoon corn syrup or honey
4 teaspoons granulated sugar
12 ounces Gatorade
10 ounces milk*
milkshake* ($\frac{2}{3}$ cup milk and $\frac{1}{4}$ cup vanilla ice cream)

Starch (15 g carbohydrate per exchange)

The following foods may be substituted for one starch exchange:
1 slice toast
$\frac{1}{2}$ cup cooked cereal
$\frac{3}{4}$ cup cream soup*
1 cup broth-based soup
6 saltines
$\frac{1}{2}$ cup vanilla ice cream*
$\frac{1}{4}$ cup sherbet
$\frac{1}{4}$ cup pudding*
$\frac{1}{2}$ cup *sweetened* gelatin

*Milk or milk-products may not be tolerated when nausea, vomiting, or diarrhea are present.

that are soft and easy to digest, such as canned fruits, eggs, toast, crackers, and hot cereal, especially if these foods are taken frequently in small amounts. If the child is unable to tolerate soft foods, a liquid diet can be used. Guidelines for these specific modifications need to be included with the individualized meal plan. The soft foods or liquids should be taken in amounts to satisfy the carbohydrate content of each meal and snack in the meal plan. Table 8–30 presents the carbohydrate content of foods that may be used during illness. Eating six to eight smaller meals, rather than three to four normal meals, is recommended.

When nausea, vomiting, or diarrhea are present, milk and milk-products may not be tolerated as well as nondairy foods and should be avoided. Caution must be exercised with the child when nausea and vomiting are present because the child may be unable to tolerate and to retain any carbohydrates, thus resulting in hypoglycemia. While water, broth, tea, or other sugar-free fluids cannot be used to replace meals and snacks, they are needed to replace fluids that are lost by diarrhea, vomiting, and fever. These fluids should be encouraged throughout the day.

It is imperative to monitor the blood sugar, regardless of the nature of the illness. The child should be in contact with his physician if the blood sugar is less than 80 mg percent in the presence of nausea or vomiting or greater than 240 mg percent on three subsequent blood sugar tests.

Physicians: How to Order Diet

The diet order should indicate a *diet for a child with diabetes mellitus.*

REFERENCES

1. Weidman W, Kwiterovich P, Jesse MJ, Nugent E. Diet in the healthy child. Circulation 1983;67:1411A–1414A.
2. Steinberg D, Chairman, Consensus Development Panel. National Institutes of Health Consensus Development Conference Statement. Lowering blood cholesterol to prevent heart disease. JAMA 1985;253:2080–2086.
3. Nuttall FQ. Diet and the diabetic patient. Diabetes Care 1983;6:197–207.
4. United States Department of Agriculture, National School Lunch Program. School lunch patterns for various age/grade groups, November, 1982.
5. Gettinger J, McConahay G, Sebastean S. Sick day management. Diabetes Forecast 1979;32:43–45.

DIARRHEA

General Description

Diarrhea has been defined as a change in stool consistency, an excessive intestinal loss of fluid and electrolytes, and an increase in frequency or volume of stool such as to make the child ill. For a child, daily fecal losses exceeding 200 ml per square meter of body surface are considered excessive. Almost all acute diarrhea in children is caused by intestinal tract infections. Approximately 50 percent of these infections are caused by human rotavirus, and the rest are caused by bacteria, food poisoning from improperly stored foods, and inflammatory bowel disorders.[1]

Chronic diarrhea is the presence of diarrhea for a period of more than 2 weeks.[2] Chronic diarrhea may be of nonspecific etiology or may result from liver disease, from hormonal disorders, from pancreatic disease such as cystic fibrosis, or from chronic diseases of the small and large intestine such as celiac disease, Crohn's disease, and ulcerative colitis.[2,3] Chronic nonspecific diarrhea has been found to be associated with inappropriately low fat diets,[4] with ingestion of apple juice,[5] and with excessive fluid intake.[6] Chronic nonspecific diarrhea may or may not be associated with malabsorption of nutrients. If diarrhea and malabsorption are severe and persistent, malnutrition may result, with complications such as loss of immunocompetence and further impairment of gastrointestinal function.

Chronic diarrhea is often associated with weight loss or with growth failure. Delayed growth is chiefly related to an inadequate supply of dietary protein and kilocalories, although zinc intake may also be crucial.[2] Inadequate intake of food because of anorexia, defective digestion and absorption of ingested food, and increased metabolic demands may contribute to nutritional deficiencies, even in the absence of malabsorption.

Indications and Rationale

An inverse relationship between the prevalence of diarrheal disease and the overall growth of children has been demonstrated in less developed countries, as well as in individual children in more developed countries.[7,8] Growth failure secondary to diarrhea has been attributed to decreased dietary intake and to impaired intestinal absorption during and after enteric infections. Younger children and those whose nutritional status is marginal are more likely to suffer nutritional consequences from diarrhea.

Various factors contribute to the vulnerability of infants and young children to diarrheal disease. First, the child's intestine lacks a full range of defense mechanisms against potential pathogens once he or she is weaned and thereby deprived of the passive protection of breast milk. Second, the impact of intestinal malfunction on acute losses of fluid from the gut is much greater in young children than in older children. This age-related difference may be in part attributable to the relative inefficiencies of most transport systems in the developing intestine. Third, the young infant's kidneys have less capacity than those of adults to adjust to fluid losses, although these infants are equipped with a relatively large volume of extracellular fluid to cushion against intestinal losses. Finally, the infant has relatively meager nutritional reserves, so that depletion of both macro- and micronutrients develops quickly when limited intake and excessive losses occur.[9] Decreased intake is likely a greater contributor to malnutrition than is malabsorption.[1,2]

Decreased mucosal surface area, alterations of the villus-crypt ratio, and decreased concentrations of the disaccharidases have all been observed during and following diarrhea. Injury to the intestinal mucosa, along with alteration in intestinal transit time, accounts for the diarrhea-related malabsorption of carbohydrate. Carbohydrate malabsorption is usually self-limited, but may continue beyond the period of diarrhea.[7]

Goals of Dietary Management

Fluid and Electrolyte Therapy.   Whenever possible, the oral route should be used for rehydration. A rehydration solution containing 75 to 90 mEq sodium to 20 to 30 mEq potassium, appropriate anions, and 20 to 22.5 g glucose per liter is recommended for treatment or for significant dehydration. Generally, a solution of this type should be administered in a hospital under medical supervision. During the rehydration phase, which should not exceed 4 to 6 hours, the oral rehydration solution should be used alone in volumes that replace the extracellular fluid losses.[10,11] The World Health Organization's Oral Rehydration Solution, which contains 90 mEq sodium, 20 mEq potassium, 80 mEq bicarbonate, and 20 g glucose per liter, is particularly useful for rapid rehydration of children with diarrhea.[9] (see *Appendix 11*).

One reason for failure of oral therapy may be vomiting, which can be severe early in the disorder. However, when the fluid is given by spooning, rather than through a nipple or from a cup, successful retention is usually obtained, despite small amounts being vomited.[11] Another reason for failure is that there may be intestinal brush border damage, thus making the solute in the solution poorly absorbed in the intestine.[11] Hyperosmolar solutions, such as fruit juices, sweetened beverage mixes, gelatins, and carbonated beverages, are not recommended because they are likely to draw additional extracellular fluid into the lumen, thus favoring additional fluid losses.[12] Parenteral fluid therapy is indicated for patients who are severely dehydrated and in shock.

A solution with 40 to 60 mEq sodium per liter of fluid is recommended to prevent dehydration, to treat mild dehydration, or to maintain hydration. This level of intake can be achieved by feeding with commercial oral electrolyte solutions designed for this purpose, or by feeding with an oral rehydration solution containing 75 to 90 mEq sodium per liter alternately (on a 1 to 1 basis) with fluids such as water, unsweetened juices, or breast milk (see *Appendix 11*). The total volume given should not exceed the individual's daily fluid requirement. If additional fluids are desired, a low solute fluid, such as water or breast milk, can be used.[10,11] There does not appear to be any advantage in delaying the introduction of food beyond 24 hours.[7,10,11]

Nutritional Therapy. Fasting is not recommended during an acute episode of diarrhea. Feeding should be encouraged for many reasons. Suboptimal absorption is better than no absorption of food. Considerable carbohydrate absorption may be possible, even when disaccharidase concentrations are reduced by diarrhea. Intestinal disaccharidase levels are dramatically reduced during fasting. Continued breast feeding during diarrhea helps to maintain the mother's ability to lactate.[7,8,13]

The patient should receive an adequate balanced nutrient intake as soon as possible. Considerable absorption of nutrients can take place in spite of malabsorption, and feeding will assist in the repair of intestinal absorptive surfaces. The Subcommittee on Nutrition and Diarrheal Disease Control of the Food and Nutrition Board reviewed the nutritional consequences of diarrhea and concluded that "continued feeding" is both safe and beneficial. In order to promote catch-up growth, the subcommittee recommended frequent feeding of small amounts of high caloric, nutrient-dense foods at levels that provide at least 25 percent more energy than the estimated mean requirement for healthy children and that provide 100 percent more protein than the RDA.[11]

The World Health Organization Program for Control of Diarrheal Diseases'[7,8,13] recommendations for feeding during diarrhea are as follows.

1. Breast feeding should be continued once rehydration, if needed, is complete.

2. Children who are fully weaned should eat their regular diet; if they are not fully weaned and are under 9 months, milk and milk-based formulas should

be diluted to at least half strength for 1 to 2 days, or a lactose-free formula should be offered.

3. Children who are 4 months of age or older should be encouraged to eat solid foods if they cannot satisfy their energy needs by breast feeding or by formula alone.

4. Children should be allowed to determine the amount of food they need. Anorexic children should not be forced to eat.

5. Children should be allowed to have extra food when the diarrhea has subsided in order to recover from any nutritional deficit caused by the illness.

6. Foods high in carbohydrate content, particularly those containing disaccharides and monosaccharides (fruits, sweet desserts), should be avoided or limited during convalescence, since they tend to overwhelm damaged absorptive mechanisms.

Avoidance of milk has mistakenly been advocated during the early phase of convalescence from diarrhea because the lactose content might exceed intestinal lactase capacity and because of possible damage to mucosa from cow's milk protein during diarrhea. However, studies involving infants with acute gastroenteritis found that recovery from mild acute gastroenteritis occurred within 2 weeks, irrespective of carbohydrate ingested.[14,15] For the rare patient who is truly intolerant of milk, special formulas prepared without milk protein or lactose may be tried on a temporary basis for 10 days to 2 weeks.[9]

Solid food has the advantage of slowing gastric emptying in the breast-fed or milk-based formula-fed infant, thus reducing the amount of lactose in the small intestine per unit of time. More frequent, smaller feedings would have the same beneficial effect on lactose digestion and on absorption.[7]

Use of the BRAT diet (consisting of bananas, rice, applesauce, and tea or toast) is not recommended. This diet is not only deficient in protein, fat, and energy, but also does not include typical foods consumed by most infants and small children. The BRAT diet usually excludes the use of any formula and can also compound caloric deficiency and lead to further nutritional decline.[16]

Chronic Diarrhea. Therapy for chronic diarrhea should first be focused on treatment of the underlying disease. If the suspected etiology for nonspecific diarrhea is dietary, the diet should be returned to a normal fat composition for age.

For most infants, the management of chronic intractable diarrhea requires parenteral nutrition. Several reports show benefits from continuing minimal oral feeding. The introduction of one new food at a time in small amounts helps to re-establish food tolerance because of the trophic effect on the small intestine. Intravenous feeding is continued until a satisfactory weight gain has been achieved and is sustained by oral intake.[2]

In rare situations, intestinal sucrase is decreased. This decrease requires the use of elemental formulas containing glucose or its polymers (Pregestimil, Nutramigen, or Carbohydrate-Free formula) to which monosaccharides can be added in sequential increments (see *Pediatric Appendices 1*, page 458, for composition). Those few children who are unable to absorb monosaccharides require parenteral nutrition.

REFERENCES

1. Hamilton JR. Acute diarrhea. In: Walker WA, Watkins WA, eds. Nutrition in pediatrics. Boston: Little, Brown and Co, 1985:529.

2. Meadows NJ, Walker-Smith JA. Chronic diarrhea. In: Walker WA, Watkins WA, eds. Nutrition in pediatrics. Boston: Little, Brown and Co, 1985:529.

3. DeBenham BJ, Ellett M, Perez RC, Clark JH. Initial assessment and management of chronic diarrhea in toddlers. Pediatr Nurs 1985;11:281–285.

4. Cohen SA, Hendricks KM, Mathis RK, Laramee S, Walker WA. Chronic nonspecific diarrhea: dietary relationships. Pediatrics 1979;64:402–407.

5. Hyams JS, Leichtner AM. Apple juice: an unappreciated cause of chronic diarrhea. Am J Dis Child 1985;139:503–505.

6. Green HL, Ghishan FK. Excessive fluid intake as a cause of chronic diarrhea in young children. J Pediatr 1983;102:836–840.

7. Brown KH, MacLean WO. Nutritional management of acute diarrhea: an appraisal of the alternatives. Pediatrics 1984;73:119–125.

8. Nutritional management of acute diarrhea. Pediatr Curr 1984;33:21–22.

9. Hamilton JR. Treatment of acute diarrhea. Pediatr Clin North Am 1985;32:419–427.

10. Committee on Nutrition American Academy of Pediatrics. Oral fluid therapy and post-treatment feeding following enteritis. In: American Academy of Pediatrics. Pediatric nutrition handbook. Elk Grove Village, Illinois: 1985:274.

11. Committee on Nutrition American Academy of Pediatrics. Use of oral fluid therapy and post-treatment feeding following enteritis in children in a developed country. Pediatrics 1985;75:358–361.

12. Stickler GB, Hick JF. Oral replacement therapy in children with acute diarrhea. In: Mellinger JF, Stickler GB, eds. Clinical problems in pediatrics. Philadelphia: Lippencott, 1983;117.

13. Feeding during diarrhea. Nutr Rev 1986;44:102.

14. Placzek M. Comparison of two feeding regimes following acute gastroenteritis in infancy. J Pediatr Gastroenterol Nutr 1984;3:245–248.

15. Groothuis JR, Berman S, Chapman J. Effect of carbohydrate ingested on outcome in infants with mild gastroenteritis. J Pediatr 1986;108:903–906.

16. Self TW. Pitfalls of the "BRAT" diet. Nutr and the M.D. 1986;12:1–3.

GLUTEN-SENSITIVE ENTEROPATHY: CELIAC DISEASE

General Description

Wheat, rye, oats, barley, and products containing these grains are omitted from the diet in order to reduce the intake of gluten, the protein found in these grains. Corn, rice, and products made from them may be used as substitutes. Other substitutes include wheat starch, tapioca, and soybean, buckwheat, arrowroot, and potato flours.

Transient lactose intolerance is commonly seen, and temporary fat intolerance sometimes occurs. Initially, lactose and fat control should be considered.

Nutritional Inadequacy

The gluten-controlled diet is adequate in nutrients when compared to the Recommended Daily Allowances (RDA). However, prior to the initiation of dietary treatment, nutrient deficiencies may be seen as a result of malabsorption and inadequate dietary intake. Water-miscible preparations of fat-soluble vitamins and a daily vitamin supplement may be indicated to correct these deficiencies. Increased absorption of nutrients occurs with dietary treatment and the resultant intestinal mucosa recovery, so supplements may no longer be routinely needed. Therefore, ongoing supplementation should be assessed for each patient individually.

If diarrhea has been severe, electolyte supplements might be needed for the first few days of therapy. With severe malabsorption, calcium and magnesium blood levels could be low and thus need to be corrected by supplementation.

Indications and Rationale

Celiac disease is one of the most common chronic intestinal diseases that causes malabsorption in childhood.[1] Symptoms often begin during the second half of the first year of life after wheat-containing foods are added to the diet. The affected child gradually becomes irritable and unwell, experiences loss of appetite, and begins to pass frequent, foul, bulky stools. Vomiting is also common. Weight gain slows during this time. Small bowel biopsy shows atrophy of intestinal mucosa, and the typical clinical findings are those of malnutrition. Diminished body weight is seen in almost all patients, especially in those with prolonged active disease; short stature is also common. These growth problems are related more closely to inadequate caloric and protein intake than to the severity of the malabsorption. In infants and children with celiac disease who follow a diet controlled in gluten, studies have shown that complete recovery in weight, height, and bone age occurs.[2]

If gluten is eliminated from the diet, patients become asymptomatic with regeneration of small bowel mucosa over a period of several months. If the disease is associated with exacerbations, one must suspect the inadvertent intake of gluten-containing foods. In only a few patients, the disease is reported to be transient and is possibly related to an infection or to another inflammatory process. The patient and the parents must be cautioned against resuming the use of gluten-containing foods in the diet when symptoms subside because mucosal damage usually recurs with the reintroduction of dietary gluten. Since the diet must be continued for life, it is important to confirm the diagnosis of celiac disease by biopsy of the small intestine before diet therapy begins.

Goals of Dietary Management

With the infant or the child with celiac disease, the goals of dietary management are to control gluten intake (see Table 6–32, sources of gluten) while providing all nutrients in quantities that are adequate to ensure that needs are met for growth, development, and activity. The infant's or the child's dietary intake should be assessed for adequacy, as well as for the presence of food intolerances. Dietary guidelines should be designed using catch-up growth energy and protein recommendations (see *Failure to Thrive*, page 322). When catch-up growth has occurred, a gluten-controlled diet that reflects normal energy and nutrient needs should be recommended.

Dietary Recommendations

Dietary management requires the use of a gluten-controlled diet (see page 154). Temporary intolerance to lactose is common, and temporary intolerance to fat is sometimes seen. Therefore, the recommended diet should be not only controlled in gluten, but initially should contain milk only if it is well-tolerated. Some control of the dietary fat content should be considered because unabsorbed long chain fatty acids may be converted to hydroxy-fatty acids, which may produce diarrhea. With control of symptoms, milk and milk products should be added back into the diet, and the level of fat can be increased.

Manufacturers' information regarding the gluten content of infant foods may be obtained when planning the diet for infants.

Physicians: How to Order Diet

The diet order should indicate *gluten-controlled diet* for a child with celiac disease.

REFERENCES

1. Hamilton JR. Gastrointestinal disease: an important cause of malnutrition in childhood. In: Suskind RM, ed. Textbook of pediatric nutrition. New York: Raven Press, 1981:465–474.
2. Barr DGD, Shmerling DH, Prader A. Catch-up growth in malnutrition studied in celiac disease after reinstitution of gluten-free diet. Pediatr Res 1972;6:521–527.

HYPERLIPIDEMIA AND HYPERTENSION

General Description

Children at risk for cardiovascular disease should be treated with a low fat, low cholesterol diet with modified sodium content as defined by a statement issued in 1983 by the Task Force Committee of the Nutrition and Cardiovascular Disease in the Young Council of the American Heart Association.[1] These "high-risk" children should be closely followed. The diet is also recommended for the general population of healthy children over the age of 2 years.

Nutritional Inadequacy

This diet is planned to meet the Recommended Daily Allowances (RDA) for calories and all nutrients. This diet may be inappropriate in children who are malnourished or who have special nutritional needs.[1]

Indications and Rationale

Atherosclerosis begins in childhood and progresses in adolescence and young adulthood, even though serious clinical manifestations usually do not appear until middle age or later.[2] The evidence that establishes a causal relationship between blood cholesterol (low-density lipoprotein cholesterol) levels and coronary heart disease comes from genetic, experimental pathologic, epidemiologic, and intervention studies. However, it is clear that an elevated blood cholesterol level is not the only cause of coronary artery disease. Factors associated with risk for developement of the disease are documented in adults. Whether or not these risk factors operate in children to exert influences over the atherosclerotic process is not firmly established.

The awareness that elevated blood pressure is a pediatric problem has increased. The evidence pertaining to blood pressure is less complete than that for hyperlipidemia, but many children have blood pressures that are high, even by adult standards.[3] It is probable that primary hypertension or its predisposition has its origin in early life.[3]

There are some risk factors that are nonalterable, such as sex and genetic differences. Risk factors potentially modifiable in childhood include cigarette smoking, sedentary lifestyle, obesity, hypertension, and elevated plasma cholesterol. Healthy food habits in early childhood are important. Unfavorable lifestyle and eating habits could be corrected more readily in youth than later in life, when both are more intractable and self-perpetuating.

Goals of Dietary Management

The primary goal is to achieve moderate changes in children's cholesterol, fat, and sodium intakes while maintaining nutritional adequacy for growth and development. Excessive weight gain is to be avoided. Emphasis is placed on substitution and modification of current dietary practices, rather than inducing a drastic change or complete elimination of favorite foods. The dietary modifications are to be made gradually over several months and at a pace identified as reasonable for each individual child and adolescent. The goal should be long-term, with emphasis on gradually setting a lifestyle that can persist into adulthood. The new eating habits must be implemented in a way that allows the child or the adolescent to maintain a good self-image and to be flexible enough to maintain a reasonable lifestyle.

Dietary Recommendations

Children at Risk for Cardiovascular Disease. Children at "high-risk" can often be identified from a family history of hypercholesterolemia, premature coronary heart disease, hypertension, or stroke.[4] These children should have one high-density lipoprotein cholesterol (HDLP) determination, and two fasting total cholesterol and total triglyceride determinations. Low-density liproprotein cholesterol (LDLC) can be calculated using the formula:

$$LDLC = \text{total cholesterol} - \left(HDLC + \frac{\text{triglycerides}}{5} \right)$$

If the LDL cholesterol is between the 75 and 90 percentile (approximately 115 to 125 mg per deciliter for ages 2 to 19 years), the child is counseled regarding diet and other cardiovascular risk factors and then followed at 1-year intervals. Those with LDL cholesterol levels above the 95 percentile (greater than 135 mg per deciliter) may have familial hypercholesterolemia. The diet described in the following section (Healthy Children Over 2 Years of Age) is used initially for all children with LDL cholesterol above the 75 percentile. Nonresponders to this diet are counseled about a more controlled diet in which 25 percent of calories are from fat (equal amounts of the three types of fatty acids), and cholesterol is controlled to a daily intake less than 200 to 250 mg. Nonresponders to the second diet are considered for treatment with a lipid-lowering agent. Again, counseling regarding cardiovascular risk factors is carried out. These children are followed at 3- to 6-month intervals.

If the child has hypertriglyceridemia, the low fat, low cholesterol diet designed with calories for weight control is planned. If the hypertriglyceridemia is not successfully treated by weight control, a no "free" sugar feature is added to the diet.

Dietary sodium recommendations are consistent with those of healthy children if the "high-risk" child is not hypertensive. In our practice, a sustained blood pressure above the 95 percentile[5] requires that dietary sodium be controlled to a daily intake of 90 to 150 mEq.

Healthy Children Over 2 Years of Age. The basic intervention is a gradual shift from the current typical diet to one that is lower in total fat, saturated fat, cholesterol, and sodium. The following guidelines are recommended by the American Heart Association for healthy children over 2 years of age.[1] (Table 8–31).

TABLE 8–31   American Heart Association Dietary Guidelines for Healthy Children Over 2 Years of Age[1]

1. The diet should be nutritionally adequate, consisting of a variety of foods.
2. Caloric intake should be based on growth rate, activity level, and content of deposits of subcutaneous fat, so as to maintain desirable body weight.
3. Total fat intake should be approximately 30 percent of kilocalories, with 10 percent or less from saturated fat, about 10 percent from monounsaturated fat, and less than 10 percent from polyunsaturated fat. The emphasis should be on the reduction of total fat and saturated fat, rather than on increasing polyunsaturated fat.
4. Daily cholesterol intake should be approximately 100 mg cholesterol per 1,000 kilocalories, not to exceed 300 mg. This allows for differences in caloric intake in various age groups.
5. Protein intake should be about 15 percent of kilocalories derived from varied sources.
6. Carbohydrate kilocalories should be derived primarily from complex carbohydrate sources to provide necessary vitamins and minerals. Thus, the total percent of kilocalories from carbohydrates would be about 55 percent.
7. Excessive salt intake may be associated with hypertension in susceptible persons. On the whole, the American diet contains excessive amounts of salt. Therefore, a limitation on most highly salted processed foods and sodium-containing condiments and the elimination of added salt at the table is recommended.

Physicians: How to Order Diet

The diet order should indicate a diet for *modified cholesterol, total fat and/ or sodium for the healthy child* or a diet for *modified cholesterol, total fat and/ or sodium for the high-risk child.* Weight control or weight reduction should also be stated in the diet order (the dietitian will determine caloric levels).

REFERENCES

1. Weidman W, Kwiterovich P, Jesse MJ, Nugent E. Diet in the healthy child. Circulation 1983;67:1411A–1414A.
2. Strong JP, McGill HC Jr. The pediatric aspects of atherosclerosis. J Atheroscler Res 1969;9:251–265.
3. Lauer RM, Connor WE, Leaverton PE, Reiter MA, Clarke WR. Coronary heart disease risk factors in school children: the muscatine study. J Pediatr 1975;86:697–706.
4. Steinberg D, Chairman, Consensus Development Panel. National Institutes of Health Consensus Development Conference Statement. Lowering blood cholesterol to prevent heart disease. JAMA 1985;253:2080–2086.
5. Blumenthal S. Report of the task force on blood pressure control in children. Pediatrics 1979;suppl No. 5:797–820.

INBORN ERRORS OF METABOLISM

General Description

Metabolic disorders are inherited traits that cause disease when the normal metabolism of a compound is impaired because of the absence or the reduced activity of a specific enzyme or cofactor.[1] Some errors of metabolism result in no serious physical or mental limitations; others lead to rapid changes in the central nervous system and to severe mental retardation; still others may be lethal shortly after birth.[2]

In many cases, nutritional treatment is available to modify the effect of the disorder by providing or by limiting the missing or inactive enzyme. Nutritional treatment can be used to restrict the amount of a substrate (A) available, to supplement the amount of product (B), to supplement the cofactor (C), or to combine two or all three of these approaches (Fig. 8–2).

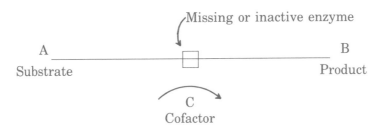

Figure 8–2 Defects seen in inborn errors of metabolism.

With permission from Trahms CM. Nutritional care for children with metabolic disorders. In: Krause MV, Mahan LK, eds. Food, nutrition and diet therapy. A textbook of nutritional care. Philadelphia: WB Saunders, 1984:802.

Table 8–32 lists examples of inborn errors of metabolism that are treated with substrate restriction.[3]

Goals of Dietary Management

The goals of nutritional therapy are to maintain biochemical equilibrium for the specific pathway, to provide adequate nutrients to support normal growth and development, and to provide support for social and emotional development.[1]

Dietary Recommendations

Dietary management is a special challenge for the dietitian, the patient, and the patient's family. Accurate calculation of the meal plan is especially critical because, in some instances, excessive intake of the restricted nutrient can lead to neurologic damage. On the other hand, insufficient amounts of kilocalories, protein, (Table 8–33) vitamins, or minerals can impair growth and development.[2] Each clinic visit should include height and weight measurements and a thorough diet history or, when possible, a food record of the preceding 3 days. Particular attention should be paid to feeding problems or to unusual food habits that might suggest noncompliance with the diet.[4]

Treatment and monitoring should be conducted at a center that has specific knowledge and experience in the evaluation and the treatment of metabolic disorders. A multidisciplinary approach is essential. The coordination of pediatric, social work, psychological, nutritional, and nursing skills, together with the assistance of a qualified biochemical laboratory, provide the resources for care of these children.[4]

A list of medical centers with expertise in the evaluation and the treatment of inborn errors of metabolism is available from the National Center for Education in Maternal and Child Health (NCEMCH).* Suggested references for these disorders that may be of benefit for both parents and health professionals follow herein.[4]

Information Sources for Parents and Health Professionals

Acosta PB. A parent's guide to the child with maple syrup urine disease. Florida State University, Center for Family Services, 103 Sandels Building, Tallahassee, Florida 32306, 1980.

Acosta PB, Elsas LJ. Dietary management of inherited metabolic disease: Phenylketonuria, galactosemia, tyrosinemia, homocystinuria, maple syrup urine disease. ACELMU Publishers, 1939 Westminister Way, Atlanta, Georgia 30307, 1976.

Bell L. Arginine equivalency system. Clinical Investigation Unit, Nutrition Division, The Hospital for Sick Children, 555 University Avenue, Toronto, Ontario, Canada M5X 1G8, 1980.

Bell L. H.S.C. equivalency system for dietary treatment of maple syrup urine disease. Clinical Investigation Unit, Nutrition Division, The Hospital for Sick Children, 555 University Avenue, Toronto, Ontario, Canada M5X 1G8, 1979.

Bell L. Low protein equivalency system. Clinical Investigation Unit, Nutrition Division, The Hospital for Sick Children, 555 University Avenue, Toronto, Ontario, Canada M5X 1G8, 1981.

Roberts RS, Meyer BA. Living with galactosemia: A handbook for families. Metabolic Unit, James Whitcomb Riley Hospital for Children, Department of Pediatrics, Indiana University School of Medicine, 702 Barnhill Drive, Indianapolis, Indiana 46223, 1983.

Lo-Pro Diet Guide. Metabolism Office, James Whitcomb Riley Hospital for Children, Room A-36, 1100 West Michigan Street, Indianapolis, Indiana 46223.

Amino acids. In: Pennington JAT, Church HN. Bowes and Church's food values of portions commonly used. 14th ed. Philadelphia: JB Lippencott Company, 1985;167.

Products for dietary management of inborn errors of metabolism and other special feeding problems. Mead Johnson & Co., Evansville, Indiana 47721, 1983.

Schuett VE. Low protein food list: For phenylketonuria and metabolic diseases requiring a low-protein diet. The Waisman Center, University of Wisconsin, 1500 Highland Avenue, Madison, Wisconsin 53706, 1981.

---

*This list is published in a booklet entitled "State treatment centers for metabolic disorders" and is available from the NCEMCH, 3520 Prospect Street, NW, Washington, D.C., or telephone (202) 625-8400.

TABLE 8–32 Hereditary Metabolic Disorders Treated by Substrate Restriction*

Disorder	Defective Pathway	Treatment	Selected Reference
Amino acids Maple syrup urine disease (branched chain ketoaciduria)	α-Keto-iscocaproic acid (α-Keto-β-methylvaleric acid α-Ketoisovaleric acid) BLOCK → α-Ketodecarboxylase +CoASH $-CO_2$ Isovaleryl CoA (α-Methylbutyryl CoA Isobutyryl CoA)	See page 381. (Nutritional therapy for classic maple syrup urine disease)	Essential amino acid requirements[4] (Table 8–33)
Hypervalinemia	Valine $-NH_2$ Valine Transaminase BLOCK α-Ketoisovaleric acid	Diet low in branched-chain amino acids	Essential amino acid requirements[4] (See Table 8–33)
Isovaleric acidemia	Isovaleryl CoA Isovaleryl CoA Dehydrogenase BLOCK β-Methylcrotonyl CoA	Low protein diet	
Leucinosis		Diet low in leucine, isoleucine, valine: milder variant responds well to massive doses of B_1, up to 20 mg/day	Essential amino acid requirements[4] (See Table 8–33)
Methylmalonic aciduria (acidemia)	Isoleucine, methionine, valine, threonine Methylmalonyl CoA → methylmalonate Cobalamin Dependent BLOCK Succinyl CoA	Dietary restriction of protein If vitamin B_{12} responsive, 1 mg/day IM Restrict protein containing isoleucine, threonine, valine, and methionine to amounts required for growth	

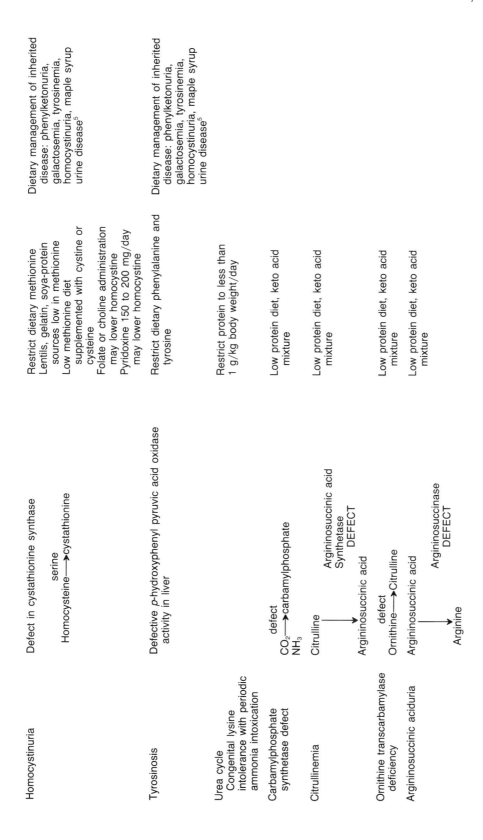

Disorder	Biochemical defect	Dietary treatment	Reference
Homocystinuria	Defect in cystathionine synthase serine Homocysteine → cystathionine	Restrict dietary methionine Lentils, gelatin, soya-protein sources low in methionine Low methionine diet supplemented with cystine or cysteine Folate or choline administration may lower homocystine Pyridoxine 150 to 200 mg/day may lower homocystine	Dietary management of inherited disease: phenylketonuria, galactosemia, tyrosinemia, homocystinuria, maple syrup urine disease[5]
Tyrosinosis	Defective p-hydroxyphenyl pyruvic acid oxidase activity in liver	Restrict dietary phenylalanine and tyrosine	Dietary management of inherited disease: phenylketonuria, galactosemia, tyrosinemia, homocystinuria, maple syrup urine disease[5]
Urea cycle Congenital lysine intolerance with periodic ammonia intoxication		Restrict protein to less than 1 g/kg body weight/day	
Carbamylphosphate synthetase defect	CO_2 NH_3 defect→ carbamylphosphate	Low protein diet, keto acid mixture	
Citrullinemia	Citrulline → Argininosuccinic acid Synthetase DEFECT Argininosuccinic acid	Low protein diet, keto acid mixture	
Ornithine transcarbamylase deficiency	defect Ornithine → Citrulline	Low protein diet, keto acid mixture	
Argininosuccinic aciduria	Argininosuccinic acid → Argininosuccinase DEFECT Arginine	Low protein diet, keto acid mixture	

TABLE 8–32 Hereditary Metabolic Disorders Treated by Substrate Restriction* (continued)

Disorder	Defective Pathway	Treatment	Selected Reference
Carbohydrates Hereditary galactokinase deficiency	Galactose → Galactose-1-P Galactokinase ATP DEFECT	Galactose-free diet	Common carbohydrate in food per 100 g edible portion (see *Pediatric Appendix 3*, page 472)
Galactosemia	Galactose-1-P + UDPG → UDP-galatose + glucose-1-P Glactose-1-P Uridyl transferase DEFECT	Galactose-free diet	Dietary management of inherited metabolic disease: phenylketonuria, galactosemia, tyrosinemia, homocystinuria, maple syrup urine disease[5]
Hereditary fructose intolerance	Fructose-1-P → Glyceraldehyde + DHAP Fructose-1-P Aldolase ALMOST ABSENT	Fructose-free diet	Common carbohydrate in foods per 100 g edible portion (see *Pediatric Appendix 3*, page 472)
Carbohydrate malabsorption Glucose-galactose malabsorption		Only fructose is tolerated Formula: protein hydrolysate, corn oil, and fructose Jerusalem artichoke is a useful carbohydrate source (contains inulin-fructose polymer)	
Sucrose-isomaltose malabsorption		Eliminate sucrose, dextrins, and starch from the diet	

Disorder	Description	Treatment
Lactose malabsorption		Remove milk, certain milk products from diet Calcium is supplied by other sources
Sucrase-isomaltase deficiency		Dietary fructose (up to 60% of total calories) as a form of therapy to increase sucrase activity Then, sucrose-restricted diet with approximately 20% of the total calories as fructose, permits occasional sucrose ingestion
Glycogen diseases Type O-glycogen synthetase deficiency	Liver has a very low glycogen content and virtual absence of glycogen synthetase	High protein diet Frequent carbohydrate feedings Extra meal at night
Type I: glucose-6-P defect (Van Creveld-Von Gierke's disease)	Glucose-6-P $\xrightarrow{\text{Glucose-6-phosphatase DEFICIENCY}}$ Glucose + P; Glycogen mobilization-inhibited	See Glycogen storage disease page 372
Type III: debrancher enzyme defect (limit dextrinosis or Forbes disease)	Deficiency in enzymes needed for degradation of glycogen: amylo-1,6-glucosidase and/or oligo-1,4 → 1,4 gluconyl-transferase	See Glycogen storage disease page 372
Type V: myophosphorylase deficiency (McArdle-Schmidt-Pearson disease)	Inability to mobilize glycogen from skeletal muscle	See Glycogen storage disease page 372
Type VI: hepatic phosphorylase deficiency glycogenosis (Hers disease)	Inability to mobilize glycogen from the liver to maintain homeostasis in glycose metabolism	See Glycogen storage disease page 372

* Reprinted with permission from Nyhan WL. Nutritional treatment of children with inborn errors of metabolism. In: Suskind RM, ed. Textbook of pediatric nutrition. New York: Raven Press, 1981:563.

TABLE 8–33 Essential Amino Acid Requirements*†

	Infants 2 to 4 Months mg/kg/day	Boys 10 to 12 Years		Young Adults	
		mg/day	mg/kg/day	mg/day	mg/kg/day
Histidine	16–34				
Isoleucine	80–100	1,000	30	250–700	10–11
Leucine	76–150	1,000–1,500	45	620–1,100	11–13
Lysine	88–103	1,200–1,600	60	300–900	9–10
Methionine—					
no cystine		400–800	27	800–1,100	11–16
cystine present	35–45			75–350	2–5
Phenylalanine—					
no tyrosine		400–800	27	800–1,100	11–16
tyrosine present	47–90			220–500	3–7
Threonine	45–87	800–1,000	35	310–500	6–7
Tryptophan	15–22	60–120	3.7	160–225	3.1–3.2
Valine	85–105	600–900	33	650–800	11–14

*Reprinted with permission from the Committee on Nutrition, American Academy of Pediatrics. Final report, task force on the dietary management of metabolic disorders. December, 1985;19–21.

†Exact information about amino acid requirements is deficient in that only three age groups have been investigated: infants under 3 months of age, boys 10 to 12 years old, and young adults of college age. Since the diets in these studies were mixtures of amino acids, they are very similar to the diets used in the treatment of metabolic errors.

The figures for the adults are a composite of several studies; the values expressed in terms of body weight have used 60 kg for female and 70 kg for male subjects. It should be noted that, expressed in terms of body weight, there is a reduction in quantities required with age. The greatest reduction occurs during the first year of life.

REFERENCES

1. Trahms CM. Nutritional care for children with metabolic disorders. In: Krause MV, Mahan LK, eds. Food, nutrition and diet therapy. A textbook of nutritional care. Philadelphia: WB Saunders, 1984;802.
2. Robinson CH, Lawler MR, Chenowether WL, Garwick AE. Normal and therapeutic nutrition. 17th ed. New York: Macmillan Publishing Company, 1986;588.
3. Nyhan WL. Nutritional treatment of children with inborn errors of metabolism. In: Suskind RM, ed. Textbook of pediatric nutrition. New York: Raven Press, 1981;563.
4. Committee on Nutrition, American Academy of Pediatrics. Final report, task force on the dietary management of metabolic disorders. December, 1985;19–21.
5. Acosta PB, Elsas LJ. Dietary management of inherited metabolic disease: phenylketonuria, galactosemia, tyrosinemia, homocystinuria, maple syrup urine disease. Atlanta: ACELMU Publishers, 1976.

Glycogen Storage Diseases

The glycogen storage diseases (GSD) are a group of disorders characterized by metabolic errors that lead to abnormal concentrations or structures of glycogen, primarily in liver or muscle tissue.

Glycogen Storage Disease Type I

General Description

Type I Glycogen Storage Disease (GSD-I) is a disorder that involves the enzyme glucose-6-phosphatase and results in difficulties in glucose synthesis from glyconeogenic precursors.[1] Frequent high starch feedings that are limited in galactose and fructose content are prescribed during the day in conjunction with continuous tube feedings during the night.

Nutritional Inadequacy

The meal plan and the nocturnal feedings provide adequate kilocalories for the child's age, size, and activity and adequate protein for growth. The diet needs to be evaluated for nutritional adequacy as compared with the Recommended Daily Allowance (RDA). Supplementation with a pediatric multivitamin-mineral supplement, including calcium, is required due to the limited intake of milk and fruit.

Indications and Rationale

The most common of the 12 recognized types of GSD is Type I Glycogen Storage Disease (GSD-I), which represents about a quarter of the patients diagnosed with GSD and which affects one child in every 200,000 births.[2] Two types of GSD-I have been identified (Type Ia and Ib) and both are thought to be autosomal recessive disorders. Type Ia results from deficient activity of hepatic, renal, and intestinal glucose-6-phosphatase, the last enzymatic step in glucose production, by the liver, from both hepatic glycogen and from the conversion of gluconeogenic precursors (such as amino acids and lactate) to glucose via gluconeogenesis.[3] Type Ib results from a defect in the transport of glucose-6-phosphate through the microsomal membrane, which is a necessary step for the substrate to gain access to glucose-6-phosphatase.

Hypoglycemia is the most prominent and life-threatening complication of Type Ia and Ib GSD and occurs within 2 to 4 hours after a meal;[1] however, the degree of hypoglycemia can be extremely variable.[4] Plasma concentrations of gluconeogenic precursors (lactate, pyruvate, and alanine) are elevated and can be associated with severe lactic acidosis. The elevation of blood lactate, rather than ketone bodies, may provide an alternate substrate for brain metabolism, since these patients do not develop significant ketosis.[3] The hypoglycemia is often asymptomatic. Plasma glucose concentrations of 5 to 10 mg glucose per deciliter (0.3 to 0.6 mM) after a 6- to 8-hour fast are not unusual.

Other abnormalities associated with GSD-I include: hypertriglyceridemia, hyperuricemia, clotting defect, hepatomegaly, growth retardation, and osteoporosis. Plasma triglyceride concentrations frequently are increased to 1,000 to 2,000 mg per deciliter[3] or more and probably are responsible for the platelet abnormalities that are seen in these patients. The hyperlipidemia is believed to be related to decreased lipoprotein lipase activity and to decreased lipogenesis.[5] Osteoporosis usually is present and may be attributable to negative calcium balance related to chronic metabolic acidosis.[4] Osteoporosis may be severe enough to cause spontaneous fractures.[3] Severe growth retardation and delayed puberty are common. If left untreated, the individual's final adult stature may be less than 5 feet. The abdomen is enlarged to accomodate a massively enlarged liver, secondary to fat accumulation within the hepatocytes. There is a tendency to adiposity with poor muscle tone and with an accumulation of fat in the buttocks, the cheeks, and the subcutaneous tissues. In untreated children, hyperuricemia may cause renal damage,[3] and hepatic adenomas may develop, usually after the age of 15.[1] In addition, patients with Type Ib have granulocytopenia, abnormal leukocyte chemotaxis, and recurrent mucocutaneous infections, which can be life-threatening.

Goals of Dietary Management

The goal of treatment is to minimize organic acidemia[6] and to maintain blood glucose levels between 80 to 100 mg per deciliter, thereby avoiding hypoglycemia from inadequate glucose (starch) intake or reactive hypoglycemia from excessive glucose intake.[1]

Dietary Recommendations

High starch feedings spaced at 2- to 4-hour intervals[7] during the day and combined with nocturnal tube feedings of liquid formulas that contain glucose polymers have been successful at improving survival and correcting abnormal growth and development.[4,5,8] Treatment has reportedly resulted in reduced hepatomegaly secondary to loss of fat accumulation, improved bone mineralization with a decreased risk of spontaneous fracture, reduced uric acid levels, correction of acidosis,[3] increased rate of protein synthesis[9] due to changes in nitrogen metabolism,[3] improvement of muscle mass and strength, reversal of adiposity,[5] and regression of hepatic adenomas.[1] The improvement in blood chemistries and the growth spurt after the initiation of treatment may be attributable to the correction of hypoglycemia and the correction of the chronic metabolic acidosis.

Patient response to treatment with frequent day-time starch feedings and with nocturnal tube feedings is variable, and most abnormalities associated with GSD-I improve, but are not corrected. Lactate and triglyceride levels continue to be mildly to moderately elevated in most patients.[3,10,11] In addition, continued abnormalities in venous CO_2, total lipids, phospholipids,[11] cholesterol,[10,11] serum uric acid,[3,8,10,11] and serum glutamic oxaloacetic transaminase (SGOT)[10,11] have been reported in some patients.

Nocturnal Tube Feedings. Night-time tube feedings need to provide exogeneous glucose at a rate that minimizes the need for the liver to produce glucose, and thereby effectively take over the main function of the missing glucose-6-phosphatase.[3] Most normal infants and children produce glucose at the rate of 5 to 8 mg per kilogram per minute.[12] The major factor in controlling blood lactate levels of these patients may be the adjustment of the rate of feeding to be equal to or slightly greater than normal hepatic glucose production.[3,13] Glucose provided at the rate of 8 to 9 mg per kilogram of body weight per minute prevent hypoglycemia and minimize organic acidemia in most GSD-I patients.[6] The infusion rate needs to be adjusted on an individualized basis and re-evaluated every 3 to 6 months.[7] Infusion rates significantly greater than this can lead to day-time anorexia,[6] to difficulty in consuming adequate carbohydrate during the day, and to inadequate protein intake.[7] Glucose can be provided by Vivonex,[7,14] by glucose polymers, or, in a less expensive form, by glucose (dextrose) that is obtained from wine-making shops or from bakery supply companies.[6] Nocturnal feedings should be continued at least until maximum growth is achieved.[1]

Providing the formula by constant, even infusion using a feeding pump with an alarm system to warn of tube occlusion or power failure is essential. Hypoglycemia occurs much more rapidly after the discontinuation of tube feedings than after a meal. This hypoglycemia is perhaps secondary to decreased circulating lactate levels, which decrease the availability of this presumed substrate for brain metabolism.[9] Deaths have occured from rapid and severe hypoglycemia in patients in whom the infusion was accidentally stopped.[3]

Most children can learn to insert their own nasogastric tubes nightly without difficulty. Parents and children need careful instruction in the use of and the care of the pump. If use of the nasogastric tube is unsuccessful, a gastrostomy tube may be inserted. However, with proper instruction most patients can be managed appropriately with nasogastric tubes.

Cornstarch Therapy. In older children, in adolescents, and in adults, uncooked cornstarch can be used as an alternative form of effective therapy for GSD-I patients.[15] Ingestion of 1.75 to 2.5 g cornstarch per kilogram of body weight every 6 hours, which provides 5.3 to 7.6 mg of glucose per kilogram per minute, has been demonstrated to maintain a relatively constant blood glucose concentration if initial blood glucose concentration was normal. The long-term cornstarch regimen has been as effective as nocturnal nasogastric infusions at maintaining commonly measured laboratory data and at promoting normal or catchup growth.[15]

Proper preparation of the cornstarch is imperative to proper management. The cornstarch must be prepared with tap water at *room temperature.* Cooked cornstarch, or cornstarch mixed with hot water or lemonade, results in a sharp rise in blood glucose followed by a rapid fall within 3 to 5 hours. Heating the cornstarch may disrupt the starch granules, thereby making them more accessible to hydrolysis by amylase. Side effects of transient diarrhea, abdominal distention, and increased flatulence are minor and resolve spontaneously.[15] Cornstarch therapy is less effective when blood glucose concentrations are low.[15]

Cornstarch therapy is not recommended for infants or for young children. Starch hydrolysis results primarily from the activity of two enzymes, pancreatic amylase and intestinal glucoamylase. By 1 month, infants have levels of glucoamylase comparable to that of young adults, but do not reach full levels of adult pancreatic amylase until 2 to 4 years.[15] In addition, the cornstarch has a granular texture, must be eaten without additives or flavorings, and, therefore, is not generally palatable to young children. This results in inconsistent intake and increases the risks and the problems associated with hypoglycemia and poor metabolic control.

Oral Feedings. The child should consume small, frequent high starch feedings every 2 to 4 hours,[7] or as often as is necessary to keep blood glucose levels between 80 to 100 mg per deciliter.[1] The first feeding of the day must be within approximately 30 minutes before, or *immediately* after, the child discontinues nocturnal tube feedings,[14] due to the rapid onset of hypoglycemia after the cessation of intragastric feedings. Five to six oral feedings are given per day, depending upon the duration of the tube feeding schedule and the individual child's needs.[14] The last evening feeding should occur within the 2- to 3-hour period before nocturnal feeding begins.

Oral feedings provide 60 to 70 percent of the kilocalories from carbohydrate, 25 to 35 percent of the kilocalories from fat, and 10 to 15 percent of the kilocalories from protein. The carbohydrate source should be primarily starch. Galactose- and fructose-containing foods, such as fruits, table sugar, and milk, are limited or avoided, since these carbohydrates must be metabolized in the liver and are converted either to glycogen or to lactate. Ingestion of large amounts of these sugars can contribute to lactic acidosis.[7] A high protein diet is not beneficial, since GSD-I patients have a limited ability to convert amino acids to free glucose.[4]

The child's meal plan provides guidelines for food intake and needs to be based on the child's food preferences and on family eating habits. Prime emphasis needs to be placed on the *frequency of feeding* and the *ingestion of the high starch feedings.* Variation from the meal plan and inclusions of small amounts of lactose or galactose are allowed, as long as the patient is able to maintain blood glucose levels within the desired range.

Food exchanges (Tables 8–34 and 8–35) that eliminate lactose, fructose, and sucrose are used in preparing a meal plan that provides small, equal-sized feedings at set intervals. Each feeding should contain, as nearly as practical to do so, the same distribution of carbohydrate and of protein. Fat should be evenly distributed when possible. The incorporation of some protein and some fat in each high starch feeding seems to help prolong the period of absorption of the glucose.[14] Some school-aged children are able to meet their needs for glucose by mixing Polycose powder (2 g carbohydrate per level teaspoon) with sugar-free carbonated beverages, or by eating cornstarch (8.3 g of carbohydrate per tablespoon).[7]

The long-term prognosis of GSD-I patients is still unclear. Patients who survive past the second decade usually have less tendency toward hypoglycemia,[2,15] and one patient has been weaned completely from nocturnal feedings and maintains normal blood glucose and other blood chemistry values.[16]

Glycogen Storage Disease Type III and VI

General Description

Glycogen Storage Disease Type III (GSD-III) is characterized by a deficiency in the hepatic debrancher enzyme (amylo-1, 6-glucosidase), which is required for the release of glucose from all but the terminal portions of the glycogen polymer.[3] Glycogen Storage Disease Type VI is characterized by a reduction of normal hepatic phosphorylase activity. The majority of patients have hepatomegaly, growth failure, and mild to moderate increases in serum lipids early in life. The clinical courses in GSD-III and GSD-VI are generally much milder than in GSD-I because severe hypoglycemia is not a problem, except with more prolonged fasting.[1]

Nutritional Inadequacy

The meal plan and the nocturnal feedings provide adequate kilocalories for the child's age, size, and activity and adequate protein for growth. The diet needs to be evaluated for nutritional adequacy as compared with the Recommended Daily Allowance (RDA). Supplementation with a pediatric multiple vitamin and mineral supplement, including calcium, is required because of the limited intake of milk and fruit.

Indications and Rationale

These patients are able to readily convert fructose, galactose, and gluconeogenic precursors (lactate, pyruvate, and amino acids) to glucose.[1,4] Patients can adapt to prolonged fasting by accelerated ketogenesis and can maintain normal blood glucose levels by gluconeogenesis when the onset of fasting is gradual.

After a high carbohydrate meal, hypoglycemia occurs before the alternate sources of fuel can be mobilized.

Dietary Recommendations

Hypoglycemia and wide swings in plasma glucose levels can be averted by a diet that is high in protein,[3,4,16] that has small, frequent feedings,[4,17] and that has a limited free sugar intake[3] (approximately 20 to 25 percent protein, 40 to 50 percent carbohydrate, 25 to 35 percent fat).[18] In addition, the high protein diet may improve the mild muscle weakness that is occasionally observed in these children.[1]

Frequent day-time feedings are usually sufficient to prevent hypoglycemia. However, some patients with GSD-III have more severe disease with myopathy and growth failure. These abnormalities may result, in part, from muscle protein degradation that occurs in order to provide adequate amino acid as a gluconeogenic substrate to maintain hepatic glucose production.[18] A high protein nocturnal tube feeding combined with a high protein diet has been demonstrated to improve muscle strength, muscle mass, endurance, and growth rates,[5,18] and to eliminate early morning hypoglycemia.[18]

After puberty, the liver decreases in size,[1,18] symptomatic hypoglycemic episodes are rare, and there is a normal growth spurt.[18] Outlook for a long life is good.[4]

Glycogen Storage Disease Type IIB

General Description

GSD Type IIB is characterized by deficient activity of α-1, 4-glucosidase (acid maltase deficiency). The disease presents in childhood or in adulthood with muscle weakness and hypotonia.[4]

Dietary Recommendations

Patients may benefit from increased protein intake.[7]

Other Types of GSD

General Description

Nutritional therapy has not proven beneficial with other types of GSD.

GSD Support Group

There is a support group for patients with GDS and their parents:

> Association for Glycogen Storage Disease
> RR #1, Box 46
> Stockton, IA 52769

Physicians: How to Order Diet

The diet order should indicate:

GDS-I: Indicate *diet for GSD-I without cornstarch* or *diet for GDS-I with cornstarch*. The type and rate of nocturnal feeding must be specified.

GSD-IIB: Indicate *diet for GDS Type IIB.*

GSD-III: Indicate *diet for GSD-III.* The type of nocturnal tube feeding (if any) must be specified.

GSD-VI: Indicate *diet for GSD-VI.*

Other GSD: No diet therapy is indicated.

TABLE 8-34 Food Exchanges for GSD-I Meal Planning*

Exchange Groups	Protein g	Fat g	Carbohydrate g
Starch	2	0	15
Meat (1/2 oz)	3	2	0
Fat	0	5	0
Vegetables (free in small amounts)	—	—	—

*Folk CC, Greene HL. Dietary management of type I glycogen storage disease. Copyright The American Dietetic Association. Reprinted with permission from Journal of the American Dietetic Association 1984;84:293.

TABLE 8-35 Exchange Lists for Glycogen Storage Disease Type I*

Starch Exchanges

Bagel	1/2 average	Crackers	
Bread	1 slice	Cheese Tid-bits§	40
Bread crumbs, dry	1/4 cup	oyster	20
Bread stuffing, dry	1/3 cup	pretzels, very thin	
Buns		sticks	60
wiener	1/2	round, thin ($1\frac{1}{2}$ inch)	6
large hamburger	1/2	saltines (2 inch square)	6
small hamburger	1	Wheat Thins§	12
Cake, angel (1/2 inch slice)	1	Starchy vegetables	
Melba toast, oblong	4	beans (lima, navy, pinto, white, lentils),	
Melba toast, round	8	dried, cooked	1/2 cup
Roll (2 inch diameter)	1	corn	
Rusk	2 slice	hominy	1/2 cup
Tortilla (6 inch diameter)	1	on the cob	1 small
Zwieback	3 slice	whole kernel	1/3 cup
Cereals		mixed vegetables	1/2 cup
All-bran†	1/3 cup	peas (black-eyed, etc.)	1/2 cup
barley	1/2 cup	potato, white	
bran flakes, raisin bran	1/2 cup	baked or boiled	1 small
cooked	1/2 cup	mashed	1/2 cup
dry (flakes or puffed)	3/4 cup	squash (acorn,	
Cornmeal (dry)	2 Tbsp	butternut, or	
Cornstarch	2 Tbsp	winter)	3/4 cup
Flour	$2\frac{1}{2}$ Tbsp	sweet potatoes or	
Grape Nuts,‡ wheat germ	1/4 cup	yams	1/4 cup
Grits, cooked	1/2 cup	Prepared foods	
Macaroni, cooked	1/2 cup	biscuit (2 inch diameter)	1
Noodles, cooked	1/2 cup	cornbread ($1\frac{1}{2}$ inch	
Popcorn (no fat added)	2 cups	cube)	1
Rice, cooked	1/2 cup	corn chips	1/3 cup
Spaghetti, cooked	1/2 cup	corn muffin (2 inch diameter)	1
		French fries	8 pieces or 1/2 cup
		pancake (5 inch diameter)	1
		potato chips	15

TABLE 8–35 Exchange Lists (continued)

Meat Exchanges

Cooked meat, fish,		Cheese	1 oz
poultry	1/2 oz	Peanut butter (no sugar)	1/2 oz
Canned fish	1/2 oz	Luncheon meat (avoid	
Egg	1/2	excessive sucrose)	1 oz

Fat Exchanges

Avocado	1/8	Bacon drippings or grease	1 tsp
Cooking oil or shortening	1 tsp	Butter	1 tsp
Margarine, diet	2 tsp	Chitterlings, boiled	1/8 cup
Margarine, regular	1 tsp	Chocolate, unsweetened	1 tsp
Mayonnaise	1 tsp	Coconut, shredded	2 Tbsp
Nuts, pecans, or walnuts	4 large halves	Cracklins	1 heaping tsp
Olives	5 small	Cream cheese	1 Tbsp
Peanuts, shelled	1 Tbsp	Cream	
Salad Dressings		heavy, unwhipped	1 Tbsp
French, Italian, oil		heavy, whipped	2 Tbsp
and vinegar, Roquefort,		Fatback (2 inch × 1 inch	
Thousand Island	2 tsp	× 1/2 inch)	1 slice
Sunflower seeds	1 Tbsp	Gravy	2 Tbsp
Tartar sauce	2 tsp	Half and half	1/4 cup
Sour cream (commercial)	2 Tbsp	Lard	1 tsp
Sour cream substitutes	2 Tbsp	Whipped topping	
bacon, crisp	1 slice	(commercial)	3 Tbsp

Vegetables

Artichoke	1 med	Onions	
Asparagus		Parsley	
Bamboo shoots		Peppers, green	
Bean sprouts		Pimiento	
Broccoli		Radishes	
Brussels sprouts		Rhubarb	
Cabbage		Romaine	
Carrots		Rutabagas	
Cauliflower		Sauerkraut	
Celery		Squash, summer	
Chicory		String beans, young	
Cucumber		Tomatoes	
Eggplant		Tomato juice	1/2 cup
Endive		Tomato paste	
Escarole		Tomato puree	
Greens		Tomato sauce	
beet, chard, collard,		Turnips	
dandelion, kale,		Vegetable juice cocktail	1/2 cup
lettuce, mustard, poke,		Watercress	
spinach, turnip		Zucchini	
Mushrooms			
Okra			

TABLE 8–35 Exchange Lists (continued)

Free Foods

Beverages
  Kool-Aid,[‡] artificially
    sweetened
  lemonade, artifically
    sweetened
  limeade, artifically
    sweetened
  sugar-free carbonated
    drinks (avoid
    caffeine)
Sauces
  catsup   1 Tbsp
  chili sauce   1 Tbsp
  hot sauce
  seafood cocktail sauce
  soy sauce
  steak sauce
Seasonings
  artificial sweeteners
  butter flavoring
  butter-flavored salt
  garlic
  herbs
  lemon
  liquid smoke
  mint
  onion
  parsley
  pepper
  salt
  seasoned salt
  spices
  tenderizers
  vanilla and other
    flavorings
  vinegar

Soups
  bouillon
  clear broth
Miscellaneous
  cranberries, fresh or
    frozen without
    sugar
  gelatin, unsweetened
    or artificially
    sweetened
  horseradish
  mustard, prepared or
    dry
  pickles, sour or
    unsweetened dill
  rennet tablets
  salad dressing,
    calorie-free
  salad dressing, low
    calorie—up to
    15 kilocalorie
  sugarless chewing
    gum
  whipped topping   1 Tbsp
  corn syrup in small
    amounts

Foods Restricted In Intake

Cakes, unless glucose is
  used
Candy
Chewing gum, regular
Coffee
Cookies, unless glucose
  is used
Condensed milk
Custards or puddings
Doughnuts
Fried foods—except if
  allowed fats are used
Fruits
Fruit juices
Fruit drink mixes, such
  as Tang[‡] and Kool-Aid[‡]
  (pre-sweetened)
Tea
Honey

Jam
Jelly
Marmalade or preserves
Milk
Milk shakes
Molasses or sorghum
Pies
Soft drinks containing
  sugar or caffeine
Sugar
Sugar-coated cereals
Sweet pickles
Sweet rolls
Syrups

---

[*] Folk CC, Greene HL. Dietary management of type I glycogen storage disease. Copyright The American Dietetic Association. Reprinted with permission from Journal of the American Dietetic Association, 1984;84:293.
[†] Kellogg Co., Battle Creek, MI
[‡] General Foods Corp, White Plains, NY
[§] Nabisco, East Hanover, NJ

REFERENCES

1. Greene HL. Glycogen storage disease. Semin Liver Dis 1982;2:291–301.
2. Greene HL, Slonim AE, Burr IM. Type I glycogen storage disease: A metabolic basis for advances in treatment. In: Barness LA, ed. Advances in pediatrics. Chicago: Year Book Medical Publishers, Inc., 1979:63.
3. Stanley CA. Intragastric feeding in glycogen storage disease and other disorders of fasting. In: Walker WA, Watkins JB, eds. Nutrition in pediatrics. Boston/Toronto: Little, Brown and Company, 1985:781.
4. Howell RR, Williams JC. The glycogen storage diseases. In: Stanbury JB, Wyngaarden JB, Fredrickson DS, Goldstein JL, Brown MS. The metabolic basis of inherited disease. 5th ed. New York: McGraw-Hill Book Company, 1983:141.
5. Daeschel IE, Janick LS, Kramish MJ, Coleman RA. Diet and growth of children with glycogen storage disease types I and III. J Am Diet Assoc 1983;83:135–141.
6. Haymond MW, Schwenk WF. Optimal rate of enteral glucose administration in children with glycogen storage disease type I. N Engl J Med 1986;314:682–685.
7. Haymond MW. Personal communication. Mayo Clinic Department of Pediatrics, 1986.
8. Greene HL, Slonim AE, O'Neill JA Jr, Burr IM. Continuous nocturnal intragastric feeding for management of type I glycogen-storage disease. N Engl J Med 1976;294:423–425.
9. Slonin AE, Lacy WW, Terry A, Greene HL, Burr IM. Nocturnal intragastric therapy in type I glycogen storage disease: effect on hormonal and amino acid metabolism. Metabolism 1979;28:707–715.
10. Greene HL, Slonim AE, Burr IM, Moran JR. Type I glycogen storage disease: five years of management with nocturnal intragastric feeding. J Pediatr 1980;96:590–595.
11. Michels VV, Beaudet AL, Potts YE, Montandon CM. Glycogen storage disease: long-term follow-up of nocturnal intragastric feeding. Clin Genet 1982:21:136–140.
12. Bier DM, Leake RD, Haymond MW, Arnold KJ, Gruenke LD, Sperling MA, Kipnis MK. Measurement of "true" glucose production rates in infancy and childhood with 6,6-dideuteroglucose. Diabetes 26:1016–1023.
13. Tsalikian E, Howard C, Gerich JE, Haymond MW. Increased leucine flux in short-term fasted human subjects: evidence for increased proteolysis. Am J Physiol 1984;247:E323–327.
14. Folk CC, Greene HL. Dietary management of type I glycogen storage disease. J Am Diet Assoc 1984;84:293–301.
15. Chen UT, Cornblath M, Sidbury JB. Cornstarch therapy in type I glycogen-storage disease. N Engl J Med 1984;310:171–175.
16. Greene HL, Parker PH, Slonim AE, Burr IM. Resolution of the need for continuous nocturnal feeding in a patient with severe type I glycogen storage disease. J Pediatr 1981;99:602–605.
17. Leonard JV, Francis DEM, Dunger DB. The dietary management of hepatic glycogen storage disease. Proc Nutr Soc 1979;38:321–324.
18. Slonim AE, Coleman RA, Moses WS. Myopathy and growth failure in debrancher enzyme deficiency: improvement with high-protein nocturnal enteral therapy. J Pediatr 1984;105:906–911.

Maple Syrup Urine Disease

General Description

Leucine, isoleucine, and valine are controlled according to individual needs. A semi-synthetic formula that is free of the branched chain amino acids provides the majority of the protein. Foods that contain small amounts of protein and branched chain amino acids make up the rest of the diet.

Nutritional Inadequacy

The meal plan needs to provide adequate kilocalories for the child's age, size, and activity and adequate amino acid intake for growth. The diet needs to be evaluated for nutritional adequacy as compared with the Recommended Daily Allowance (RDA) for age.

Indications and Rationale

Classic maple syrup urine disease (MSUD) results from the deficiency of a single common enzyme that catalyzes the oxidative decarboxylation of the branched chain amino acids (BCAA) leucine, isoleucine, and valine. The plasma concentration of leucine is significantly higher than that of the other two branched chain amino acids[1] in untreated children with MSUD. The disease is inherited as an autosomal recessive trait[1] and is estimated to occur in 1 in 225,000 newborns.[1] Often, the first clue toward diagnosis is the distinctive odor of the urine, perspiration, or ear wax towards the end of the first week of life. The substances responsible for the maple syrup odor are unknown at present; the odor is not attributable to the branched chain keto acids.[2] If untreated, MSUD leads to progressive hypoglycemia, metabolic acidosis, neurologic deterioration, coma, and death.[3] Delay in diagnosis or treatment beyond 1 week of life generally results in severe neurologic damage and mental retardation in those who survive. These problems are usually minimized or averted with early diagnosis and proper therapy. Reportedly, normal growth and a mean IQ development quotient of 101 were achieved in four patients with MSUD who were followed for 8,400 treatment days.[4]

Variants of MSUD. Other variants of MSUD are intermediate, intermittent, and thiamine-responsive in addition to classic MSUD.[5] The degree of severity and protein tolerance are related to the amount of residual enzyme activity (Table 8–36).

TABLE 8–36 Classification of MSUD by Branched Chain Ketoacid Decarboxylase Activity*

Classification	Decarboxylase Activity (percent of normal level)	Dietary Protein Tolerance
Classic	0–2	Dietary restriction of leucine, isoleucine, and valine. Nitrogen provided as L-amino acids.
Intermediate	5–25	Moderate dietary restriction of leucine, isoleucine, and valine
Intermittent	2–40	Unrestricted
Thiamine-responsive	approximately 40	Thiamine supplementation (10–1,000 mg per day); possible mild restriction of leucine, isoleucine, and valine.

*With permission from Rohr FJ, Levy HL, Shih VE. Inborn errors of metabolism. In: Walker WA, Watkins JB, eds. Nutrition in pediatrics. Boston/Toronto: Little, Brown and Company, 1985:400.

Goals of Dietary Management

Depending on the severity of the child's clinical condition, the acute phase of treatment may consist of peritoneal dialysis to remove α keto acids, infusion of high rates of intravenous glucose (10 to 15 mg per kilogram per minute) to suppress proteolysis, and initiation of a branched chain amino acid-free diet. Oral feedings can be initiated after fluid and electrolyte imbalances are corrected.[5] Anabolic requirements of the branched chain amino acids, including the requirement for growth, must be provided, yet must not permit the accumulation of precursor metabolites proximal to the deficient enzyme (BCAA and their keto acid derivatives).

Nutritional management involves assessment of growth, evaluation of nutritional adequacy of the diet, and extremely careful monitoring of blood levels of the branched chain amino acids, especially leucine, and perhaps branched chain α keto acids.[6] BCAA intake needs to be adjusted frequently to maintain plasma leucine levels between 2 to 5 mg per deciliter. Levels above 10 mg per deciliter are associated with α ketoacidemia and neurologic symptoms.[7] During illness, BCAA intake must be decreased and carbohydrates increased to suppress proteolysis. Acute infections or catabolic illnesses may lead to encephalopathy and death despite treatment.

Dietary Recommendations

The diet for MSUD necessitates the use of a semi-synthetic formula, such as MSUD diet powder. The formula contains crystalline L-amino acids except the BCAA, as well as appropriate amounts of carbohydrate, fat, minerals, and vitamins (Table 8–37). Small, carefully measured amounts of milk or regular infant formula need to be added to the MSUD formula to provide the BCAA needs of the infant. Small amounts of low protein foods are used to provide the BCAA needs of the older child.

The child's daily requirements for kilocalories, protein, leucine, isoleucine, and valine should be individually assessed. Energy requirements are normal after the acutely ill infant stabilizes and compensates from growth defects secondary to the initial illness.[5] Nutrient requirements of children and infants with MSUD are the same as those for normal children.[8] While nitrogen balance studies would be the most precise method of monitoring adequacy of the dietary protein intake, weight gain in infants is a sensitive and an easily monitored index of well-being and nutritional adequacy.[7]

The amount of MSUD diet powder to be used needs to be determined. (See Table 8–37 for composition.)

The amount of milk or regular infant formula, if any, to be added to meet the child's needs for the BCAA is also estimated. The requirements for individual amino acids are difficult to determine since normal growth and development can be achieved over a wide range of intake. The following guidelines

TABLE 8–37 Nutrient Composition of Formula* for the Treatment of Maple Syrup Urine Disease and Organic Acidemias (per 100 g Powder)

Nutrient	MSUD Diet Powder (Mead J)
Powder (g)	100
Energy (kilocalories)	470
Protein equiv. (g)	8.2
Fat (g)	20
Carbohydrate (g)	63.3

TABLE 8–37 Nutrient Composition of Formula* for the Treatment of Maple Syrup Urine Disease and Organic Acidemias (per 100 g Powder) (continued)

Nutrient	MSUD Diet Powder (Mead J)
Essential Amino acids (mg)	
Isoleucine	0
Leucine	0
Lysine	510
L-Methionine	250
Phenylalanine	550
Threonine	550
Tryptophan	200
Valine	0
Histidine	250
Non-Essential Amino Acids (mg)	
Arginine	490
Alanine	440
Asparate	1,140
Cystine	250
Glutamate	2,100
Glycine	600
Proline	890
Serine	690
Tyrosine	650
Glutamine	#N/A
Vitamins	
Vitamin A (International Units)	1,180
Vitamin D (International Units)	300
Vitamin E (International Units)	7.4
Vitamin C (mg)	38
Thiamine (μg)	370
Riboflavin (μg)	440
Pyridoxine (μg)	300
Niacin (mg)	5.9
Folic acid (μg)	74
Pantothenic acid (mg)	2.2
Choline (mg)	63
Biotin (μg)	40
Vitamin K (μg)	74
Inositol (mg)	22
Vitamin B_{12} (μg)	1.5
Minerals	
Calcium (mg)	490
Phosphorus (mg)	270
Magnesium (mg)	52
Iron (mg)	8.9
Iodine (μg)	33
Copper (μg)	430
Manganese (μg)	740
Zinc (mg)	3
Selenium (μg)	#N/A
Molybdenum (μg)	#N/A
Sodium (mEq)	8
Potassiumn (mEq)	12.5
Chloride (mEq)	10.4

* Mead Johnson & Company, Evansville, Indiana
#N/A = number not available

(Table 8–38) are often used as the basis for amino acid requirements and the prescription for nutritional therapy.[6] This table should be used only as a guide. Tolerance to BCAA varies with individual patients.

TABLE 8–38 Amino Acid Requirements for Infants and Children

Amino Acid	Unit	0–2 months	2–5 months	6–12 months	1–10 years
Leucine					
Infants	mg/kg	76–150	76–150	76–150	—
Children	mg/day	—	—	—	1,000
Isoleucine					
Infants	mg/kg	79–110	79–110	50–75	—
Children	mg/day	—	—	—	1,000
Valine					
Infants	mg/kg	65–105	65–105	50–80	—
Children	mg/day	—	—	—	400–600

With permission from Trams CM. Nutritional care for children with metabolic disorders. In: Krause MV, Mahan LK, eds. Food, nutrition and diet therapy. 7th ed. Philadelphia: WB Saunders, 1984:804–805.

The amount of water to be added to the MSUD diet powder is also determined. A 20 calorie per ounce formula can be prepared by adding 80 ml water to each firmly packed level scoop. The total amount of fluid needed should be based on the child's age, weight, and hydration status.

The amount of solid foods to include in the diet, if any, should be included into the nutritional plan. Table 8–39 provides a method of calculating daily intake of leucine, isoleucine, and valine to avoid either excessive or deficient amounts. Isoleucine and valine intakes may vary 10 to 30 percent from the prescription in the meal plan; leucine may vary 1 to 2 percent.[8] Supplementation of the diet with isoleucine and valine[8] is usually necessary in the newborn until the infant is on a mixed diet.

TABLE 8–39 Average Composition of Exchange Lists

List	Isoleucine (mg)	Leucine (mg)	Valine (mg)	Protein (g)	Energy (kilocalories)
Table Foods					
Bread/Cereals	18	35	25	0.4	25
Fats	7	10	7	0.1	70
Fruits	17	25	22	0.6	75
Vegetables	22	30	24	0.6	15
Free food A	3	5	4	0.1	50
Free food B	0	0	0	0	55

With permission and adapted from Acosta PB. Microcomputers in nutrition support of genetic disease. Tallahassee: Florida State University, 1984.

Exchange lists for MSUD are also provided in Table 8–40. It is useful to give serving portions in both household measurements and gram weights. High protein foods, ordinary breads and pasta, and foods for which the BCAA-containing ingredients cannot be determined are omitted from the diet. Even small amounts of high protein foods are excluded because imprecise measurements could result in a wide variation in intake of BCAA. Including these foods causes intake of fruits, vegetables, and cereals to be decreased and may further prove to be an undesirable temptation for the child.[1]

Parents need frequent nutritional education and counseling. Food records kept by parents before each clinic visit are essential in assessing the consistency of intake and the adequacy of the home diet. Knowledge of the child's amino acid intake can be used to assess requirements for amino acids. Frequent adjustments in the child's meal plan are needed to meet changing needs for kilocalories, protein, and the BCAA. The diet needs to be continued indefinitely without liberalization.[6]

Physicians: How to Order Diets

The diet order should indicate *diet for MSUD*. Specify the level of leucine, isoleucine, and valine to be allowed. The dietitian will determine the caloric level and adjust the nutritional care plan according to the preceding guidelines.

REFERENCES

1. Bell L, Chas E, Milne J. Dietary management of maple syrup urine disease, extension of equivalency systems. J Am Diet Assoc 1979;74:357–361.
2. Tanaka K, Rosenberg LE. Disorders of branched chain amino acid and organic acid metabolism. In: Stansbury JB, Wyngaarden JB, Fredrickson DS, Goldstein JL, Brown MS, eds. The metabolic basis of inherited disease. 5th ed. New York: McGraw-Hill, 1983:451.
3. DiGeorge AM, Rezvanic I, Garebaldi LR, Schwartz M. Prospective study of maple syrup urine disease for the first four days of life. N Engl J Med 1982;307:1492–1495.
4. Clow CL, Reade TM, Scriver CR. Outcome of early and long-term management of classical maple syrup urine disease. Pediatrics 1981;68:856–862.
5. Rohr FJ, Levy HL, Shih VE. Inborn errors of metabolism. In: Walker WA, Watkins JB, eds. Nutrition in pediatrics. Boston/Toronto: Little, Brown and Company, 1985:400.
6. Snyderman SE. Maple syrup urine disease. In: Wapnir PA, ed. Congenital metabolic diseases. New York: Marcel Dekker, Inc., 1985:153.
7. Krause MV, Mahan LK. Food, nutrition and diet therapy. 7th ed. Philadelphia: WB Saunders, 1984:818.
8. Acosta PB, Elas LJ. Dietary management of inherited metabolic disease: phenylketonuria, galactosemia, tyrosinemia, homocystinuria, maple syrup urine disease. Atlanta: Acelmu Publishers, 1976:65.

Additional References for Parents and/or Health Professionals

Acosta PB, Bell L. Branched chain amino acid content of foods: A parent's guide to the child with maple syrup urine disease. The Florida State University Center for Family Services, 103 Sandels Building, Tallahassee, Florida 32306.

Pennington JAT, Church HN. Bowes and Church's food values of portions commonly used. 14th ed. Philadelphia: JB Lippincott, 1985.

Bell L. Leucine equivalency system for dietary management of maple syrup urine disease. Nutrition Division, Clinical Investigation Unit, Room 815, The Hospital for Sick Children, 555 University Avenue, Toronto, Ontario, Canada, M5G 1X8.

TABLE 8–40 Exchange Lists for Diets Restricted in Isoleucine, Leucine, and Valine* Strained and Junior Foods (Gerber)†

Food	Measure	Weight (g)	Ile (mg)	Leu (mg)	Val (mg)	Protein (g)	Energy (Kcal)
Bread/Cereal							
Dry Cereals							
Barley	1 Tbsp	3.6	15	30	21	0.5	14
Mixed	1 Tbsp	3.6	16	35	22	0.6	14
Mixed/bananas	1 Tbsp	3.6	15	36	19	0.4	14
Oatmeal	1 Tbsp	3.6	20	39	28	0.6	14
Rice	1 Tbsp + 2 tsp	5.9	18	34	27	0.5	23
Rice/banana	1 Tbsp + 1 tsp	4.7	17	35	23	0.4	19
Jarred Cereals							
Mixed/apples & bananas							
Strained	3 Tbsp	43	18	37	25	0.7	25
Junior	2 Tbsp + 2 tsp	38	18	35	24	0.6	26
Oatmeal/apples & bananas							
Strained	2 Tbsp + 1 tsp	33	16	34	23	0.5	19
Junior	2 Tbsp + 1 tsp	33	18	36	25	0.5	18
Rice/apples & bananas	3 Tbsp	43	16	35	20	0.4	31
Rice/mixed fruit	2 Tbsp	29	17	36	22	0.5	21
Fruits and Juices							
Fruits, strained and junior							
Apricots with tapioca	9½ Tbsp	135†	16	30	18	0.5	100
Bananas with tapioca	1/2 cup	114	15	31	21	0.5	76
Bananas with pineapple and tapioca	9 Tbsp	128†	13	23	17	0.4	64
Guava	9 Tbsp	128†	14	26	13	0.4	84
Mango	9 Tbsp	128†	10	23	15	0.4	92
Peaches	5 Tbsp	72	12	24	23	0.4	52
Pears	7 Tbsp	100	15	28	20	0.6	52
Pears & pineapple	9 Tbsp	128	15	26	19	0.5	68
Juices, strained and toddler							
Mixed fruit	4.2 oz	—	15	24	20	0.5	70
Orange	4.2 oz	—	25	22	39	0.9	70
Orange-apple	4.2 oz	—	17	23	23	0.5	70

TABLE 8–40 Exchange Lists for Diets Restricted in Isoleucine, Leucine, and Valine* (continued)
Strained and Junior Foods (Gerber)†

Food	Measure	Weight (g)	Ile (mg)	Leu (mg)	Val (mg)	Protein (g)	Energy (Kcal)
Orange-apricot	3.0 oz	—	19	26	25	0.7	50
Orange-pineapple	4.2 oz	—	24	29	33	0.8	80
Vegetables							
Strained and junior							
Beets	1/3 cup	71	26	32	31	0.9	26
Carrots	7 Tbsp	100	21	29	27	0.7	24
Creamed corn	2 Tbsp	29	19	40	22	0.4	19
Creamed spinach	1 Tbsp	14	17	33	22	0.4	6
Garden vegetables	1 Tbsp + 2 tsp	24	24	39	27	0.6	8
Green beans	2 Tbsp + 2 tsp	38	21	31	26	0.5	9
Mixed vegetables	2 Tbsp + 2 tsp	38	21	33	25	0.5	16
Peas	1 Tbsp	14	20	32	23	0.5	6
Squash	1/3 cup	71	23	33	25	0.6	18
Sweet potatoes	3 Tbsp	43	24	36	34	0.5	26
Vegetable and meat combinations							
Vegetables and bacon							
Strained	2 Tbsp	29	19	31	25	0.5	22
Junior	1 Tbsp + 1 tsp	19	17	28	22	0.4	15
Vegetables and beef							
Strained	2 Tbsp	29	19	31	24	0.5	19
Junior	1 Tbsp + 1 tsp	19	19	31	23	0.5	13
Vegetables and chicken							
Strained	1 Tbsp + 1 tsp	19	19	29	22	0.4	9
Junior	1 Tbsp + 1 tsp	19	18	27	20	0.4	10

Food	Measure						
Vegetables and ham							
Strained	2 Tbsp	17	0.5	24	33	21	29
Junior	1 Tbsp	8	0.4	19	27	16	14
Vegetables and lamb							
Strained	1 Tbsp + 1 tsp	11	0.4	18	27	16	19
Junior	1 Tbsp + 2 tsp	14	0.4	20	30	18	24
Vegetables and liver							
Strained	1 Tbsp	7	0.3	20	27	15	14
Junior	1 Tbsp + 1 tsp	8	0.4	19	33	18	19
Vegetables and turkey							
Strained	1 Tbsp + 2 tsp	12	0.4	21	30	18	24
Junior	1 Tbsp + 2 tsp	13	0.4	23	31	19	24
Free Foods A							
Fruits, strained and junior							
Apple blueberry	2 Tbsp	17	0.1	4	6	3	29
Applesauce	3 Tbsp	20	0.1	4	5	3	43
Applesauce & apricots	3 Tbsp	21	0.1	5	5	4	43
Applesauce with pineapple	3 Tbsp	21	0.1	4	5	3	43
Guava & papaya	1/4 cup	38	0.1	3	5	3	57
Papaya & applesauce	1/4 cup	37	0.1	4	5	3	57
Plums with tapioca	1/4 cup	39	0.1	5	5	6	57
Prunes with tapioca	3 Tbsp	32	0.3	6	6	7	43
Juices, strained and toddler							
Apple	4.2 oz	60	0.1	5	8	5	—
Apple-banana	2.0 oz	29	0.1	6	8	4	—
Apple-grape	4.2 oz	60	0.1	5	5	3	—
Apple-peach	2.0 oz	29	0.1	6	7	4	—
Apple-plum	2.0 oz	29	0.1	4	5	4	—
Apple-prune	2.0 oz	29	0.1	4	5	4	—

† Derived from data in Nutrient Values, Gerber Baby Foods, 1981, 1982.

Table Foods

Food	Measure	Weight (g)	Ile (mg)	Leu (mg)	Val (mg)	Protein (g)	Energy (Kcal)
Bread/Cereal							
Cooked (measure after cooking)							
Corn grits, regular & quick	1 Tbsp	15	8	32	11	0.2	9
Cream of rice	3 Tbsp	46	7	33	26	0.4	24
Cream of wheat, regular	2 Tbsp	31	21	36	23	0.5	17
Cream of wheat, quick	2 Tbsp	30	20	34	22	0.4	16
Cream of wheat, instant	1 Tbsp + 2 tsp	25	210	35	22	0.4	16
Farina	2 Tbsp	29	18	32	20	0.4	14
Oats, regular, quick, & instant	1 Tbsp	15	17	29	22	0.4	9
Ralston	1 Tbsp + 1 tsp	20	20	34	22	0.4	11
Rice							
Brown	1 Tbsp + 2 tsp	15	18	33	27	0.4	18
White	2 Tbsp	19	18	32	26	0.4	20
Wheatena	1 Tbsp + 1 tsp	20	18	31	20	0.4	11
Whole wheat, hot, natural	1 Tbsp + 1 tsp	20	18	31	20	0.4	12
Ready to serve							
Alpha Bits	3 Tbsp	5	18	38	23	0.4	21
Apple Jacks	1/4 cup	7	16	38	20	0.4	28
Bran Chex	1 Tbsp	3	14	25	16	0.3	10
Cap'n Crunch	2 Tbsp	5	10	30	13	0.2	20
Cap'n Crunchberries	3 Tbsp	7	14	42	18	0.3	27
Cap'n Crunch Peanut Butter	2 Tbsp	4	13	32	16	0.3	19
Cherrios	2 Tbsp	3	20	33	25	0.4	11
Cocoa Krispies	1/4 cup	9	8	38	30	0.5	35
Cocoa Pebbles	1/4 cup	8	20	31	25	0.4	33
Cookie-Crisp	1/4 cup	8	14	36	21	0.4	30
Corn Chex	2 Tbsp	4	10	38	12	0.2	14
Corn flakes	2 Tbsp	3	9	34	11	0.2	11
Crispy rice	1/4 cup	7	8	36	28	0.4	28
Crispy Wheats 'n Raisins	3 Tbsp	8	21	37	26	0.5	28
40% Bran flakes (Post)	1 Tbsp	3	12	22	16	0.3	10
Fruit Loops	3 Tbsp	5	14	32	17	0.3	21
Frosted Rice Krinkles	1/4 cup	8	21	33	25	0.4	31
Frosted Rice Krispies	6 Tbsp	11	8	39	31	0.5	41
Fruity Pebbles	1/3 cup	10	21	34	26	0.4	41

Food	Portion					
Golden Grahams	2 Tbsp	5	12	33	15	0.3	19
Grape Nuts Flakes	2 Tbsp	4	18	31	22	0.4	15
Honeycomb	1/4 cup	6	13	40	17	0.3	22
King Vitamin	1/4 cup	5	12	35	15	0.3	21
Kix	3 Tbsp	4	13	41	17	0.3	14
Lucky Charms	3 Tbsp	6	25	42	32	0.5	23
10% Bran	1 Tbsp	4	16	31	24	0.5	11
Quisp	3 Tbsp	6	12	36	15	0.3	23
Raisin Bran (Post)	2 Tbsp	7	22	38	28	0.6	22
Rice Chex	1/3 cup	8	7	34	26	0.4	31
Rice Krispies	1/4 cup	7	8	38	30	0.5	28
Rice, puffed	1/2 cup	7	23	37	29	0.5	28
Super Sugar Crisp	1/4 cup	8	23	38	26	0.5	31
Team	3 Tbsp	8	24	43	30	0.5	31
Toasties	2 Tbsp	3	9	34	12	0.2	11
Total	3 Tbsp	6	24	43	30	0.6	22
Trix	3 Tbsp	5	12	40	15	0.3	20
Wheat, puffed	1/4 cup	3	19	32	21	0.5	11
Wheat, shredded	1/4 large biscuit	5	20	36	25	0.5	17
Wheaties	3 Tbsp	5	20	36	26	0.5	19
Cookies and crackers							
Arrowroot (Nabisco)	1 biscuit	5	16	35	22	0.4	21
Barnum's animal	4 crackers	8	18	39	25	0.5	36
Graham (Nabisco)	1 cracker	7	26	42	24	0.5	27
Ritz	2 crackers	7	21	36	23	0.5	36
Saltine	2 crackers	6	25	37	23	0.6	28
Triangle thins	2 crackers	4	20	34	22	0.4	20
Wheat thins	4 crackers	7	22	39	25	0.5	36
Miscellaneous							
Corn, canned, solids	1 Tbsp + 1 tsp	14	11	34	2	0.3	10
Macaroni, cooked tender	2 Tbsp	18	30	40	34	0.6	19
Noodles, cooked	1 Tbsp	10	32	44	39	0.7	20
Popcorn, oil added	2 Tbsp + 1 tsp	3	12	34	13	0.3	12
Potatoes, white							
Boiled in skin	1/3 medium	33	31	35	37	0.7	25
French fries	3 pieces (1/2" × 1/2" × 2")	15	28	32	33	0.6	41
Hashed brown	2 Tbsp	25	34	39	41	0.8	57
Potato chips	6 pieces (2" diam)	12	29	33	35	0.7	68
Spaghetti, cooked tender	1 Tbsp + 2 tsp	16	26	35	24	0.5	17
Sweet potatoes							
Baked in skin	1/4 small	25	25	30	39	0.5	35
Candied	1/2 potato (2" × 4")	50	31	37	49	0.6	84
Canned, syrup pack	1/2 small	50	24	29	38	0.5	57

Table Foods (continued)

Food	Measure	Weight (g)	Ile (mg)	Leu (mg)	Val (mg)	Protein (g)	Energy (Kcal)
Fats							
Butter	1 Tbsp	15	9	12	9	0.1	108
Coffee rich	1 Tbsp liquid	14	8	11	8	0.1	24
Cream, whipping, heavy	1 tsp fluid	5	6	10	7	0.1	17
French dressing	2 Tbsp	28	6	7	7	0.2	114
Margarine, regular stick or brick	1 Tbsp	14	6	12	9	0.1	101
Margarine, regular soft, tub	1 Tbsp	14	6	9	6	0.1	101
Margarine, regular, liquid, bottle	1 tsp	5	5	9	6	0.1	34
Mayonnaise	2 tsp	9	6	9	7	0.1	66
Thousand Island dressing	1 Tbsp	16	7	10	8	0.1	59
Fruits							
Apple, raw, whole	1 large	230	18	28	21	0.4	136
canned, sweetened slices	1 cup	204	14	22	16	0.4	136
dried, uncooked	1/2 cup	43	16	25	19	0.4	104
dried, cooked, sweetened	3/4 cup	210	16	26	19	0.4	174
Applesauce, canned, sweetened	1 cup	255	18	28	20	0.5	194
Apricots, raw	1 fruit	35	14	27	17	0.5	17
canned, with/without skin	1/3 cup	86	14	27	16	0.5	71
dried, uncooked	3 halves	10	12	22	14	0.4	25
dried, cooked, sweetened	2 Tbsp	34	12	23	14	0.4	38
frozen, sweetened	1/4 cup	60	12	24	15	0.4	60
nectar, canned	1/2 cup	126	14	26	16	0.5	72
Avocado, raw, all varieties	1 Tbsp + 1 tsp	19	13	23	18	0.4	31
Banana, raw	1/3 small	38	13	27	18	0.4	35
Blackberries, raw	1/2 cup	72	15	23	20	0.5	37
canned	3 Tbsp	48	18	28	24	0.6	44
Blueberries, raw	1/2 cup	72	15	29	20	0.5	41
canned	1/4 cup	64	13	25	17	0.4	66
frozen, sweetened	1/2 cup	115	14	26	20	0.4	94
Boysenberries, canned	3 Tbsp	48	14	21	18	0.5	42
Cherries, sour, red, canned	1/3 cup	85	17	28	22	0.6	72
Cherries, sweet, raw	1/3 cup	48	17	26	22	0.6	35
canned	6 Tbsp	97	17	26	22	0.6	80

Food	Serving						
Dates, natural & dry	3 dates	25	12	22	16	0.5	68
Figs, raw	1½ medium	75	18	26	21	0.6	66
canned	1/2 cup	130	16	22	18	0.5	114
dried uncooked	1 fruit	19	17	25	22	0.6	48
dried, cooked	3 Tbsp	49	19	27	24	0.6	52
Fruit cocktail	1/2 cup	130	12	22	20	0.5	93
Grapefruit, pink, red, or white	1/3 cup sections	77	14	22	18	0.5	25
canned, light syrup	1/3 cup	85	14	21	18	0.5	51
juice, canned unsweetened	1/2 cup	124	19	29	25	0.6	46
Grapes, adherent skin	1 cup	160	8	22	29	1.1	114
Thompson seedless, canned	1 cup	256	10	26	33	1.2	187
juice, canned or bottled	1 cup	253	30	25	25	1.4	155
Guava, raw	1/4 cup	41	12	23	12	0.3	21
sauce	1/2 cup	119	15	25	13	0.4	44
Mangos, raw	1/2 cup, diced	82	15	26	22	0.4	54
Melon							
cantaloupe	1/3 cup, diced	53	14	21	18	0.5	19
casaba	1/3 cup, diced	57	15	23	19	0.5	15
honeydew	2/3 cup, diced	113	14	23	18	0.5	38
Mixed fruit, canned	1/2 cup	128	14	24	21	0.5	92
Nectarines, raw	1/2 cup, sliced	69	19	29	25	0.6	34
Oranges, raw, all varieties	1/2 cup, sections	90	23	22	36	0.8	42
juice, canned,	1 cup	249	15	27	22	1.5	104
frozen, diluted	3/4 cup	187	13	24	20	1.3	84
Papaya, raw, diced	1 cup	140	11	22	14	0.9	54
Peaches, raw	1/3 cup sliced	57	11	23	22	0.4	24
canned	1/3 cup slices	85	11	22	21	0.4	63
dried, uncooked	1/2 fruit	13	14	26	26	0.5	31
frozen, sweetened	1/4 cup	62	11	22	21	0.4	59
spiced, canned	1/2 cup	121	15	28	28	0.5	90
nectar, canned	3/4 cup	187	15	29	27	0.5	100
Pears, raw	1 cup sliced	165	33	23	23	0.6	97
canned	1 cup halves	255	26	18	18	0.5	188
dried, uncooked	2 halves	35	33	23	23	0.6	92
Persimmon, Japanese, raw	1/3 fruit	56	14	24	17	0.3	39
Pineapple, raw	1 cup, diced	155	20	29	25	0.6	77
canned	3/4 cup	196	17	26	22	0.7	98
frozen chunks, sweet	1/2 cup	122	16	25	20	0.5	104

Table Foods (continued)

Food	Measure	Weight (g)	Ile (mg)	Leu (mg)	Val (mg)	Protein (g)	Energy (Kcal)
juice, canned	3/4 cup	188	20	29	25	0.6	104
juice, frozen, dilute	1/2 cup	125	16	25	20	0.5	64
Plantains, cooked	1/2 cup slices	77	17	27	22	0.6	90
Plums, raw	1 cup slices	165	35	28	31	1.3	91
canned, purple	1 cup	258	26	21	23	0.9	230
Prunes, dried uncooked	1/4 cup	40	28	23	25	1.0	96
dried, cooked, unsweetened	1/2 cup	106	33	27	30	1.2	113
juice, canned	3/4 cup	192	31	26	27	1.1	138
Raisins	4 Tbsp	40	10	27	35	0.6	120
Raspberries, raw	1/2 cup	62	16	25	21	0.6	30
canned	1/4 cup	64	15	24	20	0.5	58
frozen, red, sweet	1/3 cup	83	17	26	22	0.6	85
Rhubarb							
frozen, cooked, sweet	1/2 cup	120	14	21	18	0.5	139
Strawberries, raw	1/2 cup	75	11	23	13	0.5	22
frozen, sweet, sliced	1/3 cup	85	10	23	13	0.4	82
Tangerines, raw	2 fruit	168	28	26	46	1.1	74
canned	1 cup	252	30	28	48	1.1	153
juice, canned	1 cup	249	12	25	20	1.2	125
juice, fresh	1 cup	247	12	25	20	1.2	106
Watermelon	1 cup, diced	160	30	29	26	1.0	50
Vegetables (For cooked and canned vegetables, measurements are based on drained solids)							
Asparagus, green							
raw, cooked, or canned	1½–2 spears	33	18	32	26	0.7	9
Beans, green, snap, or yellow wax							
cooked or canned	1/4 cup	31	21	27	22	0.5	8
frozen cooked	1/4 cup	30	23	30	25	0.5	8
Bean sprouts, mung							
raw	2 Tbsp	8	17	28	18	0.3	3
cooked	2 Tbsp + 2 tsp	10	18	29	19	0.3	3
Bean sprouts, soya							
raw	2 Tbsp	12	27	32	27	0.7	6
cooked	1 Tbsp + 2 tsp	14	27	32	27	0.7	5
Beet greens							
cooked or canned	2 Tbsp	25	18	27	21	0.4	5

Food	Amount						
Beet roots							
cooked or canned	1/2 cup, diced	83	29	28	25	0.8	31
Broccoli							
cooked (fresh or frozen)	2 Tbsp	20	23	30	31	0.6	5
raw	2 Tbsp	17	23	30	31	0.6	5
Brussels sprouts							
cooked (fresh)	1 sprout	17	30	32	31	0.7	6
cooked (frozen)	1 sprout	22	30	31	31	0.7	6
raw	1 sprout	14	29	30	30	0.6	6
Cabbage, headed							
cooked	1/2 cup	70	21	30	22	0.7	14
raw	2/3 cup	55	20	29	22	0.7	14
Cabbage, red							
raw	1/3 cup	33	26	27	20	0.7	10
Carrots							
cooked (fresh or frozen)	1/2 cup	75	26	37	32	0.7	23
raw	1 small	60	25	36	31	0.7	25
Cauliflower							
cooked (fresh)	3 Tbsp	20	20	31	28	0.5	5
cooked (frozen)	3 Tbsp	23	19	30	26	0.4	5
raw	3 Tbsp	17	20	31	28	0.5	5
Celery							
cooked or raw	1/3 cup	50	17	29	21	0.4	8
Chard, Swiss							
cooked	3 Tbsp	33	26	33	24	0.6	6
raw	3 Tbsp	25	26	32	23	0.6	6
Collards							
cooked (fresh or frozen)	1 Tbsp + 1 tsp	16	14	26	23	0.5	5
Cucumber							
raw, not pared	3/4 medium	75	23	31	26	0.8	12
raw, pared	1 medium	100	19	25	21	0.6	14
Eggplant							
cooked	1/4 cup	50	25	31	30	0.5	10
Kale							
cooked	2 Tbsp	17	18	34	25	0.5	5
Lettuce							
raw	2½ large leaves	40	19	32	27	0.5	6
Mushrooms,							
sauteed or fried	1 large	23	39	27	23	0.6	26
Mustard greens							
cooked (fresh or frozen)	1/4 cup	50	36	30	51	1.1	10

Table Foods (continued)

Food	Measure	Weight (g)	Ile (mg)	Leu (mg)	Val (mg)	Protein (g)	Energy (Kcal)
Okra, cooked	2 pods	25	21	31	28	0.6	10
Onions, mature							
cooked	1/2 cup	100	18	31	26	1.2	29
raw	1/3 cup chopped	50	15	25	20	1.0	20
Peas, green							
canned	1 Tbsp + 1 tsp	11	24	33	21	0.5	10
cooked (fresh)	1 Tbsp	10	25	34	22	0.5	7
cooked (frozen)	1 Tbsp	8	20	27	17	0.4	6
Pepper, green							
cooked or raw	1 medium shell	70	30	30	21	0.8	14
Pickle, cucumber							
dill	1 large	100	22	30	24	0.7	11
sweet	1 large	100	22	30	24	0.7	146
Pumpkin							
canned or cooked	1/4 cup	58	22	32	22	0.6	19
Radish, raw	4 medium	44	22	30	29	0.4	7
Rutabagas							
cooked	6 Tbsp diced	75	16	27	16	0.7	26
raw	6 Tbsp diced	70	18	31	18	0.8	32
Sauerkraut							
canned	1/2 cup	80	31	32	24	0.8	14
Spinach							
canned	1 Tbsp + 1 tsp	15	19	31	22	0.4	4
cooked (fresh)	1 Tbsp	11	16	26	18	0.3	3
frozen (cooked)	1 Tbsp, chopped	12	18	29	21	0.4	8
raw	1 leaf & stem	12	18	29	21	0.4	8
Squash, summer							
cooked, fresh	6 Tbsp	75	22	31	25	0.7	10
cooked (frozen)	1/4 cup	50	22	32	26	0.7	10
raw	7 Tbsp	58	21	30	24	0.7	10
Squash, winter							
baked	3 Tbsp	38	22	31	25	0.7	24
boiled, mashed	3 Tbsp	50	18	25	20	0.6	19
cooked (frozen)	1/4 cup	50	19	27	22	0.6	19

Food	Measure						
Tomato							
canned	1/3 cup	62	18	26	18	0.6	13
cooked	1/4 cup	50	19	27	18	0.6	13
raw	1/2 medium	75	24	34	23	0.8	16
juice	1/2 cup	100	26	37	25	0.9	19
Turnip greens, canned	2 Tbsp	20	16	31	23	0.4	4
Turnip root							
cooked	2/3 cup diced	100	19	32	19	0.8	23
raw	2/3 cup diced	83	20	33	19	0.8	25
Soups, Condensed, Campbell's (Measure before diluting—dilute with water)							
Asparagus, Cream of	1 Tbsp + 2 tsp	26	20	34	24	0.5	18
Celery, Cream of	2 Tbsp	31	19	31	22	0.5	22
Chicken gumbo	1 Tbsp + 1 tsp	21	17	28	20	0.4	9
Chicken vegetable	1 Tbsp	15	17	29	20	0.4	9
Minestrone	1 Tbsp	15	16	30	22	0.5	10
Mushroom, Cream of	1 Tbsp + 2 tsp	26	20	33	22	0.4	27
Potato, Cream of	2 Tbsp	31	19	29	23	0.4	18
Tomato bisque	2 Tbsp	31	19	32	21	0.5	30
Tomato	2 Tbsp + 2 tsp	42	20	33	22	0.7	29
Vegetable, vegetarian	1 Tbsp + 2 tsp	25	20	30	20	0.4	15

Free Foods A

Food	Measure						
Aproten Low Protein Products‡							
Anellini, cooked	2 Tbsp	28	2	6	2	0.1	25
Ditalini, cooked	3 Tbsp	24	2	6		0.1	21
Rigatini, cooked	3 Tbsp	24	2	6	2	0.1	21
Rusks	1/2 rusk	6	2	4	2	0.1	22
Semolino, cooked	1/4 cup	67	2	5	2	0.1	23
Tagliatelle, cooked	2 Tbsp	30	2	6	2	0.1	27
Unimix bread	1 slice	20	4	5	4	0.1	44
dp Low Protein Products‡							
Bread	1/2"–1/4" slice	8	4	6	4	0.1	20
Cookies							
Butterscotch	2 cookies	28	3	4	3	0.1	140
Chocolate chip	1 cookie	14	6	10	7	0.1	70
Fruits and Juices							
Apple juice, canned	4 oz	124	3	5	4	0.1	60
Apple butter, canned	1 Tbsp + 1 tsp	20	4	6	5	0.1	37
Cranberry juice cocktail	1 cup	253	2	4	3	0.1	147
Cranberry sauce, canned	1/4 cup	69	4	6	5	0.1	104
Grapes, slip skin	1/2 cup	46	2	6	8	0.3	29
Honey	1 Tbsp	21	3	5	4	0.1	64

Table Foods *(continued)*

Food	Measure	Weight (g)	Ile (mg)	Leu (mg)	Val (mg)	Protein (g)	Energy (Kcal)
Jams, commercial							
grape	1 Tbsp + 1 tsp	20	3	5	4	0.1	55
plum	1 Tbsp + 1 tsp	20	3	5	4	0.1	59
	1 Tbsp + 1 tsp	20	3	5	4	0.1	59
Lemon juice	1 Tbsp	15	2	3	3	0.1	3
Lime juice	1 Tbsp	15	2	3	3	0.1	4
Orange marmalade	1 Tbsp	20	5	5	9	0.2	56
Papaya nectar	4 oz	125	3	5	3	0.2	72
Pear nectar	3 oz	94	3	5	3	0.1	57
Free Foods B							
Beverages							
Carbonated	4 oz	125	0	0	0	0	52
Gatorade	4 oz	125	0	0	0	0	25
Koolaid	4 oz	125	0	0	0	0	48
Lemonade	4 oz	125	0	0	0	0	53
Limeade	4 oz	125	0	0	0	0	51
Tang	4 oz	125	0	0	0	0	59
Candy							
Butterscotch	1 piece	5	0	0	0	0	21

Food	Measure					
Candy						
Fondant	1 mint	11	0	0	0	4
Gumdrop	1 large	10	0	0	0	33
Hard candy	2 rolls (1" × 1¹/₂")	10	0	0	0	36
Jelly beans	10 beans	28	0	0	0	66
Lollypop	1 medium	28	0	0	0	108
Miscellaneous						
Cornstarch	1 Tbsp	8	0	0	0	29
Rich's topping	1 Tbsp (unwhipped)	15	0	0	0	42
Shortening, vegetable	1 Tbsp	13	0	0	0	113
Sugar and Sweets						
Sugar, brown	1 Tbsp	14	0	0	0	52
Sugar, granulated	1 Tbsp	12	0	0	0	46
Sugar, powdered	1 Tbsp	11	0	0	0	59
Corn syrup	1 Tbsp	20	0	0	0	57
Danish dessert	1/2 cup	—	0	0	0	123
Fruit ices	1/3 cup	—	0	0	0	46
Jelly, commercial	1 Tbsp	20	0	0	0	50
Maple syrup	1 Tbsp	20	0	0	0	50
Molasses	1 Tbsp	20	0	0	0	50
Popsicle	1 Twin bar	—	0	0	0	95
Prono‡	1/3 cup	—	0	0	0	55

*Reprinted with permission from Acosta PB. Microcomputers in nutrition support of genetic disease. Tallahassee: Florida State University, 1984.
†Derived from data in Nutrient Values, Gerber Baby Foods, 1981, 1982.
‡Available from Dietary Specialties, P.O. Box 227, Rochester, N.Y. 14601. (716) 263-2787

General Description

Phenylalanine intake is controlled according to individual needs. The majority of the protein in the diet is provided by a product that is low in or free of phenylalanine. Foods that contain only small amounts of phenylalanine make up the rest of the diet.

Nutritional Inadequacy

Caloric, carbohydrate, fat, vitamin, and mineral requirements are the same as for children and infants without PKU. Subclinical deficiencies of zinc and copper have been reported in PKU children, but long-term consequences are not known.[1] Lofenalac, Phenyl Free, and PKU-2 contain recommended amounts of vitamins and minerals, as well as supplemental L. tyrosine, which becomes an essential amino acid for the PKU patient. These products do not contain fluoride, which may need to be supplemented. See *Pediatric Appendix 1,* page 458, for formula compositions.

Indications and Rationale

Phenylketonuria (PKU) is an autosomal recessive genetic disorder seen in 1:11,000 births in the United States. PKU is a disease primarily of Caucasians. The phenylalanine hydroxylase activity in the liver of PKU patients is approximately 0.27 percent of normal.[2] This defect causes a block in the conversion of phenylalanine to tyrosine, thereby resulting in a markedly elevated level of blood phenylalanine and the excretion of phenylalanine and its metabolites, such as phenylpyruvic acid and phenylacetic acid, in the urine. Because tyrosine formation is blocked, the production of melanin is decreased. The affected children have blue eyes and are blonder than unaffected siblings if the disease has not been treated early and if retardation has occurred.[3] Untreated patients lose 50 IQ points the first year of life and 96 to 98 percent ultimately have an IQ of less than 50.[2] The most likely mechanism for retardation is that elevated phenylalanine competes with other amino acids for transport into the neurons and creates an amino acid imbalance that inhibits protein synthesis and synaptogenesis.[2]

Classic PKU can be defined as meeting these criteria: a plasma phenylalanine level consistently above 16 to 20 mg per deciliter; blood tyrosine levels less than about 3 mg per deciliter; the presence of phenylpyruvic acid and o-hydroxyphenylacetic acid in the urine; and the inability to tolerate an oral challenge of phenylalanine. All infants with persistent hyperphenylalaninemia should have screening for the atypical PKU variants that do not respond to diet therapy alone and that need additional medical treatment.

Atypical PKU is a less severe defect of phenylalanine hydroxylation in which blood phenylalanine is not as high as in classic PKU. Phenylketones may or may not be present in the urine. Untreated atypical PKU may cause central nervous system impairment. Diet therapy is usually initiated when blood phenylalanine levels exceed 12 mg per deciliter.[4]

The older, untreated PKU patient who is difficult to manage due to hyperactivity and self-abuse may benefit from a trial of a low phenylalanine diet.[5]

Goals of Dietary Management

Nutritional therapy needs to provide sufficient amounts of the essential amino acid, phenylalanine, for proper growth and development, but to restrict intake so that high blood phenylalanine levels are reduced and mental retardation is prevented. The optimal therapeutic range for blood phenylalanine levels in persons with PKU is between 2 and 10 mg per deciliter.[6] Blood phenylalanine should be measured a minimum of one time per week during the first year of life.[2] Additional measurements should be obtained when the diet is first instituted and when the blood phenylalanine level is outside of the desired therapeutic ranges. "Over-treating" of PKU, resulting in phenylalanine deficiency, causes deficient growth, retarded bone age, hepatomegaly, repeated infections, hypoglycemia, neurologic symptoms,[2] lethargy, anorexia, rashes, anemia, and diarrhea.[3]

Elevations in blood phenylalanine levels are generally caused by (1) intake of phenylalanine in excess of the child's need for growth, (2) insufficient caloric intake[5] or protein intake,[7,8] which promotes tissue catabolism resulting in an accumulation of phenylalanine in the blood, and (3) tissue catabolism during illness.[7]

Dietary Recommendations

Special dietary products used for treating PKU are either low in or free of phenylalanine. These products need to be prescribed under the care of an experienced dietitian and physician. The patient should not start on a special formula until the initial elevated phenylalanine level is confirmed by retesting. Lofenalac (Mead Johnson and Company, Evansville, Indiana 47721) is a casein hydrolysate formula from which most of the phenylalanine has been removed. In order to meet the phenylalanine needs for growth in infancy, evaporated milk or other foods high in phenylalanine must be added to the Lofenalac. Phenyl Free (Mead Johnson and Company) and PKU-2 (Milupa Corporation, Darien, Connecticut 06820) are crystalline amino acid formulas, which contain no phenylalanine and allow more flexibility in the diet of the older child by allowing all of the phenylalanine requirements to be supplied by foods other than formula. The use of Phenyl Free has also been reported, with infants, to allow a more varied diet.[9]

The infant with PKU may be breast fed. Human milk contains approximately 13 mg phenylalanine per ounce, which is less than cow's milk (52 mg per ounce) or infant formulas (20 to 30 mg per ounce). If exclusively breast fed, the infant consumes too much phenylalanine, so breast feeding must be combined with a low phenylalanine or a phenylalanine-free formula. Based on the average phenylalanine content of the mother's milk, the infant's estimated need for calories, and the infant's tolerance for phenylalanine, a certain number of ounces of Lofenalac or Phenyl Free are planned per day. The infant is allowed to breast feed, as desired, between formula feedings. Blood phenylalanine initially needs to be measured two to three times per week and adjustments made in the amount of formula and in the frequency of breast feeding.[4]

Phenyl Free formula or PKU-2 is usually introduced into the diet when the child is 3 to 6 years old. The greater flexibility that these formulas allow in menu planning becomes important as the child enters school or other group settings. Criteria for introduction of these formulas include that the child accepts the meal plan and formula and consumes a wide variety of foods from the low phenylalanine food lists on a regular basis.[5]

Parents of children with PKU need careful nutritional education with frequent follow-up. A meal plan (page 404) provides parents with specific guidelines to follow. The parents should be able to demonstrate the ability to prepare formula correctly, to plan accurate menus, and to plan replacements for foods not eaten. To avoid conflicts over food, children should be involved at an early age in choosing appropriate foods. Diet diaries need to be kept by parents for the 3 days preceding each blood phenylalanine analysis. At each clinic visit the diet records should be evaluated for the variety of foods chosen and the adequacy of caloric, protein, phenylalanine, vitamin, and mineral intakes. These records are useful in adjusting intake if serum phenylalanine is above or below recommended values and for evaluating the accuracy and consistency of the home diet.

The artificial sweetener, aspartame (NutraSweet), contains a significant source of phenylalanine and should not be a part of the diet for the child with PKU. Foods containing NutraSweet should have the statement "Phenylketonurics: Contains Phenylalanine" near the ingredient panel. Parents need to be alerted to read labels for this statement or for the ingredients NutraSweet or aspartame.

Calculation of the Diet

The following are guidelines for determining the needed levels of phenylalanine, kilocalories, protein, and fluid. The diet should be adjusted frequently to meet the child's changing needs for kilocalories, protein, and phenylalanine and to accommodate changes in the child's eating habits.

1. Establish the child's daily requirements for kilocalories, protein, and phenylalanine. See Table 8–41 for suggested requirements. Infants with PKU have the same protein requirements as other infants, but have a higher protein intake due to the high protein content of Lofenalac. Phenylalanine intake needs to be adjusted frequently in response to blood levels.

TABLE 8–41 Suggestions for Daily Diet Prescription in PKU[4]

Age	Recommended Protein Intake	Recommended Phenylalanine Intake	Recommended Caloric Intake
0–2 months	4.2 g per kg	40–70 mg per kg	120 kilocalories per kg
3–6 months	3.0 g per kg	25–55 mg per kg	115 kilocalories per kg
6 months–1 year	2.5 g per kg	25–50 mg per kg	110–115 kilocalories per kg
1–3 years	25 g per day	20–40 mg per kg	900–1,800 kilocalories per day
4–6 years	30 g per day	10–40 mg per kg	1,300–2,300 kilocalories per day
7–10 years	35 g per day	10–40 mg per kg	1,650–3,300 kilocalories per day

2. Establish the amount of Lofenalac to be given. The amount of formula given is determined by the protein allowance. Protein intake (85 to 90 percent) must be met by Lofenalac since natural foods containing protein would be too high in phenylalanine.[7] The amount of Lofenalac is stated in measures. One measure (a packed dry scoop) equals 9.5 g (or 1 tablespoon) and contains 1.4 g of protein, 7.6 mg of phenylalanine, and 43.7 kilocalories.

3. State the amount of milk to be added, if any, to meet the child's needs

for phenylalanine. Since Lofenalac does not provide sufficient phenylalanine for growth, evaporated milk is added to the Lofenalac to maintain desired phenylalanine levels. Evaporated whole milk provides 104 mg of phenylalanine, 2.1 g of protein, and 42 kilocalories per ounce. The evaporated milk should be mixed with the Lofenalac so the child does not develop a taste for milk instead of formula.

4. State the amount of water to be added to the Lofenalac powder. The amount of water needed is determined by the child's weight, age, hydration status, preference for fluids, and taste for Lofenalac. Higher fluid intakes may be needed because of the high protein content of the diet. Because Lofenalac is a concentrated source of protein and carbohydrate, children taking this formula tend to have greater thirst than most children consuming regular milk or formulas.[7] The Lofenalac can be made into a paste with water or with apple juice and can be spoon fed, particularly if the child rejects the formula when being weaned from the bottle. Additional fluids should be offered between feedings.[7]

5. Determine the amount and type of solid foods to be given. Solid foods are introduced at about 4 to 6 months of age as with non-PKU children. To calculate the amount and type of solid foods to be in the diet, subtract the amount of phenylalanine, kilocalories, and protein provided by the Lofenalac or Phenyl Free from the diet prescription. Food lists are used that contain 0 to 30 mg phenylalanine per serving (Tables 8–42 and 8–43). Phenylalanine is 2.6 to 5.0 percent of the protein found in food.[7] A variety of foods similar to those normally eaten by infants should be given to ensure that these foods are accepted later in life, to meet increasing phenylalanine requirements and nutrient needs, to develop jaw muscles for speech, and to provide exercise for teeth and gums.[7] Free foods and special low protein breads, pastas, and baked goods provide kilocalories and variety in the diet and allow the child to eat some foods as desired.

6. Develop a meal plan that distributes the day's allowance of Lofenalac. The Lofenalac should be given with each feeding to promote effective utilization of incomplete protein sources. A meal plan can be developed using servings from the food groups (see Table 8–43) or by specifying the milligrams of phenylalanine allowed from each food group at each meal or snack.

TABLE 8–42 Food Groups for Phenylalanine Restricted Diet
Average Nutrient Content*

Food Group	Phenylalanine mg	Tyrosine mg	Protein g	Fat g	Energy Kcal
Starch	30	20	0.6	0	30
Fats	5	4	0.1	5	60
Fruits	15	10	0.5	0	60
Vegetables	15	10	0.5	0	15
Free foods A	5	4	0.2	0	65
Free foods B	0	0	0	0	55

*With permission from Acosta PB, Fernhoff PM, Rappaport A. The parents guide to the child with PKU (revised). Tallahassee: Florida State University, 1982.

Sample Calculation—Infant

Age: 2 months
Weight: 5 kg

1. Approximate daily requirement for kilocalories   600 kilocalories (120×5)
   Approximate daily allowance for protein   21 g (4.2×5)
   Approximate daily requirement for phenylalanine   300 mg (60×5)

2. Amount of protein from Lofenalac = 85 to 90% of total protein allowance: $21 \times 0.85 = 17.85$ g.
3. Amount of Lofenalac to give: Divide the grams of protein required from Lofenalac by the amount of protein per measure of Lofenalac (1.4 g protein/measure) and round up to the nearest $\frac{1}{2}$ measure: $17.85 \div 1.4 = 12.75$ (13 measures Lofenalac).
4. Amount of evaporated milk to give:
   a. Determine the amount of phenylalanine provided by the Lofenalac: 13 measures $\times$ 7.6 mg phenylalanine/measure = 99 mg phenylalanine.
   b. Determine the additional phenylalanine requirement by subtracting the phenylalanine supplied from Lofenalac from the day's phenylalanine requirement: 300 mg − 99 mg = 201 mg.
   c. Divide additional phenylalanine requirement by the phenylalanine content of 1 oz evaporated whole milk (104 mg/oz) to equal the amount of evaporated milk: 201 mg ÷ 104 mg = 1.93 (2 ounces) evaporated milk.

Formula Prescription:	Phenylalanine (mg)	Protein (g)	Energy (Kcal)
13 packed measures Lofenalac	99	18.2	568
2 oz evaporated whole milk	208	4.2	84
26 oz water*			
Totals	307	22.4	652

Phenylalanine—Controlled Diet Meal Plan[5]

Date _____ Age _____ Name _____
Weight _____ Height _____

Approximate total milligrams phenylalanine daily _____
Approximate total grams protein daily _____
Approximate total energy (kilocalories) daily _____

	Phenylalanine (mg)	Protein (g)	Energy (Kcal)
_____ measures packed dry Lofenalac	_____	_____	_____
Add _____ oz evaporated milk	_____	_____	_____
Add _____ oz water	_____	_____	_____
One oz contains			

Breakfast

_____ Lofenalac			
_____ Servings fruit	_____	_____	_____
_____ Servings starch	_____	_____	_____
_____ Servings fat	_____	_____	_____
_____ Servings free food A	_____	_____	_____
_____ Servings free food B	_____	_____	_____

Between Meals

_____ Servings _____	_____	_____	_____

Noon

_____ Lofenalac			
_____ Servings fruit	_____	_____	_____
_____ Servings vegetable	_____	_____	_____
_____ Servings starch	_____	_____	_____
_____ Servings fat	_____	_____	_____
_____ Servings free food A	_____	_____	_____
_____ Servings free food B	_____	_____	_____

Between Meals

_____ Servings	_____	_____	_____

*Normal dilution (20 kilocalories/fluid ounce): Add two ounces water to each packed level measuring scoop of Lofenalac powder.

Evening Meal

_____ Lofenalac
_____ Servings fruit
_____ Servings vegetable
_____ Servings starch
_____ Servings fat
_____ Servings free food A
_____ Servings free food B

Bedtime

_____ Servings _____
                    Total
                    Per kilogram

Comments:

Sample Calculations—Toddler

Lofenalac With Table Foods

Age: 21 months
Weight: 12.5 kg

1. Approximate daily requirement for kilocalories — 1,190 calories (basal + 70% using Table 8–41 on page 402)
   Approximate daily requirement for protein — 25 g (from Table 8–41 on page 402)
   Approximate daily requirement for phenylalanine — 375 mg (30 × 12.5)
2. Amount of protein from Lofenalac = 85 to 90% of total protein requirements: 25 × 0.85 = 21 g.
3. Amount of Lofenalac to give: Divide the grams of protein required from Lofenalac by the amount of protein per measure of Lofenalac (1.4 g/measure): 21 ÷ 1.4 = 15 measures Lofenalac.
4. Amount of water to add to Lofenalac: Water can be added to the child's taste. 2 ounces water/ measure will prepare a 20 kilocalorie/ounces formula. Additional fluid given as water or juices.
5. Amount of table foods to give: Total phenylalanine requirements per day minus phenylalanine content of the days prescription for Lofenalac equals amount of phenylalanine required from solid foods: 375 − 114 = 261 mg phenylalanine from table foods.
6. Divide phenylalanine allowance from table foods into exchange groups based on the child's eating preferences and caloric needs:

Foods	Phenylalanine (mg)	Protein (g)	Energy (Kcal)
2 vegetable servings	30	1.0	30
5 fruit servings	75	2.5	300
5 starch servings	150	3.0	150
1 fat serving	5	0.1	60
15 packed dry measures Lofenalac (add water to make 32 oz)	114	21.0	655
Total	374	27.6	1,195

Sample Menu

Breakfast
3 Tbsp banana
3 Tbsp Maltomeal
8 oz Lofenalac

Midmorning
1/2 cup pineapple juice

Noon Meal
1/2 cup sliced strawberries
1/3 cup cooked carrots
2 Tbsp macaroni, cooked
1 tsp butter
8 oz Lofenalac

Midafternoon
1/2 cup grape juice
5 animal crackers

Evening Meal
1/2 cup canned sliced peaches
1/3 cup cooked green beans
1/4 baked potato, no skin
   ($2\frac{1}{2}$" diameter)
1 tsp butter

Bedtime
8 oz Lofenalac

TABLE 8–43 Exchange List for Phenylalanine-Restricted Diets Strained and Junior Foods (Gerber)

Food	Measure	Weight (g)	Phenylalanine (mg)	Tyrosine (mg)	Protein (g)	Energy (Kcal)
Starch						
Cereal–dry						
Barley	1 Tbsp + 1 tsp	4.7	30	19	0.6	18
Mixed	1 Tbsp + 1 tsp	4.7	29	22	0.8	18
Mixed/banana	1 Tbsp + 1 tsp	4.7	27	19	0.5	18
Oatmeal	1 Tbsp	3.6	28	20	0.6	14
Oatmeal/banana	1 Tbsp	3.6	27	16	0.5	14
Rice	2 Tbsp	7.1	26	24	0.6	27
Rice/banana	2 Tbsp	7.1	31	19	0.7	28
Cereal–jarred						
Mixed/apples and bananas	3½ Tbsp	50	33	22	0.8	32
strained	3 Tbsp	43	32	23	0.6	25
junior	2 Tbsp + 2 tsp	38	30	22	0.6	21
Rice/apples and bananas	5 Tbsp + 1 tsp	76	32	33	0.7	54
Rice/mixed fruit	3½ Tbsp	50	30	34	0.8	36
Vegetables						
Creamed corn	3 Tbsp	43	30	28	0.6	27
Creamed spinach	1 Tbsp + 1 tsp	19	27	23	0.5	8
Sweet potato	2 Tbsp + 2 tsp	38	30	22	0.5	23
Fruits/Juices						
Strained and junior fruits						
Applesauce and apricots	10 Tbsp	143	15	9	0.4	74
Apricots with tapioca	7 Tbsp	100	17	9	0.4	72
Bananas with tapioca	7 Tbsp	100	14	9	0.4	67
Bananas with pineapple and tapioca	10 Tbsp	143	15	12	0.4	72
Peaches	7 Tbsp	100	19	16	0.6	73
Pears	7 Tbsp	100	13	4	0.5	52
Pears and pineapple	7 Tbsp	100	11	8	0.4	53
Plums with tapioca	10 Tbsp	143	13	5	0.6	96

Food	Measure					
Prunes with tapioca	7 Tbsp	100	13	5	0.6	72
Strained Juices						
Mixed fruit	4 oz	—	14	10	0.5	66
Orange	2 oz	—	15	8	0.5	35
Orange-apple	4 oz	—	15	10	0.5	66
Orange-apricot	2 oz	—	17	9	0.5	35
Orange-pineapple	3 oz	—	18	12	0.6	57
Vegetables						
Beets	1/3 cup	71	17	24	0.9	26
Carrots	1/3 cup	71	14	12	0.5	18
Creamed green beans	1 Tbsp + 2 tsp	24	16	14	0.3	10
Garden vegetables	1 Tbsp	14	16	12	0.3	5
Green beans	2 Tbsp	29	17	13	0.4	7
Mixed vegetables	2 Tbsp	29	19	14	0.4	12
Squash	1/4 cup	57	18	15	0.5	15
Vegetables and meat combinations, strained only						
Vegetable and bacon	2 Tbsp	29	18	16	0.5	22
Vegetable and beef	2 Tbsp	29	16	12	0.5	19
Vegetable and chicken	1 Tbsp + 1 tsp	19	17	13	0.4	9
Vegetable and ham	1 Tbsp + 1 tsp	19	12	9	0.3	11
Vegetable and turkey	1 Tbsp + 2 tsp	24	16	13	0.4	12
Free Foods						
Fruits						
Apple blueberry	1/4 cup	57	5	3	0.1	34
Applesauce	7 Tbsp	100	5	4	0.2	46
Applesauce with pineapple	7 Tbsp	100	6	5	0.2	49
Mango	1/4 cup	57	6	3	0.2	41
Papaya and applesauce	7 Tbsp	100	4	3	0.2	65
Juices						
Apple	4.2 oz	—	3	3	0.1	60
Apple-banana	3.0 oz	—	6	4	0.2	43
Apple-cherry	3.0 oz	—	5	4	0.2	43
Apple-grape	3.0 oz	—	3	3	0.1	60
Apple-peach	4.2 oz	—	7	6	0.3	60
Apple-plum	4.2 oz	—	6	4	0.3	60
Apple-prune	4.2 oz	—	6	4	0.3	60
Strained tropical fruit						
Guava	14 Tbsp	200	2	8	0.6	134
Guava and papaya	14 Tbsp	200	4	4	0.4	134

These data were derived from Nutrient Values, Gerber Baby Food, 1981 & 1982.

Table Foods

Food	Measure	Weight (g)	Phenylalanine (mg)	Tyrosine (mg)	Protein (g)	Energy (Kcal)
Starch						
Cereals, cooked						
Corn grits, regular and quick, plain	3 Tbsp	45	33	28	0.6	28
Corn grits, instant, plain	1/4 pkt	34	27	22	0.5	20
Corn grits, instant with artificial cheese flavor	1/4 pkt	36	36	29	0.7	27
Cream of Rice	1/3 cup	81	30	40	0.7	42
Cream of Wheat, regular	2 Tbsp	31	26	15	0.5	17
Cream of Wheat, quick	2 Tbsp	30	25	14	0.4	16
Cream of Wheat, instant	2 Tbsp	30	30	18	0.6	19
Cream of Wheat, mix and eat, plain	1/4 pkt	36	37	22	0.7	26
Cream of Wheat, mix and eat, flavored	1/4 pkt	38	33	20	0.6	33
Farina	3 Tbsp	44	34	20	0.6	22
Maltex	2 Tbsp	31	33	19	0.7	22
Malt-O-meal	3 Tbsp	45	31	18	0.7	23
Maypo oat cereal	2 Tbsp	30	34	20	0.7	21
Oats, regular, quick and instant	1½ Tbsp	22	31	20	0.6	14
Pettijohns	2 Tbsp	30	24	14	0.5	20
Ralston	2 Tbsp	32	32	19	0.7	17
Rice, brown	3 Tbsp	28	36	41	0.7	33
Rice, white	3 Tbsp	28	28	32	0.6	31
Roman Meal, plain	1½ Tbsp	22	31	22	0.6	14
Wheatena	2 Tbsp	30	29	17	0.6	22
Whole wheat hot natural cereal	2 Tbsp	30	29	17	0.6	19
Cereals, ready to eat						
All Bran	1 Tbsp	6	34	25	0.8	14
Alpha Bits	1/4 cup	7	29	20	0.6	28
Apple Jacks	1/3 cup	9	26	18	0.5	37
Bran Buds	1 Tbsp	6	33	24	0.8	15
Bran Chex	2 Tbsp	6	24	18	0.6	20
C.W. Post, plain	1 Tbsp	6	29	21	0.5	27

Cereal	Serving					
C.W. Post, with raisins	1 Tbsp	6	28	21	0.6	28
Cap'n Crunch	1/4 cup	9	25	19	0.5	39
Cap'n Crunch Berries	1/4 cup	9	24	18	0.4	36
Cap'n Crunch Peanut Butter	1/4 cup	9	33	26	0.6	38
Cheerios	3 Tbsp	4	35	23	0.6	17
Cocoa Krispies	1/3 cup	12	27	36	0.6	46
Cocoa Pebbles	1/2 cup	16	33	42	0.7	66
Cookie Crisp	1/2 cup	15	37	30	0.8	60
Corn Bran	1/4 cup	9	32	26	0.6	31
Corn Chex	1/4 cup	7	26	21	0.5	28
Cornflakes	1/3 cup	7	29	24	0.6	28
Crispy Rice	1/3 cup	9	26	34	0.6	37
Crispy Wheats'n Raisins	1/4 cup	11	37	21	0.8	38
Fortified Oat Flakes	1 Tbsp	3	29	21	0.6	11
40% Branflakes (Post)	2 Tbsp	6	30	20	0.7	19
Fruit Loops	1/3 cup	9	29	20	0.6	37
Frosted Mini-Wheats	1 biscuit	8	38	22	0.8	28
Frosted Rice Krinkles	1/2 cup	16	34	44	0.8	62
Frosted Rice Krispies	1/2 cup	14	28	37	0.6	54
Fruity Pebbles	1/2 cup	16	27	37	0.6	66
Golden Grahams	1/4 cup	10	28	22	0.6	38
Grape Nuts Flakes	2 Tbsp	4	22	13	0.4	15
Honey Nut Cheerios	3 Tbsp	6	35	24	0.7	23
Honeycomb	1/2 cup	11	33	26	0.6	43
King Vitamin	1/2 cup	10	28	22	0.6	42
Kix	1/3 cup	6	27	21	0.5	23
Life	1 Tbsp	3	28	21	0.5	10
Lucky Charms	3 Tbsp	6	30	20	0.5	23
Nutri-Grain Barley	2 Tbsp	5	31	19	0.6	19
Nutri-Grain Corn	3 Tbsp	8	33	27	0.6	30
Nutri-Grain Rye	3 Tbsp	8	31	14	0.7	27
Nutri-Grain Wheat	3 Tbsp	8	33	19	0.7	30
Product 19	3 Tbsp	6	30	22	0.6	24
Quisp	6 Tbsp	11	30	23	0.6	46
Raisin Bran, Post	2 Tbsp	7	26	17	0.6	22
Raisin Chex	1/2 cup	13	29	38	0.7	50
Rice Krispies	1/3 cup	9	27	36	0.6	37
Rice, puffed	3/4 cup	10	28	38	0.7	42
Special K	2 Tbsp	3	22	19	0.5	14
Sugar Pops	1/2 cup	14	36	29	0.7	54
Sugar Frosted Flakes	1/3 cup	12	31	25	0.6	44

Table Foods (continued)

Food	Measure	Weight (g)	Phenylalanine (mg)	Tyrosine (mg)	Protein (g)	Energy (Kcal)
Sugar Smacks	1/4 cup	9	32	23	0.6	34
Sugar Sparkled Flakes	1/2 cup	13	35	29	0.7	64
Super Sugar Crisp	1/4 cup	8	28	16	0.5	31
Team	1/4 cup	10	32	31	0.7	41
Toasties	1/3 cup	7	29	24	0.6	27
Total	3 Tbsp	6	30	18	0.6	22
Trix	1/3 cup	9	27	21	0.5	36
Wheat Chex	2 Tbsp	6	26	15	0.6	21
Wheat, puffed	1/3 cup	4	30	18	0.6	15
Wheat, shredded	2 Tbsp	6	30	18	0.6	20
Wheaties	1/4 cup	7	33	20	0.7	25
Crackers						
Animal crackers	5	10	33	19	0.7	43
Graham crackers	1—2″ × 2″	7	19	15	0.6	27
Ritz crackers	3	10	33	19	0.7	54
Rye Thins	3	8	27	12	0.6	39
Saltines	2	6	29	14	0.5	26
Soda crackers	1	7	35	19	0.7	30
Sugar wafers (Nabisco)	5	16	30	16	0.6	75
Tortilla, corn	1/4—6″ diameter	8	36	29	0.7	27
Tortilla, flour	1/4—6″ diameter	8	33	19	0.7	27
Vanilla wafers	4	13	32	16	0.6	60
Wheat thins	5	9	29	17	0.6	45
Miscellaneous						
Cake flour	1 Tbsp	7	28	16	0.6	29
Chocolate sauce, Hersheys	1 Tbsp	20	25	18	0.5	49
Corn, cooked	2 Tbsp	21	26	21	0.5	17
Corn-on-cob	1/6 medium ear	17	31	25	0.6	16
Jello	1/3 cup	80	30	3	0.6	65
Macaroni, cooked	2 Tbsp	18	31	16	0.6	19
Marshmallows	6 (60/pound)	45	30	6	1.2	150
Noodles, cooked	2 Tbsp	20	40	22	0.8	25
Popcorn, popped, plain	1/3 cup	5	31	16	0.6	19

Food	Measure					
Spaghetti, cooked	2 Tbsp	21	0.6	17	33	19
Potatoes						
Baked, no skin	1/4 (2½")	24	0.6	18	28	25
Boiled, in skin	1/3 (2½")	25	0.7	16	30	33
Boiled, no skin	1/3 (2½")	22	0.6	18	28	33
Chips	6 (2" diameter)	68	0.7	18	29	12
French fried	3 (½" × ½" × 2")	42	0.8	18	28	15
Panfried from raw	2 Tbsp	57	0.8	24	38	21
Sweet potatoes						
Baked in skin	1/4 small	35	0.5	13	29	25
Boiled in skin	1/4 large	43	0.6	16	38	45
Canned, syrup pack	1/2 small	57	0.5	12	28	50
Fats						
Butter	2 tsp	72	0.1	4	4	10
Dessert topping,						
frozen,	2 Tbsp	26	0.1	6	6	8
pressurized	2 Tbsp	22	0.1	4	4	8
Margarine, stick	2 tsp	68	0.1	4	4	9
Margarine, soft, tub	2 tsp	67	0.1	4	4	9
Margarine, liquid	1 tsp	34	0.1	4	4	5
Nondairy creamers	2 tsp liquid	14	0.1	4	6	10
	1 tsp powder	11	0.1	5	5	2
Salad Dressing (commercial)						
French dressing	1 Tbsp	67	0.1	3	4	16
Italian	1 Tbsp	69	0.1	3	4	15
Mayonnaise	2 tsp	66	0.1	4	5	9
Thousand Island	1 Tbsp	59	0.1	3	4	16
Fruits						
Apricots						
canned†	1/4 cup	54	0.3	8	14	64
dried	3 halves	25	0.4	9	16	10
frozen, sweet	1/4 cup	60	0.4	9	16	60
nectar	3 oz	54	0.4	8	15	94
raw	1 fruit	17	0.5	10	18	35
Avocado, mashed	1½ Tbsp	35	0.4	11	15	22
Banana, sliced	3 Tbsp	39	0.4	10	16	42
Blackberries‡						
canned†	2 Tbsp	59	0.4	8	12	32
raw	1/2 cup	37	0.5	10	15	72

Table Foods *(continued)*

Food	Measure	Weight (g)	Phenylalanine (mg)	Tyrosine (mg)	Protein (g)	Energy (Kcal)
Blueberries						
canned†	1/4 cup	64	15	5	0.4	56
frozen, sweet	1/2 cup	115	16	6	0.5	94
raw	1/2 cup	72	17	6	0.5	41
Boysenberries, canned†‡	1/4 cup	64	18	13	0.6	56
Cherries‡						
sour, red, canned†	1/4 cup	64	13	9	0.5	58
sweet, canned†	1/3 cup	86	15	10	0.5	67
raw	1/4 cup	72	13	9	0.4	26
Dates	3 fruits	25	14	8	0.5	68
Figs						
canned†	1/2 cup	130	12	20	0.5	114
dried	1 fruit	19	14	25	0.6	48
raw	1 large fruit	64	12	20	0.5	47
Fruit cocktail, canned†	1/2 cup	128	14	10	0.5	93
Fruit salad, canned†	1/2 cup	128	14	10	0.5	94
Grapefruit, red, pink & white‡						
canned§	1/3 cup	85	14	10	0.5	51
juice, canned unsweetened	4 oz	124	19	13	0.6	48
raw	1/3 cup sections	77	14	10	0.5	25
Grapes						
adherent skin, raw	3/4 cup	120	16	12	0.8	86
slip skin, raw	1 cup	92	12	10	0.6	58
Thompson seedless canned†	1/2 cup	128	13	10	0.6	94
Grape juice, canned	1/2 cup	126	15	4	0.7	78
Mango, raw	1/2 cup slices	82	14	9	0.4	54
Melon						
cantaloupe	1/3 cup cubed	53	14	9	0.5	19
casaba	1/3 cup cubed	57	15	10	0.5	15
honeydew	1/2 cup cubed	85	11	8	0.4	30
Nectarines, raw	1/2 cup slices	69	19	13	0.6	34
Orange						
juice, canned	1 cup	249	17	7	1.5	105
frozen, diluted	3/4 cup	187	15	8	1.3	84

Food	Serving					
Orange						
raw, sections	1/4 cup	45	14	7	0.4	21
Papaya, raw	1 cup cubed	140	13	7	0.9	54
Peaches						
canned†	1/2 cup slices	128	18	16	0.6	95
dried	1/2 peach	13	15	12	0.5	31
frozen, sweet	1/3 cup	83	17	13	0.5	78
nectar	3/4 cup	187	16	13	0.5	100
spiced, canned†	1/2 cup	121	16	13	0.5	90
raw	1/2 cup slices	85	18	16	0.6	37
Pears						
canned†	1 cup halves	255	13	5	0.5	188
dried	2 halves	35	17	6	0.7	92
raw	1 cup sliced	165	17	5	0.6	97
Persimmons, Japanese	1/3 fruit	56	15	9	0.4	39
Pineapple						
canned,† chunks, tidbits, crushed	3/4 cup	191	17	15	0.8	149
frozen, sweet	1/2 cup chunks	122	15	16	0.5	104
juice, canned	1/2 cup	125	13	13	0.4	70
raw	3/4 cup cubed	116	14	10	0.4	58
Plantains, cooked	1/3 cup slices	51	14	10	0.4	60
Plums						
purple, canned†	3/4 cup	194	16	6	0.7	172
raw	1/2 cup	82	14	5	0.6	46
Prunes						
dried	3 fruits	25	14	2	0.7	60
juice	1/2 cup	128	17	6	0.8	90
Raisins, seedless	2 Tbsp	18	12	10	0.6	54
Raspberries‡						
canned†	1/4 cup	64	15	11	0.5	58
frozen, red, sweetened	1/3 cup	83	17	12	0.6	85
raw	1/2 cup	62	16	11	0.6	30
Rhubarb, cooked sweetened	1/2 cup	120	14	9	0.5	139
Strawberries						
frozen, sweetened	1/3 cup sliced	85	13	15	0.5	82
raw	1/2 cup sliced	74	13	16	0.5	23
Tangerines						
canned§	1/3 cup	84	13	7	0.4	51
juice, canned, sweetened	1 cup	249	15	7	1.2	125
juice, frozen diluted	1 cup	241	12	5	1.0	110

Table Foods (continued)

Food	Measure	Weight (g)	Phenylalanine (mg)	Tyrosine (mg)	Protein (g)	Energy (Kcal)
Tangerine						
raw	1 medium fruit	84	18	9	0.5	37
Watermelon	3/4 cup diced	120	18	14	0.7	38
Vegetables (Drain before measuring or weighing)						
Asparagus						
canned, green	1 spear	19	11	8	0.4	4
canned, white	2 spears	38	19	13	0.6	7
frozen, cooked	1 spear	17	17	12	0.6	7
raw	1 spear	20	16	10	0.5	5
Beans, green						
canned	1/3 cup	42	14	11	0.6	10
frozen (cooked)		33	13	10	0.5	8
Beans, yellow wax						
canned	1/4 cup	50	17	13	0.7	12
frozen, cooked		33	14	11	0.6	9
Bean sprouts, mung						
cooked	2 Tbsp	12	19	11	0.4	4
raw	2 Tbsp	12	14	8	0.3	3
Bean sprouts, soy						
cooked	1 Tbsp	8	13	12	0.4	3
raw	1 Tbsp	6	12	11	0.4	3
Beets, red						
cooked, fresh	1/2 cup diced	83	15	15	0.9	27
canned	1/2 cup diced	83	14	14	0.8	31
pickled	1/2 cup	83	14	14	0.8	80
Beet greens, cooked	1 Tbsp	12	12	11	0.2	2
Broccoli, fresh or frozen, cooked	1 Tbsp	10	11	9	0.3	3
Brussels sprouts						
cooked (fresh)	1 Tbsp	10	14	12	0.4	4
frozen (cooked)		15	16	13	0.5	5
Cabbage						
cooked	1/3 cup	52	12	7	0.6	10
raw, shredded	1/2 cup	50	14	9	0.6	12

Food	Measure					
Cabbage, red, raw, shredded	1/3 cup	33	14	9	0.7	10
Carrots						
canned	1/3 cup	50	14	11	0.4	15
cooked	1/3 cup	50	16	13	0.5	16
raw	1/3 large	33	13	10	0.4	14
Cauliflower						
cooked	3 Tbsp	21	15	6	0.5	5
frozen (cooked)	1/4 cup	29	17	7	0.6	5
raw	3 Tbsp	30	16	6	0.8	8
Celery						
cooked	1/3 cup	33	12	3	0.3	5
raw	1/3 cup	33	14	4	0.3	6
Chard, cooked	1½ Tbsp	16	16	8	0.3	3
Collards						
cooked (fresh)	1½ Tbsp	19	16	20	0.5	6
cooked (frozen)	1 Tbsp	12	11	13	0.3	4
Cucumber						
not pared	1/2 medium	50	12	12	0.5	8
pared	1 medium	100	14	14	0.6	14
Eggplant						
cooked	3 Tbsp	38	16	15	0.4	7
Kale						
cooked (fresh)	1 Tbsp	12	15	10	0.4	8
cooked (frozen)	1 Tbsp	10	12	8	0.3	3
Lettuce	2 leaves	30	13	10	0.4	4
Mushrooms, Lactarius						
sauteed or fried	6 medium	105	15	14	2.6	117
Mustard greens						
cooked (fresh or frozen)	2 Tbsp	25	18	30	0.6	6
Okra						
cooked (fresh or frozen)	2 pods	22	17	13	0.5	7
Onions						
cooked	1/4 cup	50	17	21	0.6	15
raw, chopped	2 Tbsp	20	12	15	0.4	8
Peas, green						
canned	1 Tbsp	8	18	13	0.4	7
Peppers, green						
Baked, no filling, or raw	1/4 large shell	25	14	8	0.3	6
Pumpkin, canned	1/4 cup	58	16	16	0.6	19
Radish, red	3 small	33	15	8	0.3	6

Table Foods (continued)

Food	Measure	Weight (g)	Phenylalanine (mg)	Tyrosine (mg)	Protein (g)	Energy (Kcal)
Rutabagas						
cooked	1/2 cup	100	18	13	0.9	35
raw	—	82	18	13	0.9	38
Sauerkraut	1/4 cup	40	12	8	0.4	7
Spinach						
canned	1 Tbsp	11	13	11	0.3	3
frozen (cooked)	1 Tbsp	12	16	13	0.4	2
raw		10	14	12	0.3	3
Squash, summer						
boiled (fresh)	1/3 cup	62	15	15	0.6	9
frozen (cooked)	3 Tbsp	38	14	14	0.5	8
Squash, winter						
baked	2 Tbsp	25	12	12	0.4	16
boiled	3 Tbsp	47	14	14	0.5	18
frozen (cooked)	1/4 cup	50	16	16	0.6	19
Tomato						
canned	1/4 cup	50	14	10	0.5	10
catsup	3 Tbsp	45	16	12	0.9	48
juice	3 oz	90	16	12	0.9	18
puree	2 Tbsp	33	16	12	0.6	13
raw	1/2 small	50	16	12	0.6	11
Turnip greens, fresh or frozen,						
cooked	1 Tbsp	10	11	7	0.2	2
canned	2 Tbsp	25	17	10	0.4	4
Turnip root						
cooked	2/3 cup diced	50	14	10	0.8	23
raw	1/2 cup diced	50	12	8	0.5	15
Soups, Condensed, Campbell's (measure before diluting—prepare with equal volume of water after measuring in condensed form).						
Asparagus, cream of	1 Tbsp	16	12	9	0.3	11
Celery, cream of	2 Tbsp	32	20	14	0.4	22
Chicken gumbo	1 Tbsp	16	12	9	0.3	7
Mushroom, cream of	1 Tbsp	16	12	9	0.3	16
Potato, cream of	1 Tbsp	16	10	8	0.2	9
Tomato bisque	2 Tbsp	32	19	15	0.6	31
Tomato	2 Tbsp	32	18	11	0.5	21
Vegetarian vegetable	1 Tbsp	15	12	6	0.3	9

Free Foods A: Limit to prescribed servings

Aprotein Low Protein Products#						
dp chocolate chip cookies	2 cookies	28	4	4	0.2	140
Low protein bread	1/2-1/2" slice	16	5	4	0.1	42
Rusks	1 slice	10	2	2	0.1	43
Pastas, cooked						
Anellini	1/2 cup	110	4	3	0.2	98
Ditalini	1 cup	130	4	3	0.2	114
Rigatini	1 cup	130	4	3	0.2	114
Semolino	1 cup	267	3	2	0.1	91
Tagliatelle	1/2 cup	120	4	3	0.2	107
Fruit and Juices						
Apple	1 small	100	5	4	0.2	59
Apples, canned, sliced sweetened	1/2 cup	102	5	3	0.2	68
Apples, dehydrated	1/4 cup	15	6	4	0.2	54
Apples, dehydrated cooked	1/4 cup	48	4	3	0.1	36
Apple juice, frozen diluted	1/4 cup	120	4	3	0.2	56
Applesauce, canned sweetened	1/2 cup	128	6	4	0.2	97
Cranberry sauce, canned	1/4 cup	69	4	3	0.1	104
Lemonade	1/2 cup	125	4	2	0.1	55
Papaya nectar	6 oz	187	4	2	0.1	108
Peach nectar	2 oz	62	5	4	0.2	34
Pear nectar	6 oz	187	5	1	0.2	114

Free Foods B: These foods contain little or no phenylalanine or tyrosine. May be used as desired if child is not overweight and if they do not depress appetite for prescribed foods.

Beverages						
Apple juice, canned	4 oz	124	2	2	0.1	60
Carbonated beverage, sweetened	4 oz	113	0	0	0	52
Cranberry juice cocktail	4 oz	126	1	1	0	52
Gatorade	4 oz	126	0	0	0	25
Koolaid, sweetened	4 oz	125	0	0	0	48
Limeade, sweetened	4 oz	125	0	0	0	51
Tang	4 oz	125	0	0	0	59
Candies						
Butterscotch	1 piece	5	0	0	0	21
Fondant	1 mint	11	0	0	0	4
Gumdrop	1 large	10	0	0	0	33
Hard candy	2 rolls 1"	10	0	0	0	38
Jelly beans	10 beans	28	0	0	0	66
Lollypop	1 medium	28	0	0	0	108

Table Foods (continued)

Food	Measure	Weight (g)	Phenylalanine (mg)	Tyrosine (mg)	Protein (g)	Energy (Kcal)
Fruit and Products						
Fruit butters	1 Tbsp	20	3	2	0.1	37
Fruit ices	1/2 cup	90	0	0	tr	69
Guava, raw	1 fruit	90	2	9	0.7	45
Guava sauce	1/2 cup	119	1	5	0.4	43
Jams	1 Tbsp	20	3	2	0.1	55
Jellies	1 Tbsp	20	0	0	0	50
Miscellaneous						
Corn starch	1 Tbsp	8	0	0	tr	29
Rich's topping	1 Tbsp unwhipped	—	0	0	0	42
Shortening, vegetable	1 Tbsp	13	0	0	0	113
Wheat starch	1 Tbsp	8	1	1	tr	25
Sugar and sweets						
Corn syrup	1 Tbsp	20	0	0	0	57
Danish dessert	1/2 cup	—				123
dp cookies#						
Butterscotch Chip	1 cookie	14	0	0	0	70
Honey	1 Tbsp	20	1	1	0	64
Maple syrup	1 Tbsp	20	3	2	0.1	50
Molasses	1 Tbsp	20	0	0	0	50
Popsicle	1 twin bar		0	0	0	95
Prono#	1/3 cup	14**	0	0	0	55
Sugar, brown	1 Tbsp	14	0	0	0	52
Sugar, granulated	1 Tbsp	12	0	0	0	46
Sugar, powdered	1 Tbsp	11	0	0	0	59

* Adapted from Acosta PB, Fernhoff PM, Rappaport A. The parents' guide to the child with PKU (revised). Tallahassee: Florida State University, 1982, and with permission.

† In heavy syrup

‡ Phenylalanine calculated as 2.9%, tyrosine as 2.0% of protein

§ In light syrup

Available from Dietary Specialties, P.O. Box 277, Rochester, NY 14601. (716) 263-2787

** Weight before water added

The optimal time to discontinue the diet is controversial. Once maturation of the brain is completed, discontinuation of the low phenylalanine diet should not have a devastating effect on future intellectual ability or emotional behavior.[2] There is, however, varied response to discontinuation of dietary management of blood phenylalanine levels.[2] Some children taken off the diet at $4\frac{1}{2}$ years showed no loss in IQ scores, but others lost as many as 19 IQ points.[2] Even without loss of IQ, significant differences in spelling and reading ability[10] and in performance on neuropsychological tests[11] have been reported between groups of patients on or off a phenylalanine-controlled diet. Returning patients to a phenylalanine-controlled diet after the diet has been discontinued is difficult and often unsuccessful. The PKU diet should not be discontinued under the assumption that the diet can easily be resumed if undesirable effects of diet discontinuation occur. To test the effects of an increased phenylalanine intake, milk can be added to the child's formula before discontinuing the diet entirely. It is not clear if academic decline can be reversed by resumption of the diet.[12] Delay of diet discontinuation until 8 to 10 years of age[2] or until adolescence[10] is often recommended. Two-thirds of PKU clinics surveyed now reportedly recommend continuation of the PKU diet indefinitely.[13]

Maternal PKU. Women with PKU are at risk for bearing infants with mental retardation, microcephaly, low birth weight, and congenital heart disease and have more frequent spontaneous abortions than women without PKU. Fetal brain damage is correlated to maternal phenylalanine levels.[2] Apparently the infant is at high risk with classic maternal PKU (blood phenylalanine levels of 20 mg per deciliter or greater), and mild hyperphenylalaninemia (blood phenylalanine level less than 10 mg per deciliter) carries little or no risk to the fetus. Toxicity to the fetus is uncertain with degrees of maternal hyperphenylalaninemia between these levels.[6]

Females with PKU should maintain dietary phenylalanine restriction prior to conception and during the pregnancy to control blood phenylalanine levels between 2 and 10 mg per deciliter.[6] Diet and plasma phenylalanine levels need to be monitored as carefully as during infancy. L-tyrosine supplementation is needed to maintain the tyrosine intake at 110 mg per kilogram per day during pregnancy. Nutritional factors particularly important during pregnancy, such as kilocalories, protein, vitamins, and mineral intake, should be monitored.[6]

Since reinstitution of a PKU diet is difficult, continuing a small amount of Lofenalac in the diet of PKU females after discontinuation of the diet may help her retain a taste for the formula. Compliance with the diet during pregnancy, even for the well-motivated woman, is usually difficult and requires support of family, physician, and dietitian.

Physicians: How to Order Diet

The diet order should indicate *diet for PKU*. The level of phenylalanine should be specified.

REFERENCES

1. Acosta PB, Farnhoff PM, Warshaw HS, Hambidge KM, Ernest A, MoCahe RB, Elsas LJ. Zinc and copper status of treated children with phenylketonuria. JPEN 1981;5:406–409.
2. Tourian A, Sidbury JB. Phenylketonuria and hyperphenylalinemia. In: Stanbury JB, Wyngaarden JB, Fredrickson DS, Goldstein JL, Brown SB, eds. The metabolic basis of inherited disease. 5th ed. New York: McGraw-Hill, 1983:270.

3. Behrman RE, Vaughan VC III. Nelson textbook of pediatrics. In: Nelson WE, senior ed. 12th ed. Philadelphia: WB Saunders, 1983:424.

4. Rohr FJ, Levy HL, Shich VE. Inborn errors of metabolism. In: Walker WA, Watkins JB, eds. Nutrition in pediatrics. Boston/Toronto: Little, Brown and Company, 1985:384,391.

5. Trahms CM. Nutritional care for children with metabolic disorders. In: Krause MV, Mahan LK, eds. Food, nutrition, and diet therapy. 7th ed. Philadelphia, WB Saunders, 1984:802.

6. Committee on Nutrition, American Academy of Pediatrics. Final report, task force on the dietary management of metabolic disorders. December, 1985.

7. Acosta PB, Elsas LJ. Dietary management of inherited metabolic disease: phenylketonuria, galactosemia, tyrosinemia, homocystinuria, maple syrup urine disease. Atlanta: ACELMU Publishers, 1976:7.

8. Michels V. Personal communication. Mayo Clinic, Department of Medical Genetics.

9. Flannery DB, Hitchcock E, Mamunes P. Dietary management of phenylketonuria from birth using a phenylalanine-free product. J Pediatr 1983;103:247–249.

10. Koch R, Azan CG, Friedman EG, Williamson ML. Preliminary report of the effects of diet discontinuation in PKU. J Pediatr 1982;100:870–875.

11. Should dietary treatment of phenylketonuria be continued after infancy? Nutr Rev 1985;43:176–177.

12. Michals K, Dominck M, Schuett V, Brown E, Matalon R. Return to diet therapy in patients with phenylketonuria. J Pediatr 1985;106:933–936.

13. Schuett VE, Brown ES. Diet policies of PKU clinics in the United States. Am J Public Health 1984;74:501–503.

Additional References For Parents and/or Health Professionals

Acosta PB et al. Parents' guide to the child with PKU. Florida State University, Center for Family Services, 103 Sandels Building, Tallahassee, Florida 32306, 1980.

Acosta PB, Wenz E. Diet management of PKU for infants and preschool children. DHEW Publications No. (HSA) 78-5209, 1978.

Bell L. The phenylalanine content of foods. Clinical Investigation Unit, Nutrition Division, The Hospital for Sick Children, 555 University Avenue, Toronto, Ontario, Canada, M5X 1G8, 1980.

Ernest AE, McCabe ERB, Nerfert MR, O'Flynn ME. Guide to breast feeding the infant with PKU. Superintendent of Documents, US Government Printing Office, Washington, DC 20402.

Henderson RA et al. PKU and the schools: information for teachers, administrators, and other school personnel. DHEW Publication No. (HSA) 80-5233, 1980.

Holtzman NA. Newborn screening for genetic metabolic diseases: progress, principles and recommendations. DHEW Publication No. (HSA) 70-5207, 1977.

Levy HL, Lenke RR, Crocker AC, eds. Maternal PKU. DHHS Publication No. (HSA) 81-5299.

Management of newborn infants with phenylketonuria. DHEW Publication No. (HSA) 70-5211, 1979.

Pennington JAT, Church HN. Bowes and Church's food values of portions commonly used. 14th ed. Philadelphia: JB Lippincott Company, 1985.

PKU: phenylketonuria: a guide to dietary management. Mead Johnson & Co., Evansville, Indiana 47721, 1981.

Products for dietary management of inborn errors of metabolism and other special feeding problems. Mead Johnson & Co., Evansville, Indiana 47721, 1981.

Read E et al. The PKU cookbook. Program in Dietetics, Emory University, 2040 Ridgewood Drive N.E., Atlanta, Georgia 30322, 1976.

Schuett VE. Low protein cookery for phenylketonuria. University of Wisconsin Press, Box 1379, Madison, Wisconsin 53701, 1981.

Schuett VE. Low protein food list: for phenylketonuria and metabolic diseases requiring a low protein diet. The Waisman Center, University of Wisconsin, 1500 Highland Avenue, Madison, Wisconsin 53706, 1981.

Schuett VE, Gurda RF. Treatment programs for PKU in the United States: a survey. DHEW Publication No. (HSA) 77-5207, 1977.

Taylor M, Schuett VE. You and PKU. Waisman Center on Mental Retardation and Human Development, 1500 Highland Avenue, Madison, Wisconsin 53706, 1978.

INFLAMMATORY BOWEL DISEASE

General Description

Dietary recommendations that encourage the use of or the avoidance of specific foods for children with inflammatory bowel disease have not been shown to be effective in influencing the course of the disease. Primary emphasis should be placed on recommendations for a well-balanced diet that meets protein and caloric needs to restore normal growth and to promote catch-up growth. Enteral or parenteral routes of nutrition may be used. Vitamin and mineral supplements may be needed.

Nutritional Inadequacy

Multivitamin and mineral supplementation is often needed to prevent or to replace nutrient deficiencies in the diet. Folic acid, vitamin D, iron, calcium, magnesium, and zinc should be provided when their need is indicated by the dietary assessment or when laboratory findings are consistent with a deficiency state.[1] Drug therapy may also contribute to nutrient deficiencies. Examples are: sulfasalazine, which interferes with folate absorption; corticosteroids, which suppress calcium absorption; and cholestyramine, which impairs the absorption of fat and fat-soluble vitamins.[2] A daily multivitamin with a mineral supplement is recommended when the child is following a low-residue diet.[1]

Indications and Rationale

Chronic idiopathic inflammatory bowel disease represents two intestinal disorders of childhood—ulcerative colitis and Crohn's disease. Ulcerative colitis is an inflammatory process that is limited to the colon. In contrast, Crohn's disease may occur in any portion of the gastrointestinal tract, although more than 60 percent of patients have disease that involves primarily the terminal ileum and the colon.[3] Major symptoms commonly associated with ulcerative colitis and with Crohn's disease include diarrhea, intestinal blood and protein loss, abdominal pain, and fever. Inflammatory bowel disease in children, especially Crohn's disease, is associated with a lack of weight gain, the cessation of linear growth, a retarded bone maturation, and a delayed sexual maturation.

Growth failure represents one of the most serious complications of inflammatory bowel disease in children and is one of the most difficult to treat. The etiology of the growth failure is not known, but is considered to be multifactorial, including an inadequate dietary intake, excessive gastrointestinal losses, malabsorption, and increased nutritional requirements.[4] Nutritional deficiencies, especially energy and protein, account largely for the poor growth and the lack of weight gain in these patients.[4] Inadequate food intake often results from anorexia and from fear of postprandial abdominal pain and diarrhea. Intestinal malabsorption and enteric losses of protein, of blood, and of micronutrients put children with inflammatory bowel disease at risk for other nutritional deficiencies as well. The most common nutritional deficiencies include folate, vitamin B_{12}, vitamin D, zinc, iron, calcium, and magnesium.[3]

The need for nutritional assessment[2] in the routine management of children with inflammatory bowel disease is now apparent as the influence of early nutritional intervention on malnutrition and delayed growth is being seen.[2,5] Although nutritional considerations should be given to all patients with inflammatory bowel disease, nutritional therapy has its primary impact in the treatment of Crohn's disease, particularly in individuals with small bowel involvement.

Goals of Dietary Management

The goals of nutritional therapy are to replace the nutrient losses associated with the inflammatory processes, to correct body deficits, to provide sufficient nutrients to promote energy and nitrogen balance, to restore normal growth, and to promote catch-up growth.

Dietary Recommendations

The methods available for the treatment of nutritional disorders in inflammatory bowel disease include enteral and parenteral feeding routes.[2] No specific diet has been shown to consistently alter the course of ulcerative colitis or of Crohn's disease. The limitation of dietary choices is discouraged because this limitation usually results in further nutritional deficiencies and creates stress associated with eating for the child. There is no clear evidence that the consumption or the avoidance of specific foods induces a remission or influences the severity of the disease or the frequency of relapses.[3] For children, a balanced diet that meets caloric and protein needs (adjusted for height-age) is recommended for catch-up growth.[6] The diet should be modified accordingly when the disease is active, when specific foods exacerbate symptoms, or when laboratory tests suggest specific abnormalities, such as steatorrhea or lactose intolerance. A low fat diet supplemented with medium chain triglyceride oil may be helpful in the control of symptoms in children with steatorrhea or with diarrhea. Some patients may have secondary lymphangiectasia owing to chronic inflammation or to previous surgery and may also benefit from the use of medium chain triglyceride oil as a source of kilocalories. A low residue diet in small, frequent feedings is recommended when severe postprandial pain or partial bowel obstruction is present.

Nutritional supplementation with a liquid formula may be necessary when the child is unable to increase dietary protein and energy intakes with ordinary foods. Dietary intake suplementation may be achieved with these formulas, but sometimes children experience satiety when taking these formulas and are, therefore, not able to increase their total nutrient intake significantly. Nasogastric infusions, either continuously or intermittently, may be used in these cases and have been effective in improving the nutritional status, the growth rates, and the clinical well-being in patients with inflammatory bowel disease.[3] Nocturnal nasogastric feedings with chemically defined diets permit these children to go to school during the day.

Patients with inflammatory bowel disease who are unable to tolerate sufficient amounts of enteral feeding because of active inflammatory disease or diarrhea may receive substantial benefit from parenteral nutrition.[1]

Physicians: How to Order Diet

The diet order should indicate a diet for a child with *inflammatory bowel disease*.

REFERENCES

1. Grand RJ. Model for the treatment of growth failure in children with inflammatory bowel disease. In: Suskind RM, ed. Textbook of pediatric nutrition. New York: Raven Press, 1981:483–492.
2. Chan ATH, Fleming CR. Nutritional management in patients with Crohn's disease. IM 1983;4:65–77.
3. Motil KG, Grand RJ. Nutritional management of inflammatory bowel disease. Pediatr Clin North Am 1985;32:447–469.
4. Motil KG, Grand RJ, Maletskos CJ, Young VR. The effect of disease, drug, and diet on whole body protein metabolism in adolescents with Crohn's disease and growth failure. J Pediatr 1982;101:345–351.
5. Motil KG, Altchuler SI, Grand RJ. Mineral balance during nutritional supplementation in adolescents with Crohn's disease and growth failure. J Pediatr 1985;107:473–479.
6. Peterson KE, Washington J, Rathbun JM. Team management of failure to thrive. J Am Diet Assoc 1984;84:810–815.

Fat Absorption Test Diet

General Description

The diet is generally planned to provide 100 g of fat in adults, but in children estimates of actual fat intake are made since many children are not able to consume this amount of fat. Therefore, interpretation of the test results according to the actual fat intake is permitted.

Indications and Rationale

The test diet is used to determine if steatorrhea is present. Steatorrhea is an indication of gastrointestinal maldigestion or malabsorption.

Stools are collected during a 3-day period while the patient's dietary intake is being recorded. Ordinarily, the test is done in the hospital or in a facility that allows outpatients to be served accurately measured diets. With children, however, the estimates of actual fat intake are done based on a 3-day food record, so the test can be done at home. The patient and the parents are instructed to keep a 3-day food record during the time of the stool collection. The actual amount of fat ingested can be determined from the 3-day food record, and this information can be used to interpret results of the stool fat collection by the following formula:

$$(0.021 \times \text{grams of dietary fat per 24 hours}) + 2.93$$

$$= \text{grams of fecal fat per 24 hours.}$$

According to this formula, a stool fat of 3.98 g would be expected after a dietary fat intake of 50 g.

REFERENCE

Chapter 9, *Diets in Preparation for Diagnostic Tests–Fat Absorption* (page 513).

KETOGENIC DIET

General Description

The ketogenic diet is used in the prophylactic treatment of some types of epilepsy in children. All foods are weighed. The diet is high in fat and low in carbohydrates and is planned to produce ketosis by reversing the usual ratio of dietary carbohydrate and fat. The diet may be planned with or without medium chain triglyceride (MCT) oil.

Nutritional Inadequacy

A multivitamin and a calcium and an iron supplement should be prescribed, since this diet does not meet the Recommended Dietary Allowances (RDA) for these nutrients for children.

Indications and Rationale

The diet is designed to produce ketone bodies as a result of the incomplete oxidation of fat. Ketone bodies (acetone, acetoacetic acid, and β-hydroxybutyric acid) are thought to have an anticonvulsant action.

The diet is planned to provide adequate calories for normal growth, development, and activity. The amount of fat in the diet is gradually increased, and the carbohydrate content is decreased. The amount of protein stays at the level recommended for the individual (see RDA page 39). The diet is thought to be most effective in children under 10 years of age.[1] There is usually a period of 10 to 21 days after initiation of the diet before complete seizure control is achieved.[2] Some data suggest that the diet is an ineffective treatment; if the diet does not control seizures within 3 months,[1] it should be discontinued.

This dietary program is used when drug therapy is not fully effective in controlling seizures.[3] Although several new and useful anticonvulsant drugs have become available in recent years, some patients have incomplete control of seizures or have unpleasant side effects with drug therapy, but obtain a therapeutic effect from the diet. The drugs are ordinarily continued with the diet, but the dose can often be reduced, and sometimes the drugs can be discontinued.

Goals of Dietary Management

The goal of the ketogenic diet is to produce and to maintain a ketotic state in a child by gradually reversing the usual amounts of dietary fat and carbohydrate while meeting the child's kilocalorie and protein needs.

Dietary Recommendations

A 3:1 ratio of ketogenic to antiketogenic substances must be achieved* to produce ketosis of sufficient degree to have beneficial control of seizures. The time usually required to reverse the usual ratio (1:3) to the 3:1 ratio is 4 days. A further increase in the amount of fat and a decrease in the amount of carbohydrate may be necessary if this diet does not produce ketosis.

Tests of the urine should show the presence of ketones consistently and

---

*For the purpose of calculating this ratio, it is assumed that glucose is antiketogenic and fatty acids are ketogenic and that 100 g of dietary carbohydrate yields 100 g of glucose, 100 g of dietary fat yields 10 g of glucose and 90 g of fatty acids, and 100 g of dietary protein produces 58 g of glucose and 46 g of fatty acids. Then the ketogenic to antiketogenic ratio may be calculated by dividing the sum of 90 percent of dietary fat and 46 percent of dietary protein by the sum of 100 percent of dietary carbohydrate, 10 percent of fat and 58 percent of protein. All terms in this calculation are in grams of carbohydrate, protein, or fat.

definitely when the desired state of ketosis has been achieved. Children on a ketogenic diet tend to excrete ketones at a maximal rate in the midafternoon and at a minimal rate in the early morning hours. Hence, it is usually sufficient to test the urine only on arising.

An abrupt change in a ketogenic diet may cause nausea or even vomiting. The practice is to alter the ratio of ketogenic to antiketogenic substances over a 4-day period in order to avoid these symptoms. If nausea or vomiting occurs, one or two meals should be omitted and small amounts of fruit juice should be given before the ketogenic diet is resumed.

A diet containing medium chain triglyceride oil can be used to produce ketosis, instead of the standard ketogenic diet (see Table 8–50). Because medium chain triglycerides are said to be more ketogenic than other dietary fats, the diet can include a greater proportion of foods containing carbohydrate and protein, while maintaining adequate levels of ketosis. This dietary regime is usually more effective in controlling seizures than is the standard ketogenic diet. However, the diet is usually not as well accepted by the patient and the family.[3]

Calculation of Ketogenic Diet Without Medium Chained Triglyceride (MCT) Oil

Ratio of Ketogenesis to Antiketogenesis (K:AK). In 4 days the ratio of protein and carbohydrate to fat can be reversed. The ratio of ketogenic (K) to antiketogenic (AK) materials can be altered as suggested in Table 8–44. The physician may indicate a different rate of progression and ratio if desired.

TABLE 8–44   Alteration of K:AK Ratio

Day	K:AK
First	1.1:1
Second	1.6:1
Third	2.2:1
Fourth	2.8:1

The 4-day dietary regimen of fat (F) and of protein and carbohydrate (P + C) can be calculated as in Table 8–45.

TABLE 8–45   Calculation of the 4-Day Dietary Regimes

Day	K:AK Ratio	Calculation		
First	1.1:1	1 g F 1 g P + C	= 9 Kcal × 1.1 = = 4 Kcal × 1.0 =	9.9 Kcal 4.0 Kcal 13.9 Kcal per unit
Second	1.6:1	1 g F 1 g P + C	= 9 Kcal × 1.6 = = 4 Kcal × 1.0 =	14.4 Kcal 4.0 Kcal 18.4 Kcal per unit
Third	2.2:1	1 g F 1 g P + C	= 9 Kcal × 2.2 = = 4 Kcal × 1.0 =	19.8 Kcal 4.0 Kcal 23.8 Kcal per unit
Fourth	2.8:1	1 g F 1 g P + C	= 9 Kcal × 2.8 = = 4 Kcal × 1.0 =	25.2 Kcal 4.0 Kcal 29.2 Kcal per unit

Kilocalories, Protein, Fat, and Carbohydrates. Protein, fat, and carbohydrate can be calculated as follows (also see example on page 427):

1. Determine the total kilocalorie requirement of the child.

The kilocalorie needs of the child are determined primarily from current dietary intake obtained by a thorough dietary history. Recommended Dietary Allowances and caloric requirements that are determined by the *Nomogram for Estimating Caloric Requirements, (Appendix 6)* and the estimated level of activity are additional sources of data for calculating kilocalorie needs.

2. Divide total kilocalories by kilocalories per unit:

$$\frac{\text{Total kilocalories}}{\text{Kilocalories per unit}} = \text{Total units per day}$$

3. For grams of fat, multiply the number of units by the K value in the ratio of ketogenesis to antiketogenesis:

$$\text{Number of units} \times \text{K} = \text{grams of fat}$$

4. For grams of protein and carbohydrate, multiply the number of units by the AK value in the ratio of ketogenesis to antiketogenesis:[4]

$$\text{Number of units} \times \text{AK} = \text{grams of protein plus carbohydrate}$$

5. For grams of protein, a patient 3 years of age or younger needs 1.5 g of protein per kilogram of weight for height and age. A patient older than 3 years needs 1 g of protein per kilogram of weight for height and age.

6. For grams of carbohydrate, subtract the grams of protein in the diet from the total units per day:

$$\text{Total units per day} - \text{grams of protein} = \text{grams of carbohydrate.}$$

The carbohydrate level should not be reduced below 10 g. For some patients, it may be necessary to decrease the carbohydrate content at a slower rate if an intolerance to fat is exhibited.

The diet may be planned with three meals or three meals and snacks as desired by the patient. Each meal and snack *must* have fat exchanges and/or cream to maintain the ratio. Each meal should consist of one-third of the total fat in the diet. If snacks are planned, each meal is planned with the remaining fat divided into thirds.

Sample Determination of the Ketogenic Diet Without MCT Oil

Calculation of the diet, composition of the diet (Table 8–46), sample daily food exchanges (Table 8–47), and a sample menu pattern (Table 8–48) are given for the following child.

TABLE 8–46 Calculated Values of the Dietary Program

Day	Protein g	Fat g	Carbohydrate g	Kilocalories	K:AK Ratio	Kilocalories Per Unit*
First	18	121	92	1,529	1.1:1	13.9
Second	18	133	65	1,529	1.6:1	18.4
Third	18	141	46	1,525	2.2:1	23.8
Fourth	18	146	34	1,522	2.8:1	29.2

*The procedure for calculation is on page 425.

Age: 5-year old male
Height: 110 cm
Weight: 18 kg
Kilocalories: 1,530 (18 kg × 85 Kcal)
The values for the 4-day dietary regimen are calculated as follows:

First Day			*Second Day*	
1,530 Kcal ÷ 13.9 Kcal	= 110 units		1,530 Kcal ÷ 18.4 Kcal	= 83 units
F 110 × 1.1	= 121 g		F 83 × 1.6	= 133 g
P + C = 110 × 1.0	= 110 g		P + C = 83 × 1.0	= 83 g
P (1 g/kg)	= 18 g		P (1 g/kg)	= 18 g
C (110-18)	= 92 g		C (83-18)	= 65 g

Third Day			*Fourth Day*	
1,530 Kcal ÷ 23.8 Kcal	= 64 units		1,530 Kcal ÷ 29.2 Kcal	= 52 units
F 64 × 2.2	= 141 g		F 52 × 2.8	= 146 g
P + C = 64 × 1.0	= 64 g		P + C = 52 × 1.0	= 52 g
P (1 g/kg)	= 18 g		P (1 g/kg)	= 18 g
C (64-18)	= 46 g		C (52-18)	= 34 g

TABLE 8–47   Sample Daily Food Exchanges

Day	Meat	Fat	Whipping Cream	Bread	Bread Product	Vegetable	Fruit
First	1½	14	3	1	5	1	10
Second	1½	12	4	—	4	1	8
Third	1½	14	4	—	4	1	5
Fourth and subsequent	1½	15	4	—	3	1	3

TABLE 8–48   Sample Meal Plan

Foods	Number of Servings*			
	First Day	Second Day	Third Day	Fourth Day
Breakfast				
Fruit	3	1	1	—
Starch	1	—	—	—
Bread product	2	2	2	1
Fat	5	2	2	4
Whipping cream	1	2	2	2
Noon Meal				
Meat	1/2	1/2	1/2	1/2
Starch	—	—	—	—
Bread product	1	1	1	1
Vegetable	1/2	1/2	1/2	1/2
Fat	5	5	6	5
Whipping cream	1	1	1	1
Fruit	4	4	2	1½
Evening Meal				
Meat	1	1	1	1
Starch	—	—	—	—
Bread product	2	1	1	1
Vegetable	1/2	1/2	1/2	1/2
Fat	4	5	6	6
Whipping cream	1	1	1	1
Fruit	3	3	2	1½

* All food is weighed.

The composition of the diet varies slightly from the calculated values according to the foods included in the diet.

Alternative Method of Calculation

Instead of calculating each diet individually, Table 8–49 may be used. Proceed as follows:

1. Determine the kilocalorie and the protein requirement.
2. Check the ratio to be used.
3. Grams of fat are given in column F.
4. Grams of carbohydrate and protein are given in column C + P.
5. Subtract the number of grams of protein required by the patient from the total number of C + P. The remaining number equals the number of grams of carbohydrate.

TABLE 8–49   Ketogenic Calculation Table

| | Ratio of Ketogenesis to Antiketogenesis | | | | | | | |
| | 1.1:1 | | 1.6:1 | | 2.2:1 | | 2.8:1 | |
Kilocalories	F g	C + P g	F g	C + P g	F g	C + P g	F g	C + P g
800	64	58	69	43	73	33	76	27
900	72	65	78	49	84	38	87	31
1,000	79	72	87	54	92	42	96	32
1,100	87	79	96	60	102	46	105	38
1,200	95	86	104	65	111	50	115	41
1,300	103	94	113	71	120	55	125	45
1,400	111	101	122	76	129	59	134	48
1,500	119	108	130	82	139	63	144	51
1,600	127	115	139	87	148	67	153	55
1,700	135	122	148	92	158	71	163	58
1,800	143	130	157	98	167	76	173	62
1,900	151	137	165	103	176	80	182	65
2,000	159	144	174	109	185	84	192	68
2,100	166	151	183	114	194	88	201	72
2,200	174	159	191	120	203	92	211	75

F = fat; C + P = carbohydrate plus protein.

TABLE 8–50   Calculation of Ketogenic Diet with MCT Oil[5]

Component	Comments
Kilocalories	Determined primarily from current dietary intake obtained by a thorough diet history. RDA for calories and basal caloric requirement determined by Nomogram and the estimated level of activity are additional sources for estimating caloric needs.
Protein	Approximately 10 percent of kilocalories Children 3 years old and younger 1.5 g/kg* Children older than 3 years of age 1.0 g/kg*
Carbohydrate	18 percent of kilocalories
Fat	12 percent of kilocalories Include a source of linoleic acid, such as corn or safflower oil
MCT Oil	60 percent of kilocalories MCT oil contains 8.3 kilocalories per gram

*Weight for height and age

The MCT oil should be introduced slowly, beginning with approximately 10 or 15 ml per day and increasing by 10 or 20 ml daily.

The patient may have diarrhea, vomiting, and abdominal pain during the introduction of the MCT oil. These symptoms usually begin when one-half the oil has been introduced. The gradual increase of the MCT oil can be continued if the symptoms are not distressing. If the patient becomes ill, reduce the MCT oil by one-half, and slowly begin to increase to the required amount again. The full allowance of food should not be given until the required amount of MCT oil has been reached.

Each of three meals should consist of one-third of the MCT oil planned in the diet. The equal distribution of MCT oil and its slow ingestion may be helpful in alleviating side effects.

Physicians: How to Order Diet

The diet order should indicate *ketogenic diet* or *ketogenic diet with MCT.* The diet will be planned without medium chain triglyceride oil, unless it is re-

Exchange List for Ketogenic Diet

Foods to Avoid

The following foods contain a substantial and a variable amount of carbohydrate and should be *avoided.*

Cake	Molasses
Candy	Pastries
Carbonated beverages	Pies
Catsup	Pudding
Chewing gum	Sherbet
Cookies	Sugar
Cough drops or syrups that	Sweet rolls
contain sugar	Sweetened condensed milk
Honey	Syrup
Ice cream, commercial	All breads, bread products, and
Jam	cereals, unless they are
Jelly	calculated into the meal plan
Marmalade	

Foods to Use as Desired

The following foods contain negligible amounts of protein, fat, and carbohydrate and may be used as desired without calculation into the meal plan.

Bouillon, broth, or consomme	Herbs
Chives	Horseradish, without sugar
Cocoa powder, unsweetened (limit	Mustard, dry
to 1 teaspoon each day)	Parsley
Coffee	Pepper
Decaffeinated coffee	Salt
Flavoring extracts	Tea
Gelatin, unsweetened, unflavored	Vinegar

quested. The dietitian will determine content and kilocalorie level according to principles outlined herein.

Use of Products Prepared with Artificial Sweeteners

Products made with non-nutritive artificial sweeteners contain minimal (less than 0.5 g per serving) or no carbohydrate. Products made with nutritive artificial sweeteners may contain from 0.5 g of carbohydrate to 12 g of carbohydrate per serving.

The ketogenic diet should not include more than 1 g carbohydrate (4 kilocalories) from artificially sweetened products. A choice of *one* product in the *amount* given is allowed each day. (Table 8–51)

TABLE 8–51   Caloric Content of Artificially Sweetened Products

Artificially Sweetened Products	Amount	Kilocalories per Serving
Carbonated beverage	6 oz	1
Lemonade prepared from dry mix	6 oz	3
Gelatin dessert prepared from mix	1/4 cup	4
Granulated tabletop artificial sweetener	2 tsp	4

Food Exchange List for Ketogenic Diet Without MCT Oil

This exchange list differs from the other exchange lists in the manual. Only this exchange list should be used in planning menus for a ketogenic diet. Accuracy in portion sizes is important; foods should be weighed. Table 8–52 summarizes the composition of each of the food exchange lists.

TABLE 8–52

Food Exchange List	Weight g	Kilocal-ories	Protein g	Fat g	Carbohydrate g
Meat	30	73	7	5	—
Fat	5	36	—	4	—
Whipping cream	60	187	2	19	2
Starch	varies	68	2	—	15
Bread products	2	7	—	—	1.6
Fruit	varies	24	—	—	6
Vegetable					
Group 1	100	16	1	—	3
Group 2	50	16	1	—	3

Meat Exchange

One meat exchange is equivalent to the weight listed and contains 7 g of protein, 5 g of fat, and 73 kilocalories.

Medium fat meat

Bacon (omit 2 fat exchanges)	30 g
Beef, lamb, pork, veal	30 g
Liver (add 1 fat exchange and omit 50 g of group 1 vegetable)	30 g
Pork sausage (omit 2 fat exchanges)	40 g
Dried beef (add 1 fat exchange)	20 g
Cold cuts: bologna, luncheon meat, minced ham, liverwurst (all meat, no cereal)	45 g
Salami (omit 1 fat exchange)	30 g
Frankfurters or wieners (all meat, no cereal) (omit 1 fat exchange)	50 g

Fowl

Chicken, duck, goose, turkey	30 g

Egg	one

Fish

Salmon or tuna, canned	30 g
Sardines	35 g
Clams (add 1 fat exchange and omit 100 g of group 1 vegetable)	50 g
Lobster (add 1 fat exchange)	40 g
Oysters (add 1 fat exchange and omit 100 g of group 1 vegetable)	70 g
Scallops (add 1 fat exchange)	50 g
Shrimp (add 1 fat exchange)	30 g

Cheese

American, brick, cheddar, Roquefort, Swiss, or processed cheese (omit 1 fat exchange)	30 g
Cottage cheese, creamed (add 1 fat exchange and omit 50 g of group 1 vegetable)	50 g

Fat Exchange

One fat exchange is equivalent to the weight listed and contains 4 g of fat and 36 kilocalories.

Almonds, slivered	5 g
Avocado (omit 50 g of group 1 vegetable)	30 g
Bacon	5 g
Butter or margarine	5 g
Cooking fats	5 g
Mayonnaise	5 g
Olives, green or ripe	30 g
Pecans, shelled	5 g
Salad oils	5 g
Walnuts, shelled	5 g

Whipping Cream Exchange
One whipping cream exchange is 60 g and contains 2 g of protein, 19 g of fat, 2 g of carbohydrate, and 187 kilocalories. Whipping cream that is at least 32 percent fat should be used. One whipping cream exchange (60 g) may be exchanged for 65 g of group 1 vegetable and 5 fat exchanges.

Whipping cream (32 percent fat)	60 g

Starch Exchange
One starch exchange is equivalent to the weight listed and contains 2 g of protein, 15 g of carbohydrate, and 68 kilocalories.

Bread	25 g
Melba toast	20 g
Saltines	20 g
White potato	100 g

Bread Products
One bread product contains 1.6 g of carbohydrate and 7 kilocalories.

Low calorie rice wafer	2 g

Fruit Exchange
One fruit exchange is equivalent to the weight listed and contains 6 g of carbohydrate and 24 kilocalories.

Apple			Cherries	
Fresh	40 g		Canned	60 g
Juice	60 g		Fresh	40 g
Sauce	60 g			
			Dates	
Apricots			Pitted	8 g
Canned	60 g			
Dried	10 g		Figs	
Fresh	60 g		Canned	60 g
Nectar	40 g		Dried	8 g
			Fresh	30 g
Banana				
Whole	30 g		Fruit cocktail	
			Canned	60 g
Berries, fresh				
Blackberries	50 g		Grapefruit	
Blueberries	40 g		Fresh	60 g
Boysenberries	60 g		Juice	60 g
Cranberries	50 g		Nectar	40 g
Gooseberries	60 g		Sections, canned	75 g
Loganberries	50 g			
Raspberries	50 g		Grapes	
Strawberries	75 g		Canned	40 g
			Fresh	40 g

Juice		Dried	10 g
Bottled	30 g	Fresh	60 g
Frozen	40 g	Pear	
Lemon juice	75 g	Canned	60 g
Lime juice	65 g	Dried	10 g
Mandarin orange		Fresh	40 g
Canned	100 g	Pineapple	
Mango		Canned	60 g
Fresh	35 g	Fresh	40 g
Melon		Juice	40 g
Cantaloupe	100 g	Plums	
Honeydew	100 g	Canned	60 g
Watermelon	100 g	Fresh	40 g
Nectarine		Prunes	
Fresh	40 g	Juice	30 g
Orange		Whole	8 g
Fresh, whole	50 g	Raisins	8 g
Juice	60 g	Rhubarb	
Sections, fresh or canned	50 g	Raw	160 g
Papaya		Tangerine	
Fresh	60 g	Fresh, whole	50 g
Peach		Juice	60 g
Canned	60 g	Sections	50 g

Vegetable Exchange

One serving of group 1 vegetable or group 2 vegetable contains 1 g of protein, 3 g of carbohydrate, and 16 kilocalories.

Group 1 Vegetable, 100 g

Asparagus	Chinese cabbage	Peppers, green or red
Bean sprouts	Collards	Radishes
Beans, green or wax	Cucumber	Sauerkraut
Beet greens	Dill pickle	Spinach
Broccoli	Eggplant	Summer squash
Cabbage	Endive	Tomato juice
Cauliflower	Garden cress	Tomatoes
Celery	Lettuce	Turnip greens
Chard, Swiss	Mushrooms	Turnips
	Mustard greens	Watercress

Group 2 Vegetable, 50 g

Artichokes	Dandelion greens	Okra
Beets	Kale	Onions
Brussels sprouts	Kohlrabi	Pumpkin
Carrots	Leeks	Rutabaga
		Winter squash

Food Exchange List for the Ketogenic Diet With MCT Oil

These additional food exchange lists are needed when planning the diet with MCT oil. Use these lists in addition to the previous ketogenic exchange lists.

Skim Milk Exchanges

One milk exchange is equivalent to 120 g of milk and contains 4 g protein, 6 g carbohydrate, and 40 kilocalories.

Buttermilk, fat free	120 g
Skim milk, fat free	120 g

MCT Oil (Medium Chain Triglycerides) Exchange

MCT oil contains 8.3 kilocalories per gram (ml). The MCT oil can be combined with the allowance of skim milk. The two ingredients can be mixed in a blender. Chipped ice, non-caloric carbonated beverages, fruit allowance, or tomato juice from Vegetable A allowance may be added for flavor. The beverage with MCT oil should be sipped slowly.

Starch Exchange

One starch exchange is equivalent to the weight listed and contains 2 g of protein, 1 g of fat, 15 g of carbohydrate, and 77 kilocalories.

Breads

Bread	25 g
Cornbread	35 g
Roll	25 g
Bun, hamburger, or frankfurter	30 g
Pancake	45 g

Cereals

Cooked	140 g
Dry, flake	20 g
Dry, puffed	20 g
Shredded wheat	20 g

Crackers

Graham	20 g
Melba toast	20 g
Oyster	20 g
Ritz, plain or cheese	20 g
Ry-krisp	30 g
Saltines	20 g
Soda	20 g

Desserts

Commercial-flavored gelatin	100 g
Sherbet	50 g
Sponge or angel food cake	25 g
Vanilla wafers	15 g

Flour products

Macaroni, cooked	50 g
Noodles, cooked	50 g
Rice, cooked	50 g
Spaghetti, cooked	50 g

Starchy Vegetables

Beans

Baked (no pork), cooked	90 g
Kidney, cooked	90 g
Lima, cooked	90 g
Navy, cooked	90 g
Pinto, cooked	90 g
White marrow, cooked	90 g

Corn

Canned or frozen	80 g
Fresh on cob	50 g

Hominy	100 g
Parsnips	100 g

Peas

Canned, fresh or frozen	100 g
Dry, split, cooked	90 g

Popcorn (without butter)	15 g

Potatoes

White, baked or boiled	100 g
White, mashed	100 g
Sweet or yams	50 g

REFERENCES

1. Huttenlocher PR. Ketonemia and seizures: metabolic and anticonvulsant effects of two ketogenic diets in childhood epilepsy. Pediatr Res 1976;10:536–540.

2. Dodson WE, Prensky AL, DeVivo DC, Goldring S, Dodge PR. Management of seizure disorders: selected aspects. J Pediatr 1976;89:695–703.

3. Signore JM. Ketogenic diet containing medium-chain triglycerides. J Am Diet Assoc 1973;62:285–290.

4. Keith HM. Convulsive disorders in children with reference to treatment with ketogenic diet. Boston: Little, Brown & Company, 1963.

5. Clark BJ, House FM. Medium-chain triglyceride oil ketogenic diets in the treatment of childhood epilepsy. J Hum Nutr 1978;32:111–116.

RENAL DISEASE

Chronic Renal Failure

General Description

The diet for the child with chronic renal failure is controlled in protein, sodium, potassium, and phosphorus. The primary goals of treatment include (1) adequate kilocalories for growth, (2) protein control to minimize uremic symptoms resulting from an accumulation of nitrogenous waste products, yet to provide adequate protein to promote growth, (3) addition or restriction of sodium to control blood pressure and to regulate fluid balance with regard to edema or dehydration, and (4) moderation of dietary phosphorus intake in order to minimize secondary hyperparathyroidism.

Nutritional Inadequacy

Potential deficiencies of pyridoxine, folic acid, and trace minerals exist with the renal failure diet. A pediatric multiple vitamin and folic acid are recommended for diets providing less than 2/3 of the Recommended Dietary Allowances (RDA) for age (see page 39). The diet is low in calcium because of restricted protein and phosphorus. Calcium supplements may be necessary.

Indications and Rationale

Poor growth typically occurs in children with renal failure. The etiology for growth retardation is multifactorial and includes inadequate energy intake, secondary hyperparathyroidism, abnormal vitamin D metabolism, acidosis, and metabolic imbalances of electrolytes, enzymes, and hormones.[1] The use of National Center for Health Statistics charts for assessment of growth prior to and during nutritional therapy is essential (see *Pediatric Appendices 4* and *5*, pages 480 and 488.).[2]

Weight to height ratio is frequently a more accurate measure of nutritional state than either weight or height alone. Care must be taken to correct for altered body water content.[3] Height-age should be used as a basis to estimate and to evaluate caloric and nutritional needs.[4] An adequate caloric intake is essential to maximize growth, to reduce alterations in body composition, and to promote a sense of well-being.[1] Patients and parents must be reminded that it is essential to maintain an adequate caloric intake. Nasogastric feedings may be necessary if appetite or growth do not improve.

Dietary Management

The rationale and indications for dietary management of renal failure are similar for children and adults (see *Renal Disease,* page 212).

Energy.   Growth retardation occurs when the caloric intake of children with chronic renal failure falls below 70 to 80 percent of the recommended allowance for height-age.[5] Caloric recommendations should be equal to Recommended Dietary Allowances for the child's height-age as shown in Table 8–53. The greater the amount of energy over and above maintenance requirements, the more energy there is available for growth. The average caloric cost for growth is about 5 kilocalories per gram of weight gain.[5] When protein is restricted, kilocalories must be provided from other sources. Fats, carbohydrates, low protein products, and carbohydrate supplements provide non-protein caloric sources for the uremic child.

Protein.   Protein restriction is used to decrease the accumulation of nitrogenous products and to minimize, and even decrease, uremic symptoms. Severe protein restriction is usually not recommended because of concerns regarding growth. In addition, severe restriction of protein limits the kinds of foods allowed and results in decreased caloric intake, which can lead to body tissue catabolism. The protein requirement for children with chronic renal failure has not been established.[7] Generally, the protein intake should not be reduced below 1 g per kilogram of body weight per day. Current recommendations are summarized in Table 8–53. The majority of the protein in the diet should be of high biologic value, with a goal of approximately 70 percent.[4,8] At the present time, preparations of essential amino acids or keto-acid mixtures are not recommended.

TABLE 8–53   Guidelines for Dietary Management of Infants, Children, and Adolescents in Chronic Renal Failure (Recommendations based on height-age*)

Component	Comments	
Kilocalories	Infants	105 to 115 kilocalories per kg
	1–3 years	100 kilocalories per kg
	4–10 years	85 kilocalories per kg
	11–14 years, male	60 kilocalories per kg
	11–14 years, female	48 kilocalories per kg
	15–18 years, male	42 kilocalories per kg
	15–18 years, female	38 kilocalories per kg
Protein[6]	Birth to 1 year	2 to 3 g per kg of actual body weight
	1 to 2 years	2 g per kg of actual body weight
	2 years to adolescence	1 g per kg of actual body weight
	Adolescent	1 g per kg of actual body weight
Sodium	Infants: 1 to 3 mEq per kg per day	
	Children and adolescents: No extra salt	
	(Actual intake varies with caloric intake)	
Fluid	Not restricted unless severe edema present. Increased fluid may be necessary for children with a renal concentrating defect.	
Potassium	Infants: 1 to 3 mEq per kg per day. 40 to 60 mEq potassium if serum level is elevated.	
	Potassium binder may be necessary	
Calcium and phosphorus	Calcium supplements generally prescribed to meet RDA. Restrict high phosphorus foods or use phosphate binders if serum phosphorus elevated.	
Vitamins and minerals	Pediatric one-a-day type multivitamin recommended daily.	
	50 µg folic acid is recommended for infants receiving a liquid multivitamin.	

* Height-age: Age for which child's height is equal to the 50th percentile of National Center for Health Statistics growth chart (see *Pediatric Appendices 4* and *5,* pages 480 and 488).

Sodium. Sodium control in children is individualized according to the etiology of renal failure. In children with renal dysplasia or with obstructive uropathy, there may be excessive sodium losses in the urine, and the child may crave salt. Chronic sodium depletion may also adversely affect growth.

Salt depletion may occur with vomiting and the resulting dehydration. In such circumstances, a more generous allowance of sodium, rather than a restriction, may be needed. Measurements of 24-hour urinary sodium excretion can aid in deciding how much sodium should be provided.

If hypertension and/or edema are present, a "no extra salt" restriction is recommended. The actual amount of sodium in the diet varies with the caloric intake of the child. A more limited sodium intake may be necessary if the edema or hypertension is severe. For infants, a sodium intake of 1 to 3 mEq per kilogram per day is usually recommended.

Fluid. During the predialysis period, fluid restriction is imposed only if edema is severe or if dilutional hyponatremia is a major clinical problem. Children with renal concentration defects, such as with nephrogenic diabetes insipidus, may require large daily oral fluid volumes. In order to monitor fluid balance, weighing the child daily is encouraged.

Potassium. Children and adolescents who are approaching end-stage renal disease may have hyperkalemia. Generally, as the dietary protein decreases, the potassium content of the diet decreases. Recommendations for potassium control can range from the avoidance of foods containing high amounts of potassium to the specification of a range of 40 to 60 mEq of potassium per day. An ion exchange resin may be prescribed if a more rigid potassium restriction is necessary.

Calcium and Phosphorus. Calcium and phosphorus balance must be maintained prior to the need for dialysis and/or transplantation. Secondary hyperparathyroidism is frequent in children with chronic renal failure and may cause serious bone disease (see *Chronic Renal Failure,* page 216). Generally, the phosphorus content of the diet is low because of the protein restriction, but milk and milk products may also need to be strictly controlled in order to avoid excessive phosphorus intake. The need for further restriction of high phosphorus foods is determined by careful monitoring of laboratory tests. Phosphate binders, such as calcium carbonate, aluminum carbonate, or aluminum hydroxide, may be necessary to prevent high serum levels of phosphorus. Calcium carbonate is preferred[9] since infants and young children may be at particular risk of aluminum accumulation. In addition, the calcium carbonate improves calcium intake. Calcium intake is frequently inadequate and should be supplemented if the total intake from diet and medications is less than 2/3 of the Recommended Dietary Allowance.

Vitamins and Minerals. A one-a-day type of pediatric multivitamin is recommended for children whose current intake and diet limit the variety of food choices with subsequent nutritional inadequacy. Infants who receive a liquid multivitamin should also be supplemented with 50 μg of folic acid daily. Iron supplementation is given when indicated.

Table 8–53 summarizes the guidelines for dietary management of renal failure in infants, children, and adolescents. For infants, the use of whole cow's milk is not recommended owing to its high renal solute load. Generally, breast milk or a formula that is low in sodium and low in phosphorus (such as Similac PM 60/40 or SMA) is recommended until at least 1 year of age. Solid foods should be introduced as for a normal infant. The caloric density of the formula may need to be increased by the addition of Polycose and of fat in order to achieve adequate caloric intake. For children and adolescents, the diet is planned using the dietary exchanges for renal diets on page 235.

Physicians: How to Order Diet

The diet order should indicate specific *levels of protein, sodium, fluid, potassium, calcium, and phosphorus.*

REFERENCES

1. Wassner SJ. The role of nutrition in the care of children with renal insufficiency—symposium on pediatric nephrology. Pediatr Clin North Am 1982;29:973–990.
2. National Center of Health Statistics: NCHS growth curves for children 0–18 years, United States Vital and Health Statistics, Series 11, No. 165, Washington, D.C., Health Resources Administration, U.S. Government Printing Office, 1977.
3. Sharer K, Guilio G. Growth in children with chronic renal insufficiency. In: Fine RN, Gruskin AB, eds. End stage renal disease in children. Philadelphia: WB Saunders, 1984:271.
4. Nelson P, Stover J. Principles of nutritional assessment and management of the child with ESRD. In: Fine RN, Gruskin AB, eds. End stage renal disease in children. Philadelphia: WB Saunders, 1984:209.
5. Chantler C. Nutritional assessment and management of children with renal insufficiency. In: Fine RN, Gruskin AB, eds. End stage renal disease in children. Philadelphia: WB Saunders, 1984:193.
6. Milliner DS, Pediatric Nephrologist, Mayo Clinic. Personal communication.
7. Chantler C, El Bishti M, Counaham R. Nutritional therapy in children with chronic renal failure. Am J Clin Nutr 1984;33:1682–1689.
8. Spinozzi NS, Grupe WE. Nutritional implications of renal disease. J Am Diet Assoc 1977;70:493–497.
9. Committee on Nutrition. Aluminum toxicity in infants and children. Pediatrics 1986;78:1150–1154.

Hemodialysis

General Description

The diet for the child who is receiving hemodialysis is controlled in protein, sodium, potassium, and fluid in order to minimize interdialytic abnormalities and weight changes. The diet should provide adequate kilocalories, protein, and other nutrients for growth and to replace losses in the dialysate.

Nutritional Inadequacy

The pediatric dialysis patient is at risk for deficiencies of water-soluble vitamins, particularly pyridoxine, ascorbic acid, and folic acid.[1] A daily pediatric multivitamin and folic acid should be given. A multivitamin containing fat-soluble vitamins may be necessary for the young child. Routine iron supplementation is not necessary, except when serum ferritin levels are low.[1]

The potential also exists for amino acid deficiencies, since they are lost in the dialysate. Adequate protein intake is essential, but may be difficult to obtain owing to taste alterations and to nausea and vomiting from the dialysis procedure itself.

Water-soluble vitamins lost in the dialysate need to be replaced. A multivitamin containing ascorbic acid, pyridoxine, and folic acid and fortified with calcium and iron should be taken daily.

Indications and Rationale

Flexibility in planning the nutritional management of children and adolescents on dialysis is a key component. The diet must be tailored to the individual's needs and must include nutritional requirements for growth as discussed on page 437 of *Chronic Renal Failure*. Many of the nutritional principles employed for the adult on hemodialysis also apply to children and to adolescents. (See *Hemodialysis,* page 220.)

Dietary Management

The goals for the nutritional management of the child or the adolescent on hemodialysis include (1) an adequate caloric intake to promote growth, (2) an adequate protein intake to prevent negative nitrogen balance by replacing amino acids lost in the dialysate and to promote growth, (3) the control of sodium intake to regulate blood pressure and fluid balance and to decrease thirst, (4) the control of potassium intake to prevent cardiac dysrhythmias, and (5) control of fluid intake to prevent water accumulation manifested by hyponatremia and by interdialytic weight gains. Water-soluble vitamins lost in the dialysate, especially ascorbic acid, pyridoxine, and folic acid, need to be replaced. A one-a-day type of pediatric multivitamin and 1 mg folic acid should be taken daily. Calcium and iron may also need to be supplemented.

Energy. Adequate intake of kilocalories continues to be essential once dialysis is initiated. Non-protein kilocalories from fat and from carbohydrate are the primary sources of energy that spare protein as an energy source, that prevent an accumulation of urea, and that provide the energy required for growth. A balanced diet and an adequate intake can usually be achieved without supplements, since the diet is liberalized in protein compared to predialysis. Currently, nutritional supplements to increase kilocalories are not encouraged. Rather, the goal is to aim for adherence and compliance to a diet that uses carbohydrate-containing foods, such as hard candy, sugar, jelly, syrups, and popsicles.[1] The child or the adolescent is also encouraged to drink liquids that contain kilocalories, such as fruit drinks and carbonated beverages. In practice, special caloric supplements are not well-tolerated, but are used if necessary to assure adequate caloric intake.

Protein. The recommended intake of protein for the infant and the young child receiving dialysis is the same as it is predialysis. However, for children ages 2 years through adolescence, consumption of 1.5 g of protein per kilogram per day is recommended.[2] Approximately 70 percent of the total protein should be from high biologic value protein sources.

Urea kinetic modeling (see section on kinetic modeling, in *Hemodialysis,* page 220) aids in individualizing the dialysis treatment and the patient's diet.[3] Urea kinetic modeling can serve as an early indicator for nutritional intervention and is also useful in determining whether or not to modify the patient's protein intake. Four-day food records are kept, in conjunction with the kinetic modeling program.

Sodium. Sodium control for the child and the adolescent on hemodialysis is similar to predialysis. (See *Chronic Renal Failure,* page 436). Sodium restriction lessens thirst, prevents fluid accumulation manifested by excess inter-dialytic weight gain, and aids in regulating blood pressure. Careful monitoring of urinary sodium output is essential in the child who has significant urinary losses.[4]

If the appetite is poor, liberalization of dietary sodium may be necessary in order to increase food intake and to improve adherence to diet. For certain patients, foods with greater amounts of sodium may be allowed during the 8 to 10 hours before dialysis to encourage greater caloric and protein consumption. However, a high sodium intake just prior to dialysis causes excess fluid weight gain and elevated blood pressure. Thus, this practice is discouraged for the majority of patients.

Potassium. Potassium intake is determined by the frequency of dialysis, the concentration of potassium in the dialysate, and the urinary potassium losses. The size of the child also determines intake. In our experience, for the small child weighing less than 20 kg, a restriction of 40 to 60 mEq of potassium per day has maintained serum potassium levels within acceptable ranges. For the child and the adolescent weighing more than 20 kg, 60 to 70 mEq of potassium per day is typically provided.

Kayexalate, an ion-exchange resin, may improve overall dietary intake by permitting the incorporation of certain high potassium foods in limited quantities.[4] Kayexalate can be taken as a candy, baked into cookies, or mixed with sweetened beverages.

Calcium and Phosphorous. Dietary management of calcium and of phosphorous for infants, children, and adolescents on dialysis is the same as predialysis (see *Chronic Renal Failure,* page 436). Phosphorous intake and the use of phosphate binders should be distributed throughout the day.[4]

Fluid. The fluid allowance is based on insensible losses plus urine output. Insensible losses in children are approximately 30 to 35 ml per 100 kilocalories of intake each day. Interdialytic weight gain of not more than 5 percent of estimated dry weight is acceptable and can be used to adjust the fluid allowance.[4] Those foods that are liquid at room temperature are included in the fluid allowance.

Vitamins. Children receiving hemodialysis require vitamin supplementation owing to dietary restrictions that may prevent adequate intake of all vitamins, to poor appetite, to iatrogenic dysgeusia, which may limit or eliminate certain groups of foods from the diet, and to loss of water-soluble vitamins in the dialysate. Supplements of 1.2 to 2 mg pyridoxine, 50 to 100 mg ascorbic acid, and 1 mg of folacin are recommended daily, plus supplements of other B-complex vitamins.[4] A pediatric one-a-day multivitamin plus 1 mg of folacin is recommended daily for all infants and children under 11 years of age. Adolescents should be given the same multivitamin as adults. (See *Chronic Renal Failure* and *Hemodialysis,* pages 216 and 220).

Cholesterol and Triglycerides. Currently, serum lipids are monitored, but dietary treatment of hypercholesterolemia and of hypertriglyceridemia is a lower priority, since fats and simple carbohydrates are essential in the diet as caloric sources. Therefore, severe restriction is not possible. Polyunsaturated fats should be encouraged, but a high total fat intake is unavoidable in the diet.

Again, it is important to keep in mind that an adequate caloric intake by the child and the adolescent on hemodialysis is the priority.

Table 8–54 summarizes the guidelines for dietary management for infants, children, and adolescents receiving hemodialysis. The diet is planned using the dietary exchanges for renal diets on page 235. The *Calcium and Phosphorus Content of Foods, Appendix 12,* may also be helpful.

TABLE 8–54 Guidelines for Dietary Management of Infants, Children, and Adolescents on Hemodialysis
(Recommendations based on height-age* and dry weight†)

Component	Comments	
Kilocalories	Infants	105–115 kilocalories per kg
	1–3 years	100 kilocalories per kg
	4–10 years	85 kilocalories per kg
	11–14 years, male	60 kilocalories per kg
	11–14 years, female	48 kilocalories per kg
	15–18 years, male	42 kilocalories per kg
	15–18 years, female	38 kilocalories per kg
	No less than 70 to 80 percent of RDA for height-age	
Protein	Birth to 1 year	2 to 6 g per kg of dry body weight
	1 to 2 years	2 g per kg of dry body weight
	2 years through adolescence	1.5 g per kg of dry body weight
	70 percent of total protein should be of high biologic value Amount of protein may be individually adjusted with results of urea kinetic modeling	
Sodium	Infants: 1 to 3 mEq per kg per day Children and adolescents: No extra salt (actual intake varies with caloric intake)	
	Monitor urinary sodium in salt-wasting syndrome. May need to restrict or to add sodium in diet, depending on interdialytic weight gain	
Potassium	Infants: 1 to 3 mEq per kg per day Children: Less than 20 kg of body weight, 40 to 60 mEq potassium per day Greater than 20 kg of body weight, 60 to 70 mEq potassium per day	
	Check concentration of potassium in dialysate	
Calcium and phosphorus	Calcium supplements generally prescribed to meet RDA. Restrict high phosphorus foods and/or implement use of phosphorus binders if serum phosphorus elevated	
Fluid	Insensible loss (30 to 35 ml per 100 kilocalories per day) plus urine output	
Vitamins and minerals	Infant or pediatric one-a-day type multivitamin plus 1 mg folic acid for patients up to 11 years of age Adolescents: Adult multivitamin supplement that contains 1 mg folic acid and calcium	

* Height-age: Age for which child's height is equal to the 50th percentile of NCHS growth graph (see *Pediatric Appendix 4*, page 480).
† Dry Weight: The weight immediately following dialysis.

Physicians: How to Order Diet

The diet order should indicate the *specific levels of protein, sodium, potassium, calcium, phosphorous, and fluid*. The dietitian will establish the caloric level.

REFERENCES

1. Berger M. Dietary management of children with uremia. J Am Diet Assoc 1977;70:498–505.
2. Milliner DS, Pediatric Nephrologist, Mayo Clinic. Personal communication.
3. Harmon WE, Spinozzi N, Meyer A, Grupe WE. Use of protein catabolic rate to monitor pediatric hemodialysis. Proc Eur Dial Transplant Assoc 1981;10:324–330.
4. Nelson P, Stover J. Principles of nutritional assessment and management of the child with ESRD. In: Fine RN, Gruskin AB, eds. End-stage renal disease in children. Philadelphia: WB Saunders, 1984:221.

Continuous Ambulatory Peritoneal Dialysis

General Description

The diet emphasizes an adequate protein intake to offset loss of protein in the dialysate, an adequate caloric intake to promote growth, a mild sodium restriction, and a moderate potassium restriction.

Nutritional Inadequacy

As with hemodialysis, the patient undergoing continuous ambulatory peritoneal dialysis (CAPD) is at risk for deficiencies of amino acids, water-soluble vitamins, and minerals. The extent of losses are unknown, and recommendations for levels of vitamins and minerals for children have not been established. Therefore, a pediatric one-a-day type multiple vitamin and 1 mg of folic acid are recommended. Iron is not routinely supplemented, unless serum ferritin levels are low.[1] Calcium may need to be supplemented if intake is less than 2/3 of Recommended Dietary Allowance (RDA).

Indications and Rationale

Continuous ambulatory peritoneal dialysis (CAPD) is the preferred treatment of renal failure in pediatric patients since it allows greater flexibility in planning daily routines of school and of extracurricular activities. CAPD offers liberalization of dietary restrictions and a continuous source of kilocalories from carbohydrate to promote growth.

Dietary Management

The nutritional goals of CAPD are (1) an adequate caloric intake for growth, (2) an adequate protein intake to prevent negative nitrogen balance by replacing amino acids lost in the dialysate and to promote growth, (3) an appropriate intake of sodium to control blood pressure and to prevent excess weight gain, (4) a mild to moderate potassium restriction, (5) the use of complex carbohydrates, rather than simple carbohydrates, to minimize hypertriglyceridemia, (6) the use of polyunsaturated fats to minimize hypercholesterolemia, and (7) an adequate intake of water-soluble vitamins to replace dialysate losses. Fluid restriction is generally not necessary.

Energy. Caloric requirements are based upon the RDA for patients' height-age, although actual requirements may be higher.[1] Early satiety and inadequate energy intake are common problems. Small, frequent meals are recommended to overcome a sense of fullness. Unlike the adult patient on CAPD, obesity has not been seen in the pediatric patient.[1] In some cases, fat and carbohydrate supplements may be necessary to increase total caloric intake.[2]

Theoretically, the total dietary kilocalories required can be determined by subtracting the kilocalories contributed by the dialysate from the total caloric requirements based on height-age (see *Continuous Ambulatory Peritoneal Dialysis,* page 224). However, it is not known what percent of the dialysate is absorbable, nor what effect the smaller volume of infused dialysate has on the number of kilocalories actually contributed by the dialysate in children.

Protein. Currently, protein requirements of children or of adolescents on peritonal dialysis have not been determined. However, protein intake should be higher than predialysis. Such losses can average 0.3 g per kilogram per day in infants and in young children up to 6 years of age.[1] It is suggested that 3 to 4 g of protein per kilogram per day for infants and for children up to age 5 years is required for growth and to replace amino acids lost in the dialysate. However, protein intake should be individualized. Dialysate losses of protein can average 4 to 8 g per day for older children more than 5 years of age. Current recommendations for protein are adapted from adult recommendations and are summarized in Table 8–55.

Seventy percent of the dietary protein must be from high biologic value (HBV) sources, such as meat, egg, fowl, and fish.

Sodium. Generally, sodium intake can be liberalized with peritoneal dialysis, but a "no extra salt diet" is usually recommended for children and for adolescents. The actual sodium level of the diet varies with the caloric level of the diet. The maximum is 90 to 150 mEq each day. Sodium supplementation is generally necessary for infants on CAPD. Other factors to be considered are the size of the child, the type of kidney disease, and the residual kidney function.[1] Dietary compliance is frequently facilitated if a more liberal sodium intake is allowed. Sodium may need to be restricted more severely in cases of severe hypertension or edema. Sodium intake is liberalized in the child or the adolescent who has a salt-wasting syndrome.

Potassium. Potassium restriction is individualized, depending on serum levels. In our experience, however, children and adolescents do need to restrict potassium, and hyperkalemia can occur. Usually, a mild potassium restriction of 60 to 80 mEq per day is recommended.

Calcium and Phosphorus. Dietary management of calcium and of phosphorus is similar to that for adults on CAPD. Generally, milk or milk products are limited to 1 cup per day. This amount of dairy products may be increased if appetite is poor and if the child or the adolescent is unable to increase protein intake from other food sources.

Calcium supplements generally are necessary, as well as phosphate binders, to maintain calcium and phosphorus balance (see *Continuous Ambulatory Peritoneal Dialysis,* page 224 for additional information).

Vitamins and Minerals. Vitamin and mineral needs of the pediatric population on CAPD have not been established.[1] Generally, guidelines used for adults on CAPD are followed. The loss of water-soluble vitamins in the dialysate may result in deficiencies. Currently, a pediatric one-a-day type multiple vitamin and 1 mg of folic acid are recommended daily.

Fluid. A fluid restriction is not necessary, unless edema is considered a clinical problem.

Cholesterol and Triglycerides. An elevation in serum lipids occurs in children receiving CAPD, as it occurs in adults. The emphasis in the diet is to decrease simple dietary carbohydrates and to increase food sources of complex car-

TABLE 8–55 Guidelines for Dietary Management of Infants, Children, and Adolescents Receiving Continuous Ambulatory Peritoneal Dialysis (Recommendations based on height-age* and dry weight†)

Component	Comments	
Kilocalories	Infants	105–115 kilocalories per kg
	1–3 years	100 kilocalories per kg
	4–10 years	85 kilocalories per kg
	11–14 male	60 kilocalories per kg
	11–14 female	48 kilocalories per kg
	15–18 years, male	42 kilocalories per kg
	15–18 years, female	38 kilocalories per kg
	Dietary kilocalories = total caloric requirement (above) minus kilocalories from dialysate	
Protein	Infants	3–4 g per kg
	1 to 5 years	3 g per kg
	5 to 10 years	2.5 g per kg
	10 to 12 years	2 g per kg
	>12 years	1.5 g per kg
	70 percent of protein should be high biologic value	
Sodium	Infants: May require sodium supplementation	
	Children and adolescents: No extra salt (actual intake varies with caloric intake)	
Potassium	Use high potassium foods in moderation	
	If serum potassium elevated, restrict potassium to 60 to 80 mEq per day	
Calcium and phosphorus	Calcium supplements generally prescribed to meet RDA	
	Avoid very high phosphorus foods, except meat; limit milk and milk products to $\frac{1}{2}$ to 1 cup per day	
Vitamins and minerals	Infant or pediatric one-a-day type multivitamin plus 1 mg folic acid for patients up to 11 years of age	
	Adolescents: adult multivitamin supplement that contains 1 mg folic acid and calcium to equal the RDA	
Fluid	Generally not restricted	
Simple carbohydrates	Restrict intake if hypertriglyceridemia exists	
Saturated fat	Use polyunsaturated fats rather than saturated fats if hypercholesterolemia exists	
Cholesterol	If hypercholesterolemia exists, restrict only if able to consume adequate protein from low cholesterol sources	

*Height-age: Age for which child's height is equal to the 50th percentile of National Center for Health Statistics (see *Pediatric Appendices 4* and *5*, pages 480 and 488).
†Dry weight: The weight immediately following dialysis.

bohydrates. Use of more polyunsaturated fats, rather than saturated fats, is also recommended.

Table 8–55 summarizes the guidelines for dietary management for infants, children, and adolescents receiving CAPD. The diet is planned using the renal diet exchange lists on page 235. The table *Calcium and Phosphorus Content of Foods (Appendix 12)* may also be helpful.

Physicians: How to Order Diet

The diet order should indicate *diet for CAPD*. The number of dialysis exchanges and the concentrations of the dialysate should also be specified. The dietitian will follow the preceding guidelines for modification of kilocalories and of other dietary constituents.

REFERENCES

1. Nelson P, Stover J. Principles of nutritional management of the child with ESRD. In: Fine RN, Gruskin AB. End-stage renal disease in children. Philadelphia: WB Saunders, 1984:209.
2. Salvsky IB, Lucullo L, Nelson P, Fine RN. Continuous ambulatory peritoneal dialysis in children. Pediatr Clin North Am 1982;29:1005–1012.

WEIGHT CONTROL

General Description

A weight control program for children and for adolescents provides sufficient energy to allow for weight stabilization or for gradual weight reduction and adequate nutrients so that growth and development are not compromised. The focus is on the modification of present inappropriate eating and activity behaviors to ones more appropriate for weight control.

Nutritional Inadequacy

This diet can be designed to meet the Recommended Dietary Allowances (RDA) for nutrients, unless the child or the adolescent has food dislikes or aversions that greatly limit the variety of foods that are eaten or unless the diet provides less than 1,200 to 1,400 calories. A multiple vitamin supplement would then be indicated.

Indications and Rationale

From 5 percent to 25 percent of children and of adolescents in the United States are obese. Childhood obesity is associated with decreased growth hormone release, with hyperinsulinemia, with hyperlipidemia, with hypertension, and with carbohydrate intolerance. There is some evidence that obesity in children is an independent risk factor for later coronary heart disease, and that many atherogenic serum lipid disorders originate in childhood. Even without primary medical implications, the psychological and the social consequences of childhood and adolescent obesity are profound.

Obesity that begins during childhood is likely to persist into adulthood. The chances are one to four against the achievement of normal body weight if a child enters adolescence being obese. The chances increase to 28 to 1 against achieving a normal body weight as an adult if a child is still obese at the end of adolescence.[1] Early intervention may help influence the development of eating and activity patterns and of attitudes. Intervention may also result in satisfactory weight control during the critical years when body image is forming.

The problem of dietary control for obesity is more complicated in children and in adolescents than in adults. In children, sufficient kilocalories and protein must be provided to allow for growth and for development of lean body mass while achieving a decrease in depot fat. The extent to which diet is responsible for these changes depends on the age at which the diet is started. The period of adolescence includes a growth spurt, the intensity of which is exceeded only by the fetus and the infant during the first year. Since caloric and most nutritional needs parallel the growth rate, the adolescent's needs are higher in relation to body size than those of younger or of older people. There is considerable difference between the nutritional needs of boys and of girls during this time because growth begins earlier in girls and is less rapid than for boys. There is also considerable individual variation among adolescents with respect to the age of onset, the intensity, and the duration of the growth spurt. The growth period is more closely related to the stage of sexual maturation than to chronologic age. The stage of growth and of maturation needs to be considered when formulating a kilocalorie-controlled diet for adolescents. Therefore, caution must be exercised when kilocalories are controlled in children and in adolescents, and linear growth rates need to be monitored regularly. Energy expenditure from activity can safely enhance the effects of kilocalorie-controlled intake and can serve to encourage the formation of an active life-style.

Weight control measures in the young child are directed toward the education of the family about the child's energy and nutrient needs and about the importance of regular exercise. In older children and in adolescents, the success of weight control measures depends on the motivation of the patient.

Goals of Dietary Management

Rather than loss of body weight per se, the primary goal of weight management in children and in adolescents is to aid the patient in becoming aware of inappropriate eating and activity patterns and to provide support for gradually modifying these behaviors to ones that result in achieving and in maintaining an appropriate body weight. This concept needs to be described to the patient and the parents so that they have reasonable expectations for their efforts.

Dietary Recommendations

Assessment. Management of the obese child or adolescent initially involves an assessment of the current diet, both amount and kind of foods eaten, and an inventory of family dietary patterns. The use of school lunches, fast foods, convenience foods, and restaurant meals should be identified and discussed so that the diet plan can be tailored. Identification of parental interest, patient interest, and potential for support within the family is helpful. Present activity level and activity preferences and availability also need to be assessed.

Children. The degree of obesity needs to be considered when designing a kilocalorie-controlled diet for a child. This determination is most easily made by use of growth charts (*Pediatric Appendices 4* and *5*, pages 480 and 488). A child who is 120 to 139 percent of the predicted weight for height and age would be considered mildly obese. A child who is 140 to 159 percent of the predicted weight for height and age would be considered moderately obese, and a child 160 percent or greater of the predicted weight for height and age would be considered severely obese.[2] For example, if an 8-year-old boy is 127 cm tall and weighs 31 kg, his height is at the 50 percentile and his weight is at the 90 percentile. A weight at the 50 percentile would be 25 kg. Therefore, his present weight is 124 percent of the predicted weight for height and age, and he is considered mildly obese. If this boy were to maintain his present weight for approximately 2 years, his height and weight would be proportional (see *National Center for Health Statistics [NCHS] Growth Graphs, Pediatric Appendix 4,* page 480).

In our experience with mildly overweight children, basal calories that are determined from the *Nomogram for Estimating Caloric Requirements* (see *Appendix 6*) for present weight, height, and age are appropriate for weight control. This caloric level should result in stabilizing the child's weight and in achieving an appropriate weight with growth. In moderately or severely obese children, basal kilocalories, determined from the Nomogram for weight at present height and age using the growth charts, can be used to determine the caloric level of the weight control diet. The moderately and severely obese children have medically significant obesity, and gradual weight reduction is indicated. This caloric allowance results in gradual, yet consistent, weight loss.

A caloric increment for activity (Table 8–56) may have to be added to the basal kilocalories to achieve the desired weight change goals if the child is more than normally active. This need for change in the caloric prescription is most appropriately identified at follow-up visits when caloric intake and weight change can be assessed.

TABLE 8–56 Increase in Caloric Needs for Activity[3]

Activity	Percent Above Basal
Bed rest (eating and reading)	10
Very light (sitting, playing musical instrument, working with hands)	30
Light (playing, standing, walking, volleyball)	40 to 60
Moderate (cycling, fast walking, dancing)	60 to 80
Heavy (vigorous playing or working)	100

Efforts to bring about rapid weight reduction by strenuous diets are rarely justified and are even more rarely successful. Instead, a program of caloric control accompanied by an increase in activity and augmented by growth is encouraged.

Adolescents. During adolescence, the relatively uniform growth of childhood is suddenly altered by an increased velocity of development. This growth period is more closely related to the stage of sexual maturation than to chronologic age. A scale for the stage of sexual maturation has been developed by Tanner[4] and is summarized in Table 8–57.

TABLE 8–57   Tanner Rating Stages of Maturity

Stage	Boys	Girls
I	Prepubertal	Prepubertal
II	First visible signs of sexual maturation	Peak height velocity begins
III	Peak height velocity begins	Peak height velocity continues
IV	Peak height velocity continues; facial, axillary and extremity hair growth; voice changes	Menarche
V	Adulthood	Axillary hair growth; adulthood

In girls, peak height velocity occurs at approximately midpoint between stages III and IV, while peak height velocity for boys occurs just prior to stage IV. Therefore, adolescents in stages, I, II, and III should have kilocalories identified for weight control that result in weight stabilization with sufficient kilocalories to cover the approaching growth spurt. Adolescents in stages IV and V can safely experience gradual weight loss[5] after having gone through the stage of peak demand for kilocalories that is associated with height increase. In general, the weight control diet for adolescents in stages I, II, and III can be determined in a manner similar to that for the mildly obese child. Kilocalories prescribed for adolescents in stages IV and V are determined in a manner similar to that for the moderately or severely obese child.

Again, if the adolescent is more than normally active, additional kilocalories need to be prescribed to cover this activity. This need can best be determined by assessing the activity pattern and the weight response at follow-up sessions.

Activity.   There has been continued debate about whether obesity in children is attributable to excessive ingestion of energy or to too low levels of energy expenditure. Generally, both areas need to be addressed for weight control. An activity program should be defined for the individual with self-improvement as the goal, rather than the absolute duration or the extent of exercise. The individual needs suggestions for ways of being active within the limits of the excess weight. Activities that the individual would enjoy, as well as those that are easily accessible, should be identified.

Role of Family.   The role of the family in the genesis and the treatment of obesity varies and is often difficult to assess. In younger obese children, difficulty in parental control or in the setting of limits for the child may contribute to the problem. Assisting such parents with general techniques of behavior modification may help in modifying the child's eating behavior. The problem of obesity is frequently a source of disagreement and dissention between older obese children and their parents. In such instances, the dietitian and the physician may assume the role of enforcer to relieve intra-family conflict.

Continuing Care.   Follow-up is essential and is done by return visits to the physician and dietitian. Food and activity records are used at various times to help identify areas where the greatest attention should be directed. Discussions centered around the use of school lunches, favorite foods, fast foods, restaurant meals, convenience foods, and party and holiday foods are an important part of these follow-up sessions, with weight change being of secondary importance. Caloric intake and weight change should be assessed at these sessions so that the need for caloric revision can be identified. Height should also be monitored at these follow-up sessions.

Guidelines for Long-Term Weight Control

When the patient has achieved a weight that is acceptable for height and age, dietary guidelines should be formulated with the kilocalorie content adjusted for size, age, and activity. At this time, it is helpful to discuss with the child or the adolescent how their weight will continue to change as growth and development proceeds. The patient needs to understand that this weight change is normal as long as an appropriate height change occurs with it. The importance of an active life-style for successful weight control needs to be reinforced. The support and the guidance that follow-up visits provide is also useful during this time.

Physicians: How to Order Diet

The diet order should indicate diet for *weight control*. The dietitian will determine the caloric level according to the preceding guidelines.

REFERENCES

1. Stunkard A, Burt V. Obesity and body image. II. Age at onset of disturbances in the body image. Am J Psychiatry 1967;123:1443–1447.
2. Children and weight: changing perspectives 1985. Nutr Communications Associates, Berkeley, CA.
3. Mahan LK, Rees JM. Nutrition in adolescence. St. Louis: Times Mirror/Mosley College Publishing, 1984:311.
4. Tanner JM. Growth at adolescence. 2nd ed. Oxford, England: Blackwell Scientific Publications, 1962.
5. Carruth BR, Iszler J. Assessment and conservative management of the overfat adolescent. J Adolesc Health Care 1981;1:289–299.

SPECIALIZED NUTRITIONAL SUPPORT

ENTERAL NUTRITION

Enteral alimentation is the most acceptable and effective nutritional support method for maintaining and for repleting nutrition in the pediatric patient who has a functional gastrointestinal tract. Enteral feedings are accompanied by fewer complications, are relatively easy to administer, and are lower in cost when compared with parenteral nutrition.[1] Nasogastric feedings are manageable for short-term therapy; however, in those patients requiring long-term support, a feeding gastrostomy can offer several advantages.[2] Techniques and formulas used for adults need to be adapted to provide safe and optimal nutritional support in children. Growth and biochemical status must be monitored carefully.

Criteria for Selection of Tube Feeding

Selection of tube feeding for infants, children, and adolescents should be based on a careful assessment of the patient's energy, nutrient, and fluid needs, the gastrointestinal tract function, the site of tube placement, and the medical and nutritional status, including biochemical and anthropometric indices. Feeding concentration and volume should be individualized. Supplementary vitamins and minerals are frequently necessary, since the feeding volume that is needed to meet energy and protein requirements may not contain adequate vitamins and minerals for growing children. Most often inadequate are Vitamin D, calcium, phosphorous, and iron. (See page 287 for *Pediatric Nutritional Assessment.*

Infant formulas (see *Pediatric Appendix 1,* page 458 to 469) are the most suitable tube feedings for infants (less than 1 year of age). For the young child (1 to 3 years of age), either a tube feeding used for adults (preferably a commercially prepared nutritional formula at 1 Kcal per milliliter, page 264) or an infant formula may be appropriate. Enteral formulas used for adults with additional vitamin and mineral supplements are acceptable after 3 years of age. The selection of a particular formula should be based on nutrient composition, renal solute load, and the patient's ability to concentrate urine.[2] At times, diarrhea can be a limiting factor in the use of formulas, and close attention needs to be given to the osmolality and the carbohydrate content of the formulas. Frequent determination of the stool pH or of the content of reducing substance helps. The application of tube feeding in the short bowel syndrome has recently received much interest, and in this instance, not only the osmolality and the carbohydrate content need to be watched carefully, but also the volume. A combination of enteral feeding and parenteral feeding is often initially necessary.

Administration

Feedings may be administered by constant drip or by intermittent gavage. The method depends on the child's age, the length of time without adequate food intake, the severity of the illness, and the type of feeding being used. In general, tube feeding is best tolerated and most effective if initiated by constant drip. However, intermittent feedings have been claimed to be more "physiologic." The volume of intermittent feeding is large, and, since children require more nutrients per kilogram of body weight than adults, the risk of inducing cramping and diarrhea is greater. Mechanical pumps improve the tolerance of many tube-fed patients and are essential for patients who do not tolerate fluctuations in volume of intake or for patients who undergo continuous nocturnal feedings (see *Enteral Nutrition Support of Adults,* page 261). When selecting a pump, it is important to choose one that enables the infusion rate to be adjusted in small increments.

The institution of tube feeding should proceed cautiously, and tolerance should be monitored carefully. Individual tolerance determines how rapidly feedings can be advanced. Following are guidelines for initiating tube feeding.

Guidelines for Initiating Tube Feeding[3]

1. Begin 1 to 2 ml per kilogram per hour by constant drip or by frequent intermittent feedings. Intermittent feedings should be administered by slow drip or by gravity over 15 to 30 minutes and never forced by syringe.

2. Initially, use formulas of no greater than isotonic concentration (300 mM). Initial feedings should have a concentration no greater than 0.5 kilocalories per milliliter for patients who have not been fed for more than 3 days or who are critically ill.

3. Increase volume and concentration separately. Increase to 1/3 to 1/2 of desired total volume, and then begin to increase feeding to desired concentration. Gradually increase to full volume.

4. Changes are usually made every 24 hours, depending on tolerance, but may be made as frequently as every 8 to 12 hours.

5. Regress to the most recent administration schedule that was tolerated if signs of intolerance (vomiting, diarrhea, or excessive residual volume) develop. Later, advance the administration schedule more slowly.

6. Supplemental fluid and electrolyte sources may be needed when these guidelines are used.

There are several formulas for estimating water requirements. Most give similar results. Patients receiving enteral nutrition usually tolerate additional water, but, parenteral supplementation may be needed if the patient takes less than the recommended amount (Table 8–58).

TABLE 8–58 General Guidelines for Maintenance Water Requirements[4]

Patient Weight	Water Requirement
0.5–3 kg	120 ml per kg per day
3–10 kg	100 ml per kg per day
10–20 kg	1,000 ml + 50 × (weight in kg − 10) ml per day
above 20 kg	1,500 ml + 20 × (weight in kg − 20) ml per day

Monitoring

Monitoring of nutritional status and of tolerance of tube feeding is mandatory and should include (1) the daily evaluation and documentation of caloric, protein, and fluid intake, (2) the use and intake of vitamin and mineral supplements, (3) the daily weight of the infant or child, (4) a review of intake and output for indications of intolerance (aspiration, vomiting, diarrhea, constipation) and of fluid balance, and (5) a review of serum electrolytes, glucose, albumin, urea, hematocrit, and other biochemical parameters specific to the patient's medical condition.

Common complications of tube feeding include vomiting, diarrhea, and constipation. Table 8–59 covers the usual causes.

TABLE 8–59 Common Tube Feeding Problems and Causes

Problem	Cause
Vomiting	Improper tube placement
	Tube too large
	Rate of feeding too fast
	Residual volume from previous feeding too great
	Osmolality of feeding too high
	Medication given with feeding
Diarrhea	Rate of feeding too fast
	Osmolality of feeding to high
	Intolerance to formula ingredients (e.g., lactose)
	Medications (e.g., antibiotics)
	Severe protein and caloric malnutrition
	Malabsorption
	Bacterial overgrowth
Constipation	Lack of fiber in the formula
	Inadequate fluid
	Lack of activity

REFERENCES

1. Leheiko NS, Murray C, Munio HN. Enteral support of the hospitalized child. In: Suskind R, ed. Textbook of pediatric nutrition. New York: Raven Press, 1981:357.
2. Benkou KJ, Kazlow PG, Waye JD. Percutaneous endoscopic gastrostomies in children. Pediatrics 1986;77:248–250.
3. Kennedy-Caldwell C, Caldwell M. Pediatric enteral nutrition. In: Rombeau J, Caldwell M, eds. Enteral and tube feeding. Philadelphia: WB Saunders, 1984:434.
4. Robbin S, Thorap JW, Wadsworth C. Tube feeding of infants and children. Washington D.C.: Am Soc Parenteral Enteral Nutr, 1982.

PARENTERAL NUTRITION

Parenteral nutritional support is appropriate only when the gastrointestinal tract cannot be used. In infants and in children the parenteral nutrition solution should be based on the assessed nutritional needs of the individual (see *Pediatric Nutritional Assessment,* page 287).

This institution has developed a pediatric parenteral nutrition order sheet (Forms 1 and 2), which outlines the procedures for identifying the nutritional needs of parenteral support.

The following are selected readings for pediatric parenteral nutritional support.

SUGGESTED READINGS

1. Kerner JA. Manual of pediatric parenteral nutrition. New York: John Wiley & Sons, 1983.
2. Filler RM. Parenteral support of the surgically ill child. In: Suskind RM, ed. Textbook of pediatric nutrition. New York: Raven Press, 1981:341.
3. American Academy of Pediatrics, Committee on Nutrition. Commentary on parenteral nutrition. Pediatrics 1983;71:547.
4. A statement by an expert panel. Guidelines for essential trace element preparations for parenteral use. JAMA 1979;241:2051–2054.
5. Rombeau JL, Caldwell MD, eds. Clinical nutrition volume 2: parenteral nutrition. Philadelphia: WB Saunders, 1986:680.

Form 1. PHYSICIAN'S PEDIATRIC PARENTERAL NUTRITION ORDER SHEET

(Use a new sheet for each daily order)

For more detailed information, see Pediatric Parenteral Nutrition guidelines (see Form 2)

CLINIC NUMBER
NAME
ROOM NUMBER

PATIENT'S WEIGHT _____ kg.

PATIENT'S AGE _____

PARENTERAL NUTRITION SOLUTION COMPOSITION

Dextrose _____ %
Amino Acids _____ g/kg/day
Other _____ g/kg/day
Sodium _____ mEq/kg/day
Potassium _____ mEq/kg/day
Calcium _____ mEq/kg/day
Magnesium _____ mEq/kg/day
Phosphorus _____ mmol/kg/day
Chloride (select one)

☐ Sodium = Chloride (Anions are added as chloride to equal the amount of sodium)

☐ Minimal Chloride (Anions are added as acetate to minimize amount of chloride)

☐ Minimal Acetate (Anions are added as chloride to minimize amount of acetate)

☐ Chloride _____ mEq/kg/day

Heparin Sodium _____ Units/ml. (Final Conc.)

_____
_____
_____

INTRAVENOUS FAT EMULSION

☐ 10% Fat Emulsion (1.1 Kcal/ml)

☐ 20% Fat Emulsion (2.0 Kcal/ml)

_____ g/kg/day
or
_____ ml/day
at
_____ ml/hr

OTHER FLUIDS
Oral or NG

_____
_____
_____
_____ ml/kg/day
or
_____ ml/day

☐ Standard Pediatric Multivitamin Injection to one bottle daily
☐ Patient on warfarin (no Vitamin K, see Form 2)
☐ Standard Pediatric Trace Element Injection to one bottle daily

VOLUME (specify one)
_____ ml/kg/day
_____ ml/day

NOTE: The parenteral nutrition solution ordered above is the amount the patient will receive daily. All other forms of fluid intake will be **in addition** to these amounts.

ROUTE OF ADMINISTRATION (select one)

☐ Central   ☐ Umbilical   ☐ Peripheral

Estimated Kilocalories from Parenteral Nutrition:
_____ Kcal/kg/day or _____ Kcal/day

TIME NEEDED (Nurse) _____

Date _____   Time _____   Dr. _____

Meds Solution
_____
_____
at _____ ml/hr

Other IV #1
_____
_____
at _____ ml/hr

Other IV #2
_____
_____
at _____ ml/hr

SPECIAL INSTRUCTIONS
_____
_____

Form 2. INTRAVENOUS NUTRIENT RECOMMENDATIONS FOR NEONATES, INFANTS, AND CHILDREN*

NUTRIENT	PRE-TERM NEONATE (<3 kg)	FULL-TERM NEONATE & INFANTS (>3 kg)	CHILDREN
Total Kilocalories†	Start at 60–80 Kcal/kg/day (maintenance), increase progressively as glucose and/or fat tolerance permits to 100–120 Kcal/kg/day	100–120 Kcal/kg/day	1–7 yr: 75–90 Kcal/kg/day 7–12 yr: 60–75 Kcal/kg/day 12–18 yr: 30–60 Kcal/kg/day
Protein‡	0.5 g/kg/day, increase to 2.5 g/kg/day with increase in nonprotein kilocalories	2.0–2.5 g/kg/day	1.5–2.5 g/kg/day
Fat§	For Kilocalories: 0.5–1.0 g/kg/day, increase by 0.5 g/kg/day to a maximum of 2.5 g/kg/day. For EFA Supplementation only: 0.5 g/kg/day	For Kilocalories: 1.5 g/kg/day, increase by 0.5–1.0 g/kg/day to a maximum of 3 g/kg/day. For EFA Supplementation only: 0.5–1.0 g/kg/day or 2.0 g/kg twice a week	For Kilocalories: 1.5 g/kg/day, increase by 0.5–1.0 g/kg/day to a maximum of 3 g/kg/day. For EFA Supplementation only: 0.5–1.0 g/kg/day or 2.0 g/kg twice a week
Na & Cl	3–4 mEq/kg/day or slightly higher when newborn	3–4 mEq/kg/day	3–4 mEq/kg/day
K	2–3 mEq/kg/day or slightly lower when newborn	2–3 mEq/kg/day	2–3 mEq/kg/day
Ca	1–2 mEq/kg/day, increase to 2–4 mEq (425–850 mg Ca Gluconate)/kg/day as protein and kilocalories are increased	1–2 mEq (212–425 mg Ca Gluconate)/kg/day	0.5–1.0 mEq (106–212 mg Ca Gluconate)/kg/day
P	0.5 mmol/kg/day, increase to 1.0–1.3 mmol/kg/day as protein and kilocalories are increased	1.0 mmol/kg/day	1.0–1.3 mmol/kg/day
Mg	0.5 mEq/kg/day	0.5 mEq/kg/day	0.25–0.5 mEq/kg/day

*The recommendations represent intakes appropriate for the metabolically stable patient. Other patients may require alterations of the above intakes.

†Caloric Values
Amino Acids: 4 Kcal/g   10% Fat Emulsion: 1.1 Kcal/ml
IV Dextrose: 3.4 Kcal/g   20% Fat Emulsion: 2.0 Kcal/ml

‡ A ratio of 160–200 nonprotein kilocalories per g of nitrogen (or 25–32 nonprotein kilocalories per g of protein) is needed for protein anabolism.

§Do not begin until bilirubin is less than 3 mg/dl.

Vitamins

Vitamins	Standard Daily Dose			
	(<1 kg)	(≥1 kg and <3 kg)	(≥3 kg. and <11 years)	(≥11 years)
A, IU	690 IU/day	1495 IU/day	2300 IU/day	3300 IU/day
D, IU	120 IU/day	260 IU/day	400 IU/day	200 IU/day
E, IU	2.1 IU/day	4.55 IU/day	7 IU/day	10 IU/day
C, mg	24 mg/day	52 mg/day	80 mg/day	100 mg/day
Folic Acid, µg	42 µg/day	91 µg/day	140 µg/day	400 µg/day
Thiamine, mg	0.36 mg/day	0.78 mg/day	1.2 mg/day	3 mg/day
Riboflavin, mg	0.42 mg/day	0.91 mg/day	1.4 mg/day	3.6 mg/day
Pyridoxine, mg	0.3 mg/day	0.65 mg/day	1.0 mg/day	4 mg/day
Niacin, mg	5.1 mg/day	11.05 mg/day	17 mg/day	40 mg/day
B_{12}, µg	0.3 µg/day	0.65 µg/day	1 µg/day	5 µg/day
Dexpanthenol, mg	1.5 mg/day	3.25 mg/day	5 mg/day	15 mg/day
Biotin, µg	6 µg/day	13 µg/day	20 µg/day	60 µg/day
K_1, mg	0.06 mg/day	0.13 mg/day	0.2 mg/day	0.2 mg/day*

Trace Elements	Standard Daily Dose	Max. Daily Dose
Zinc	100 µg/kg/day (≥3 kg) or 300 µg/kg/day (<3 kg)	Zinc 4000 µg
Copper	20 µg/kg/day	Copper 800 µg
Manganese	5 µg/kg/day	Manganese 200 µg
Chromium	0.17 µg/kg/day	Chromium 6.8 µg

(Note: these are general recommendations and may not be applicable for some patients.)

* Delete when checked on Order Sheet (see front)

PEDIATRIC APPENDICES

APPENDIX 1

INFANT FORMULAS

Name	Company	Classification	Food Source	Use	Form* Available	Kcal/oz Normal Dilution	Protein g/% Kcals	Fat g/% Kcals	Carbohy-drate g/% Kcals	Cal-cium (mg)
									Composition	
Enfamil with or without iron	Mead Johnson	Infant formula	Reduced mineral whey, nonfat milk; lactose, mono- and digly-cerides; soy and coconut oils	Infant feeding	Ready-to-feed; con-centrate; powder	20	15/9	38/50	69/41	458
Enfamil Pre-mature For-mula	Mead Johnson	Premature infant formula	Nonfat milk, whey protein concen-trate; corn syrup solids, lactose; medium chain tri-glycerides, soy and coconut oils	For growing healthy, low-birth-weight infants (<2000 g)	Ready-to-feed	24	24/12	41/43	89/45	938
Lofenalac	Mead Johnson	Modified infant formula	Casein hydroly-sate processed to remove most of the phenylala-nine; corn syrup solids, modified tapioca starch; corn oil	For infants with phenylketonuria	Powder	20	22/13	26/35	88/51	625
Low Methio-nine Diet Powder	Mead Johnson	Modified infant formula	Soy protein iso-late; corn syrup solids; corn and coconut oils	For infants with homocystinuria	Powder	20	20/12	36/48	66/39	573
Low Phe/Tyr Diet Powder	Mead Johnson	Modified infant formula	Casein hydroly-sate processed to remove most of the phenylala-nine; corn syrup solids, modified tapioca starch; corn oil	For infants with hereditary tyrosi-nemia	Powder	20	22/13	26/35	86/51	688
Milk, cow's		Natural food	Cow's milk	Infant feeding af-ter 6 months of age	Ready-to-feed	20	33/21	37/52	48/29	1208
Milk, evapo-rated (Re-constituted 1:1)	Several brands	Natural Food	Cow's milk	Infant feeding	Concentrate	21	36/20	40/50	53/30	1371

* R–Ready-to-feed
  C–Concentrate; Normal Dilution 1:1 with water
  P–Powder; Normal Dilution 1 scoop:2 oz. water
†–With or without iron

AND FEEDINGS[1,2,3]

per 1000 ml normal dilution												Approximate Solute Load	
Phosphorus (mg)	Iron† (w/wo) (mg)	Sodium (mEq)	Potassium (mEq)	Vitamin A (I.U.)	Vitamin D (I.U.)	Thiamin (mg)	Riboflavin (mg)	Niacin (mg)	Ascorbic Acid (mg)	Other	Miscellaneous Information	Renal mOsm/kg H_2O	GI mOsm/kg H_2O
312	12/1	9	17	2074	415	0.5	1	8	54	Other vitamins and minerals	60:40 whey:casein ratio. Powder contains corn oil instead of soy oil. For hospital use only. Also available as 13 and 24 Kcal/oz formula with appropriate adjustments in all nutrients	100	300
469	2	14	23	9583	2604	2.0	2.8	32	281	Other vitamins and minerals in amounts to meet estimated needs of premature infants except for iron and possibly Vitamin E	60:40 whey:casein ratio. Also available as 20 Kcal/oz formula	220	300
469	12	14	17	1667	415	0.5	0.6	8	54	Other vitamins and minerals	Needs to be supplemented with appropriate amounts of phenylalanine according to patient tolerance	134	360
417	12	11	15	1667	415	0.5	0.6	8	54	Other vitamins and minerals	Contains ~30 mg methionine/100 g powder, which is usually sufficient for growth. Plasma amino acids should be monitored	120	168
469	12	14	17	1667	415	0.5	0.6	8	54	Other vitamins and minerals	Needs to be supplemented with appropriate amounts of phenylalanine and tyrosine according to patient tolerance	130	420
946	0.5	22	39	1404	415	0.38	1.6	0.8	17	Other vitamins and minerals. Inadequate in Vitamin C, iron, and fluoride	Not appropriate for infants <6 mo of age. Approximate composition	240	288
1063	1	24	41	1275	415	0.25	1.7	0.8	8	Other vitamins and minerals. Inadequate in Vitamin C, iron, and fluoride	Values are for normal dilution (1:1). Requires added carbohydrate for infant feeding	N/A	N/A

INFANT FORMULAS

Name	Company	Classification	Food Source	Use	Form* Available	Kcal/oz Normal Dilution	Composition				
							Protein g/% Kcals	Fat g/% Kcals	Carbohy-drate g/% Kcals	Cal-cium (mg)	
Milk, human		Natural food	Human milk	Infant feeding	Ready-to-feed	20–21	10/6	47/57	70/38	333	
Milk, goat's		Natural food	Goat's milk	Infant feeding	Ready-to-feed	23	36/21	42/54	45/26	1340	
Milk, evaporated goat (reconstituted 1:1)	Myenberg	Natural food	Goat's milk	For people allergic to cow's milk	Concentrate	20	33/20	33/46	54/33	1192	
Mono- and Disaccharide-Free Diet Powder	Mead Johnson	Formula base	Hydrolyzed casein; modified tapioca starch; corn oil, medium chain triglycerides	For children with disaccharidase deficiencies, impaired glucose transport or study of fructose utilization; intractable diarrhea of infancy	Powder	10‡	19/NA	28/NA	§	625	
MSUD Diet Powder	Mead Johnson	Modified infant formula	Amino acids (except leucine, isoleucine and valine); corn syrup solids, modified tapioca starch; corn oil	For infants and children with maple syrup urine disease or other disorders in branched chain amino acid metabolism	Powder	20	11/7	28/39	89/54	688	
Nursoy	Wyeth	Infant formula	Soy protein isolate; sucrose; oleo, oleic, coconut, soy oils	For infants allergic or sensitive to cow's milk protein or lactose; galactosemia	Ready-to-feed; concentrate; powder	20	21/13	36/48	69/41	600	
Nutramigen	Mead Johnson	Modified infant formula	Hydrolyzed casein; sucrose; modified tapioca starch; corn oil	For infants with sensitivity to intact proteins or severe food allergies; diarrhea, colic, or other gastrointestinal disturbances	Powder; Ready-to-feed (for hospital use only)	20	22/13	26/35	88/52	625	

* R–Ready-to-feed
  C–Concentrate; Normal Dilution 1:1 with water
  P–Powder; Normal Dilution 1 scoop:2 oz. water
† –With or without iron
‡ Normal dilution without added carbohydrate.
§ Glucose, fructose, sucrose, and/or Polycose should be added in step-wise increments according to tolerance.

AND FEEDINGS[1,2,3] (continued)

per 1000 ml normal dilution

Phosphorus (mg)	Iron† (w/wo) (mg)	Sodium (mEq)	Potassium (mEq)	Vitamin A (I.U.)	Vitamin D (I.U.)	Thiamin (mg)	Riboflavin (mg)	Niacin (mg)	Ascorbic Acid (mg)	Other	Miscellaneous Information	Approximate Solute Load	
												Renal mOsm/kg H2O	GI mOsm/kg H2O
133	2	7	14	2467	20	0.21	0.3	3	33	Other vitamins and minerals. May need to be supplemented with Vitamin D, fluoride, and iron after 6 mo of age	Composition only approximate because of maternal individual differences, maternal diet, length of laction	80	300
1110	0.5	22	53	1879	21	0.5	1.6	3	13	Other vitamins and minerals. Inadequate in Vitamins D, C, folacin, iron, and fluoride	Composition only approximate. Fat is higher in essential fatty acids and short and medium chained fatty acids than cow's milk	N/A	N/A
1054	1	22	26	1950	410	0.3	1.7	58	0.5	Other vitamins and minerals. Contains 104 μg/L of folic acid. Inadequate in Vitamin C, iron, and fluoride and requires supplementation when used as only source of nutrition	Approximate Composition based on 1:1 dilution. Requires added carbohydrate for infant feeding	N/A	N/A
415	12	12	19	2500	500	0.5	0.6	8	78	Other vitamins and minerals	Adequate carbohydrate must be supplied	124	250‡
375	12	11	18	1666	410	0.5	0.6	8	54	Other vitamins and minerals	Needs to be supplemented with appropriate amounts of leucine, isoleucine, and valine according to patient tolerance	90	360
420	11.5	8.7	18	2000	400	0.67	1.0	5	55	Other vitamins and minerals	Lower in sodium than other soy formulas. Nursoy powder contains corn syrup solids and sucrose	122	296
470	12	14	17	1665	415	0.5	0.6	8	54	Other vitamins and minerals		130	480

INFANT FORMULAS

Name	Company	Classification	Food Source	Use	Form* Available	Kcal/oz Normal Dilution	Composition Protein g/% Kcals	Fat g/% Kcals	Carbohy- drate g/% Kcals	Cal- cium (mg)
Phenyl-Free	Mead Johnson	Phenylalanine- free food	Amino acids (no phenylalanine); sucrose, corn syrup solids, modified tapioca starch; corn and coconut oils	For children with phenylketonuria	Powder	25	43/21	14/14	140/66	1040
Portagen	Mead Johnson	Modified infant formula	Sodium casein- ate; corn syrup solids, sucrose; medium chain tri- glycerides, corn oil	For infants, chil- dren, or adults with fat malab- sorption such as cystic fibrosis, in- testinal resection, steatorrhea, pan- creatic insuffi- ciency, celiac dis- ease, bile acid deficiency, lym- phatic anomalies	Powder	20	24/14	32/40	78/46	625
Pregestimil	Mead Johnson	Modified infant formula	Hydrolyzed cas- ein; corn syrup solids, modified tapioca starch; corn oil and me- dium chain tri- glycerides.	For infants with malabsorption disorders, intract- able diarrhea, se- vere allergies or sensitivity to in- tact protein, cys- tic fibrosis, intes- tinal resections, steatorrhea, lac- tase or sucrase deficiency	Powder	20	19/11	27/35	91/54	625
ProSobee	Mead Johnson	Infant formula	Soy protein iso- late; syrup solids; coconut and soy oils	For infants al- lergic or sensitive to cow's milk or lactase; galacto- semia; temporary feeding following diarrhea until lac- tase regenerates; sucrose intoler- ance	Ready-to- feed; con- centrate; powder	20	20	36	69	625
Ross Carbo- hydrate-Free (RCF) Low- Iron Soy Protein For- mula Base	Ross	Protein-fat- vitamin-mineral module	Soy protein iso- late; soy and co- conut oils	For infants intole- rant to all types of carbohydrate; intractable diar- rhea	Concentrate	12‡	20	36	—‡	710

* R—Ready-to-feed
  C—Concentrate; Normal Dilution 1:1 with water
  P—Powder; Normal Dilution 1 scoop:2 oz. water
† —With or without iron
‡ Normal dilution without carbohydrate.

AND FEEDINGS[1,2,3] *(continued)*

Phos-phorus (mg)	Iron[†] (w/wo) (mg)	Sodium (mEq)	Potas-sium (mEq)	Vita-min A (I.U.)	Vita-min D (I.U.)	Thia-min (mg)	Ribo-flavin (mg)	Nia-cin (mg)	Ascor-bic Acid (mg)	Other	Miscel-laneous Information	Renal mOsm/kg H₂O	GI mOsm/kg H₂O
1040	25	36	72	2500	310	1.2	2.1	17	108	Other vitamins and minerals	Not an infant formula. Designed to complement the remainder of the diets of children 2 yr and older. Not intended to be the sole source of nutrition	340	870
470	12	13	21	5200	520	1.0	1.0	13	54	Other vitamins and minerals	Fat content is approximately 85% medium chain triglycerides and 15% corn oil (to supply essential fatty acids)	150	200
415	12	13	20	2000	400	0.5	0.6	8	54	Other vitamins and minerals	Fat content is 40% medium chain triglycerides and 60% corn oil	120	350
495	12	12	20	2080	415	0.5	0.6	8	54	Other vitamins and minerals	Powder contains corn oil instead of soy oil	130	200
510	1.5	14	20	2030	410	0.4	0.6	9	60	Other vitamins and minerals	Carbohydrates added according to tolerance. A carbohydrate concentration of at least 2% is needed to prevent hypoglycemia and ketosis. IV glucose should be used as a supplement until then. Use only under medical supervision	131	64 (no carbohydrate added)

per 1000 ml normal dilution

Approximate Solute Load

INFANT FORMULAS

Name	Company	Classification	Food Source	Use	Form* Available	Kcal/oz Normal Dilution	Protein g/% Kcals	Fat g/% Kcals	Carbohydrate g/% Kcals	Calcium (mg)
									Composition	
SMA with or without iron	Wyeth	Infant formula	Nonfat cow's milk and partially demineralized whey; lactose; coconut oleic, oleo, and soybean oils	Infant feeding; use for infants with cardiac or renal problems who could benefit from reduced sodium or renal solute load	Ready-to-feed use; concentrate; powder	20	15/9	36/48	72/43	420
SMA "Premie"	Wyeth	Premature infant formula	Nonfat cow's milk, partially demineralized whey; lactose, glucose polymers; medium chain triglycerides, oleo, oleic, coconut, and soy oils	For growing healthy low birth weight infants (<2000 g).	Ready-to-feed use (hospital use only)	24	20/10	44/47	86/43	750
Similac with or without iron	Ross	Infant formula	Nonfat cow's milk; lactose; coconut and soy oils	Infant feeding	Ready-to-feed use; concentrate; powder	20	15/9	36/48	72/43	510
Similac With Whey + Iron	Ross	Infant formula	Nonfat cow's milk, whey protein concentrate; lactose; soy and coconut oils	Infant feeding	Ready-to-feed use; concentrate; powder	20	15/9	36/48	72/43	400
Advance	Ross	Infant formula	Nonfat cow's milk, soy protein isolate; lactose, corn syrup; soy and coconut oils	Transitional beverage between infant formula and cow's milk for the older infant	Ready-to-feed use; concentrate	16	20/15	27/45	55/41	510
Isomil	Ross	Infant formula	Soy protein isolate; sucrose, corn syrup; soy and coconut oils	For infants allergic or sensitive to cow's milk protein or lactose; galactosemia; temporary feeding following diarrhea until lactase regenerates	Ready-to-feed use; concentrate; powder	20	18/11	37/49	68/40	710
Isomil SF	Ross	Infant formula	Soy protein isolate; corn syrup solids; soy and coconut oils	For infants allergic or sensitive to cow's milk protein, lactose or sucrose; temporary feeding following acute diarrhea	Ready-to-feed use; concentrate	20	20/12	36/48	68/40	710

* R—Ready-to-feed
  C—Concentrate; Normal Dilution 1:1 with water
  P—Powder; Normal Dilution 1 scoop:2 oz. water
† —With or without iron

AND FEEDINGS[1,2,3] *(continued)*

per 1000 ml normal dilution												Approximate Solute Load	
Phos-phorus (mg)	Iron[†] (w/wo) (mg)	Sodium (mEq)	Potas-sium (mEq)	Vita-min A (I.U.)	Vita-min D (I.U.)	Thia-min (mg)	Ribo-flavin (mg)	Nia-cin (mg)	Ascor-bic Acid (mg)	Other	Miscel-laneous Information	Renal mOsm/kg H_2O	GI mOsm/kg H_2O
280	12/1.5	7	14	2000	400	0.67	1.0	5	55	Other vitamins and minerals	60:40 whey:casein ratio. For hospital use only: 24 Kcal/ounce with proportional adjustments in all nutrients	91	300
400	3	14	19	2400	480	0.8	1.3	6	70	Other vitamins and minerals. Needs to be supplemented with vitamins and minerals, when used for infants <2000 g	60:40 whey:casein ratio	175	280
390	12/1.5	10	21	2030	410	0.8	1.0	7	60	Other vitamins and minerals	For hospital use only: available as 13, 24, and 27 Kcal per ounce with proportional adjustments in all nutrients. Powder contains corn oil instead of soy oil	105	290
300	12	10	19	2030	410	0.7	1.0	7	60	Other vitamins and minerals	60:40 whey:casein ratio. Powder contains corn oil instead of coconut oil	101	300
390	10	9	24	2160	410	0.8	0.9	10	50	Other vitamins and minerals		128	200
510	12	14	24	2030	410	0.4	0.6	9	60	Other vitamins and minerals		122	250
510	12	14	20	2030	410	0.4	0.6	9	60	Other vitamins and minerals		131	150

INFANT FORMULAS

Name	Company	Classification	Food Source	Use	Form* Available	Kcal/oz Normal Dilution	Protein g/% Kcals	Fat g/% Kcals	Carbohy-drate g/% Kcals	Cal-cium (mg)
									Composition	
Similac LBW	Ross	Premature infant formula	Nonfat cow's milk; corn syrup solids, lactose; medium chain tri-glycerides, soy and coconut oils	For rapidly grow-ing healthy low birth weight (<2500 g) in-fants	Ready-to-feed (hospi-tal use only)	24	22/11	45/47	85/42	730
Similac Natu-ral Care	Ross	Human milk sup-plement	Nonfat cow's milk, whey pro-tein concentrate; hydrolyzed corn starch, lactose; medium chain tri-glycerides, soy and coconut oils	To fortify human milk for prema-ture infants	Ready-to-feed (hospi-tal use only)	24	22/11	44/47	86/42	1710
Similac PM 60/40	Ross	Infant formula	Demineralized whey solids, so-dium caseinate; lactose; corn and coconut oils.	For infants whose renal or cardio-vascular system might be taxed by a sodium or solute load greater than that of human milk or who have hyper-phosphotemia	Ready-to-feed (for hospital use only); Pow-der	20	16/9	38/50	69/41	380
Similac Spe-cial Care	Ross	Premature infant formula	Nonfat cow's milk, whey pro-tein concentrate; corn syrup solids, lactose; medium chain triglycer-ides, soy and co-conut oils	For growing healthy low birth weight (<2000 g) infants	Ready-to-feed (hospi-tal use only)	24	22/11	44/47	86/42	1460
Soyalac	Loma Linda	Infant formula	Soy protein solids (whole bean); dextrins, maltose, dextrose, su-crose; soy oil	For infants al-lergic or sensitive to cow's milk pro-tein or lactose; galactosemia	Ready-to-feed use; concentrate; powder	20	20/12	37/49	66/39	634
I-Soyalac	Loma Linda	Infant formula	Soy protein iso-late; sucrose, tapioca starch; soy oil.	For infants al-lergic or sensitive to cow's milk pro-tein or lactose; galactosemia	Ready-to-feed use; concentrate	20	20/12	37/49	66/39	690

* R–Ready-to-feed
  C–Concentrate; Normal Dilution 1:1 with water
  P–Powder; Normal Dilution 1 scoop:2 oz. water
† –With or without iron

AND FEEDINGS[1,2,3] (continued)

per 1000 ml normal dilution												Approximate Solute Load	
Phos-phorus (mg)	Iron[†] (w/wo) (mg)	Sodium (mEq)	Potas-sium (mEq)	Vita-min A (I.U.)	Vita-min D (I.U.)	Thia-min (mg)	Ribo-flavin (mg)	Nia-cin (mg)	Ascor-bic Acid (mg)	Other	Miscel-laneous Information	Renal mOsm/kg H_2O	GI mOsm/kg H_2O
570	3.0	16	31	2440	490	1.0	1.2	8.5	100	Other vitamins and minerals	Requires supplements to meet estimated dietary needs for most vitamins and minerals for premature infants use; casein predominant protein	160	290
850	3.0	18	29	5520	1220	2.0	5.0	40	300	Other vitamins and minerals	Mix 50:50 with human milk; 60:40 whey:casein ratio. May require supplementation with some nutrients to meet estimated needs of premature infants	156	300
190	1.5	7	15	2030	410	0.7	1.0	7	60	Other vitamins and minerals	60:40 whey:casein ratio. May be necessary to supplement with electrolytes or minerals for the premature infant or when there is abnormally high losses. Ready-to-feed formula contains corn instead of soy oil	95	260
730	3.0	18	29	5520	1220	2.0	5.0	40	300	Other vitamins and minerals in amounts to meet estimated needs of premature infants, except for iron and possibly vitamins D and E	60:40 whey:casein ratio. Also available in 20 Kcal/ounce with proportional adjustments in all nutrients	156	300
528	10	15	24	2114	423	0.5	0.6	8.5	63	Other vitamins and minerals		129	210
480	13	12	20	2114	423	0.5	0.6	8.5	63	Other vitamins and minerals		134	280

Feeding Supplements

Name	Company	Food Source	Use	Form Available	Kilocalories	Protein g
Casec	Mead Johnson	Calcium caseinate	Protein supplement; to increase protein for low sodium and low fat diets	Powder	370	88
Enfamil Human Milk Fortifier	Mead Johnson	Whey protein concentrate, casein, corn syrup solids, lactose	To fortify human milk for premature infants	Powder	14[†]	0.7[†]
MCT oil	Mead Johnson	Lipid fraction of coconut oil	Supplement for people who cannot digest and absorb long chain fats	Liquid	821	—
Moducal	Mead Johnson	Glucose polymers from hydrolyzed corn starch	Carbohydrate supplement	Powder	380	—
Polycose	Ross	Glucose polymers from hydrolysis of corn starch	Carbohydrate supplement	Powder	380	—
				Liquid	200	—
Pro Mod	Ross	D-whey protein concentrate; soy lecithin	Protein supplement	Powder	424	76
Protein-Free Diet Powder (Product 80056)	Mead Johnson	Corn syrup solids, modified tapioca starch; corn oil	Protein-free formula base for infants who require specific mixtures of amino acids such as with hyperlysinemia, isovaleric acidemia, propionic aciduria, urea cycle disorders, B_{12} independent methylamalonic aciduria, arginemia, gyrate atrophy, histidinemia	Powder	490	—

* Manufacturer's information.
[†] Per 4 packets (3.8 g) which should be mixed with 100 ml human milk.

REFERENCES

1. Agricultural Handbook No. 8-1, Composition of Foods: Dairy and Egg Products, Raw ° Processed ° Prepared. 1976.
2. Manufacturer's information.
3. Lammi-Keefe CJ, RG Jensen. Fat soluble vitamins in human milk. Nutr Rev 1984;42:365–371.

and Modules*

							Composition Per 100 Grams	
Fat g	Carbo-hydrate g	Calcium mg	Phos-phorus g	Iron mg	Sodium mEq	Potas-sium mEq	Other	Miscellaneous Information
2	—	1600	800	—	6.5	0.25	10 mg chloride per 100 g	
0.05[†]	2.7[†]	60[†]	30[†]	—	0.3[†]	0.4[†]	Other vitamins and minerals in amounts to nearly meet estimated needs of premature infants except for iron and possibly, Vitamin E	Mix 1 packet with 25 ml human milk
100	—	—	—	—	—	—		
—	95	—	—	—	3	0.13	4.8 mEq chloride	Osmolality is approximately 1/6 of a glucose solution
—	94	30	5	—	4.8	0.3	6.3 mEq chloride	Osmolality is approximately 1/6 of a glucose solution
—	50	20	3	—	3	0.15	3.0 mEq chloride	Osmolality of liquid polycose 835 mOsm/kg H_2O
9	10	348	333	—	8.6	25		1 scoop = 6.6 g and contains 5 g protein
22.5	72	540	300	11	3	8.7	Other vitamins and minerals	Adequate protein and sodium must be added

APPENDIX 2

EXCHANGE VALUES FOR COMMERCIAL BABY FOODS*

Meat Group

Each exchange contains 7 g of protein, 3 g of fat, and 55 kilocalories.

Item	Amount	Brand[†]
Strained Beef	3 Tbsp (1/2 of $3\frac{1}{2}$ oz jar)	G,H,B
Strained Chicken[‡]	3 Tbsp (1/2 of $3\frac{1}{2}$ oz jar)	G,H,B
Strained Ham	3 Tbsp (1/2 of $3\frac{1}{2}$ oz jar)	G
Strained Lamb	3 Tbsp (1/2 of $3\frac{1}{2}$ oz jar)	G,H,B
Strained Liver	3 Tbsp (1/2 of $3\frac{1}{2}$ oz jar)	G,H
Strained Pork	3 Tbsp (1/2 of $3\frac{1}{2}$ oz jar)	G
Strained Turkey	3 Tbsp (1/2 of $3\frac{1}{2}$ oz jar)	G,H,B
Strained Veal	3 Tbsp (1/2 of $3\frac{1}{2}$ oz jar)	G,H,B
Chicken Sticks	4 sticks	G
Meat Sticks	4 sticks	G
Turkey Sticks	5 sticks	G

* Actual composition of an exchange may vary up to 10 percent from stated averages
[†] Brand: B-Beechnut G-Gerber H-Heinz
[‡] Contains 70 kilocalories per exchange—7 g protein, 4 g fat

Starch Group

Each exchange contains 2 g of protein, 1 g of fat, 15 g of carbohydrates, and 80 kilocalories.

Item	Amount	Brand*
Dry Infant Cereal (barley, mixed, oatmeal, rice)	5 Tbsp	B,G,H
Dry Infant Cereal with Fruit (all varieties)	5 Tbsp	B,H
Infant cereal with fruit (wetpack)	6 Tbsp	B,G,H
Arrowroot Biscuit	4	Nabisco
Arrowroot Cookies	3	G
Toddler Biter	$1\frac{1}{2}$	G
Toasted Oat Rings	2/3 cup	G

* Brand: B-Beechnut G-Gerber H-Heinz

Vegetable Group

Each exchange contains 2 g of protein, 5 g of carbohydrates, and 25 kilocalories.

Item	Amount	Brand*
Beets	$3\frac{1}{2}$ Tbsp	G,H
Carrots	6 Tbsp	G,H
Carrots	4 Tbsp	B
Carrots, dry	$2\frac{1}{2}$ Tbsp	H
Corn, creamed	2 Tbsp	B,G,H
Corn, dry	$2\frac{1}{2}$ Tbsp	H
Garden Vegetables	3 Tbsp	B,G
Green Beans	4 Tbsp	B,G
Green Beans	6 Tbsp	H
Green Beans, dry	2 Tbsp	H
Green Beans, creamed	$3\frac{1}{2}$ Tbsp	H
Mixed Vegetables	$3\frac{1}{2}$ Tbsp	B,G,H
Mixed Vegetables, dry	2 Tbsp	H
Peas, plain or creamed	3 Tbsp	B,G,H
Peas, creamed, dry	$2\frac{1}{2}$ Tbsp	H
Peas and Carrots	3 Tbsp	B
Peas and Carrots dry	$2\frac{1}{2}$ Tbsp	H
Spinach, creamed	$2\frac{1}{2}$ Tbsp	G
Squash	5 Tbsp	B,G,H
Squash, dry	$2\frac{1}{2}$ Tbsp	H
Sweet Potatoes	2 Tbsp	B,G,H
Sweet Potatoes, dry	2 Tbsp	H

* Brand: B-Beechnut G-Gerber H-Heinz

Fruit Group
Each exchange contains 15 g of carbohydrates and 60 kilocalories.

Item	Amount	Brand*
Apples, dry	$3\frac{1}{2}$ Tbsp	H
Applesauce	7 Tbsp	B,G,H
Apples/Apricots	7 Tbsp	B,G,H
Apples/Apricots, dry	$3\frac{1}{2}$ Tbsp	H
Apples/Blueberry	6 Tbsp	G
Applesauce/Cherries	7 Tbsp	B
Apples/Cranberry/Tapioca	4 Tbsp	H
Applesauce/Banana	7 Tbsp	B
Apples/Grapes	4 Tbsp	B
Apples/Mandarin Oranges/Banana	$4\frac{1}{2}$ Tbsp	B
Apples/Peaches, dry	$3\frac{1}{2}$ Tbsp	H
Apples/Peaches/Strawberries	4 Tbsp	B
Apples/Pears	6 Tbsp	H
Apples/Pears, dry	$3\frac{1}{2}$ Tbsp	H
Apples/Pears/Bananas	4 Tbsp	B
Applesauce/Pineapple	7 Tbsp	G
Apples/Strawberries	4 Tbsp	B
Apricots/Pears/Applesauce	6 Tbsp	B
Apricots/Pears/Bananas, dry	$3\frac{1}{2}$ Tbsp	H
Apricots/Tapioca	4 Tbsp	G
Apricots/Tapioca	6 Tbsp	H
Bananas, dry	$3\frac{1}{2}$ Tbsp	H
Bananas/Pears/Applesauce	$4\frac{1}{2}$ Tbsp	B
Bananas/Pineapple/Tapioca	6 Tbsp	G,H
Bananas/Tapioca	4 Tbsp	B,G,H
Mixed Fruit, dry	$3\frac{1}{2}$ Tbsp	H
Peaches	5 Tbsp	G,H
Peaches	7 Tbsp	B
Peaches, dry	$3\frac{1}{2}$ Tbsp	H
Peaches/Pears, dry	$4\frac{3}{4}$ Tbsp	H
Pears	6 Tbsp	B,G,H
Pears, dry	$4\frac{3}{4}$ Tbsp	H
Pears/Applesauce	5 Tbsp	B
Pears/Pineapple	6 Tbsp	G,H
Pears/Pineapple	4 Tbsp	B
Pears/Pineapple, dry	$3\frac{1}{2}$ Tbsp	H
Plums/Rice	4 Tbsp	B
Plums/Tapioca	4 Tbsp	G
Prunes/Pears	$4\frac{1}{2}$ Tbsp	B
Prunes/Tapioca	4 Tbsp	G
Fruit juices†		
Apple, Apple/Banana	4 to 4.2 ounces	B,G,H
Apple/Cherry, Apple/Grape		
Apple/Peach, Apple/Plum		
Apple/Pear, Apple/Cranberry		
Apple/Prune, Apple/Apricot		
Apple/Pineapple		
Grape	3 ounces	B
Mixed Fruit	4.2 ounces	B,G,H
Orange	$3\frac{1}{2}$ ounces	G
Orange	4.2 ounces	B,H
Orange/Apple	$3\frac{1}{2}$ ounces	G
Orange/Apple/Banana	4.2 ounces	H
Orange/Apricot	$3\frac{1}{2}$ ounces	G
Orange/Pineapple	$3\frac{1}{2}$ ounces	G
Pear	4.2 ounces	B

*Brand: B-Beechnut   G-Gerber   H-Heinz

†Juice portion sizes are based on actual small bottle sizes, which vary slightly.

PEDIATRIC APPENDIX 3

COMMON CARBOHYDRATES IN FOODS (Per 100 G Edible Portion**)

Food	Mono-Saccharides		Reducing Sugars* (g)	Disaccharides			Polysaccharides					
	Fructose (g)	Glucose (g)		Lactose (g)	Maltose (g)	Sucrose (g)	Cellulose (g)	Dextrins (g)	Hemicellulose (g)	Pectin (g)	Pentosans (g)	Starch (g)
Fruits												
Agave juice	17.0		19.0									
Apple	5.0	1.7	8.3	†		3.1	0.4		0.7	0.6		0.6
Apple juice			8.0			4.2						
Apricots	0.4	1.9				5.5	0.8		1.2	1.0		
Banana												
Yellow green			5.0			5.1						8.8
Yellow			8.4			8.9						1.9
Flecked	3.5	4.5				11.9						1.2
Powder			32.6			33.2		9.6				7.8
Blackberries	2.9	3.2				0.2						
Blueberry juice, commercial			9.6									
Boysenberries			5.3			1.1				0.3		
Breadfruit												
Hawaiian			1.8			7.7						
Samoan			4.9			9.7						
Cherries												
Eating	7.2	4.7	12.5			0.1						
Cooking	6.1	5.5	11.6			0.1						
Cranberries	0.7	2.7				0.1				0.3		
Currants												
Black	3.7	2.4				0.6						
Red	1.9	2.3				0.2						
White	2.6	3.0										
Dates												
Invert sugar, seedling type	23.9	24.9	16.2			0.3						
Deglet Noor						45.4						

Egyptian	3.0					48.5	35.8		
Figs, Kadota									
Fresh	0.1					0.9		9.6	8.2
Dried	0.3					0.1		42.0	30.9
Gooseberries						0.7		4.4	4.1
Grapes									
Black						0.2		8.2	7.3
Concord						0.2	9.5	4.8	4.3
Malaga							22.2	8.1	
White		1.3						2.0	8.0
Grapefruit						2.9	4.4		1.2
Guava						1.9			
Lemon									
Edible portion		0.7	3.0			0.2	1.3		
Whole						0.4		1.4	1.4
Juice						0.1		0.5	0.9
Peel						0.1	3.4		
Loganberries						0.2		1.9	1.3
Loquat									
Champagne						0.8		12.0	
Thales						0.9		9.0	
Mango	0.3		0.3			11.6	3.4		
Melon									
Cantaloupe						4.4	2.3	1.2	0.9
Cassaba,									
Vine ripened						6.2	2.8		
Picked green						3.9	3.2		
Honeydew									
Vine ripened						7.4	3.3		
Picked green						3.3	3.6		
Yellow					0.3	1.4		2.1	1.5
Mulberries								4.4	3.6
Orange									
Valencia (Calif)			0.3			4.2	4.7	2.4	2.3
Composite values				0.3		4.6	5.0	2.5	1.8
Juice									
Fresh						4.7	5.1	2.4	2.4
Frozen, reconstituted						3.2	4.6		
Palmyra palm, tender kernal						0.4		3.2	1.5
Papaw (Asimina triloba) (North America)						2.7	5.9		

474 / MAYO CLINIC DIET MANUAL

COMMON CARBOHYDRATES IN FOODS (Per 100 G Edible Portion**) (continued)

Food	Mono-Saccharides		Reducing Sugars*	Disaccharides			Polysaccharides					
	Fructose (g)	Glucose (g)		Lactose (g)	Maltose (g)	Sucrose (g)	Cellulose (g)	Dextrins (g)	Hemicellulose (g)	Pectin (g)	Pentosans (g)	Starch (g)
Fruits (continued)												
Papaya (Carica papaya) (Tropics)			9.0			0.5						1.8
Passion fruit juice	3.6	3.6				3.8						
Peaches	1.6	1.5	3.1			6.6		0.7		0.7		
Pears												
Anjou	5.0	2.5	7.6			1.9				0.7		
Bartlett	6.5	2.6	8.0			1.5				0.6		
Bosc						1.7				0.6		
Persimmon			17.7									
Pineapple												
Ripened on plant	1.4	2.3	4.2			7.9						
Picked green			1.3			2.4						
Plums												
Damson	3.4	5.2	8.4			1.0				0.9		
Green gage	4.0	5.5				2.9				1.0		
Italian prunes			4.6			5.4				1.0		
Sweet	2.9	4.5	7.4			4.4		0.5			0.1	
Sour	1.3	3.5				1.5						
Pomegranate			12.0			0.6						
Prunes, uncooked	15.0	30.0	47.0			2.0	2.8		10.7	0.9	2.0	0.7
Raisins, Thompson seedless			70.0									
Raspberries	2.4	2.3								1.0		
Sapote	3.8	4.2	5.0			1.0				0.8		
Strawberries				0.7								
Ripe	2.3	2.6				1.4						
Medium ripe			3.8			0.3						
Tangerine	4.8	1.6	3.4			9.0						
Tomatoes												
Canned	1.2		3.0			0.3	0.2		0.3	0.3		
Seedless pulp			6.5			0.4	0.4			0.5		

Watermelon										
Flesh red and firm, ripe			3.8	4.0				0.1		
Red, mealy, overripe			3.0	4.9				0.1		
Vegetables										
Asparagus, raw			1.2				0.3			
Bamboo shoots			0.5	0.2	1.2					
Beans										
Lima										
Canned				1.4						
Fresh				1.4						
Snap, fresh			1.7	0.5	0.5	0.3	1.0	0.5	1.2	2.0
Beets, sugar				12.9	0.9		0.8			
Broccoli,					0.9		0.9		0.9	1.3
Brussels sprouts					1.1		1.5			
Cabbage, raw			3.4	0.3	0.8		1.0			
Carrots, raw			5.8	1.7	1.0		1.7	0.9		
Cauliflower		2.8		0.3	0.7		0.6			
Celery										
Fresh			0.3	0.3						
Hearts			1.7	0.2						
Corn										
Fresh		0.5		0.3	0.6	0.1	0.9		1.3	14.5
Bran							77.1		4.0	
Cucumber			2.5	0.1						
Eggplant			2.1	0.6			0.5			
Lettuce			1.4	0.2	0.4		0.6			
Licorice root		1.4		3.2						22.0
Mushrooms, fresh			0.1		0.9		0.7			2.5
Onions, raw			5.4	2.9			0.3	0.6		
Parsnips, fresh				3.5						7.0
Peas, green				5.5	1.1		2.2			4.1
Potatoes, white	0.1	0.1	0.8	0.1	0.4		0.3			17.0
Pumpkin			2.2	0.6			0.5			0.1
Radishes			3.1	0.3			0.3	0.4		
Rutabagas		5.0		1.3					0.8	
Spinach			0.2		0.4		0.8			
Squash										
Butternut	0.2	0.1		0.4						2.6
Blue hubbard	1.2	1.1		0.4	0.7					4.8

COMMON CARBOHYDRATES IN FOODS (Per 100 G Edible Portion**) (continued)

| Food | Mono-Saccharides | | Reducing Sugars* (g) | Disaccharides | | | Polysaccharides | | | | | |
	Fructose (g)	Glucose (g)		Lactose (g)	Maltose (g)	Sucrose (g)	Cellulose (g)	Dextrins (g)	Hemicellulose (g)	Pectin (g)	Pentosans (g)	Starch (g)
Vegetables (continued)												
Golden crookneck			2.8			1.0						
Sweet potato												
Raw	0.3	0.4	0.8			4.1	0.6		1.4	2.2		16.5
Baked			14.5		1.6	7.2						4.0
Mature Dry Legumes												
Beans												
Mung												
Black gram						1.6						
Green gram						1.8						
Navy						7.2	3.1	3.7	6.4		8.2	35.2
Soy			1.6			1.5	2.6	1.4	6.6		4.0	1.9
Cow pea						2.4	5.4		4.8			
Garbanzo (chick peas)												
Garden pea (Pisum sativum)‡						6.7	5.0		5.1			38.0
Horse gram (Dolichos biplorus)						2.7						
Lentils						2.1						28.5
Pigeon pea (red gram)						1.6						
Soybean												
Flour						6.8						
Meal						6.8						
Milk and Milk Products												
Buttermilk												
Dry				39.9								

Fluid, genuine and cultured								
Casein	0.1		5.0					
Ice cream (14.5% cream)		3.6	4.9	16.6				
Milk								
Ass			6.0					
Cow			4.9					
Dried								
Skim			52.0					
Whole			38.1					
Fluid								
Skim			5.0					
Whole			4.9					
Sweetened, condensed			14.1	43.5				
Ewe			4.9					
Goat			4.7					
Human								
Colostrum			5.3					
Mature			6.9					
Whey			4.9					
Yogurt			3.8					

Nuts and Nut Products

Almonds, blanched		0.2		2.3			2.1	
Chestnuts								
Virginia		2.2		3.6		0.3	1.2	18.0
French		1.2		8.1			2.8	18.6
Coconut milk, ripe		3.3		3.6	1.2		2.5	33.1
Copra meal, dried	1.2			2.6	15.6			
Macadamia nut		0.3		14.3		0.6	2.2	0.9
Peanuts		0.2		5.5		2.5		
Peanut butter		0.9		4.5	2.4	3.8		4.0
Pecans				1.1			0.2	5.9

COMMON CARBOHYDRATES IN FOODS (Per 100 G Edible Portion**) (continued)

Food	Mono-Saccharides Fructose (g)	Glucose (g)	Reducing Sugars*	Disaccharides Lactose (g)	Maltose (g)	Sucrose (g)	Polysaccharides Cellulose (g)	Dextrins (g)	Hemicellulose (g)	Pectin (g)	Pentosans (g)	Starch (g)
Cereals and Cereal Products												
Barley												
Grain, hulled							2.6		6.0		8.5	62.0
Flour											1.2	69.0
Corn, yellow						3.1	4.5		4.9		6.2	62.0
Flaxseed							1.8		5.2			
Millet grain									0.9		6.5	56.0
Oats, hulled											6.4	56.4
Rice												
Bran			1.4			10.6	11.4		7.0		7.4	69.7
Brown, raw		2.0	0.1			0.8		2.1			2.1	
Polished, raw			trace§			0.4	0.3	0.9			1.8	72.9
Polish			0.7								3.8	
Rye												
Grain							3.8		5.6		6.8	57.0
Flour											4.1	71.4
Sorghum grain											2.5	70.2
Soya-wheat (cereal)											3.3	46.4
Wheat												
Germ, defatted						8.3					6.2	
Grain			2.0			1.5	2.0	2.5	5.8		6.6	59.0
Flour, patent			2.0		0.1	0.2		5.5			2.1	68.8
Spices and Condiments												
Allspice (pimenta)			18.0			3.0						
Cassia			23.3									
Cinnamon			19.3									2.7
Cloves			9.0									

Nutmeg			17.2						14.6
Pepper, black			38.6						34.2

Syrups and Other Sweets

Corn Syrup		21.2			26.4		34.7		
High conversion		33.0			23.0		19.0		
Medium conversion		26.0			21.0		23.0		
Corn sugar		87.5			3.5		0.5		
Chocolate, sweet dry			37.5			56.4			
Golden syrup						31.0			
Honey	40.5	34.2				1.9	1.5		
Invert sugar			74.0			6.0			
Jellies, pectin						40–65			
Royal jelly	11.3	9.8				0.9			
Jellies, starch						25–60	7=12		
Maple syrup			1.5			62.9			
Milk chocolate				8.1		43.0			
Molasses	8.0	8.8				53.6			
Blackstrap	6.8	6.8	26.9			36.9			
Sorghum syrup			27.0			36.0			

Miscellaneous

Beer			1.5				2.8	0.3	
Cacao beans, raw, Arriba	0.6	0.5	1.1		1.9				
Carob bean									
Pod			11.2		23.2	1.4			
Pod and seeds			11.1		19.4				
Soy Sauce	0.9								

* Mainly monosaccharides plus the disaccharides, maltose and lactose.
† Blanks indicate lack of acceptable data.
‡ Also known as Alaska pea, field pea, and common pea.
§ Trace = less than 0.05 g.
** From: Hardinge MG, Swarner JB, Crooks H. Carbohydrate in foods. Copyright The American Dietetic Association. Reprinted by permission from Journal of the American Dietetic Association 1965;46:197.

NATIONAL CENTER FOR HEALTH STATISTICS (NCHS) GROWTH GRAPHS

BOYS: BIRTH TO 36 MONTHS
PHYSICAL GROWTH
NCHS PERCENTILES

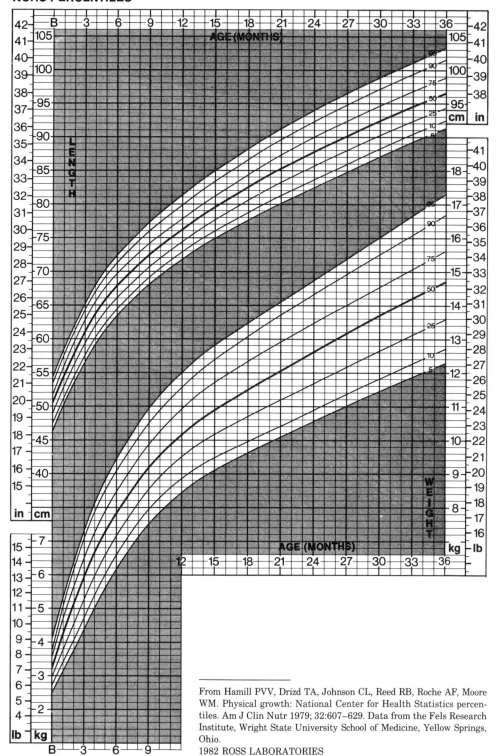

From Hamill PVV, Drizd TA, Johnson CL, Reed RB, Roche AF, Moore WM. Physical growth: National Center for Health Statistics percentiles. Am J Clin Nutr 1979; 32:607–629. Data from the Fels Research Institute, Wright State University School of Medicine, Yellow Springs, Ohio.
1982 ROSS LABORATORIES

**BOYS: BIRTH TO 36 MONTHS
PHYSICAL GROWTH
NCHS PERCENTILES**

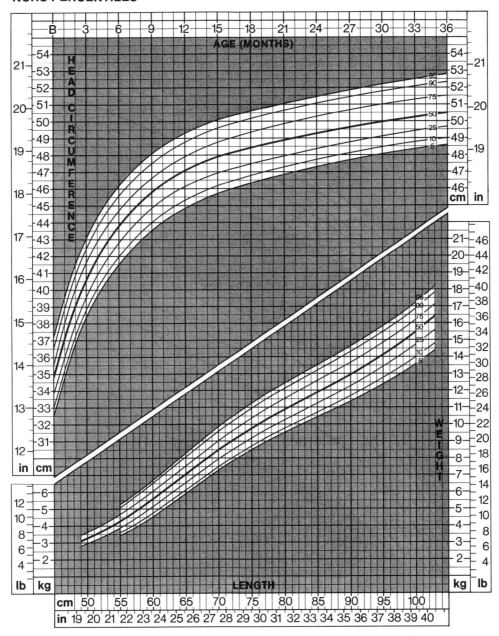

From Hamill PVV, Drizd TA, Johnson CL, Reed RB, Roche AF, Moore WM. Physical growth: National Center for Health Statistics percentiles. Am J Clin Nutr 1979; 32:607–629. Data from the Fels Research Institute, Wright State University School of Medicine, Yellow Springs, Ohio.
1982 ROSS LABORATORIES

GIRLS: BIRTH TO 36 MONTHS
PHYSICAL GROWTH
NCHS PERCENTILES

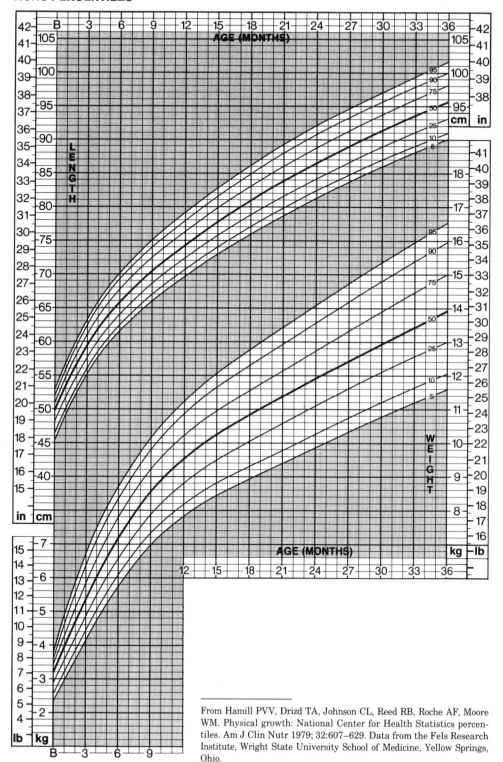

From Hamill PVV, Drizd TA, Johnson CL, Reed RB, Roche AF, Moore WM. Physical growth: National Center for Health Statistics percentiles. Am J Clin Nutr 1979; 32:607–629. Data from the Fels Research Institute, Wright State University School of Medicine, Yellow Springs, Ohio.

1982 ROSS LABORATORIES

GIRLS: BIRTH TO 36 MONTHS
PHYSICAL GROWTH
NCHS PERCENTILES

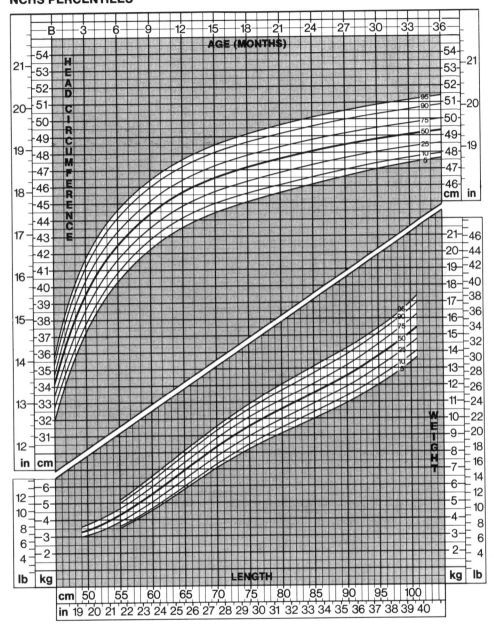

From Hamill PVV, Drizd TA, Johnson CL, Reed RB, Roche AF, Moore WM. Physical growth: National Center for Health Statistics percentiles. Am J Clin Nutr 1979; 32:607–629. Data from the Fels Research Institute, Wright State University School of Medicine, Yellow Springs, Ohio.
1982 ROSS LABORATORIES

BOYS: 2 TO 18 YEARS
PHYSICAL GROWTH
NCHS PERCENTILES

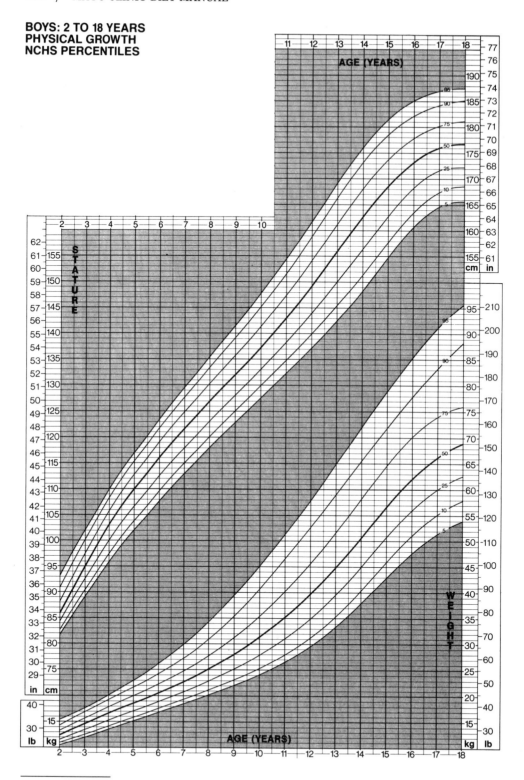

From Hamill PVV, Drizd TA, Johnson CL, Reed RB, Roche AF, Moore WM. Physical growth: National Center for Health Statistics percentiles. Am J Clin Nutr 1979; 32:607–629. Data from the Fels Research Institute, Wright State University School of Medicine, Yellow Springs, Ohio.
1982 ROSS LABORATORIES

**BOYS: PREPUBESCENT
PHYSICAL GROWTH
NCHS PERCENTILES**

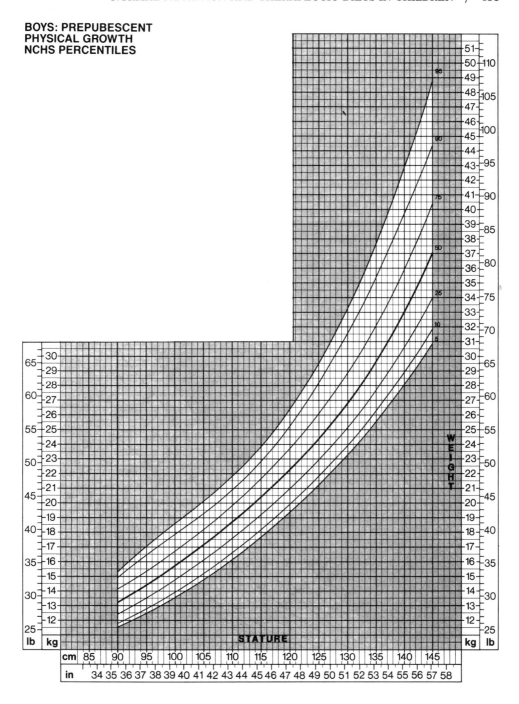

From Hamill PVV, Drizd TA, Johnson CL, Reed RB, Roche AF, Moore WM. Physical growth: National Center for Health Statistics percentiles. Am J Clin Nutr 1979; 32:607–629. Data from the Fels Research Institute, Wright State University School of Medicine, Yellow Springs, Ohio.
1982 ROSS LABORATORIES

GIRLS: 2 TO 18 YEARS
PHYSICAL GROWTH
NCHS PERCENTILES

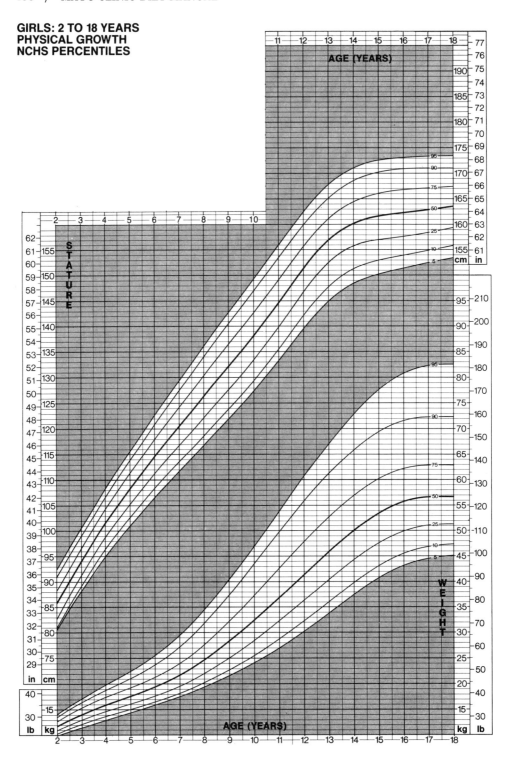

From Hamill PVV, Drizd TA, Johnson CL, Reed RB, Roche AF, Moore WM. Physical growth: National Center for Health Statistics percentiles. Am J Clin Nutr 1979; 32:607–629. Data from the Fels Research Institute, Wright State University School of Medicine, Yellow Springs, Ohio.
1982 ROSS LABORATORIES

**GIRLS: PREPUBESCENT
PHYSICAL GROWTH
NCHS PERCENTILES**

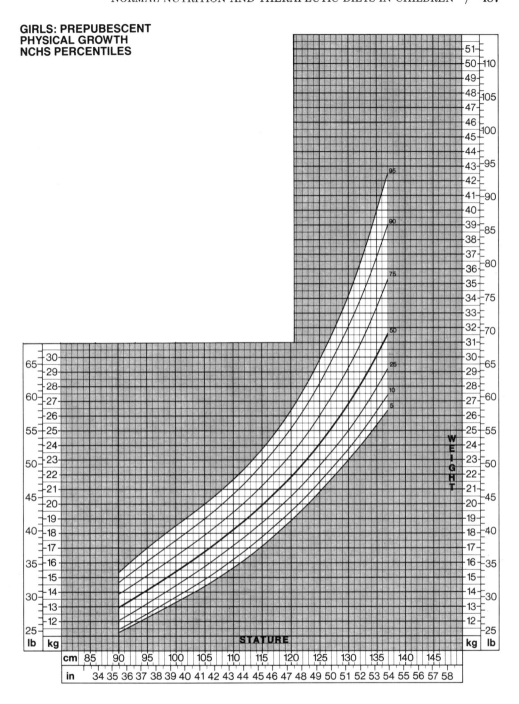

From Hamill PVV, Drizd TA, Johnson CL, Reed RB, Roche AF, Moore WM. Physical growth: National Center for Health Statistics percentiles. Am J Clin Nutr 1979; 32:607–629. Data from the Fels Research Institute, Wright State University School of Medicine, Yellow Springs, Ohio.
1982 ROSS LABORATORIES

APPENDIX 5

NATIONAL CENTER FOR HEALTH STATISTICS (NCHS) GROWTH TABLES*

PERCENTILES OF RECUMBENT LENGTH BY SEX AND AGE, BIRTH TO 36 MONTHS

Sex and age	Smoothed percentile						
	5th	10th	25th	50th	75th	90th	95th
Male	Recumbent length in centimeters						
Birth	46.4	47.5	49.0	50.5	51.8	53.5	54.4
1 month	50.4	51.3	53.0	54.6	56.2	57.7	58.6
3 months	56.7	57.7	59.4	61.1	63.0	64.5	65.4
6 months	63.4	64.4	66.1	67.8	69.7	71.3	72.3
9 months	68.0	69.1	70.6	72.3	74.0	75.9	77.1
12 months	71.7	72.8	74.3	76.1	77.7	79.8	81.2
18 months	77.5	78.7	80.5	82.4	84.3	86.6	88.1
24 months	82.3	83.5	85.6	87.6	89.9	92.2	93.8
30 months	87.0	88.2	90.1	92.3	94.6	97.0	98.7
36 months	91.2	92.4	94.2	96.5	98.9	101.4	103.1
Female							
Birth	45.4	46.5	48.2	49.9	51.0	52.0	52.9
1 month	49.2	50.2	51.9	53.5	54.9	56.1	56.9
3 months	55.4	56.2	57.8	59.5	61.2	62.7	63.4
6 months	61.8	62.6	64.2	65.9	67.8	69.4	70.2
9 months	66.1	67.0	68.7	70.4	72.4	74.0	75.0
12 months	69.8	70.8	72.4	74.3	76.3	78.0	79.1
18 months	76.0	77.2	78.8	80.9	83.0	85.0	86.1
24 months	81.3	82.5	84.2	86.5	88.7	90.8	92.0
30 months	86.0	87.0	88.9	91.3	93.7	95.6	96.9
36 months	90.0	91.0	93.1	95.6	98.1	100.0	101.5

PERCENTILES OF WEIGHT BY SEX AND AGE, BIRTH TO 36 MONTHS

Sex and age	Smoothed percentile						
	5th	10th	25th	50th	75th	90th	95th
Male	Weight in kilograms						
Birth	2.54	2.78	3.00	3.27	3.64	3.82	4.15
1 month	3.16	3.43	3.82	4.29	4.75	5.14	5.38
3 months	4.43	4.78	5.32	5.98	6.56	7.14	7.37
6 months	6.20	6.61	7.20	7.85	8.49	9.10	9.46
9 months	7.52	7.95	8.56	9.18	9.88	10.49	10.93
12 months	8.43	8.84	9.49	10.15	10.91	11.54	11.99
18 months	9.59	9.92	10.67	11.47	12.31	13.05	13.44
24 months	10.54	10.85	11.65	12.59	13.44	14.29	14.70
30 months	11.44	11.80	12.63	13.67	14.51	15.47	15.97
36 months	12.26	12.69	13.58	14.69	15.59	16.66	17.28
Female							
Birth	2.36	2.58	2.93	3.23	3.52	3.64	3.81
1 month	2.97	3.22	3.59	3.98	4.36	4.65	4.92
3 months	4.18	4.47	4.88	5.40	5.90	6.39	6.74
6 months	5.79	6.12	6.60	7.21	7.83	8.38	8.73
9 months	7.00	7.34	7.89	8.56	9.24	9.83	10.17
12 months	7.84	8.19	8.81	9.53	10.23	10.87	11.24
18 months	8.92	9.30	10.04	10.82	11.55	12.30	12.76
24 months	9.87	10.26	11.10	11.90	12.74	13.57	14.08
30 months	10.78	11.21	12.11	12.93	13.93	14.81	15.35
36 months	11.60	12.07	12.99	13.93	15.03	15.97	16.54

*From Hamill PVV, Drizd TA, Johnson CL, et al. NCHS growth curves for children birth–18 years. Vital Health Stat No. 165 1977, 11:1–74.

PERCENTILES OF STATURE BY SEX AND AGE, 2 THROUGH 24 YEARS

Sex and age	N	Observed percentile						
		5th	10th	25th	50th	75th	90th	95th
Male		Stature in centimeters						
2.00-2.25 years	419	82.6	83.5	86.1	87.8	90.3	91.9	97.3
2.25-2.75 years	945	86.1	87.0	89.0	91.2	93.8	97.3	98.3
2.75-3.25 years	785	88.9	90.5	92.4	95.1	97.2	100.1	101.2
3.25-3.75 years	857	92.1	93.3	95.7	98.2	101.1	102.8	104.4
3.75-4.25 years	856	96.2	97.3	100.0	102.6	105.3	107.5	110.8
4.25-4.75 years	937	98.0	100.2	103.4	105.8	108.6	111.8	113.2
4.75-5.25 years	874	100.7	103.2	105.5	108.8	112.4	115.4	116.5
5.25-5.75 years	878	106.2	107.7	110.1	113.5	116.1	118.2	119.5
5.75-6.25 years	908	108.5	110.1	112.8	117.0	119.4	122.2	123.1
6.25-6.75 years	1,033	108.9	110.0	114.8	118.2	121.9	125.0	127.1
6.75-7.25 years	988	114.1	115.6	118.5	122.3	125.9	128.3	129.8
7.25-7.75 years	1,120	115.6	118.3	120.8	174.5	127.9	131.4	133.4
7.75-8.25 years	1,014	119.3	121.0	123.8	127.9	131.7	134.9	138.0
8.25-8.75 years	902	121.2	123.4	126.2	129.6	133.2	136.4	138.8
8.75-9.25 years	943	121.1	124.5	127.5	132.8	136.3	139.4	141.9
9.25-9.75 years	958	125.2	127.7	131.2	135.0	138.7	142.7	144.7
9.75-10.25 years	1,030	127.3	130.0	133.7	138.6	142.1	145.9	149.0
10.25-10.75 years	1,070	130.5	132.5	135.8	139.4	144.1	148.4	151.4
10.75-11.25 years	1,052	132.5	135.3	138.7	143.5	147.9	151.4	154.0
11.25-11.75 years	952	135.1	138.0	141.4	145.8	150.8	154.5	156.1
11.75-12.25 years	1,010	138.5	140.1	144.1	148.6	153.7	159.4	162.6
12.25-12.75 years	1,092	139.3	141.8	146.4	152.1	157.2	162.6	165.5
12.75-13.25 years	1,155	142.2	144.8	149.7	154.8	159.6	165.3	167.8
13.25-13.75 years	1,056	145.6	148.6	153.6	160.0	166.5	172.2	175.5
13.75-14.25 years	954	149.2	153.0	157.7	164.4	169.9	175.1	177.6
14.25-14.75 years	1,019	152.9	156.4	161.1	167.6	173.1	177.8	179.4
14.75-15.25 years	1,112	155.0	157.6	163.0	169.4	173.8	178.2	181.8
15.25-15.75 years	914	158.8	161.4	166.6	171.6	175.4	180.4	183.4
15.75-16.25 years	1,051	160.5	164.3	169.0	173.5	177.8	181.5	185.8
16.25-16.75 years	876	163.8	165.5	170.6	174.9	179.5	183.3	186.4
16.75-17.25 years	1,054	164.4	166.2	170.7	176.8	181.8	184.6	187.3
17.25-17.75 years	935	163.3	167.7	172.1	176.4	181.0	185.0	187.8
17.75-18.25 years	866	166.5	170.1	173.1	176.0	180.2	186.1	187.3
18.25-19.00 years	1,067	166.8	169.3	172.0	175.8	180.1	185.9	186.8
19.00-20.00 years	1,770	162.8	166.9	171.6	177.2	180.8	185.0	186.2
20.00-21.00 years	1,668	159.4	168.4	172.2	177.4	181.2	183.6	185.8
21.00-22.00 years	1,703	166.2	168.3	172.5	177.3	181.1	184.8	190.0
22.00-23.00 years	1,662	167.2	167.7	171.3	177.1	180.6	187.1	192.0
23.00-24.00 years	1,589	161.3	165.3	172.3	176.8	183.0	188.5	189.2
24.00-25.00 years	1,595	165.4	168.5	172.9	178.1	183.0	186.7	189.5

PERCENTILES OF STATURE BY SEX AND AGE, 2 THROUGH 24 YEARS (Continued)

Sex and age	N	Observed percentile						
		5th	10th	25th	50th	75th	90th	95th
Female		Stature in centimeters						
2.00-2.25 years	440	81.3	82.5	84.6	86.8	89.9	93.6	94.6
2.25-2.75 years	972	84.2	85.3	87.1	90.3	93.4	94.8	96.4
2.75-3.25 years	622	90.2	90.7	92.7	95.3	96.7	99.1	100.6
3.25-3.75 years	887	91.8	92.8	95.0	97.4	99.8	102.1	103.6
3.75-4.25 years	775	94.8	96.2	97.9	100.5	103.8	106.0	108.2
4.25-4.75 years	848	96.8	97.6	100.5	103.8	106.2	109.4	112.0
4.75-5.25 years	876	99.1	101.1	105.2	108.1	111.6	113.7	114.7
5.25-5.75 years	890	103.8	106.1	108.4	111.8	115.5	118.7	121.3
5.75-6.25 years	866	107.1	109.0	111.9	115.4	118.8	122.1	124.6
6.25-6.75 years	1,025	109.3	111.6	114.3	117.7	121.7	125.2	126.9
6.75-7.25 years	945	111.7	113.2	117.4	120.8	124.3	126.8	128.6
7.25-7.75 years	952	115.8	117.2	120.0	123.7	127.9	131.7	134.2
7.75-8.25 years	1,004	117.8	119.5	122.8	127.5	130.6	132.9	134.6
8.25-8.75 years	968	118.9	121.4	124.4	129.2	133.4	135.8	138.0
8.75-9.25 years	988	122.2	124.8	128.4	132.7	137.7	141.0	142.3
9.25-9.75 years	885	126.6	127.6	131.1	135.1	139.8	144.4	147.6
9.75-10.25 years	1,092	129.0	130.3	134.4	138.5	143.0	147.0	149.8
10.25-10.75 years	1,086	129.4	131.1	135.2	140.6	144.7	149.8	152.4
10.75-11.25 years	870	132.1	134.8	139.5	143.9	148.8	153.7	157.0
11.25-11.75 years	862	134.5	135.8	141.7	147.3	152.6	157.1	158.8
11.75-12.25 years	1,082	139.4	142.2	146.7	151.8	156.4	161.4	165.9
12.25-12.75 years	1,019	141.7	145.9	150.8	154.8	159.7	164.0	165.7
12.75-13.25 years	1,058	143.7	147.7	153.0	157.5	161.4	165.5	167.4
13.25-13.75 years	1,120	149.4	151.6	155.4	159.6	163.8	165.9	169.2
13.75-14.25 years	1,080	149.8	151.6	155.7	160.0	163.4	167.1	168.7
14.25-14.75 years	951	150.3	153.2	157.4	161.6	165.4	169.5	171.1
14.75-15.25 years	1,012	151.5	153.3	157.2	161.2	166.3	171.2	174.9
15.25-15.75 years	980	152.6	154.8	157.9	162.9	167.6	172.1	176.2
15.75-16.25 years	959	152.5	154.8	158.2	163.6	167.7	170.7	172.3
16.25-16.75 years	836	150.7	153.3	157.6	162.1	166.5	171.5	172.6
16.75-17.25 years	1,108	151.8	154.6	158.0	161.8	166.5	171.6	173.8
17.25-17.75 years	810	150.7	154.3	158.0	162.6	166.6	170.0	172.5
17.75-18.25 years	826	152.2	155.5	159.8	163.9	168.0	171.0	171.8
18.25-19.00 years	1,420	154.9	157.8	161.2	165.3	167.2	172.4	174.2
19.00-20.00 years	1,384	155.0	155.9	159.9	163.0	166.8	170.6	173.1
20.00-21.00 years	1,771	152.3	155.1	159.0	163.2	168.8	172.4	175.3
21.00-22.00 years	1,818	152.0	154.6	158.5	162.5	167.0	170.8	173.0
22.00-23.00 years	1,734	150.4	153.0	156.9	162.8	167.2	171.2	174.5
23.00-24.00 years	1,800	154.2	156.0	158.6	163.1	166.8	170.5	172.6
24.00-25.00 years	1,796	152.3	155.4	158.3	162.3	167.4	170.4	171.6

PERCENTILES OF WEIGHT BY SEX AND AGE, 2 THROUGH 24 YEARS

Sex and age	N	Observed percentile						
		5th	10th	25th	50th	75th	90th	95th
Male		Weight in kilograms						
2.00-2.25 years	419	9.97	11.10	11.63	12.67	14.05	14.85	15.47
2.25-2.75 years	945	11.31	11.89	12.63	13.53	14.57	15.69	16.80
2.75-3.25 years	785	12.28	12.84	13.55	14.43	15.34	16.39	17.37
3.25-3.75 years	857	12.70	13.34	14.33	15.39	16.46	17.77	18.63
3.75-4.25 years	856	13.83	14.70	15.46	16.64	17.85	18.87	20.62
4.25-4.75 years	937	14.42	15.09	16.02	17.71	19.17	20.45	21.51
4.75-5.25 years	874	14.99	15.52	16.91	18.47	20.22	21.02	22.59
5.25-5.75 years	878	17.01	17.31	18.33	19.88	21.39	23.21	25.32
5.75-6.25 years	908	16.87	17.80	19.53	21.21	22.85	24.98	26.40
6.25-6.75 years	1,033	17.21	17.82	19.70	21.59	23.41	26.21	28.18
6.75-7.25 years	992	18.59	19.39	21.37	22.93	25.22	28.74	30.72
7.25-7.75 years	1,120	18.76	20.07	22.04	24.33	26.48	29.08	32.31
7.75-8.25 years	1,014	20.20	21.47	23.47	25.65	28.70	31.36	35.15
8.25-8.75 years	902	21.71	22.63	24.35	26.31	29.27	33.08	34.96
8.75-9.25 years	943	22.01	22.98	25.13	27.89	31.75	36.62	40.23
9.25-9.75 years	958	23.11	24.30	26.40	29.65	33.63	38.58	45.67
9.75-10.25 years	1,030	24.40	25.63	27.98	31.83	36.09	41.08	43.69
10.25-10.75 years	1,070	26.09	27.73	29.49	32.57	36.39	40.75	45.66
10.75-11.25 years	1,052	27.98	28.79	31.23	35.86	39.68	44.71	51.83
11.25-11.75 years	952	28.17	30.14	34.07	37.48	41.94	47.16	52.45
11.75-12.25 years	1,010	30.10	31.18	34.21	38.75	46.43	55.24	62.43
12.25-12.75 years	1,092	31.72	32.98	36.18	41.98	47.30	54.05	58.45
12.75-13.25 years	1,155	32.17	34.61	38.43	43.62	50.17	59.22	64.29
13.25-13.75 years	1,056	36.24	37.80	42.92	49.23	58.38	63.44	68.39
13.75-14.25 years	954	38.25	41.47	46.98	51.65	60.77	67.04	76.61
14.25-14.75 years	1,019	40.52	43.64	49.70	55.32	62.62	72.69	77.03
14.75-15.25 years	1,112	42.14	44.93	50.35	56.35	63.63	71.27	76.91
15.25-15.75 years	914	46.26	49.12	54.29	58.92	66.68	75.40	81.81
15.75-16.25 years	1,051	46.83	51.29	55.79	61.74	69.33	76.78	86.07
16.25-16.75 years	876	50.46	53.22	56.77	64.71	72.28	81.62	87.57
16.75-17.25 years	1,054	52.15	55.42	60.65	65.90	73.76	81.72	91.23
17.25-17.75 years	935	51.80	55.53	60.81	66.64	75.36	83.35	92.16
17.75-18.25 years	866	54.76	58.18	62.04	68.96	75.49	88.36	94.71
18.25-19.00 years	1,067	54.96	60.35	63.62	69.88	78.67	92.66	99.60
19.00-20.00 years	1,770	55.40	57.38	65.91	70.66	76.43	87.01	96.48
20.00-21.00 years	1,668	55.86	57.71	65.04	71.89	78.44	88.86	94.84
21.00-22.00 years	1,703	52.66	58.17	65.29	72.12	80.96	89.04	96.13
22.00-23.00 years	1,662	55.02	59.14	65.09	71.77	79.66	90.57	96.93
23.00-24.00 years	1,589	59.16	60.69	65.54	74.71	82.44	94.05	105.35
24.00-25.00 years	1,595	60.87	63.96	67.96	79.37	85.69	97.60	103.19

PERCENTILES OF WEIGHT BY SEX AND AGE,
2 THROUGH 24 YEARS (Continued)

Sex and age	N	Observed percentile						
		5th	10th	25th	50th	75th	90th	95th
Female		Weight in kilograms						
2.00-2.25 years	440	10.06	10.66	11.41	12.21	12.86	13.84	14.57
2.25-2.75 years	972	10.77	11.20	11.98	12.76	13.94	14.74	15.09
2.75-3.25 years	622	12.14	12.40	13.12	13.93	15.61	16.84	17.74
3.25-3.75 years	887	12.29	13.03	13.58	14.60	15.93	17.54	18.28
3.75-4.25 years	775	13.13	13.63	14.51	15.68	17.15	18.22	18.94
4.25-4.75 years	848	13.45	14.05	15.04	16.57	17.78	19.35	20.26
4.75-5.25 years	876	14.33	15.21	16.48	17.73	19.66	21.23	22.10
5.25-5.75 years	890	15.18	16.20	17.47	18.92	20.96	23.44	25.01
5.75-6.25 years	866	15.99	17.09	18.21	20.19	22.39	24.88	28.71
6.25-6.75 years	1,025	17.02	17.71	19.24	21.06	23.55	26.17	27.89
6.75-7.25 years	945	17.86	18.74	20.20	22.13	23.98	26.91	29.58
7.25-7.75 years	952	18.84	19.60	21.33	23.72	26.54	29.61	31.55
7.75-8.25 years	1,004	20.11	20.79	22.49	24.89	27.73	32.63	35.20
8.25-8.75 years	968	20.47	21.50	23.30	26.39	29.69	33.65	36.45
8.75-9.25 years	988	22.20	23.17	25.27	28.79	33.40	39.66	42.69
9.25-9.75 years	885	23.29	24.72	26.92	30.26	34.54	39.87	43.62
9.75-10.25 years	1,092	24.34	25.25	28.03	31.68	36.38	43.16	45.92
10.25-10.75 years	1,086	25.28	26.69	29.42	33.00	37.63	45.90	48.37
10.75-11.25 years	870	26.73	28.32	32.09	36.13	42.27	47.72	54.49
11.25-11.75 years	862	27.44	29.45	32.88	37.97	44.38	50.77	58.09
11.75-12.25 years	1,082	29.72	32.74	36.42	41.70	48.78	57.77	64.79
12.25-12.75 years	1,019	32.59	34.97	39.46	45.37	51.40	58.10	63.21
12.75-13.25 years	1,058	34.21	37.17	41.44	47.06	54.79	62.20	66.61
13.25-13.75 years	1,120	37.72	39.45	45.00	50.30	56.81	67.05	75.78
13.75-14.25 years	1,080	37.74	39.86	44.86	50.22	56.44	66.44	74.70
14.25-14.75 years	951	40.77	42.96	47.21	53.03	60.95	68.88	78.43
14.75-15.25 years	1,012	41.14	43.65	47.48	53.29	59.72	71.57	75.36
15.25-15.75 years	980	42.99	46.11	48.98	55.25	60.80	71.45	77.78
15.75-16.25 years	959	43.64	45.74	49.22	54.92	61.58	67.70	78.03
16.25-16.75 years	836	43.86	45.69	49.46	54.97	62.64	72.37	83.10
16.75-17.25 years	1,108	43.87	45.57	50.76	56.49	62.22	72.45	84.19
17.25-17.75 years	810	42.90	45.36	50.56	55.23	61.59	70.62	84.82
17.75-18.25 years	826	45.05	47.89	52.68	57.68	62.32	69.62	75.86
18.25-19.00 years	1,420	44.83	45.89	51.03	56.97	63.16	72.62	78.70
19.00-20.00 years	1,384	48.65	48.83	51.62	57.24	63.48	76.33	83.48
20.00-21.00 years	1,771	44.40	47.23	51.70	57.22	63.94	72.15	75.89
21.00-22.00 years	1,818	46.08	48.54	52.15	58.36	64.64	72.88	81.76
22.00-23.00 years	1,734	42.86	46.18	51.35	58.82	67.38	75.54	85.35
23.00-24.00 years	1,800	45.59	47.77	52.16	59.87	64.64	72.80	84.62
24.00-25.00 years	1,796	46.65	48.13	52.06	58.88	66.33	77.17	86.04

PERCENTILES OF WEIGHT BY SEX AND STATURE

Sex and stature	N	Observed percentile						
		5th	10th	25th	50th	75th	90th	95th
Male, 2-11.5 years		Weight in kilograms						
90-92 centimeters	330	12.02	12.22	12.81	13.80	14.90	15.56	15.79
92-94 centimeters	451	12.06	12.22	12.71	13.51	14.61	15.51	15.81
94-96 centimeters	451	12.31	12.66	13.68	14.66	15.46	15.94	16.61
96-98 centimeters	555	12.31	13.08	14.28	15.04	15.80	17.12	17.77
98-100 centimeters	359	13.70	14.05	14.50	15.26	16.10	18.04	19.06
100-102 centimeters	557	13.92	14.20	14.82	15.87	17.12	17.88	18.96
102-104 centimeters	414	14.31	14.64	15.63	16.66	17.51	18.19	19.30
104-106 centimeters	561	14.45	14.91	16.14	17.16	18.30	19.33	19.67
106-108 centimeters	553	15.51	15.83	16.56	17.70	18.98	19.76	20.53
108-110 centimeters	702	16.20	16.43	17.10	18.31	19.77	22.13	23.16
110-112 centimeters	641	16.15	16.50	17.57	18.83	19.91	21.50	22.37
112-114 centimeters	706	16.94	17.78	18.66	19.85	21.27	22.63	23.85
114-116 centimeters	912	18.04	18.32	19.16	20.41	21.39	21.98	23.22
116-118 centimeters	1,013	18.36	18.80	20.06	21.03	22.01	23.41	23.88
118-120 centimeters	1,284	18.43	19.01	20.29	21.43	22.81	23.76	24.64
120-122 centimeters	1,194	19.49	20.23	21.31	22.85	24.40	25.76	26.85
122-124 centimeters	1,430	20.42	21.12	22.42	23.62	25.19	26.78	27.95
124-126 centimeters	647	21.50	22.19	22.95	24.33	26.15	27.80	30.14
126-128 centimeters	1,565	22.30	22.92	24.31	25.55	27.31	29.91	31.05
128-130 centimeters	1,277	22.84	23.91	24.79	26.22	28.32	31.31	34.33
130-132 centimeters	1,524	23.96	24.35	25.41	27.29	29.35	31.17	31.96
132-134 centimeters	1,443	24.45	25.33	26.74	28.54	31.33	34.75	35.82
134-136 centimeters	1,554	24.65	25.46	27.45	29.55	32.18	37.22	39.83
136-138 centimeters	1,281	26.47	27.21	28.68	30.52	33.40	36.53	37.73
138-140 centimeters	1,184	28.11	28.48	29.59	31.91	33.85	37.25	39.62
140-142 centimeters	1,356	28.65	29.46	31.19	33.87	36.81	40.96	48.32
142-144 centimeters	1,043	29.82	31.10	32.82	35.24	38.80	42.37	44.39
144-146 centimeters	709	30.45	31.47	34.24	37.28	40.89	44.51	48.88
Female, 2-10 years								
90-92 centimeters	332	11.73	12.08	12.46	13.08	13.70	14.71	15.84
92-94 centimeters	429	12.04	12.19	12.66	13.45	14.51	15.51	15.85
94-96 centimeters	566	12.08	12.30	12.97	14.09	15.25	15.94	16.49
96-98 centimeters	608	13.08	13.22	13.66	14.53	15.49	16.35	17.21
98-100 centimeters	522	12.49	12.99	14.20	15.17	16.33	17.57	17.99
100-102 centimeters	421	14.03	14.26	14.95	16.12	17.36	18.79	22.16
102-104 centimeters	425	14.14	14.38	15.09	16.32	17.62	18.92	19.50
104-106 centimeters	524	14.38	14.95	16.19	17.00	17.81	19.08	19.66
106-108 centimeters	522	14.81	15.73	16.47	17.34	18.46	19.51	19.86
108-110 centimeters	533	14.55	15.40	16.42	17.33	18.55	19.78	20.87
110-112 centimeters	651	16.09	16.36	17.16	18.42	19.51	20.64	21.45
112-114 centimeters	793	16.28	16.92	18.30	19.41	20.89	22.04	23.14
114-116 centimeters	909	17.35	18.13	18.81	19.95	21.34	22.70	23.79
116-118 centimeters	1,099	18.09	18.37	19.23	20.63	21.93	23.65	25.07
118-120 centimeters	1,162	18.39	18.86	20.15	21.40	23.18	25.02	25.90
120-122 centimeters	1,277	19.43	20.16	21.09	22.56	23.90	25.65	27.36
122-124 centimeters	1,246	19.96	20.39	21.59	23.02	24.61	26.58	28.67
124-126 centimeters	1,319	20.47	21.47	22.59	23.77	25.72	27.74	29.72
126-128 centimeters	1,219	21.53	22.25	23.28	25.35	27.42	29.51	31.19
128-130 centimeters	1,327	22.52	23.28	24.62	26.21	28.73	31.21	33.04
130-132 centimeters	1,102	23.66	24.30	25.39	27.20	29.73	33.45	35.21
132-134 centimeters	1,088	24.47	25.30	26.67	28.42	32.47	35.43	38.82
134-136 centimeters	969	25.25	26.30	28.18	30.51	33.03	36.17	39.20
136-138 centimeters	667	26.05	26.75	28.47	30.70	34.32	37.65	42.36
138-140 centimeters	...	...	...	...	...	...	...	...
140-142 centimeters	...	...	...	...	...	...	...	...
142-144 centimeters	...	...	...	...	...	...	...	...
144-146 centimeters	...	...	...	...	...	...	...	...

APPENDIX 6
BALDWIN-WOOD TABLES

Weight-for-Height in older children

Height (cm)	8	9	10	11	12	13	14	15	16	17	18	19
						MALES						
140	*31.6	31.6	32.2	32.2	32.4	32.4	*32.5					
141	*32.1	32.3	32.9	32.8	32.9	33.2	*33.1					
142	*32.6	33.1	33.7	33.5	33.4	34.0	*33.7					
143		*33.6	34.1	34.2	34.1	34.7	34.5	*35.3				
144		*34.1	34.4	35.0	34.7	35.2	35.5	*35.8				
145		*35.6	34.9	35.7	35.4	35.8	36.3	*36.3				
146		*36.3	35.7	36.2	36.2	36.5	36.9	*37.0				
147		*34.0	36.5	36.7	36.9	37.1	37.4	*37.7				
148			37.0	37.2	37.6	37.8	38.0	38.2				
149			37.5	37.8	38.2	38.4	38.6	38.7				
150			38.1	38.5	39.0	39.1	39.3	39.3	39.2			
151			*38.7	39.2	39.5	39.7	40.0	40.3	40.3			
152			*39.4	39.9	40.0	40.3	40.7	41.3	41.5			
153				40.5	40.6	41.1	41.6	42.1	42.6			
154				41.0	41.4	41.9	42.5	42.8	43.7			
155				41.5	42.1	42.7	43.4	43.5	44.8	*46.3		
156				*42.3	42.9	43.4	44.0	44.2	45.5	*47.2		
157				*43.2	43.8	44.1	44.7	44.9	46.3	48.1		
158				*44.0	44.6	44.9	45.5	45.8	47.3	49.2	*51.3	
159				*44.9	45.4	45.8	46.4	46.9	48.6	50.3	*52.6	
160				*45.8	46.2	46.7	47.4	48.0	49.8	51.5	53.9	*55.4
161					47.4	47.3	48.1	48.8	50.2	52.0	54.4	*55.9
162					48.7	48.0	48.8	49.6	50.6	52.5	54.9	*56.4
163					49.4	48.8	49.6	50.5	51.2	53.2	55.5	*57.0
164					*49.6	49.9	50.5	51.4	52.1	54.1	56.3	*57.7
165					*49.7	50.9	51.4	52.3	53.1	55.1	57.1	58.3
166						51.4	52.1	53.2	54.1	56.1	57.9	59.3
167						51.8	52.9	54.0	55.1	57.0	58.7	60.3
168						52.3	53.7	54.8	56.1	57.8	59.4	61.0
169						*53.1	54.7	55.7	57.1	58.5	60.0	61.4
170						*53.9	55.6	56.5	58.1	59.1	60.5	61.7
171							56.7	57.3	58.8	59.9	61.2	62.5
172							57.8	58.0	59.5	60.9	62.0	63.4
173							58.7	58.7	60.2	61.8	62.8	64.2
174							59.2	59.6	61.1	62.7	63.8	65.1
175							59.7	60.4	61.9	63.5	64.7	65.9
176							60.5	61.2	62.5	64.0	65.3	66.5
177							61.4	62.0	62.9	64.3	65.7	67.2
178							62.4	62.8	63.4	64.7	66.1	67.8
179							*63.3	63.9	64.5	65.4	66.6	68.4
180							*64.2	65.1	65.7	66.1	67.1	68.8
181								65.8	66.4	66.7	67.7	69.6
182								66.3	67.0	67.3	68.3	70.4
183								66.9	67.6	68.0	69.0	71.2
184								*67.5	68.6	69.1	70.1	71.8
185								*68.2	69.5	70.3	71.3	72.5
186								*68.8	70.3	71.3	72.2	73.2
187								*69.3	71.0	72.3	73.1	73.8
188								*69.8	71.7	73.3	73.9	74.4

Starred (*) figures represent values based on theoretical computations rather than on exact ages. Age is taken at the nearest birthday, height at the nearest centimeter, and weight at the nearest tenth of a kilogram.

With permission from Jellifee DB. The assessment of the nutritional status of the community. Monograph No. 53. Geneva: World Health Organization, 1966.

PEDIATRIC APPENDIX 6

BALDWIN-WOOD TABLES

Weight-for-Height in older children

Height (cm)	8	9	10	11	12	13	14	15	16	17	18	19
						FEMALES						
138	*30.9	31.6	31.6	31.9	32.0	32.8						
139	*31.4	32.3	32.3	32.5	32.6	33.4						
140		32.9	32.9	33.1	33.2	34.1	*34.8					
141		33.3	33.6	33.7	34.0	34.9	*35.6					
142		33.6	34.4	34.3	34.8	35.8	*36.5					
143		*34.2	35.1	35.0	35.5	36.3	*37.4					
144		*34.9	35.9	35.6	36.0	36.7	*38.4					
145			36.6	36.4	36.6	37.2	39.3	*41.1				
146			36.8	37.3	37.3	38.0	40.3	*42.0				
147			37.1	38.2	37.9	38.8	41.4	*42.8				
148			37.6	38.9	38.6	39.5	42.0	*43.5	*45.1			
149			38.2	39.5	39.2	40.3	42.5	*44.0	*45.5			
150			38.8	40.2	39.9	41.1	43.0	44.6	*45.9	*46.4		
151			*39.5	41.0	40.8	41.9	43.8	45.5	*46.8	47.3		
152			*40.2	41.8	41.7	42.7	44.6	46.4	*47.7	48.1		
153				42.6	42.7	43.5	45.4	47.1	48.6	*48.9	*49.9	
154				43.4	43.8	44.2	46.2	47.6	49.4	49.7	*50.7	
155				44.0	44.8	45.0	47.0	48.1	50.2	50.4	51.4	
156				*44.1	45.5	45.7	47.5	48.9	50.7	51.1	51.7	
157				*44.2	46.2	46.5	48.1	49.8	51.1	51.8	52.0	
158					47.0	47.4	48.7	50.5	51.4	52.2	52.4	
159					47.9	48.3	49.2	51.0	51.7	52.5	52.7	
160					48.9	49.2	49.8	51.5	51.9	52.8	53.1	
161					*49.6	49.9	50.7	52.1	52.6	53.3	53.6	
162					*50.3	50.6	51.5	52.7	53.2	53.7	54.0	
163					*51.0	51.4	52.3	53.3	53.8	54.2	54.6	
164					*51.7	52.2	53.2	53.7	54.3	54.8	55.3	
165					*52.4	53.1	54.0	54.2	54.8	55.4	55.9	
166						54.0	54.5	54.6	55.7	56.1	56.6	
167						54.9	54.9	55.0	56.6	56.9	57.4	
168						*55.6	55.5	55.7	57.4	57.6	58.2	
169						*56.2	56.6	56.9	58.2	58.2	59.2	
170						*56.8	57.6	58.0	58.9	58.9	60.1	
171						*57.2	58.2	58.8	59.5	59.7	60.7	
172						*57.8	58.7	59.5	60.0	60.7	61.1	
173							59.1	60.1	60.5	61.4	61.6	
174							*59.6	*60.5	*60.9	*61.8	*62.3	
175							*60.0	*60.8	*61.2	*62.1	*62.9	
176							*60.2	*61.0	*61.6	*62.5	*63.4	
177							*60.4	*61.2	*62.0	*62.8	*63.7	
178							*60.6	*61.5	*62.4	*63.2	*64.0	
179							*60.9	*61.8	*62.7	*63.5	*64.2	
180							*61.3	*62.2	*63.0	*63.9	*64.4	

Starred (*) figures represent values based on theoretical computations rather than on exact ages. Age is taken at the nearest birthday, height at the nearest centimeter, and weight at the nearest tenth of a kilogram.

With permission from Jelliffe DB. The assessement of the nutritional status of the community. Monograph No. 53. Geneva: World Health Organization, 1966.

APPENDIX 7

GROWTH CHARTS FOR CHILDREN WITH DOWN SYNDROME

GIRLS WITH DOWN SYNDROME PHYSICAL GROWTH 1 TO 36 MONTHS

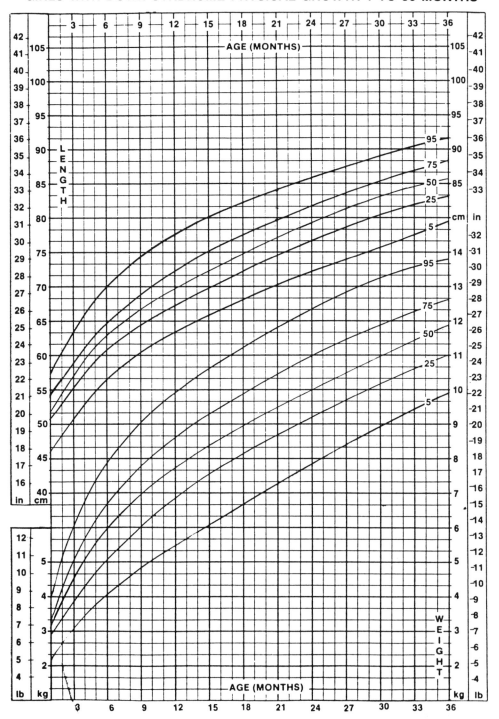

Growth Charts for Girls with Down Syndrome
1 to 36 Months

This chart provides reference percentiles for girls with Down syndrome birth to 36 months of age. It is based on mixed longitudinal data on approximately 300 girls with Down syndrome born between 1960 and 1986 and reared at home. Children with congenital heart disease are included in the sample. The centile rank for a given child indicates the relative position she would hold in a series of 100 girls with Down syndrome. For example, a girl at 10th centile is larger than 10% and smaller than 90% of girls her age with Down syndrome. Fiftieth (50th) centile is the midposition, and equivalent to "average" height or weight for a girl with Down syndrome.

These charts correct for both the smaller size and slower growth rate of girls with Down syndrome and a girl with Down syndrome would be expected to conform better to centile channels on this chart than those on the NCHS charts. However, because deficiencies in growth velocity occur at varying times, and are of widely different magnitudes, a child may not remain in a single growth channel on this chart. Downward centile shifts are common between 6 and 36 months of age.

Children with moderate or severe heart disease show greater growth deficiencies than those without or with only mild heart disease during the first three years of life. On the average girls with significant cardiac disease are 1.5 cm smaller than those without or with only mild disease beginning in the first six months of life. As with normal children with heart disease, catch-up growth may occur following surgical repair or spontaneous closure of the lesion.

Weight gain for children with Down syndrome is more rapid than height growth. This often results in overweight by 36 months of age. The etiology of this problem is not well understood, but may relate to decreased activity level and/or appetite disorder. Because the present chart reflects this tendency to overweight, it should always be used in conjunction with charts for normal children when assessing body weight.

Growth Record

Date	Age	Height	Weight	Date	Age	Height	Weight

Based on data from the Developmental Evaluation Clinic of the Children's Hospital, Boston, The Child Development Center of Rhode Island Hospital, and the Clinical Genetics Service of the Children's Hospital of Philadelphia
© C.E. Cronk, A.C. Crocker, S.M. Pueschel and E. Zachai

Girls with Down Syndrome Physical Growth: 2 to 18 Years

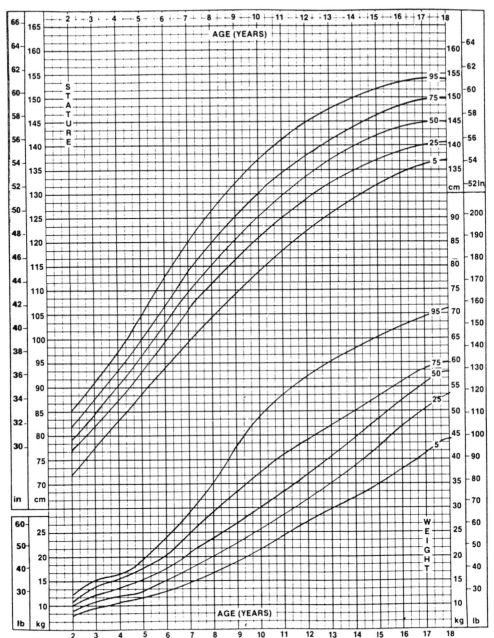

Growth Charts for Girls with Down Syndrome
2 to 18 Years

This chart provides reference percentiles for girls with Down syndrome 2 to 18 years of age. It is based on mixed longitudinal data on approximately 300 girls with Down syndrome born between 1960 and 1984 and reared at home. Children with congenital heart disease are included in the sample. The centile rank for a given child indicates the relative position she would hold in a series of 100 girls with Down syndrome. For example, a girl at 10th centile is larger than 10% and smaller than 90% of girls her age with Down syndrome. Fiftieth (50th) centile is the midposition, and equivalent to "average" height or weight for a girl with Down syndrome.

These charts correct for both the smaller size and slower growth rate of girls with Down syndrome and a girl with Down syndrome would be expected to conform better to centile channels on this chart than those on the NCHS charts. During the childhood years, girls with Down syndrome grow very similarly to normal girls. However at adolescence, their growth spurts tend to occur slightly later than normal, and are not as dramatic as those seen in normal girls. Some girls with Down syndrome do not exhibit an adolescent growth spurt.

Children with moderate or severe heart disease show greater growth deficiencies than those without or with only mild heart disease. On the average girls with significant cardiac disease are 1.5 cm smaller than those without or with only mild disease beginning in the first six months of life and continuing up through the adolescent period. As with normal children with heart disease, catch-up growth may occur following surgical repair or spontaneous closure of the lesion.

Weight gain for children with Down syndrome is more rapid than height growth. This often results in overweight by 36 months of age which is often enhanced during adolescence. The etiology of this problem is not well understood, but may relate to decreased activity level and/or appetite disorder. Because the present chart reflects this tendency to overweight, particularly in values for the 90th and 95th centiles, it should always be used in conjunction with charts for normal children when assessing body weight.

Growth Record

Date	Age	Height	Weight	Date	Age	Height	Weight

Based on data from the Developmental Evaluation Clinic of the Children's Hospital, Boston, The Child Development Center of Rhode Island Hospital, and the Clinical Genetics Service of the Children's Hospital of Philadelphia
© C.E. Cronk, A.C. Crocker, S.M. Pueschel and E. Zachai
Supported by March of Dimes grant 6-449.

Boys with Down Syndrome Physical Growth: 1 to 36 Months

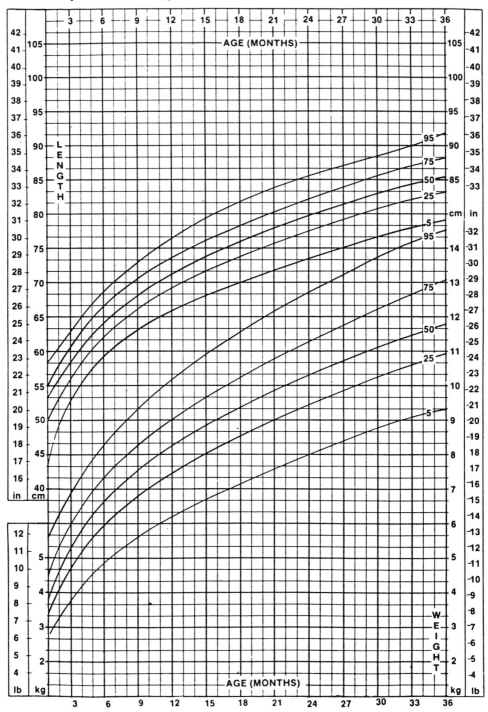

Growth Charts for Boys with Down Syndrome
1 to 36 Months

This chart provides reference percentiles for boys with Down syndrome birth to 36 months of age. It is based on mixed longitudinal data for approximately 400 boys with Down syndrome born between 1960 and 1986 and reared at home.

Children with congenital heart disease are included in the sample. The centile rank for a given child indicates the relative position he would hold in a series of 100 boys with Down syndrome. For example, a boy at 10th centile is larger than 10% and smaller than 90% of boys his age with Down syndrome. Fiftieth (50th) centile is the midposition, and equivalent to "average" height or weight for a boy with Down syndrome.

These charts correct for both the smaller size and slower growth rate of boys with Down syndrome and a boy with Down syndrome would be expected to conform better to centile channels on this chart than those on the NCHS charts. However, because deficiencies in growth velocity occur at varying times, and are of widely different magnitudes, a child may not remain in a single growth channel on this chart. Downward centile shifts are common between 6 and 36 months of age.

Children with moderate or severe heart disease show greater growth deficiencies than those without or with only mild heart disease during the first three years of life. On the average boys with significant cardiac disease are 2 cm smaller than those without or with only mild disease beginning in the first six months of life. As with normal children with heart disease, catch-up growth may occur following surgical repair or spontaneous closure of the lesion.

Weight gain for children with Down syndrome is more rapid than height growth. This often results in overweight by 36 months of age. The etiology of this problem is not well understood, but may relate to decreased activity level and/or appetite disorder. Because the present chart reflects this tendency to overweight, it should always be used in conjunction with charts for normal children when assessing body weight.

Growth Record

Date	Age	Height	Weight	Date	Age	Height	Weight

Based on data from the Developmental Evaluation Clinic of the Children's Hospital, Boston, The Child Development Center of Rhode Island Hospital, and the Clinical Genetics Service of the Children's Hospital of Philadelphia
© C.E. Cronk, A.C. Crocker, S.M. Pueschel and E. Zachai
Supported by March of Dimes grant 6-449.

Boys with Down Syndrome Physical Growth: 2 to 18 Years

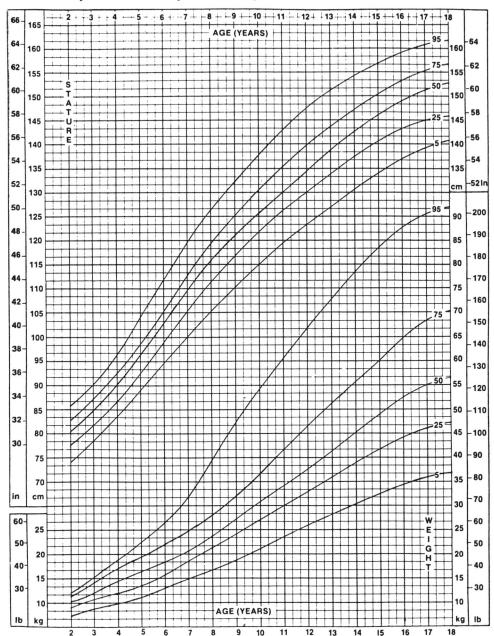

Growth Charts for Boys with Down Syndrome
2 to 18 Years

This chart provides reference percentiles for boys with Down syndrome 2 to 18 years of age. It is based on mixed longitudinal data for approximately 400 boys with Down syndrome born between 1960 and 1984 and reared at home. Children with congenital heart disease are included in the sample. The centile rank for a given child indicates the relative position he would hold in a series of 100 boys with Down syndrome. For example, a boy at 10th centile is larger than 10% and smaller than 90% of boys his age with Down syndrome. Fiftieth (50th) centile is the midposition, and equivalent to "average" height or weight for a boy with Down syndrome.

These charts correct for both the smaller size and slower growth rate of boys with Down syndrome and a boy with Down syndrome would be expected to conform better to centile channels on this chart than those on the NCHS charts. During the childhood years, boys with Down Syndrome grow very similarly to normal boys. However at adolescence, their growth spurts tend to occur slightly later than normal, and are not as dramatic as those seen in normal boys. A small percentage of boys with Down syndrome do not have an adolescent growth spurt.

Children with moderate or severe heart disease show greater growth deficiencies than those without or with only mild heart disease during the first three years of life. On the average boys with significant cardiac disease are 2 cm smaller than those without or with only mild disease beginning in the first six months of life and continuing up through the adolescent period. As with normal children with heart disease, catch-up growth may occur following surgical repair or spontaneous closure of the lesion.

Weight gain for children with Down syndrome is more rapid than height growth. This often results in overweight by 36 months of age which is often enhanced during adolescence. The etiology of this problem is not well understood, but may relate to decreased activity level and/or appetite disorder. Because the present chart reflects this tendency to overweight, particularly in values for the 90th and 95th centiles, it should always be used in conjunction with charts for normal children when assessing body weight.

Growth Record

Data	Age	Height	Weight	Date	Age	Height	Weight

Based on data from the Developmental Evaluation Clinic of the Children's Hospital, Boston, The Child Development Center of Rhode Island Hospital, and the Clinical Genetics Service of the Children's Hospital of Philadelphia
© C.E. Cronk, A.C. Crocker, S.M. Pueschel and E. Zachai
Supported by March of Dimes grant 6-449.

APPENDIX 8

GROWTH CHART FOR PREMATURE INFANTS*
Birth to 1 Year Sexes Combined

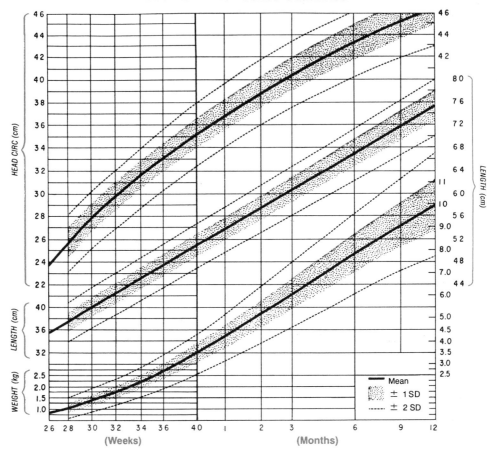

*Adapted with permission from Babson SG, Benda GI. Growth graphs for the clinical assessment of infants of varying gestational age. J. Pediatr 1976; 89:814–820.
1985 Ross Laboratories.

APPENDIX 9

TRICEPS SKIN FOLD PERCENTILES*

Percentiles for triceps skinfold for whites, ages 1 through 18, of the United States Health and Nutrition Examination Survey I of 1971 to 1974

	Triceps Skinfold Percentiles (mm²)														
Age group	n	5	10	25	50	75	90	95	n	5	10	25	50	75	90	95
	Males								Females							
1–1.9	228	6	7	8	10	12	14	16	204	6	7	8	10	12	14	16
2–2.9	223	6	7	8	10	12	14	15	208	6	8	9	10	12	15	16
3–3.9	220	6	7	8	10	11	14	15	208	7	8	9	11	12	14	15
4–4.9	230	6	6	8	9	11	12	14	208	7	8	8	10	12	14	16
5–5.9	214	6	6	8	9	11	14	15	219	6	7	8	10	12	15	18
6–6.9	117	5	6	7	8	10	13	16	118	6	6	8	10	12	14	16
7–7.9	122	5	6	7	9	12	15	17	126	6	7	9	11	13	16	18
8–8.9	117	5	6	7	8	10	13	16	118	6	8	9	12	15	18	24
9–9.9	121	6	6	7	10	13	17	18	125	8	8	10	13	16	20	22
10–10.9	146	6	6	8	10	14	18	21	152	7	8	10	12	17	23	27
11–11.9	122	6	6	8	11	16	20	24	117	7	8	10	13	18	24	28
12–12.9	153	6	6	8	11	14	22	28	129	8	9	11	14	18	23	27
13–13.9	134	5	5	7	10	14	22	26	151	8	8	12	15	21	26	30
14–14.9	131	4	5	7	9	14	21	24	141	9	10	13	16	21	26	28
15–15.9	128	4	5	6	8	11	18	24	117	8	10	12	17	21	25	32
16–16.9	131	4	5	6	8	12	16	22	142	10	12	15	18	22	26	31
17–17.9	133	5	5	6	8	12	16	19	114	10	12	13	19	24	30	37

*With permission from Frisancho AR. New norms of upper limb fat and muscle areas for assessment of nutritional status. Am J Clin Nutr 1981;34:2540–2545.

APPENDIX 10

NOMOGRAM FOR ANTHROPOMETRY FOR CHILDREN*

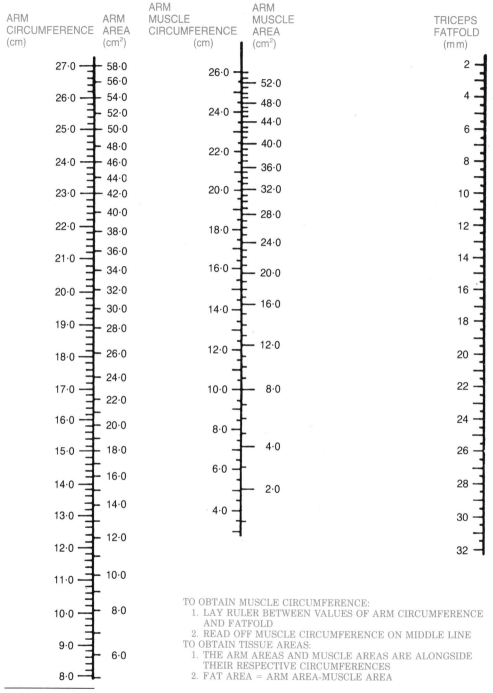

ARM CIRCUMFERENCE (cm)

ARM AREA (cm²)

ARM MUSCLE CIRCUMFERENCE (cm)

ARM MUSCLE AREA (cm²)

TRICEPS FATFOLD (mm)

TO OBTAIN MUSCLE CIRCUMFERENCE:
1. LAY RULER BETWEEN VALUES OF ARM CIRCUMFERENCE AND FATFOLD
2. READ OFF MUSCLE CIRCUMFERENCE ON MIDDLE LINE
TO OBTAIN TISSUE AREAS:
1. THE ARM AREAS AND MUSCLE AREAS ARE ALONGSIDE THEIR RESPECTIVE CIRCUMFERENCES
2. FAT AREA = ARM AREA-MUSCLE AREA

*With permission from Gurney JM, Jelliffe DM. Arm anthropometry in nutritional assessment: nomogram for rapid calculation of muscle circumference and cross-sectional muscle and fat areas. Am J Clin Nutr 1973;26:912–915.

APPENDIX 11

ARM AND ARM MUSCLE CIRCUMFERENCE PERCENTILES*

Percentiles of upper arm circumference (mm) and estimated upper arm muscle circumference (mm) for whites, ages 1 through 18, of the United States Health and Nutrition Examination Survey I of 1971 to 1974

Age group	Arm circumference (mm)							Arm muscle circumference (mm)						
	5	10	25	50	75	90	95	5	10	25	50	75	90	95
Males														
1–1.9	142	146	150	159	170	176	183	110	113	119	127	135	144	147
2–2.9	141	145	153	162	170	178	185	111	114	122	130	140	146	150
3–3.9	150	153	160	167	175	184	190	117	123	131	137	143	148	153
4–4.9	149	154	162	171	180	186	192	123	126	133	141	148	156	159
5–5.9	153	160	167	175	185	195	204	128	133	140	147	154	162	169
6–6.9	155	159	167	179	188	209	228	131	135	142	151	161	170	177
7–7.9	162	167	177	187	201	223	230	137	139	151	160	168	177	190
8–8.9	162	170	177	190	202	220	245	140	145	154	162	170	182	187
9–9.9	175	178	187	200	217	249	257	151	154	161	170	183	196	202
10–10.9	181	184	196	210	231	262	274	156	160	166	180	191	209	221
11–11.9	186	190	202	223	244	261	280	159	165	173	183	195	205	230
12–12.9	193	200	214	232	254	282	303	167	171	182	195	210	223	241
13–13.9	194	211	228	247	263	286	301	172	179	196	211	226	238	245
14–14.9	220	226	237	253	283	303	322	189	199	212	223	240	260	264
15–15.9	222	229	244	264	284	311	320	199	204	218	237	254	266	272
16–16.9	244	248	262	278	303	324	343	213	225	234	249	269	287	296
17–17.9	246	253	267	285	308	336	347	224	231	245	258	273	294	312
Females														
1–1.9	138	142	148	156	164	172	177	105	111	117	124	132	139	143
2–2.9	142	145	152	160	167	176	184	111	114	119	126	133	142	147
3–3.9	143	150	158	167	175	183	189	113	119	124	132	140	146	152
4–4.9	149	154	160	169	177	184	191	115	121	128	136	144	152	157
5–5.9	153	157	165	175	185	203	211	125	128	134	142	151	159	165
6–6.9	156	162	170	176	187	204	211	130	133	138	145	154	166	171
7–7.9	164	167	174	183	199	216	231	129	135	142	151	160	171	176
8–8.9	168	172	183	195	214	247	261	138	140	151	160	171	183	194
9–9.9	178	182	194	211	224	251	260	147	150	158	167	180	194	198
10–10.9	174	182	193	210	228	251	265	148	150	159	170	180	190	197
11–11.9	185	194	208	224	248	276	303	150	158	171	181	196	217	223
12–12.9	194	203	216	237	256	282	294	162	166	180	191	201	214	220
13–13.9	202	211	223	243	271	301	338	169	175	183	198	211	226	240
14–14.9	214	223	237	252	272	304	322	174	179	190	201	216	232	247
15–15.9	208	221	239	254	279	300	322	175	178	189	202	215	228	244
16–16.9	218	224	241	258	283	318	334	170	180	190	202	216	234	249
17–17.9	220	227	241	264	295	324	350	175	183	194	205	221	239	257

*With permission from Frisancho AR. New norms of upper limb fat and muscle areas for assessment of nutritional status. Am J Clin Nutr 1981;34:2540–2545.

APPENDIX 12

ARM FAT AREA AND ARM MUSCLE AREA PERCENTILES*

Percentiles for estimates of upper arm fat (mm²) and upper arm muscle area (mm²) for whites, ages 1 through 18, of the United States Health Examination Survey I of 1971 to 1974

Age group	Arm muscle area percentiles (mm²)							Arm fat area percentiles (mm²)						
	5	10	25	50	75	90	95	5	10	25	50	75	90	95
Males														
1–1.9	956	1014	1133	1278	1447	1644	1720	452	486	590	741	895	1036	1176
2–2.9	973	1040	1190	1345	1557	1690	1787	434	504	578	737	871	1044	1148
3–3.9	1095	1201	1357	1484	1618	1750	1853	464	519	590	736	868	1071	1151
4–4.9	1207	1264	1408	1579	1747	1926	2008	428	494	598	722	859	989	1085
5–5.9	1298	1411	1550	1720	1884	2089	2285	446	488	582	713	914	1176	1299
6–6.9	1360	1447	1605	1815	2056	2297	2493	371	446	539	678	896	1115	1519
7–7.9	1497	1548	1808	2027	2246	2494	2886	423	473	574	758	1011	1393	1511
8–8.9	1550	1664	1895	2089	2296	2628	2788	410	460	588	725	1003	1248	1558
9–9.9	1811	1884	2067	2288	2657	3053	3257	485	527	635	859	1252	1864	2081
10–10.9	1930	2027	2182	2575	2903	3486	3882	523	543	738	982	1376	1906	2609
11–11.9	2016	2156	2382	2670	3022	3359	4226	536	595	754	1148	1710	2348	2574
12–12.9	2216	2339	2649	3022	3496	3968	4640	554	650	874	1172	1558	2536	3580
13–13.9	2363	2546	3044	3553	4081	4502	4794	475	570	812	1096	1702	2744	3322
14–14.9	2803	3147	3586	3963	4575	5368	5530	453	563	786	1082	1608	2746	3508
15–15.9	3138	3317	3788	4481	5134	5631	5900	521	595	690	931	1423	2434	3100
16–16.9	3625	4044	4352	4951	5753	6576	6980	542	593	844	1078	1746	2280	3041
17–17.9	3998	4252	4777	5286	5950	6886	7726	598	698	827	1096	1636	2407	2888
Females														
1–1.9	885	973	1084	1221	1378	1535	1621	401	466	578	706	847	1022	1140
2–2.9	973	1029	1119	1269	1405	1595	1727	469	526	642	747	894	1061	1173
3–3.9	1014	1133	1227	1396	1563	1690	1846	473	529	656	822	967	1106	1158
4–4.9	1058	1171	1313	1475	1644	1832	1958	490	541	654	766	907	1109	1236
5–5.9	1238	1301	1423	1598	1825	2012	2159	470	529	647	812	991	1330	1536
6–6.9	1354	1414	1513	1683	1877	2182	2323	464	508	638	827	1009	1263	1436
7–7.9	1330	1441	1602	1815	2045	2332	2469	491	560	706	920	1135	1407	1644
8–8.9	1513	1566	1808	2034	2327	2657	2996	527	634	769	1042	1383	1872	2482
9–9.9	1723	1788	1976	2227	2571	2987	3112	642	690	933	1219	1584	2171	2524
10–10.9	1740	1784	2019	2296	2583	2873	3093	616	702	842	1141	1608	2500	3005
11–11.9	1784	1987	2316	2612	3071	3739	3953	707	802	1015	1301	1942	2730	3690
12–12.9	2092	2182	2579	2904	3225	3655	3847	782	854	1090	1511	2056	2666	3369
13–13.9	2269	2426	2657	3130	3529	4081	4568	726	838	1219	1625	2374	3272	4150
14–14.9	2418	2562	2874	3220	3704	4294	4850	981	1043	1423	1818	2403	3250	3765
15–15.9	2426	2518	2847	3248	3689	4123	4756	839	1126	1396	1886	2544	3093	4195
16–16.9	2308	2567	2865	3248	3718	4353	4946	1126	1351	1663	2006	2598	3374	4236
17–17.9	2442	2674	2996	3336	3883	4552	5251	1042	1267	1463	2104	2977	3864	5159

*With permission from Frisancho AR. New norms of upper limb fat and muscle areas for assessment of nutritional status. Am J Clin Nutr 1981;34:2540–2545.

PEDIATRIC APPENDIX 13

SELECTED REFERENCES FOR PEDIATRIC LABORATORY VALUES

Normal ranges for laboratory tests in pediatric patients are in the process of being developed at the Mayo Clinic. The following are two sources of published pediatric normal laboratory values.

1. Rowe PC. Johns Hopkins Hospital, The Harriet Lane Handbook: A manual for pediatric house officers. 11th ed. Chicago: Year Book Medical Publishers, 1987:349.
2. Nelson WE, Behrman RE, Vaughan VC III. Nelson textbook of pediatrics. 12th ed. Philadelphia: WB Saunders, 1983:1827.

CHAPTER 9

DIETS IN PREPARATION FOR DIAGNOSTIC TESTS

The breath hydrogen analysis test is used in the study of carbohydrate maldigestion and malabsorption and, most commonly, in the assessment of lactose intolerance. In addition, this test can indicate the presence of small bowel bacterial overgrowth or of intestinal stasis syndromes, as in pseudo-obstruction.[1,2]

Ordinarily, lactose is broken down by small intestine enzymes into galactose and glucose, and these are absorbed. When maldigestion exists, ingested lactose is not absorbed, and bacteria in the colon metabolize the lactose to form hydrogen. The hydrogen is then absorbed into the bloodstream and, finally, expired in the breath. The appearance of hydrogen in any significant amount in expired air is abnormal and is a useful indication of lactose (or other carbohydrate) malabsorption.

Hydrogen breath analysis is performed after an overnight fast. Individuals are instructed not to eat or to drink anything except water after midnight. For the test, oral lactose (or other carbohydrate) is given, and serial samples of breath are collected and measured for hydrogen.

Studies have shown that the fasting breath hydrogen concentration can be affected by the meal preceding the fast.[3] As little as 100 g of breadstuffs or pastas made from wheat flour can significantly elevate breath hydrogen concentration for up to 10 hours postprandially.[4] Legumes contain substantial amounts of carbohydrates that cannot be digested and absorbed in the small intestine, but that are fermented by bacteria in the colon. As little as 2 to 5 g of these carbohydrates can elevate breath hydrogen.

Patients scheduled for hydrogen breath testing should be instructed to avoid dietary sources of breath hydrogen that may interfere with test results. The meal preceding the fast should not contain the following foods:

Wheat-Containing Foods

Breads	Spaghetti
Rolls	Noodles

Breadsticks
Crackers
Macaroni

Breaded items, such as
breaded fish
Desserts, such as cake
and cookies

Legumes

Beans such as butter beans, navy, pinto, and kidney beans, baked beans, string beans, soya and mung beans
Peas such as garden peas, chick and split peas
Peanuts
Lentils

Physicians: How to Order Diet

The diet order should indicate *diet for breath hydrogen test.*

REFERENCES

1. Calloway DH, Murphy EL, Bauer D. Determination of lactose intolerance by breath analysis. Am J Dig Dis 1969;14:811–815.
2. Levitt MD, Donaldson RM. Use of respiratory hydrogen (H_2) excretion to detect carbohydrate malabsorption. J Lab Clin Med 1970;75:937–945.
3. Perman JA, Modler S, Barr RG, Rosenthal P. Fasting breath hydrogen concentration: Normal values and clinical application. Gastroenterology 1984;87:1358–1363.
4. Anderson IH, Levine AS, Levitt MD. Incomplete absorption of the carbohydrate in all-purpose flour. N Engl J Med 1981;304:891–892.

CARBOHYDRATE METABOLISM

Patients scheduled for glucose tolerance testing (oral and intravenous) or for tolbutamide response testing should receive a diet with ample carbohydrate for at least 3 days before the test is performed. The diet should contain adequate protein, adequate kilocalories (for weight maintenance), and at least 150 g of carbohydrate. Although 300-g carbohydrate diets have traditionally been used in preparation for tests of carbohydrate metabolism, valid testing results have been reported with intakes of 150 to 200 g.[1]

The purpose of the diet is to condition the insulin-releasing mechanism and the glucose-disposing enzyme systems to respond fully to a glucose or a tolbutamide challenge. This diet also helps assure adequate stores of hepatic glycogen to provide a source of glucose for restoration of plasma glucose levels after the initial hypoglycemic response to tolbutamide. The response to challenge by a glucose load or by tolbutamide may be abnormal in normal persons who have fasted, who have missed meals during the several days before testing, or who have followed a diet very low in carbohydrate.[2] Results of glucose tolerance tests in hospitalized patients are commonly invalid because of the stress of current or recent illness, inactivity, drugs, or the supine position during the test.

Hospitalized patients are served a general diet (which contains 200 to 300 g of carbohydrate) or a modified diet with at least 150 g of carbohydrate. The physician should be notified if the patient's intake is inadequate.

Outpatients should be advised to eat their usual diet and some additional sweets and desserts. It is particularly important that a dietitian discuss with the patient an appropriate diet to follow in preparation for the test if the patient has been following a weight reduction diet, a diet very low in carbohydrate, or other unusual dietary practices.

Physicians: How to Order Diet

The diet order should indicate *diet in preparation for glucose tolerance test.*

REFERENCES

1. Wilkerson HLC, Hyman H, Kaufman M, McCuistion AC, Francis JOS. Diagnostic evaluation of oral glucose tolerance tests in nondiabetic subjects after various levels of carbohydrate intake. N Engl J Med 1960;262:1047–1053.
2. Marble A, Ferguson BD. Diagnosis and classification of diabetes mellitus and the nondiabetic melituria. In: Marble A, Kroll LP, Bradley RF, Christlieb AR, Soeldner JS, eds. Joslin's diabetes mellitus, 12th ed. Philadelphia: Lea & Febiger, 1985:339.

FAT ABSORPTION

The test diet is used to determine the presence of steatorrhea, an indication of gastrointestinal maldigestion or malabsorption. Fat intake is controlled, and stools are collected during the test period, usually 48 to 72 hours.

In the hospital setting, food intake is monitored, and fat intake can be accurately estimated. In the outpatient setting, patients are advised to control fat intake as closely as possible. However, there is likely to be greater variance in the diet owing to inaccuracies in fulfilling instructions coupled with difficulties in tolerating a daily intake of 100 g of fat. Actual fat consumption can be estimated through diet recall.

The diet is generally planned to provide 100 g of fat per day. An average intake of 100 ± 10 g of fat is usually considered acceptable. Ordinarily, stool fat for normal adult subjects who are consuming the 100-g fat test diet is 4 to 5 g per day.[1] A value greater than 7 g per day is considered to indicate steatorrhea.* Because of the large variation in total fecal solids, fat excretion expressed as a percentage of the dry weight of the stool is not a satisfactory measure of steatorrhea. Average stool fat increases with increased dietary fat. Some patients find it extremely difficult to eat a diet containing 100 g of fat. In some instances, it may be more reasonable to set a goal of 60 to 80 g of fat. Normal standards for the lower fat intake are then computed by the following formula:

---

* In children, steatorrhea is defined as fecal fat excretion of 5 g or more per day with a diet containing 40 to 65 g of fat. See page 423 for additional guidelines for test diets for steatorrhea in children.

$$(0.021 \times \text{grams of dietary fat per 24 hours}) + 2.93$$

$$= \text{grams of fecal fat per 24 hours}^\dagger$$

This formula may permit the interpretation of fecal fat analysis, even when fat intake differs considerably from that in the standard test diet. The dietitian can determine the expected average amount of stool fat for this level of intake in addition to reporting the amount of fat actually consumed.

Stool nitrogen remains remarkably constant over a wide range of protein intake, although a high fiber diet tends to increase stool nitrogen somewhat. Mean stool nitrogen on the standard 100-g fat test diet was 1.7 g per 24 hours (a range of 0.8 to 2.5 g) in the studies by Wollaeger, et al.[1,2] Other studies suggest a somewhat lower range, with means of 1.2 to 1.3 g of nitrogen per 24 hours.[2,3] Stool nitrogen, like stool fat, is increased in malabsorption and in maldigestion and can be used to confirm stool fat data.

Stool fat and nitrogen data should be viewed, not only as numbers to confirm or to disprove a diagnosis, but also as a means of assessing the nutritional consequences of an intestinal disorder. Stool fat in excess of 7 g per day can be multiplied by the factor of 9 Kcal per gram to obtain kilocalories wasted by steatorrhea. Stool nitrogen in excess of 2 g per day multiplied by the factor of 6.25 g of protein per gram of nitrogen gives the equivalent amount of protein wasted. This figure multiplied by the factor of 4 Kcal per gram yields protein kilocalories wasted by malabsorption or by maldigestion.

Physicians: How to Order Diet

The diet order should indicate *test diet for steatorrhea or 100-g fat test diet* and the date the diet is to begin. The dietitian will calculate the normal value for fat excretion based on the estimated fat consumption if actual fat intake is outside the range of 100 ± 10 g per day.

Suggestion for Meal Planning

When portion sizes can be measured reliably, any food may be served as long as fat content can be determined. In an outpatient setting, the diet may be more accurately fulfilled if fat free and low fat foods are used and if measured amounts of fat are added. Table 9–1 gives three examples of daily meal plans that allow for 100 g of fat. The *Food Exchange Lists* see page 114, can be used as a tool for meal planning.

TABLE 9–1 Three Possible Meal Plans to Achieve a Daily Intake of 100 Grams of Fat

Whole Milk	Skim Milk	Vegetable	Fruit	Bread	Meat*	Fat	Low Fat Dessert	Low Fat Sweets
2	—	Ad lib	Ad lib	Ad lib	6	10	Ad lib	Ad lib
—	2	Ad lib	Ad lib	Ad lib	6	14	Ad lib	Ad lib
—	—	Ad lib	Ad lib	Ad lib	8	12	Ad lib	Ad lib

*Calculations are based on values for medium-fat meats

---

† According to this formula, an average amount stool fat of 5.03 grams would be expected after a dietary fat intake of 100 grams, and a stool fat of 3.98 grams would be expected after a dietary fat intake of 50 grams. Example: $(0.021 \times 50 \text{ grams of dietary fat}) + 2.93 = 3.98$ grams of stool fat.

REFERENCES

1. Wollaeger EE, Comfort MW, Osterberg AE. Total solids, fat and nitrogen in the feces: III. A study of normal persons taking a test diet containing a moderate amount of fat; comparison with results obtained with normal persons taking a test diet containing a large amount of fat. Gastroenterology 1947;9:272–283.
2. Wollaeger EE, Comfort MW, Weir JF, Osterberg AE. The total solids, fat and nitrogen in the feces: I. A study of normal persons and of patients with duodenal ulcer on a test diet containing large amounts of fat. Gastroenterology 1946;6:83–92.
3. Reifenstein EC Jr, Albright F, Wells SL. The accumulation, interpretation and presentation of data pertaining to metabolic balances, notably those of calcium, phosphorous and nitrogen. J Clin Endocrinol Metab 1945;5:367–395.

5-HIAA

The presence of 5-HIAA (5-hydroxyindoleacetic acid) in the urine is an indication of an abnormal production of serotonin. An excess of 5-HIAA may indicate that the patient has a carcinoid tumor. For 24 hours before urine collection, patients scheduled for 5-HIAA testing should avoid ingesting exogenous sources of serotonin, which increase urinary 5-HIAA, and medications that interfere with the test.

Foods to Avoid[1,2,3]

Avocado	Pecans
Bananas	Plantain
Butternuts	Plums
Eggplant	Tomatoes
Hickory nuts	Walnuts, black and English
Kiwi fruit	Alcohol
Pineapple	

Medications to Avoid

Cough syrup containing glyceryl guaiacolate
Acetaminophen (Tylenol)
Phenacetin

Physicians: How to Order Diet

This diet may be ordered as *diet in preparation for 5-HIAA testing.*

REFERENCES

1. Wegener LT. 5-Hydroxyindoleacetic acid (S-HIAA), urine. In: Wegener LT, ed. Mayo medical laboratories handbook. Rochester, MN: Mayo Clinic, 1983:116.
2. Feldman JM, Lee EM. Serotonin content of foods: effect on urinary excretion of 5-hydroxyindoleacetic acid. Am J Clin Nutr 1985;42:639–643.
3. Feldman JM, Lee EM, Castleberry CA. Catecholamine and serotonin content of foods: effect on urinary excretion of homovanillic and 5-hydroxyindoleacetic acid. J Am Diet Assoc 1987;87(8):1031–1035.

STANDARDS OF PRACTICE

NUTRITIONAL SUPPORT DIETITIAN*

Introductory Note

The Standards of Practice for Nutritional Support Dietitians should be utilized in conjunction with the following A.S.P.E.N. publications:

Standards for Nutrition Support, Hospitalized Patients, 1984.

Standards for Nutrition Support, Home Patients, 1985.

Standards of Practice, Nutrition Support Nursing, 1985.

These Standards of Practice for Nutritional Support Dietitians should be utilized in conjunction with the following American Dietetic Association publications:

Standards of Practice for the Profession of Dietetics (A.D.A. Council on Practice, The American Dietetic Association, February 1984)

These standards are provided for the general guidance of health professionals. Their application in any individual case should be determined by the best judgment of the professional.

Scope of Practice

Background

It is widely accepted that optimum nutrition plays an important role in good health. Historically, the dietitian has been the health care professional charged with the task of ensuring that diets are adequate for patients with various disease states. The advent and sophistication of specialized nutritional support—enteral and parenteral therapies—have allowed the health care professional to ensure that even patients who are unable to eat will receive adequate nutrition. As the importance of specialized nutritional support has become recognized and techniques for the delivery of enteral and parenteral therapies have evolved, nutritional support has become an established area of dietetic practice.

---

*With permission from the American Society for Parenteral and Enteral Nutrition. From: Nutrition in Clinical Practice 1986;1:216–220.

517

Role

The Nutritional Support Dietitian, in conjunction with other health care professionals, including a physician director, registered nurse, and registered pharmacist, shall participate in the provision of specialized nutritional support. If a formal nutritional support service has not been established, the Nutritional Support Dietitian shall function, along with other appropriate health care professionals, as a member of the nutritional support committee or subcommittee.

The Nutritional Support Dietitian works specifically with enteral, parenteral, modular, and transitional nutritional therapies. The Nutritional Support Dietitian is a registered dietitian with clinical expertise in specialized nutritional support obtained through education and specialized training or experience in this field. With this, the role of the dietitian should include ongoing nutritional assessment and planning, as well as monitoring and documentation of the response of the patient to specialized nutritional support. Other activities include facilitating both a smooth transition to an oral diet and the termination of enteral and parenteral therapies when appropriate. Last, the Nutritional Support Dietitian educates patients, families, and other health care professionals concerning principles of nutritional therapy.

Goals

Utilizing current knowledge of nutritional therapy and scientific theory, the Nutritional Support Dietitian strives to provide optimal nutritional support for all patients. Specific goals include:

Identification of patients at nutritional risk

Provision of appropriate nutritional therapy to such patients

Performance of periodic nutritional assessments of patients undergoing nutritional support

Assurance of smooth and adequate transitional feedings

Documentation of nutritional care plans

The Nutritional Support Dietitian actively pursues new knowledge in nutritional support. When appropriate, the Nutritional Support Dietitian assists in and/or initiates nutritional support and is an active participant in local, regional, and national educational programs. Through these endeavors, the Nutritional Support Dietitian shares expertise, knowledge, and investigational findings with other health care professionals.

Definitions

Diet. A prescribed allowance of nutrients provided via the oral route.

Enteral Nutrition. Nutrition provided through or via the gastrointestinal tract.

Oral: enteral nutrition taken through or via the mouth

Tube: enteral nutrition provided through a tube that delivers nutrients distal to the oral cavity

Feeding Formulation. A ready-to-administer mixture of nutrients.

Malnutrition. Any disorder of nutrition, either an excess or deficiency of nutrient intake, or impaired nutrient metabolism.

Modular Enteral Feeding. The combination of sources of nutrients so that an existing formula is modified or a new formula is created.

Nutrient. Protein, carbohydrate, lipids, vitamins, electrolytes, minerals, and water.

Nutritional Support Service. A multidisciplinary group of health care professionals who aid in the provision of specialized nutrition support.

Parenteral Nutrition. Nutrients provided by means other than the gastrointestinal tract

Central: parenteral nutrition delivered through a large diameter vein, usually the subclavian or superior vena cava, that empties directly into the heart

Peripheral: parenteral nutrition delivered through a smaller vein, usually in the hand or forearm

Specialized Nutritional Assessment. A comprehensive approach to defining nutrition status that employs clinical and dietary histories, physical examination, anthropometric measurements, and laboratory data.

Specialized Nutritional Support. Provision of specially formulated and/or delivered parenteral or enteral nutrients to prevent or to treat malnutrition.

Transitional Feeding. Progression from one mode of feeding to another, while attempting to maintain/achieve estimated nutrient requirements.

Assessment

Standard A: Nutritional Status

The nutritional support dietitian, in conjunction with other appropriate health care professionals, shall establish criteria for the identification of a patient who either is, or may become, malnourished.

Rationale. Nutritional assessment can assist in the identification of patients who are or may become malnourished. Prevention or correction of malnutrition can contribute to a more positive outcome from medical or surgical intervention.

Criteria. Evaluation and/or documentation of nutritional status in the medical record, which may include the following:

1. History of nutrient intake
2. Weight history and growth history (when appropriate)
3. Anthropometrics
4. Age
5. Sex
6. Clinical signs of malnutrition
7. Biochemical indices of nutritional status and urine determinations
8. Mechanical, physiological, or psychological problems which interfere with ingestion, digestion, absorption, or metabolism of nutrients

Standard B: Guidelines for the Use of Specialized Nutritional Support

The nutritional support dietitian, in conjunction with other appropriate health care professionals, shall participate in the establishment and modification of guidelines for the use of specialized nutritional support.

Rationale. Well-defined guidelines should prevent the under- or over-utilization of specialized nutritional support.

Criteria. Documentation of:

1. Formalized guidelines for the use of specialized nutritional support
2. Participation in the establishment and modification of these guidelines
3. Willingness of the patient, family, or significant other to agree with the therapeutic plan and/or ability to cooperate in the therapy when appropriate

Standard C: Determination of Nutrient Requirements

The nutritional support dietitian, in conjunction with other appropriate health care professionals, shall determine the nutrient requirements of the patient prior to the initiation of specialized nutritional support.

Rationale. The determination of nutrient requirements is often complex and may require specialized multidisciplinary expertise. Insufficient nutrient provision results in less than optimum repletion or maintenance of nutritional status. Over- and underfeeding can affect nutrient requirements. Overfeeding provides no additional therapeutic benefit, can result in complications, and is not cost-effective.

Criteria. Documentation of:

1. Nutrient requirements based on calculated or measured needs
2. Modification of nutrient needs of the patient based on the specific disease state, the proposed medical/surgical therapy, the nutritional status, the duration of anticipated inadequate intake

Therapeutic Plan

Standard A: Objective

The nutritional support dietitian, in conjunction with other appropriate health care professionals, shall determine and document the rationale and objective(s) for specialized nutritional support.

Rationale. Clearly formulated rationale and objectives should improve the likelihood that therapy will meet the specific nutrient needs of the patient and prevent misuse.

Criteria. Documentation of:

1. Proposed immediate, intermediate, and end outcomes of specialized nutritional support
2. Anticipated duration of time receiving specialized nutritional support
3. Discharge planning and/or home training when appropriate

Standard B: Mode

The nutritional support dietitian, in conjunction with other appropriate health care professionals, shall provide input into the selection of the appropriate route(s) by which nutritional support is administered.

Rationale. The access route(s) selected to provide nutritional support should be appropriate to the medical problems of the patient and permit delivery of his nutrient requirements. The safest, most cost-effective route should be utilized whenever possible. When adequately functioning, the gastrointestinal tract should be utilized. If adequate nutritional support can be achieved only by central venous nutrition, then central venous nutrition should be implemented. The optimal mode may change from a venous route to an enteral route as the clinical condition of the patient progresses.

Criteria. Documentation that the nutritional support dietitian provides input into the selection of the route(s) for nutritional support based upon:

1. Medical condition of the patient
2. Assessed nutrient requirements
3. Therapeutic objectives
4. Safety
5. Cost effectiveness

Standard C: Diets and Feeding Formulations

The nutritional support dietitian, in conjunction with other health care professionals, shall participate in the identification and selection of diet and feeding formulations (enteral and parenteral) appropriate to the disease process and compatible with the access route.

Rationale. The diets and feeding formulations (enteral and parenteral) selected should be appropriate to the disease process and compatible with the access route.

Criteria. Assistance in determination and documentation of:

1. The ability of the patient to tolerate various modes of feeding
2. Adequacy of intake
3. Evaluation factors which may affect nutrient intake, digestion, absorption, and assimilation
4. Calculated nutrient requirements
5. A nutritional care plan, with recommendations for specific nutrition intervention (supplements, diet modification, diet instruction, and enteral, modular and parenteral feeding)

Implementation

Standard A: Product Preparation

The nutritional support dietitian, in conjunction with other appropriate health care professionals, shall verify that enteral formulations are prepared according to established guidelines for safe and effective nutritional therapy.

Rationale. Enteral feeding formulations should be prepared accurately, with attention to the feeding prescription, the prevention of contamination, the compatibility of ingredients, and the appropriateness of packaging and labeling.

Criteria. Establishment and/or verification of:

1. Adequate written guidelines for the preparation of enteral feeding formulas
2. Dietary quality assurance monitoring to ensure that guidelines are being met
3. Documentation in the medical record that the product meets the nutrient needs of the patient

4. Written policies specifying that the actual contents of compounded formulations are accurate

Standard B: Diet and Feeding Formulation Administration

The nutritional support dietitian, in conjunction with other appropriate health care professionals, shall verify that specialized nutritional support is administered, in accordance with the prescribed therapeutic plan, and consistent with tolerance of the patient, after an appropriate access has been established and verified.

Rationale. Accurate administration of diet, enteral, and parenteral feeding formulations promotes safe and effective nutritional support.

Criteria. Verification and/or documentation that the appropriate health care professional:

1. Has verified that enteral feeding tubes are properly placed prior to instituting specialized nutritional support

2. Routinely checks the labels of feeding formulations of patients, and reports discrepancies to the appropriate personnel

3. Cooperates with other disciplines to minimize errors in formula administration

4. Maintains current knowledge of feeding formulations and feeding access methods

5. Recommends the rate of administration and concentration for initiation of feeding formulation

6. Recommends the rate of administration and concentration during progression of the feeding formulation to levels meeting the nutrient needs of the patient

7. Monitors and records nutrient intake during the administration of the feeding formulations

8. Recognizes signs and symptoms of feeding formulation intolerance

9. Recommends modification of the feeding formulation to minimize intolerance

Standard C: Quality Assurance for Implementing Nutritional Support

The nutritional support dietitian, in conjunction with other appropriate health care professionals, shall establish protocols for implementing specialized nutritional support.

Rationale. Protocols should be established in order to ensure safe and effective delivery of specialized nutritional support.

Criteria. Establishment of written protocols regarding:

1. Administration of specialized nutritional support

2. Monitoring of specialized nutritional support

3. Infection control

4. Documentation in the medical record

Patient Monitoring

Standard A: Monitoring Nutrition Response

The nutritional support dietitian, in conjunction with other health care professionals, shall monitor the response of the patient to specialized nutritional support, to provide a basis for adjusting therapy.

Rationale. The effectiveness and safety of nutritional support requires routine monitoring which can measure success or adverse effects.

Criteria. Monitoring and documentation of:

1. Actual nutrient delivery during nutritional support
2. Biochemical and other pertinent laboratory data; nonroutine analyses if appropriate
3. Weight or other appropriate indices of body composition
4. The implications of any nutrient-drug interactions
5. Intolerance to therapy which may include gastrointestinal complications, fluid, and electrolyte imbalances
6. Signs and symptoms of nutrient deficiencies or excesses
7. The clinical course of the patient, including indices of major organ functions
8. The psychosocial adjustment of the patient when appropriate
9. Alterations or changes in nutrient requirements based on changes in clinical status

Transitional Feeding

Standard A: Transition from Parenteral Nutrition

The nutritional support dietitian, in conjunction with other health care professionals, shall establish criteria to evaluate adequacy of the enteral intake prior to the discontinuation of parenteral nutrition.

Rationale. Parenteral nutrition should not be discontinued until estimated nutrients are tolerated by the gastrointestinal tract. Parenteral nutrient formulation should be discontinued over time while enteral or oral feedings are increased. Documentation of ingestion of adequate nutrients via the gastrointestinal tract should be made in the medical record.

Criteria. Evaluation and documentation of:

1. Nutrient intake
2. Tolerance of enteral intake which may include assessment of gastrointestinal status including diarrhea, residuals, distention, nausea, vomiting, swallowing, aspiration, and absorption problems

Standard B: Transition from Enteral Tube Feedings

The nutritional support dietitian, in conjunction with other health care professionals, shall verify adequate oral intake prior to discontinuation of enteral tube feedings.

Rationale. Enteral tube feedings should not be discontinued until estimated nutrient requirements are met by oral intake. Tube feedings should be discontinued over time while oral intake increases, to avoid periods of nutritional compromise.

Criteria. Verification and documentation of:

1. Oral nutrient intake

2. Tolerance to oral intake, which may include assessment of gastrointestinal status including diarrhea, gastric residuals, distention, nausea, vomiting, swallowing, aspiration, and absorption problems

3. Tolerance to individual foods

4. Diet prescription based on medical diagnosis

INTERACTIONS BETWEEN DRUGS, NUTRIENTS,

AND NUTRITIONAL STATUS*

The interactions between drugs and nutrient intake and the nutritional status of the individual is becoming more appreciated. Drugs can influence nutrient absorption, metabolism, or excretion; the effects may alter nutritional status. On the other hand, specific nutrients, foods, or beverages interact with drug metabolism, action, or excretion. The dietitian must be attentive to the interactions of drugs and nutrients and to the effect on nutritional status.

---

*Smith CH, Bidlack WR. Dietary concerns associated with the use of medications. Copyright The American Dietetic Association. Reprinted by permission from JOURNAL OF THE AMERICAN DIETETIC ASSOCIATION 1984;84:901.

TABLE 1. Dietary Suggestions Associated with Drugs that Alter Nutrient Absorption

Drug (Usage)	Nutritional Implications		Dietary Suggestions
	Gastrointestinal Side/Adverse Effects	Other Reactions	
Aluminum hydroxide gel (antacid, phosphate binder)	bloating, constipation, fecal impaction, nausea or vomiting, stomach cramps	Phosphate malabsorption, hypophosphatemia, vitamin A malabsorption, thiamin destruction, loss of appetite, unpalatable (chalky)	*Ulcer therapy—Drug:* Take between meals, chew chewable tablets until thoroughly wetted, then follow with 125 ml water. *Diet Rx:* Teach dietary principles associated with treatment of ulcer disease. *Phospate-binding therapy—Drug:* Take at mealtime with 250 ml water or fluids indicated for patients with renal disease. *Diet Rx:* Dietary phosphate restriction may be prescribed. If permissable, include a high-bulk diet to counter constipation. *Other:* Prolonged usage or large doses, especially with a low-phosphate diet, may result in hypophosphatemic osteomalacia. Decreased absorption of fat-soluble vitamins (especially vitamin A) may be due to precipitated bile acids.
Bisacodyl (laxative)	Belching, mild cramping, diarrhea, nausea	Fluid and electrolyte loss, hypokalemia (long use)	*Drug:* Take on empty stomach with at least 250 ml water and at least 1 hr away from milk. (Milk may dissolve enteric coating, causing gastric irritation.) Swallow tablet whole (do not chew or crush). *Diet Rx:* Drink at least 6 to 8 glasses of 250 ml fluid/day to aid stool softening. Teach the importance of diet, increased fluid intake, and exercise. See Table 8. *Other:* Prolonged usage or large doses may result in nutrient loss, fluid and electrolyte disturbances, and dependence on drug for bowel function.
Cholestyramine (antihyperlipemic, bile acid sequestrant)	Belching, bloating, constipation, flatulence, heartburn, nausea or vomiting, steatorrhea, stomach pain	Malabsorption of fat, iron, carotene, vitamins A, D, and K, and folacin; hypoprothrombinemia; gritty texture; unpalatable taste	*Drug:* Thoroughly hydrate drug with at least 120 to 180 ml water, milk, fruit juice, or noncarbonated or other beverages prior to ingestion; disguise gritty texture and unpalatable taste by mixing with highly flavored liquids, thin soups, milk in cereals, or pulpy fruits (applesauce, crushed pineapple). *Diet Rx:* If permissible, include a high bulk diet with increased fluid intake to counter constipation. During long-term therapy, supplementation with a water-soluble (or parenteral) form of vitamins A and D may be prescribed. Parenteral or oral administration of vi-

TABLE 1. Dietary Suggestions Associated with Drugs that Alter Nutrient Absorption (continued)

Drug (Usage)	Nutritional Implications		Dietary Suggestions
	Gastrointestinal Side/Adverse Effects	Other Reactions	
			tamin K may also be considered if hypoprothrombinemia occurs. Folacin supplementation may be prescribed for patients with reduced serum or red cell folacin. *Other:* Prior to drug therapy, control of serum cholesterol is attempted by diet therapy. During drug therapy, advise patient of the importance of following a prescribed diet.
Colchicine (antigout)	Diarrhea (may be severe), nausea or vomiting, abdominal pain	Malabsorption of sodium, potassium, fat, carotene, and vitamin B_{12} due to altered mucosal function; decreased lactase activity; loss of appetite	*Drug:* Take with water immediately before, with, or after meals to reduce gastric irritation. *Diet Rx:* May indicate increased intake of alkaline ash foods or beverages and low purine foods, no alcoholic beverages, and a high fluid intake of >2,000 ml/day. *Other:* Gradual weight reduction may be suggested. Alert physician if patient reports any gastrointestinal side/adverse effects.
Mineral oil (laxative)	Flatulence, indigestion, nausea or vomiting (with long use)	Malabsorption of carotene, vitamins A, D, E, and K, calcium, and phosphorus; tasteless and odorless (when cold); disagreeable consistency; loss of appetite and of weight; hypokalemia (with long use)	*Drug:* Take at least 2 hr away from food (to avoid delayed digestion and movement of chyme from stomach). May mix with or follow by orange juice to counter consistency. *Diet Rx:* See bisacodyl. Concurrent use with fat-soluble vitamins may interfere with vitamin absorption. Do not use in the preparation of low calorie salad dressings. *Other:* See bisacodyl.
Phenolphthalein (laxative)	(See bisacodyl)	Malabsorption of vitamin D, calcium, and other minerals; hypokalemia (long use); may be excreted in breast milk	*Drug:* Take on empty stomach. Chew chewable tablets or wafers well before swallowing. Chew gum well. (Do not swallow gum.) *Diet Rx:* See bisacodyl. *Other:* See bisacodyl.
Sulfasalazine (anti-inflammatory)	Diarrhea, gastric distress, nausea or vomiting	Impaired folacin absorption, loss of appetite, excreted in breast milk	*Drug:* Take with 250 ml water or after meals or with food to minimize gastric irritation. *Diet Rx:* Ensure adequate fluid intake to maintain at least 1,200 to 1,500 ml urine output/day. Encourage the intake of foods high in folacin.

TABLE 2. Dietary Suggestions Associated with Drugs That Alter Nutrient Metabolism

Drug (Usage)	Nutritional Implications		Dietary Suggestions
	Gastrointestinal Side/Adverse Effects	Other Reactions	
Hydralazine (antihypertensive)	Diarrhea, nausea or vomiting, constipation (rare)	Vitamin B_6 antagonism (may result in peripheral neuropathy), sodium and water retention (long-term therapy), loss of appetite	*Drug:* Intake with food may increase bioavailability of drug. Consistently take with food. *Diet Rx:* If appropriate, teach and emphasize the importance of dietary modifications associated with treatment of hypertension. May also indicate a sodium-restricted diet, weight reduction and monitoring, and alcoholic beverage restriction. Vitamin B_6 supplementation may be prescribed if symptoms of peripheral neuropathy develop. *Other:* Avoid over the counter (OTC) preparations that contain indirect acting sympathomimetics, especially those advertised for weight control, unless discussed with physician.
Isoniazid (antitubercular)	Epigastric distress, nausea or vomiting (may be signs of hepatotoxicity)	Vitamin B_6 antagonism (may result in peripheral neuropathy), tyramine-type reactions with certain foods, dry mouth, loss of appetite, excreted in breast milk	*Drug:* Take with 250 ml water on an empty stomach, as food decreases drug absorption. If gastrointestinal irritation occurs, drug may be taken with food to lessen that effect. *Diet Rx:* May indicate avoidance of alcoholic beverages and foods high in pressor amines. Vitamin B_6 supplementation may be prescribed for the malnourished or for those patients predisposed to vitamin B_6 deficiency or exhibiting signs of peripheral neuropathy. *Other:* Alert physician if patient reports loss of appetite, nausea, or vomiting.
Methotrexate (antineoplastic, antipsoriatic)	Abdominal distress, diarrhea, GI ulceration and bleeding, nausea or vomiting	Folacin antagonist (irreversibly binds with dihydrofolate reductase); malabsorption of folacin, vitamin B_{12}, and fat; hyperuricemia; loss of appetite; altered taste acuity; sore mouth and lips	*Drug:* To reduce nausea and to help foster compliance. See Table 8. Absorption may be decreased by milky meals. See Table 5. *Diet Rx:* May indicate increased intake of alkaline ash foods and beverages and the ingestion of ~2,000 ml water/day to aid in excretion of uric acid. Patients should avoid the use of alcoholic beverages. Caution patient against self medication with OTC preparations, especially the use of supplements that contain para-aminobenzoic acid and folacin. See Table 7. *Other:* Alert physician if patient reports diarrhea, abdominal distress, bloody vomit, or black tarry stools.
Penicillamine (chelating agent, antiarthritic, antiurolithic, heavy metal antagonist)	Diarrhea, epigastric pain, nausea or vomiting	Inhibits pyridoxal-dependent enzymes; chelates copper, iron, and zinc; unpleasant taste; decreased taste acuity (salt, sweet); loss of appetite	*Wilson's disease—Drug:* Take on an empty stomach 30 min to 1 hr before and at least 2 hr after meals. *Diet Rx:* A low copper diet (<2 mg/day) may be prescribed. Advise patient to drink demineralized drinking water if local water supply contains >100 µg copper/L. *Cystinuria—Diet Rx:* May indicate a low methionine diet (not for children) and a high fluid intake (3 to 4 L/day), with some intake during the night. *Rheumatoid arthritis—Drug:* Take with water on an empty stomach at least 1 hr apart from any meals, food, milk, or snacks. *Lead poisoning—Drug:* Take with water on an empty stomach 2 hr before and at least 3 hr after meals. *Other:* Diet Rx may include pyridoxine supplementation for patients with rheumatoid arthritis, cystinuria, and Wilson's disease. Drug should be taken away from iron and other mineral supplements. See Table 7.

TABLE 2. Dietary Suggestions Associated with Drugs That Alter Nutrient Metabolism (continued)

Drug (Usage)	Nutritional Implications		Dietary Suggestions
	Gastrointestinal Side/Adverse Effects	Other Reactions	
Phenobarbital (anticonvulsant, sedative-hypnotic)	Nausea or vomiting	Hepatic microsomal enzyme induction increases inactivation of 25-OH vitamin D and may result in rickets or osteomalacia; may decrease serum folacin, vitamin B_{12}, pyridoxine, calcium, and magnesium; appetite changes; excreted in breast milk	*Drug:* Swallow extended-release tablet whole. Take oral solution straight or mix with water, milk, or juice. *Diet Rx:* Emphasize the importance of good dietary habits with adequate intake of vitamin D-containing foods. Serum folacin, calcium, or 25-OH vitamin D levels as well as indexes of bone resorption may be monitored in patients on prolonged therapy (especially children and those concomitantly prescribed phenytoin) prior to vitamin D supplementation. Avoid alcoholic beverages.
Phenytoin (anticonvulsant, antiarrhythmic)	Constipation, nausea or vomiting	Hepatic microsomal enzyme induction increases inactivation of 25-OH vitamin D and may result in rickets or osteomalacia; may decrease serum folacin levels and result in megaloblastic anemia; decreased taste acuity; possible weight changes; serum levels of minerals and other vitamins may be altered; excreted in breast milk	*Drug:* Take with food or immediately after meals to minimize gastric irritation. *Diet Rx:* May include information that concerns hydration status, alcoholic beverage restriction, and the importance of consistent caloric intake. Emphasize the importance of good dietary and health habits, especially the intake of vitamin D-containing foods. If folacin or pyridoxine supplementation is indicated, vitamins must be administered cautiously. See Table 7.
Pyrimethamine (antimalarial)	Vomiting (dose related)	Inhibits dihydrofolate reductase (inhibitory potential greater on the intact microorganisms than on host); megaloblastic anemia (large doses); loss of appetite (large doses); excreted in breast milk	*Drug:* Take with meals or snacks to minimize gastric irritation. *Diet Rx:* May indicate concomitant administration of preformed folic acid (folinic acid) to prevent anemia; caution against the use of para-aminobenzoic acid supplements. See Table 7.
Triamterene (potassium-sparing diuretic)	Diarrhea, gastric upset, nausea or vomiting	Weak folacin antagonist, electrolyte imbalance (possible hyperkalemia), dry mouth, increased thirst, excreted in breast milk.	*Drug:* Take with or after meals to minimize gastric irritation. Dosing information may indicate to take drug with or after breakfast or no later than 6 P.M. *Diet Rx:* If appropriate, teach and emphasize the importance of dietary modifications associated with treatment of hypertension. May also indicate allowable fluid and sodium intake and caution against the use of potassium-containing salt substitutes, low salt foods with high potassium content, and intake of potassium-rich foods or potassium supplements. *Other:* Drug should be cautiously used in patients with poor nutritional status. May decrease serum folacin. Alert physician if patient reports dry mouth, increased thirst, or severe nausea, vomiting, or diarrhea (may indicate or contribute to fluid and electrolyte imbalance).

TABLE 3. Dietary Suggestions Associated with Drugs that Alter Nutrient Excretion

Drug (Usage)	Nutritional Implications		Dietary Suggestions
	Gastrointestinal Side/Adverse Effects	Other Reactions	
Aspirin (analgesic, antipyretic, anti-inflammatory)	Gastric pain or bleeding, heartburn, nausea or vomiting	Increased ascorbic acid excretion and potassium depletion (large doses), iron-deficiency anemia (long use or overuse), salicylate excreted in breast milk	*Drug:* Take with 250 ml water (for rapid analgesia) or food to reduce gastric irritation. (However, drug absorption may be delayed when aspirin is taken with food.) Swallow enteric tablets whole. Some buffered preparations contain sodium and may be contraindicated for patients on sodium-restricted diets. *Diet Rx:* May caution against concomitant intake with alcoholic beverages; may indicate the need for adequate fluid intake and emphasize the intake of foods rich in ascorbic acid. Ascorbic acid supplementation may be prescribed for ascorbic acid-depleted patients who receive large doses of the drug. *Other:* Drug should be cautiously used in patients prone to vitamin K deficiency. Drug-induced gastric bleeding may contribute to or aggravate iron-deficiency anemia.
Furosemide (potassium-depleting diuretic)	Constipation (or diarrhea), nausea or vomiting, stomach distress	Enhances the excretion of potassium, calcium, magnesium, sodium, chloride, and water; fluid and electrolyte disturbances; dry mouth; increased thirst; loss of appetite; excreted in breast milk	*Drug:* Intake with food may slow the rate of drug absorption without altering the bioavailability of drug. To minimize the effect of increased urinary output at night, take single daily dose early in the morning. *Diet Rx:* If appropriate, teach and emphasize the importance of dietary modifications associated with treatment of hypertension. May also indicate the need for a sodium-restricted diet, a high intake of potassium and magnesium-rich foods (especially in patients taking digitalis), weight reduction and monitoring, and alcoholic beverage restriction. Limit the intake of natural licorice. See Table 6.

TABLE 3. Dietary Suggestions Associated with Drugs that Alter Nutrient Excretion (continued)

Drug (Usage)	Nutritional Implications		Dietary Suggestions
	Gastrointestinal Side/Adverse Effects	Other Reactions	
			Other: See hydralazine. (Table 2) Alert physician if patient reports dry mouth, increased thirst, or severe nausea, vomiting, or diarrhea (may indicate or contribute to fluid and electrolyte imbalance).
Spironolactone (potassium-sparing diuretic)	Abdominal cramps, diarrhea, nausea or vomiting	Enhances the excretion of sodium, chloride, and water; fluid and electrolyte disturbances; dry mouth; increased thirst; loss of appetite; canrenone (metabolite) in breast milk	Drug: Take with food to minimize gastric irritation. Diet Rx: See triamterene (Table 2) Other: See hydralazine (Table 2). Alert physician if patient reports dry mouth, increased thirst, or severe nausea, vomiting, or diarrhea (may indicate or contribute to fluid and electrolyte imbalance).
Thiazide (potassium-depleting diuretic)	Constipation (or diarrhea), nausea or vomiting, upset stomach or cramping	Enhances the excretion of potassium, magnesium, sodium, and water; fluid and electrolyte disturbances; decreased urinary calcium excretion; dry mouth; increased thirst; loss of appetite; excreted in breast milk	Drug: Take after food to lessen gastric irritation. To minimize the effect of increased urinary output at night, take single dose early in the morning. Diet Rx: If appropriate, teach and emphasize the importance of dietary modifications associated with treatment of hypertension. May also indicate the need for a sodium-restricted diet, a high intake of potassium- and magnesium-rich foods, weight reduction and monitoring, alcoholic beverage restriction, and limited intake of natural licorice. See Table 6. Other: See furosemide.

TABLE 4. Dietary Suggestions Associated with Selected Drugs That May Produce Fluid or Electrolyte Disturbances

Drug (Usage)	Nutritional Implications		Dietary Suggestions
	Gastrointestinal Side/Adverse Effects	Other Reactions	
Adrenal corticosteroids	Bloating, indigestion, nausea or vomiting, ulcerogenic potential	Fluid and electrolyte disturbances; negative nitrogen balance; protein catabolism; lipolysis with possible redistribution of body fat; antivitamin D activity (inhibits calcium absorption); appetite stimulation; weight gain; excreted in breast milk	*Drug:* Take with food or low-sodium snack to minimize gastric irritation. *Diet Rx:* May include the need for a sodium-restricted diet, a diet high in potassium and protein, and caloric restriction or weight monitoring (especially during long-term therapy). Adequate intake of vitamin D–containing foods may be indicated. Advise patient that alcohol may enhance ulcerogenic potential of drug.
Anabolic steroids	Abdominal fullness, nausea or vomiting, stomach pain	Fluid and electrolyte retention, edema, weight gain (large doses), burning tongue, possible appetite stimulation	*Diet Rx:* Drug effectiveness (improved nitrogen balance) may depend on a diet high in calories and protein. May indicate the need for weight monitoring and a sodium-restricted diet to control edema. (Concurrent diuretic therapy may be prescribed.) *Other:* Drugs may exert a placebo effect in athletes. Enlargement of muscles is believed to be caused by cells retaining water, thus adding bulk but not fiber. Risk of various side or adverse effects may outweigh beneficial effects.
Clonidine (antihypertensive)	Constipation, nausea or vomiting	Salt and fluid retention, dry mouth (common), loss of appetite, weight gain (edema)	*Diet Rx:* If appropriate, teach and emphasize the importance of dietary modifications associated with treatment of hypertension. May also indicate the need for a sodium-restricted diet, weight reduction and monitoring, and alcoholic beverage restriction. (Concurrent diuretic therapy may be prescribed.) *Other:* See hydralazine (Table 2).
Estrogens	Abdominal cramping, diarrhea (mild), nausea or vomiting	Salt and fluid retention, loss of appetite, weight gain (edema), excreted in breast milk (inhibits lactation)	*Drug:* Take with or immediately after food to minimize nausea. *Diet Rx:* May indicate the need for a sodium-restricted diet and weight monitoring. Probable effectiveness in the treatment of estrogen-deficient osteoporosis may also depend on diet, calcium balance, and good health habits.

TABLE 4. Dietary Suggestions Associated with Selected Drugs That May Produce Fluid or Electrolyte Disturbances (continued)

Drug (Usage)	Nutritional Implications		Dietary Suggestions
	Gastrointestinal Side/Adverse Effects	Other Reactions	
Guanethidine (antihypertensive)	Diarrhea, nausea or vomiting	Sodium and fluid retention (with continuing use), dry mouth, taste disturbances, weight gain (edema)	*Diet Rx:* See clonidine. *Other:* See hydralazine (Table 2).
Indomethacin (anti-inflammatory, analgesic)	Bloating, constipation (or diarrhea), heartburn or indigestion, nausea or vomiting, stomach pain, ulcerogenic potential	Sodium and fluid retention, (mild) weight gain (edema), excreted in breast milk	*Drug:* Even though food may slightly delay or reduce absorption, take drug after meals or with food to reduce gastric irritation. (An antacid may be prescribed.) *Diet Rx:* Inform patient to avoid alcoholic beverages. Even though salt and fluid retention effects are less pronounced than with phenylbutazone, a sodium-restricted diet may be indicated. *Other:* Drug-induced gastric bleeding may contribute to or aggravate iron-deficiency anemia.
Methyldopa (anti-hypertensive)	Diarrhea, nausea or vomiting	Salt and fluid retention, dry mouth, weight gain (edema), excreted in breast milk	*Diet Rx:* See clonidine. *Other:* See hydralazine (Table 2). Also see Tables 5 and 7 with regard to protein and amino acid effects on drug action.
Phenylbutazone (anti-inflammatory)	Constipation (or diarrhea), heartburn or indigestion; nausea or vomiting, ulcerogenic potential	Salt and fluid retention, weight gain (edema), excreted in breast milk	*Drug:* Take with meals to minimize gastric irritation. *Diet Rx:* May indicate the need for a sodium-restricted diet. Instruct patient to avoid alcoholic beverages. *Other:* See indomethacin.
Sodium polystyrene sulfonate (antihyperkalemic, cation-exchange resin)	Constipation, fecal impaction, nausea or vomiting	Sodium retention, hypokalemia, hypocalcemia, hypomagnesemia, loss of appetite	*Drug:* Mix oral dose with food or suspend in water or other fluids appropriate for patients with renal disease. May be mixed with sorbitol. *Diet Rx:* May indicate sodium restriction, as drug contains about 100 mg sodium/g. (Drug is usually administered with sorbitol to hasten elimination of potassium, prevent constipation, and reduce tendency toward fecal impaction.)

TABLE 5. Effects of Various Foods and Beverages on Drug Absorption

Food or Beverage	Drug	Effect
Coffee and tea	Neuroleptic agents (fluphenazine, haloperidol)	Mixing drug with coffee or tea can precipitate the drug, prevent absorption, and impede its therapeutic effects.
Fiber bran pectin(?) or high carbohydrate meal	Digoxin Acetaminophen	May reduce drug absorption. May depress rate of drug absorption.
Food (in general)	Chlorothiazide Propranolol Nitrofurantoin Cimetidine Aspirin Antimicrobial agents (cephalexin, penicillin G, erythromycin stearate, penicillin V, tetracycline)	May increase drug absorption. May increase drug absorption. Increases bioavailability of the drug. Delayed absorption may benefit patient by maintaining blood concentration of drug between meals. May decrease drug absorption and absorptive rate. May reduce drug absorption.
High fat meal	Griseofulvin	Increases drug absorption.
High protein diets	Levodopa, methyldopa	Amino acids from dietary protein inhibit absorption of drugs.
Milk and milk products	Tetracycline	Calcium inhibits drug absorption.
Milky meal[†]	Methotrexate	May inhibit drug absorption.

[†] Milky meal contained milk, corn flakes, white bread, butter, and sugar.

TABLE 6. Effects of Various Foods and Beverages on Drug Action

Food or Beverage	Drug	Effect
Beverages coffee, tea, and other caffeine-containing beverages	Theophylline	Increased intake may enhance drug side effects (nervousness, insomnia).
	Neuroleptic agents (fluphenazine, haloperidol)	Increased intake may result in a large variation in plasma concentration of drug and may reduce its clinical effectiveness.
citrus juices	Quinidine	Excessive intake may increase blood levels of drug (alkalinization of urine).
Licorice	Antihypertensive agents, diuretics	Glycyrrhizic acid in natural licorice tends to induce hypokalemia and sodium retention; ingestion in large amounts may complicate antihypertensive drug therapy.
	Digoxin	Licorice-induced hypokalemia may enhance the action of digitalis and result in drug toxicity.
Protein or charcoal-broiled meats	Theophylline	High protein or low carbohydrate diet or ingestion of charcoal broiled meats may decrease plasma half-life of drug.
Salty foods, sodium (salt)	Lithium	Increased intake of sodium may reduce therapeutic response to drug. Low-salt diets may enhance drug activity.
Vegetables boiled or fried onions	Warfarin	May increase fibrinolytic activity of drug.
broccoli, turnip greens, lettuce, cabbage	Warfarin	Vegetables rich in vitamin K may inhibit hypoprothrombinemic response to oral anticoagulants.

**TABLE 7.   Vitamins, Minerals, and Other Supplements
That Affect Drug Action**

Supplement	Drug	Effect
Vitamins		
vitamin A	Alcohol	Hypervitaminosis A may enhance hepatotoxicity of alcohol.
	Isotretinoin	Additive toxic effects may result from combination therapy with vitamin A or other supplements containing vitamin A.
	Tetracycline	Combination therapy may enhance drug-induced intracranial hypertension (severe headache).
vitamin D	Digoxin	Vitamin D-induced hypercalcemia may potentiate the effects of the drug and result in cardiac arrhythmias.
vitamin E	Warfarin	May enhance anticoagulant response to warfarin.
vitamin K	Warfarin	Vitamin K in liquid food supplements may inhibit the hypoprothrombic effect of drug.
ascorbic acid	Fluphenazine	Large doses may interfere with drug absorption and result in a return of manic behavior.
	Warfarin	Megadoses may decrease prothrombin time.
folacin	Methotrexate	Folacin or its derivatives in vitamin preparations may alter responses to drug.
	Phenytoin	May decrease anticonvulsant action of drug.
pyridoxine	Levodopa	Reverses the antiparkinsonism effect of drug.
	Phenytoin	Large doses may reduce phenytoin levels.
	Hydralazine, isoniazid, penicillamine	May correct drug-induced peripheral neuropathy.
Minerals		
calcium, iron, magnesium, zinc	Tetracycline	Concurrent use may decrease drug absorption.
iron	Penicillamine	Concurrent use may decrease drug effectiveness.
Other supplements		
para-aminobenzoic acid	Methotrexate	?May increase toxicity by displacing drug from plasma protein binding (*in vitro study*).
	Pyrimethamine	?May interfere with drug action against toxoplasmosis.
protein or amino acids	Levodopa, methyldopa, theophylline	?May inhibit drug absorption. ?May decrease plasma half-life of drug.
tryptophan	Monoamine oxidase inhibitors	May cause a deterioration in mental status.
yeast extracts	Monoamine oxidase inhibitors	Concomitant intake may produce significant hypertension.

TABLE 8. Dietary and Other Suggestions to Aid in the Relief of Unpleasant Side Effects of Drugs

Drug-induced Side Effects	Suggestions*
Loss of appetite	Question patient regarding factors contributing to appetite loss. Determine food likes and dislikes. Serve favorite or special snack foods. Inform patient that food interests tend to diminish as the day progresses (breakfast may be an important first meal). Provide variety in color, texture, and temperature of food at each meal or snack. Offer small, frequent, attractive meals or snacks in a pleasant environment. Enhance food flavors by using various seasonings. Marinate meats in sauces, wines, or fruit juices. Advise patient to maintain adequate fluid intake. Instruct patient to avoid excessive alcohol intake.
Appetite stimulation or weight gain	Encourage the intake of low calorie foods, beverages, and snacks. Evaluate the intake of various beverages used to counter dry mouth. Alert patients that certain drugs may increase desire for sweets and other foods. Instruct patient or food provider to control access to various foods, snacks, or beverages.
Altered taste perception, bitter taste, or aftertaste	If permissable, advise patients to mask taste of drug with food, pulpy fruits (applesauce, crushed pineapple), fruit juices, or milk. Unless otherwise indicated, urge patient to take medication with adequate fluid. To improve taste, suggest the use of sugarless gum or water or lemon juice as mouth rinses. Encourage good oral hygiene.
Dry or sore mouth	Counsel patient to moisten (dunk) dry foods in beverages or to swallow foods or snacks with a beverage. Decrease the use of dry (or salty) foods or snacks. Offer moist, soft-textured foods (mashed potatoes or pureed vegetables, milk toast without crust, custards or puddings, fruit whips, creamed ground meat, or fish). Advise patient to avoid spicy, rough textured, or highly acidic foods or snacks. Add milk-flavored sauces, gravies, or syrups to food. Suggest the patient lick or suck on ice chips. Incorporate cold foods or beverages into meals or snacks (sherbets, ice or cold milk, ice cream, melons, fruit ices). Avoid overuse of calorie-containing fluids (weight gain may occur). Suggest the use of sugarless gum. Caution patient that the use of hard candies may increase the incidence of dental caries. Advise patient to maintain adequate fluid intake. Encourage good oral hygiene. Inquire about the use of artificial saliva.

TABLE 8. Dietary and Other Suggestions to Aid in the Relief of Unpleasant Side Effects of Drugs *(continued)*

Drug-induced Side Effects	Suggestions*
Nausea	Offer small quantities of easily digestible foods at frequent intervals.
	Reduce food volume at meals; serve beverages after meals or limit beverage intake with meals.
	Suggest the intake of toasted or dry enriched white bread, crackers, or cooked or dry ready-to-eat cereals.
	Serve cold, clear beverages or juices.
	Instruct the patient to avoid any fried, greasy, or fatty foods.
	Inform the patient or food provider that aromas from hot food may aggravate nausea.
	Reschedule mealtimes if nausea occurs at consistent times each day.
	Evaluate discomfort as a possible side effect of drug (nausea in a digitalized patient may be a possible indication of drug toxicity, especially in the elderly).
	Suggest that patient take deep breaths or find other distractions to relieve nausea.
Heartburn	Question patient regarding factors that may contribute to heartburn.
	Offer small quantities of food at frequent intervals. Advise patient to avoid overeating.
	Instruct the patient not to homogenize, mince, or puree food (may stimulate acid secretion).
	Control the use of alcohol; coffee, tea, and other caffeine-containing beverages; decaffeinated coffee; chocolate or peppermint; and pepper.
	Avoid serving orange and citric juices, tomato products and other highly acidic foods, and concentrated fruit beverages if they are found to cause heartburn.
	Advise patient to avoid spicy, greasy, fried, or fatty foods.
	Evaluate the intake of milk or cream (may stimulate acid secretion).
	Urge patient to avoid eating before bedtime.
	If patient is overweight, advise patient to decrease food intake sensibly to lose weight.
Constipation	Question patient about the prolonged use or overuse of cathartics or laxatives.
	Incorporate sources of bulk or fiber in diet (include raw vegetables and fruits high in fiber, whole grain breads and cereals, bran or pulpy fruit, and vegetable juices).
	Advise patient to maintain adequate fluid or water intake.
	Encourage a daily program of exercise, if permissible.
	Inform patient about the importance of good health habits—regular meals, defecation reflex recognition (usually active after meals), and regularity in defecation time.

TABLE 8. Dietary and Other Suggestions to Aid in the Relief of Unpleasant Side Effects of Drugs *(continued)*

Drug-induced Side Effects	Suggestions*
Diarrhea	Focus on fluid and electrolyte replacement. Maintain adequate fluid intake and encourage the intake of juices high in postassium.
	Urge patient to drink a variety of beverages betweeen meals to counter dehydration.
	Serve small quantities of food at frequent intervals.
	Suggest the incorporation of pectin-containing foods in the diet (applesauce, grated raw apple).
	Let hot foods cool slightly before eating; cold foods or beverages may also aggravate diarrhea.
	Evaluate the intake (and amount) of foods high in fiber, caffeine-containing beverages, alcohol, milk products, or other foods which may be contributing to the diarrhea.
Flatulence	Question patient regarding factors that may contribute to flatulence.
	Encourage patient to avoid gas-forming foods (a matter of individual response).
	Advise patient to chew food slowly with mouth closed.

*Suggestions are intended to reinforce rather than replace any information in the diet prescription provided by the physician.

NUTRITIVE VALUE OF ALCOHOLIC AND CARBONATED BEVERAGES

Beverage	Amount	Kilo-calories	Carbo-hydrate, (g)	Alcohol,* (g)
Alcoholic beverages				
Beer	8 oz	100	9	9
Brandy	Brandy glass	75	. . .	11
Gin, rum, vodka, whiskey	1 jigger			
80 proof		70	. . .	10
90 proof		80	. . .	11
100 proof		90	. . .	13
Liqueurs, average	Cordial glass	65	6	7
Wines	3 1/2 oz			
Champagne		75	3	10
Muscatel		160	14	15
Sauterne		85	4	10
Table wine		85	. . .	10
Vermouth, French		105	1	15
Vermouth, Italian		165	12	18
Carbonated beverages	8 oz			
Carbonated waters				
(sweetened quinine soda)		75	19	. . .
Colas		95	24	. . .
Ginger ale		75	19	. . .
Root beer		100	25	. . .
Soda, cream or fruit-flavored		105	26	. . .

*Alcohol calculated as 7 kilocalories per gram.

Caloric Value of Alcoholic Beverages

The caloric contribution of an alcoholic beverage can be estimated by multiplying the number of ounces by the proof and then again by the factor 0.8. For beers and wines, kilocalories can be estimated by multiplying ounces by percentage of alcohol and then by the factor 1.6.

SUGGESTED READINGS

Adams CF. Nutritive value of american foods in common units. In: Agriculture handbook, No. 456. Washington, D.C.: United States Department of Agriculture, 1975.

Gastineau CF. Alcohol and calories. Mayo Clin Proc 1976; 51:88.

Pennington JAT, Church HN. Alcoholic beverages—caloric, carbohydrate and alcohol content. In: Pennington JAT, Church HN, eds. Bowes and Church's food values of portions commonly used. 14th ed. Philadelphia: JB Lippincott, 1985;196–197.

METROPOLITAN WEIGHT* AND HEIGHT† TABLES (1983)[1]

WOMEN				HEIGHT		MEN			
WEIGHT						WEIGHT			
Pounds		Kilograms				Pounds		Kilograms	
Av-erage	Range	Av-erage	Range	Feet	Centi-meters	Av-erage	Range	Av-erage	Range
117	102–131	53.2	46.4–59.5	4'9"	145	—	—	—	—
119	103–134	54.1	46.8–60.9	4'10"	147	—	—	—	—
121	104–137	55.0	47.3–62.3	4'11"	150	—	—	—	—
123	106–140	56.0	48.2–63.6	5'0"	152	—	—	—	—
126	108–143	57.3	49.1–65.0	5'1"	155	139	128–150	63.2	58.2–68.2
129	111–147	58.6	50.5–66.8	5'2"	158	142	130–153	64.5	59.1–69.5
133	114–151	60.5	51.8–68.6	5'3"	160	144	132–156	65.5	60.0–70.1
136	117–155	61.8	53.2–70.4	5'4"	163	147	134–160	66.8	60.1–72.7
140	120–159	63.6	54.5–72.3	5'5"	165	150	136–164	68.2	61.8–74.5
143	123–163	65.0	55.9–74.1	5'6"	168	153	138–168	69.5	62.3–76.4
147	126–167	66.8	57.3–75.9	5'7"	170	156	140–172	70.9	63.6–78.2
150	129–170	68.2	58.6–77.3	5'8"	173	159	142–176	72.3	64.5–80.0
153	132–173	69.5	60.0–78.6	5'9"	175	162	144–180	73.6	65.4–81.8
156	135–176	70.9	61.4–80.0	5'10"	178	165	146–184	75.0	66.4–83.4
159	138–179	72.3	62.7–81.4	5'11"	180	169	149–188	76.8	67.7–85.4
—	—	—	—	6'0"	183	172	152–192	78.2	69.1–87.3
—	—	—	—	6'1"	185	176	155–197	80.0	70.4–89.5
—	—	—	—	6'2"	188	180	158–202	81.8	71.8–91.8
—	—	—	—	6'3"	191	185	162–207	84.1	73.6–94.1

*Weights are at ages 25 to 59 yr based on lowest mortality. Weight is in pounds (indoor clothing weighing 3 lb for women, 5 lb for men).
†The table is adjusted to reflect subject without shoes for height measurement.

REFERENCE

1. Adapted with permission from: 1979 Build Study Society of Actuaries and Association of Life Insurance Medical Directors of America, 1980. Courtesy of Metropolitan Life Insurance Company.

MAYO CLINIC NORMAL PHYSIOLOGIC VALUES

Blood or Serum Values	Normal Ranges
Ascorbic acid (vitamin C)	0.6–2.0 mg/dl
Bleeding time—Simplate	3–11 min
Calcium, total	8.9–10.1 mg/dl
Carotene	48–200 μg/dl
Chloride	100–108 mEq/liter
Copper	0.75–1.45 μg/ml
Erythrocyte count	M, 4.5–6.2 × 10^6/μl
	F, 4.2–5.4 × 10^6/μl
Ferritin	Newborn: 25–200 μg/L
	1 mo: 200–600 μg/L
	2–5 mo: 50–200 μg/L
	6 mo–15y: 7–142 μg/L
	M, 20–300 μg/L
	F, 20–120 μg/L
Folate (serum)	2–20 μg/ml
Glucose, fasting	70–100 mg/dl
Glycosylated hemoglobin	4.0–7.0%
Hematocrit	M, 38.6–48.0%
	F, 34.5–43.9%
Hemoglobin	M, 12.9–16.6 g/dl
	F, 11.6–14.9 g/dl
Iron	M, 75–175 μg/dl
	F, 65–165 μg/dl
Iron binding capacity, total	240–450 μg/dl
Iron binding capacity, % saturation	18–50%

Lipids	Male (mg/dl)	Female (mg/dl)
Cholesterol		
upper 90th percentile	6 yr: 187	189
	10 yr: 196	203
	15 yr: 190	199
	20 yr: 204	197
	25 yr: 222	207
	30 yr: 238	217
	35 yr: 250	228
	40 yr: 258	239
	45 yr: 264	251
	50 yr: 270	263
	55 yr: 275	276
	60 yr: 278	290

MAYO CLINIC NORMAL PHYSIOLOGIC VALUES *(continued)*

Blood or Serum Values			Normal Ranges
		Male (mg/dl)	Female (mg/dl)
HDL cholesterol (for males and females > 20 yr, values 30–37 mg/ dl are considered "marginally low")	<20 yr:	30–65	30–70
	20–29 yr:	30–70	30–75
	30–39 yr:	30–70	35–80
	40–49 yr:	30–70	35–85
	50–59 yr:	30–70	35–85
	>60 yr:	30–70	35–85
Triglicerides upper 95th percentile	6 yr:	102	76
	10 yr:	103	121
	15 yr:	124	122
	20 yr:	137	97
	25 yr:	157	100
	30 yr:	171	106
	35 yr:	182	110
	40 yr:	189	117
	45 yr:	193	122
	50 yr:	195	128
	55 yr:	197	134
	60 yr:	198	140
Magnesium			1.7–2.1 mg/dl
Osmolality			275–295 mOsm/kg
Phosphorus			2.5–4.5 mg/dl
Potassium			3.6–4.8 mEq/L
Prealbumin			16.6–40.2 mg/dl
Protein, total			6.3–7.9 g/dl
Protein electrophoresis			
Albumin			3.1–4.3 g/dl
Alpha-1 globulin			0.1–0.3 g/dl
Alpha-2 globulin			0.6–1.0 g/dl
Beta-globulin g/dl			0.7–1.4 g/dl
Gamma globulin			0.7–1.6 g/dl
Prothrombin time			10.9–12.85
Sodium			135–145 mEq/L
Urea			M, 17–51 mg/dl
			F, 13–45 mg/dl
Uric acid			M, 4.3–8.0 mg/dl
			F, 2.3–6.0 mg/dl
Vitamin A			360–1,200 μg/L
Vitamin B_{12}			F, 190–765 ng/L
			M, <29y: 281–1079 ng/L
			30–39y: 248–965 ng/L
			40–49y: 218–863 ng/L
			50–59y: 191–770 ng/L
			60–69y: 168–687 ng/L
			>70y: 152–630 ng/L
Vitamin E			5.5–17.0 mg/L
1,25 Dihydroxy vitamin D			15–60 pg/ml
25-hydroxy vitamin D			Winter 14–42 ng/ml
			Summer 15–80 ng/ml
Zinc			0.66–1.10 μg/ml

Urine Values	Normal Ranges
Ammonia	36–86 mEq/24 hr
Calcium	M, 25–300 mg/24 hr
	F, 20–275 mg/24 hr
Chromium	<8 μg/24 hr
Creatinine clearance	M (20y), 90 ml/min/SA
	F (20y), 84 ml/min/SA
	(decreased by 6 ml/min/ decade)

MAYO CLINIC NORMAL PHYSIOLOGIC VALUES *(continued)*

Urine Values	Normal Ranges
Osmolality	300–800 mOsm/kg <100, mOsm/kg overhydrated >800 mOsm/kg dehydrated
Oxalate	M, 20–60 mg/24 hr F, 20–55 mg/24 hr
Potassium	30–90 mEq/24 hr
Protein, total	M, 0–150 mg/24 hr F, 27–93 mg/24 hr
Renal clearance—standard	
Glomerular filtration rate (inulin or iothalamate[125]I)	90–130 ml/min/surface area* at age 20 (decreased by 4 ml/min/decade)
Effective renal plasma flow (PAH)	400–700 ml/min/surface area* at age 20 (decreased by 17 ml/min/decade)
Filtration fraction	18–22%
Renal clearance—short	
Glomerular filtration rate (iothalamate[125]I)	110 ml/min/surface area* at age 20 (decreased by 4 ml/min/decade)
Glomerular filtration rate (creatinine)	See creatinine clearance
Sodium	40–217 mEq/24 hr
Uric acid	<750 mg/24 hr
Zinc	300–600 μg/24 hr

Miscellaneous Values	Normal Ranges
Basal metabolism rate	−10 to +10%
Stool examination	
Fat, quantitative	2–7 g/24 hr
Fat, percent	0–20%
Nitrogen	1–2 g/24 hr
Vitamin B_{12} absorption (Schilling test)	≥8% excretion

*Surface area is a standard measure of body surface area; 1.73 m^2.

Directions for Estimating Caloric Requirement:

To determine the desired allowance of kilocalories, proceed as follows: 1. Locate the ideal weight on Column I by means of a common pin. 2. Bring edge of one end of a 12 or 15-inch ruler against the pin. 3. Swing the other end of the ruler to the patient's height on Column II. 4. Transfer the pin to the point where the ruler crosses Column III. 5. Hold the ruler against the pin in Column III. 6. Swing the left hand end of the ruler to the patient's sex and age (measured from last birthday) given in Column IV (these positions correspond to the Mayo Clinic's metabolism standards for age and sex). 7. Transfer the pin to the point where the ruler crosses Column V. This gives the basal kilocaloric requirement (basal kilocalories) of the patient for 24 hours and represents the kilocalories required by the fasting patient when resting in bed. 8. To provide the extra kilocalories for activity and work, the basal kilocalories are increased by a percentage. To the basal kilocalories for adults add: 50 to 80 per cent for manual laborers, 30 to 40 per cent for light work or 10 to 20 per cent for restricted activity such as resting in a room or in bed. To the basal kilocalories for children add 50 to 100 per cent for children ages 5 to 15 years. This computation may be done by simple arithmetic or by the use of Columns VI and VII. If the latter method is chosen, locate the "per cent above or below basal" desired in Column VI. By means of the ruler connect this point with the pin on Column V. Transfer the pin to the point where the ruler crosses Column VII. This represents the calories estimated to be required by the patient.

W. M. Boothby and J. Berkson
October, 1933
Copyright, 1959
Mayo Association

MC-702 Rev. 10-59

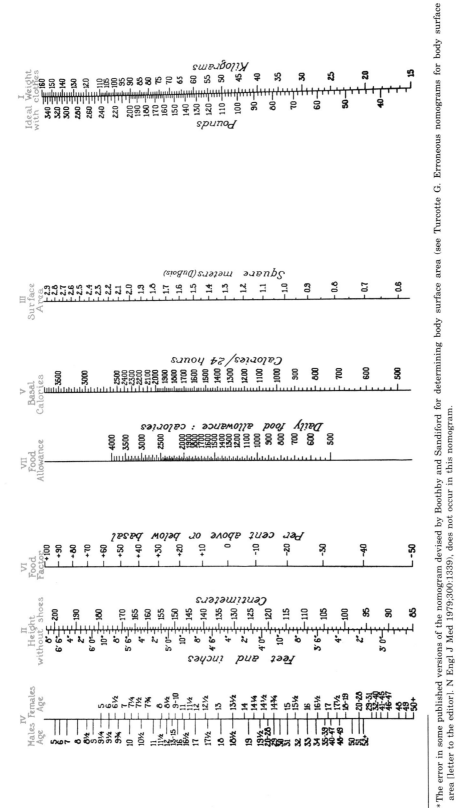

*The error in some published versions of the nomogram devised by Boothby and Sandiford for determining body surface area (see Turcotte G. Erroneous nomograms for body surface area [letter to the editor]. N Engl J Med 1979;300:1339), does not occur in this nomogram.

NOMOGRAM FOR BODY MASS INDEX

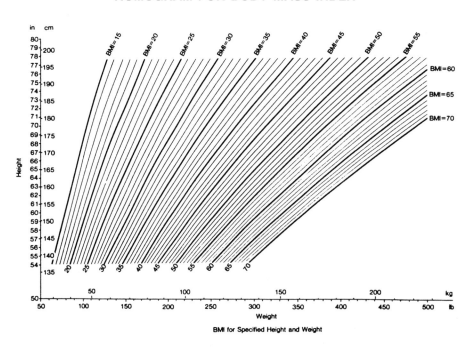

BMI for Specified Height and Weight

Body mass index (BMI) (body weight in kilograms/height in meters^2) for specified height and weight, barefoot and unclothed. A woman with a BMI over 27.3, or a man with a BMI over 27.8, is at increased risk of the health complications of obesity

Reproduced with permission from the Portland Health Institute, Portland, Oregon.

SUGGESTED READING

Frankel HM. Determination of body mass index. JAMA 1986;255:1292.

A dietetic product is one in which some ingredient has been restricted or changed and a substitution has been made. The Food and Drug Administration has labeling regulations for food manufacturers making nutritional claims. The following are commonly used labeling terms and their definitions.

Low Calorie: No more than 40 Kcal per serving with a caloric density of no more than 0.4 Kcal per gram as consumed. Foods naturally low in kilocalories must be labeled so this fact is clear.

Reduced Kilocalorie: Foods must be at least one-third lower in caloric content than a similar food. The label must describe the comparison on which the reduced kilocalories claim is based.

Diet, Dietetic, Artificially Sweetened: These terms may be used if a food item qualifies as a low caloric or reduced caloric food.

Sugar Free, Sugarless, No Sugar: These terms may be used if a food item is labeled as low kilocalorie or reduced kilocalorie unless used for purposes other than weight control.

Light or Lite: There are no labeling regulations for this term. The dictionary defines light as less than the usual weight, amount, or intensity. Generally, the term is used for a food that is reduced in kilocalories, fat, or sodium.

Nutritive and Non-nutritive Alternative Sweeteners: The presence of sweeteners must be indicated on the label.

Sodium Free: Less than or equal to 5 mg of sodium per serving.

Very Low Sodium: Less than or equal to 35 mg of sodium per serving.

Low Sodium: Less than or equal to 140 mg of sodium per serving.

Reduced Sodium: At least a 75 percent reduction in the usual level of sodium in the food.

Unsalted: No salt added during processing to a food normally processed with salt.

Extra Lean: Less than or equal to 5 percent fat than a comparable product.

Lean and Low Fat: Less than or equal to 10 percent fat than a comparable product.

Light, Lite, Leaner and Lower Fat: At least 25 percent less fat than similar products.

549

Pending Ammendment

Cholesterol Free: Less than or equal to 2 mg of cholesterol per serving.
Low Cholesterol: Less than or equal to 20 mg of cholesterol per serving.
Reduced Cholesterol: At least a 75 percent reduction in cholesterol content compared with the food it replaces.

REFERENCES

1. Food labeling. Fed Regist Jan 19, 1973;38:2124.
2. Food labeling; declaration of sodium content of foods and label claims for foods on the basis of sodium content; extension of effective date. Fed Regist July 1, 1985;50:26984.
3. Food labeling; definitions of cholesterol free, low cholesterol and reduced cholesterol. Fed Regist Nov 25, 1986;51:42584.
4. USDA policy memos 070A and 071A. Washington D.C.: U.S. Department of Agriculture, Food Safety and Inspection Service, Printing and Distribution Section, Room 0151—South Building, 1986.

AMERICAN HEART ASSOCIATION THREE PHASE APPROACH TO DIET

Nutrient	Phase I	Phase II	Phase III
Cholesterol	≤300 mg/day	200–250 mg/day	100 mg/day
Total Kilocalories	Reduction to achieve and/or to maintain ideal weight	Reduction to achieve and/or to maintain ideal weight	Reduction to achieve and/or to maintain ideal weight
Total fat (% of Kilocalories)	30–35	25–30	20–25
Saturated	10–15	8	7
Monounsaturated	10	8	7
Polyunsaturated	10	8	7
P:S Ratio	1.4–1.2	1.5–1.1	1.5–1.1
Carbohydrate (% of Kilocalories)	45–50	50–55	55–65
Starch	30–25	increased more	40
Simple sugar	10	decreased more	minimal
Protein (% of Kilo-calories)	20–24	19–25	18–25
Sodium	decreased	decreased indirectly	76–100 mEq
Potassium	increased indirectly	increased indirectly	120–150 mEq
Dietary Fiber	increased indirectly	increased indirectly	48–60 g
Alcohol	Limit to 0 to 1 drink per day	Limit to 0 to 1 drink per day	Limit to 0 to 1 drink per day

NUTRITIVE AND NON-NUTRITIVE SWEETENERS

Nutritive Sweeteners				
Sweetener	*Derivation*	*Sweetness*	*Description*	*Use*
Sucrose	Dissaccharide fructose and glucose (derived—sugar cane and beets)	Used as standard for sweeteners, therefore, is assigned the number, 1	Requires insulin for metabolism; causes rise in blood glucose 4 Kcal/g	Table top sweetner, foods beverages, drugs Cariogenic
Fructose or Levulose	Monosaccharide	1.1–1.7 times sweeter than sucrose	Metabolized in liver, thus does not require insulin to enter liver cells. With insulin insufficiency, glycogen synthesis is impaired and a rise in blood glucose can occur. Has affected triglyceride levels in some diabetics. 4 Kcal/g	Table top sweetener, foods, beverages, drugs, occurs naturally in fruits Cariogenic
Sorbitol, Mannitol	Reduction of glucose polyalcohol	0.5–0.7 times the sweetness of sucrose	Metabolized same pathway as fructose. Osmotic diarrhea can occur with ingestion of 30–50 g sorbitol or 20 g of mannitol 4 Kcal/g	Sugarless gum and candies Noncariogenic
Xylitol	Reduction of xylose polyalcohol	1 times sweeter than sucrose	Limited impact on blood sugar. Osmotic diarrhea can occur with ingestion of 30–40 g 4 Kcal/g	Question potential toxicity. Use in U.S. discontinued until results of FDA study completed. Noncariogenic
Dextrose	Starch hydrolysate	0.7 times the sweetness of sucrose	Similar to sucrose 4 Kcal/g	Used in foods with liquid base Cariogenic
Polydextrose	Polymer dextrose	Less sweet than sucrose	Unclear how it affects blood sugar 1 Kcal/g	Replaces sucrose Approved in 1981 by FDA
High Fructose Corn Syrup	Fructose and dextrose		High fructose content. Same effect on blood glucose as for fructose	
Extraction 55%		1 times sweeter than sucrose		
Extraction 90%		1.5 times sweeter than sucrose		
Not Available in U.S. Maltitol	Reduction Maltose Polyalcohol	0.9 times the sweetness of sucrose		Controversy whether caloric or non-caloric sweetener. Not approved for use in U.S. although used widely in Japan Noncariogenic

NUTRITIVE AND NON-NUTRITIVE SWEETENERS *(continued)*

Non-nutritive Sweeteners

Sweetener	Derivation	Sweetness	Description	Use
Available in U.S.				
Aspartame (Equal, Nutra-sweet)	Dipeptide	180–200 times sweeter than sucrose	Metabolized in a similar manner as protein. 4 Kcal/g Unstable when heated	Questions of safety, therefore moderate ingestion recommended. Used in foods, beverages, drugs, table top sweetner. Noncariogenic
Saccharin	Phthalic anhydride derivative	300–400 times sweeter than sucrose	Essentially no kilocalorie value. Bitter after-taste	Questions of safety, therefore moderate ingestion recommended. Used in foods, beverages, drugs, table top sweetener. Noncariogenic
Not Available in U.S. Currently				
Cyclamates	Sulfonated cyclohexylamine	30 times sweeter than sucrose	Free of aftertaste	Banned in 1969 by FDA as cancer risk. Used in some countries including Canada. ? Noncariogenic
Thaumatin (Talin)	Extract from Thaumatoccus danielli plant of West Africa	2,000–3,000 times sweeter than sucrose	Protein Flavor & aroma enhancer Unstable when heated Licorice aftertaste	Used as substitute for saccharin Widely used in Japan since 1979 Unknown if cariogenic
Stevioside	Extract from leaves of stevia rebaldiana plant	300 times sweeter than sucrose		Used as substitute for saccharin Widely used in Japan Non-cariogenic
Acesulfame-K	Acetoacetic acid derivative	130–200 times sweeter than sucrose	Not metabolized Does not lose sweetness	In the process of passing qualification tests for marketing.
Glycyrrhizin	Licorice root extract	50–100 times sweeter than sucrose	Licorice flavor	Used as flavoring for tobacco and pharmaceuticals. Foaming agent in soft drinks. Undergoing evaluation by FDA as a sweetener

Adapted from Wylie-Rosett J, EdD RD. Alternative sweeteners For diabetics. Cardiovascular Reviews and Reports 1982;3:1386–1391.

ORAL REHYDRATION SOLUTIONS

Solution*	Electrolyte Concentration
Rehydralyte™ (Ross Laboratories)	Na⁺ 75 mEq/L Na^+ 75 mEq/L

Solution*	Electrolyte Concentration
Rehydralyte™ (Ross Laboratories)	Na^+ 75 mEq/L K^+ 20 mEq/L Cl^- 65 mEq/L Glucose 25 g/L
World Health Organization Formula[1] 3.5 g Table Salt (NaCl) 2.5 g Baking Soda (NaHCO₃) 1.5 g Potassium Chloride (KCl) 20.0 g Glucose (2%) 960 g Water	*Electrolyte Concentration* Na^+ 90 mM HCO_3 30 mM K^+ 20 mM Cl^- 80 mM Glucose 111 mM

*To improve palatability, noncaloric flavoring can be added (e.g., commercial enteral formula flavor packets, unsweetened or artificially sweetened beverage mixes).

REFERENCE

1. MacMahon RA. The use of the World Health Organization's oral rehydration solution in patients on home parenteral nutrition. JPEN 1984;8:720–721.

CALCIUM AND PHOSPHORUS CONTENT OF FOODS[1]

Food	Amount	Calcium (mg)	Phosphorus (mg)
Meat, fish, poultry			
Beef	1 oz	4	70
Pork	1 oz	4	100
Chicken	1 oz	4	75
Liver	1 oz	2	100
Fish, average	1 oz	15	75
Tuna in oil—Albacore	1/4 cup	2	78
Sardines, canned, with bones	1 oz	86	250
Salmon, pink, canned	1 oz	78	114
Luncheon meat	1 oz	3	35
Bacon, strip	1–5 g	1	11
Meat substitutes			
Eggs, poached, large	1	28	90
Dried beans, average, cooked	2/5 cup	44	144
Lentils, cooked	2/3 cup	25	119
Peanuts and peanut butter	1 Tbsp	11	60
Milk			
Whole milk	1 cup	290	227
2% milk	1 cup	297	232
Skim milk	1 cup	302	247
Buttermilk	1 cup	285	219
Chocolate milk—2%	1 cup	284	254
Hot cocoa with whole milk	1 cup	298	270
Other dairy products			
Yogurt, plain, low fat	8 oz	415	326
Cheddar cheese	1 oz	206	146
Swiss cheese	1 oz	272	171
Processed American cheese	1 oz	174	211
Cottage cheese, creamed	1/4 cup	31	69
Half and half	2 Tbsp	32	28
Vanilla ice cream	1/2 cup	88	67
Sherbet	1/2 cup	48	38
Cereal and grain products			
Bread, white	1 slice	30	26
Bread, whole meat	1 slice	17	63
Bread products made from white flour			
Biscuit, homemade	1	34	49

CALCIUM AND PHOSPHORUS CONTENT OF FOODS[1] (continued)

Food	Amount	Calcium (mg)	Phosphorus (mg)
Biscuit, mix	1	58	128
Doughnut, cake	1 average	11	55
Doughnut, raised, yeast	1 average	11	23
Pancake, batter mix	1 medium	22	110
Sweet roll	1 average	11	30
Waffle, frozen	5-in diameter, 1 waffle	85	135
Cereal, refined	1/2 cup cooked	49	73
Cereal, refined	3/4 cup dry	7	41
Cereal, whole grain	1/2 cup cooked;	19	94
Cereal, whole grain	3/4 cup dry	13	114
Crackers, saltines	5 2-in squares	10	15
Crackers, graham	2 2½ in squares	5	17
Macaroni, spaghetti, noodles	1/2 cup cooked	8	47
Rice, white	1/2 cup cooked	5	17
Vegetables	100 g, about 1/2 cup cooked (unless otherwise indicated)		
Artichokes		51	69
Asparagus		21	50
Bean sprouts		17	48
Broccoli		88	62
Brussels sprouts		32	72
Cabbage		44	20
Corn, frozen, yellow		5	72
Cress		61	48
Greens			
Beet greens		99	25
Collards		152	39
Dandelion greens		140	42
Kale	3/4 cup	134	46
Mustard greens		138	32
Spinach		83	33
Swiss chard		73	24
Turnip greens	2/3 cup	184	37
Leeks	3–4 medium	52	50
Lima beans	5/8 cup	47	121
Mushrooms	raw ~ 10 small	6	116
Okra	8–9 pods	92	41
Parsnips		45	62
Peas, whole, mature		19	102
Potatoes, white, baked	1 medium	9	65
Rutabagas		59	31
Winter squash, baked		28	48
Other vegetables, average		25	26
Fruit			
Blackberries	1/2 cup	23	15
Orange, Valencia	1 medium	48	21
Raspberries	1/2 cup	13	7
Rhubarb	1/2 cup	174	10
Tangerine	1 medium	12	8
Fresh fruit, average	1/2 cup or 1 medium	16	20
Canned fruit, average	1/2 cup	10	12
Fruit juice	1/2 cup	8	10
Fats and Oils			
Butter or margarine	1 tsp	1	1
Nondairy cream substitute, nondairy powder	1 tsp	Tr	8
French dressing	1 Tbsp	2	2
Gravy	1 Tbsp	0	Tr
Mayonnaise	1 tsp	1	1

CALCIUM AND PHOSPHORUS CONTENT OF FOODS[1] *(continued)*

Food	Amount	Calcium (mg)	Phosphorus (mg)
Sweets			
Candy, sugar	1/2 oz	0	0
Candy, milk chocolate	1/2 oz	22	45
Honey	1 Tbsp	1	1
Jelly	1 Tbsp	4	1
Sugar, white	1 Tbsp	0	0
Sugar, brown	1 Tbsp	11	5
Syrup, maple	1 Tbsp	33	3
Desserts			
Assorted cookies	1 2-in.	7	15
Cake, white, mix	1 piece, 2 in by 3 in by 2 in	34	115
Pie, cream	1/8 of 9-in pie	62	88
Pie, fruit	1/8 of 9-in pie	10	25
Snack foods			
Popcorn	1 cup	2	39
Potato chips	5	4	14
Beverages			
Beer	8 oz	9	33
Carbonated beverages			
Colas, average	8 oz	8	35
Ginger ale, average	8 oz	7	0
Coffee, brewed	6 oz	13	4
Tea	6 oz	4	8

REFERENCE

1. Pennington JAT, Church HN. Bowes and Church's food values of portions commonly used. 14th ed. Philadelphia: JB Lippincott, 1985.

ENTERAL NUTRITION

Polymeric Formulas—

| Formula | Caloric Density (Kcal/ml) | Nutrients per 1,000 Milliliters | | | | | |
		Protein (g) (% Kcal)	Fat (g) (% Kcal)	Carbo-hydrate (g) (% Kcal)	Non-protein Kcal:N	mOsm/kg	Sodium (mg/mEq)
Complete Regular (Sandoz)	1.07	43 (16%)	43 (36%)	128 (48%)	131:1	405	1,300/56
Complete-Modified (Sandoz)	1.07	43 (16%)	37 (30%)	141 (54%)	131:1	300	670/29
Vitaneed (Sher-wood)	1.0	35 (14%)	40 (36%)	125 (50%)	154:1	310	500/22

* Reprinted with permission from: Nelson JK. Home enteral nutrition. In: Spittell JA, ed. Clinical Medicine. Vol 9,
† Characteristics: Contain nondigestible residue; ± lactose; require intact bowel function
        Protein, fat, carbohydrate—based on blended mix of food
        Not intended for oral use

FORMULAS*

Blended Foodstuffs[†]

Potassium (mg/mEq)	Vol (ml) to meet Vitamin Requirements	Protein Sources	Fat Sources	Carbohydrate Sources
1,400/36	1,500	Beef puree, nonfat dry milk	Beef puree, corn oil	Maltodextrins, vegetables, lactose (24 g), fruit
1,400/36	1,500	Beef puree, calcium caseinate	Beef puree, corn oil	Maltodextrins, vegetables, fruit
1,250/32	2,000	Beef, sodium, and calcium caseinates	Soy oil, beef puree	Maltodextrins, pureed fruit and vegetables

Philadelphia: Harper and Row, 1985:25.

Polymeric Formulas—

		Nutrients per 1,000 Milliliters					
Formula	Calorie Density (Kcal/ml)	Protein (g) (% Kcal)	Fat (g) (% Kcal)	Carbo-hydrate (g) (% Kcal)	Non-protein Kcal:N	mOsm/kg	Sodium (mg/mEq)
CIB (Carnation)	1.1	60 (21%)	36 (29%)	136 (50%)	92:1	677–715	966/42
Meritene Liquid (Sandoz)	0.96	58 (24%)	32 (30%)	110 (46%)	79:1	505+	880/38
Meritene Powder (Sandoz)	1.0	69 (26%)	34 (29%)	119 (45%)	71:1	690	1,100/48
Sustacal Powder (Mead Johnson)	1.33	77 (24%)	34 (22%)	180 (54%)	80:1	700–1,010	1,200/54
Sustagen (Mead Johnson)	1.7	111 (24%)	16 (8%)	312 (68%)	77:1	1,100	1,270/55

* Characteristics: Moderate to low residue; milk base
Protein—intact: semipurified isolates; high molecular weight
Carbohydrate—lactose, sucrose, corn syrup solids
Hyperosmolar
Palatable, designed as oral supplement

Polymeric Formulas—

		Nutrients per 1,000 Milliliters					
Formula	Caloric Density (Kcal/ml)	Protein (g) (% Kcal)	Fat (g) (% Kcal)	Carbo-hydrate (g) (% Kcal)	Non-protein Kcal:N	mOsm/kg	Sodium (mg/mEq)
Hypercaloric							
Sustacal HC (Mead Johnson)	1.5	61 (16%)	58 (34%)	190 (50%)	134:1	650	840/37
Isocal HCN (Mead Johnson)	2.0	75 (15%)	91 (40%)	225 (45%)	145:1	690	800/35
Travasorb MCT (Travenol)	1.5	74 (20%)	50 (30%)	185 (50%)	100:1	488	524/23
Ensure Plus HN (Ross)	1.5	63 (17%)	50 (30%)	200 (53%)	125:1	650	1,184/51
Ensure Plus (Ross)	1.5	55 (15%)	53 (32%)	200 (53%)	146:1	600	1,141/50
Magnacal (Bio-search)	2.0	70 (14%)	80 (36%)	250 (50%)	154:1	590	1,000/44
TwoCal HN (Ross)	2.0	83 (17%)	90 (40%)	216 (43%)	126:1	740	1,052/46
Normocaloric							
Osmolite (Ross)	1.06	37 (14%)	38 (31%)	145 (55%)	153:1	300	634/28

Lactose Containing*

Potassium (mg/mEq)	Vol (ml) to meet Vitamin Require-ments	Protein Sources	Fat Sources	Carbohydrate Sources
2,808/72	1,373	Nonfat milk, soy protein, sodium caseinate	Milk fat	Sucrose, corn syrup solids, lactose (96 g)
1,600/41	1,250	Concentrated sweet skim milk	Corn oil	Lactose (55 g), corn syrup solids, sucrose
2,800/72	1,040	Nonfat dry milk, whole milk	Milk fat	Lactose (104 g), sucrose, corn syrup solids
3,400/87	800	Nonfat milk	Whole milk	Lactose (86 g), sucrose, corn syrup solids
3,380/87	1,030	Nonfat milk, whole milk, calcium caseinate	Milk fat	Corn syrup solids, lactose (96 g), dextrose

Lactose Free*

Potassium (mg/mEq)	Vol (ml) to meet Vitamin Require-ments	Protein Sources	Fat Sources	Carbohydrate Sources
1,480/38	1,200	Calcium and sodium caseinates	Soybean oil	Corn syrup solids, sucrose
1,400/36	1,500	Calcium and sodium caseinates	Soybean oil (70%), MCT (30%)	Corn syrup solids
1,480/38		Casein, lactalbumin, whey proteins	MCT (80%) safflower oil (20%)	Maltodextrin
1,818/47	947	Sodium and calcium caseinates, soy protein isolates	Corn oil	Corn syrup solids, sucrose
2,113/55	1,600	Sodium and calcium caseinates, soy protein isolates	Corn oil	Corn syrup solids, sucrose
1,250/32	1,000	Calcium and sodium caseinates	Soy oil	Maltodextrin, sucrose
2,316/59	950	Sodium and calcium caseinates, soy isolates	Corn oil, MCT	Hydrolyzed corn starch, sucrose
1,014/26	1,887	Sodium and calcium caseinates, soy protein isolate	MCT (50%), Corn and soy oil (50%)	Hydrolyzed cornstarch

Polymeric Formulas—

Formula	Caloric Density (Kcal/ml)	Nutrients per 1,000 Milliliters					
		Protein (g) (% Kcal)	Fat (g) (% Kcal)	Carbo-hydrate (g) (% Kcal)	Non-protein Kcal:N	mOsm/kg	Sodium (mg/mEq)
Normocaloric (continued)							
Isocal (Mead Johnson)	1.06	34 (13%)	44 (37%)	132 (50%)	167:1	300	530/23
Precision Isotonic (Sandoz)	1.0	29 (12%)	30 (28%)	144 (60%)	183:1	300	770/34
Fortison (Sher-wood)	1.0	35 (14%)	40 (36%)	125 (50%)	131:1	300	500/22
Ensure (Ross)	1.06	37 (14%)	38 (31%)	145 (55%)	153:1	450	845/37
Enrich (Ross)	1.06	40 (14%)	37 (31%)	162 (55%)	148:1	480	845/37
Travasorb Liquid (Travenol)	1.06	35 (14%)	35 (32%)	136 (55%)	154:1	488	738/32
Precision LR (San-doz)	1.1	26 (10%)	1.6 (1%)	248 (89%)	239:1	530	700/30
High Nitrogen and Normocaloric							
Precision HN (Sandoz)	1.05	44 (17%)	1.3 (1%)	216 (82%)	125:1	525	980/43
Ensure HN (Ross)	1.06	44 (17%)	36 (30%)	141 (53%)	125:1	470	930/40
Osmolite HN (Ross)	1.06	44 (17%)	37 (30%)	141 (53%)	124:1	310	930/40
Isotein HN (San-doz)	1.2	68 (23%)	34 (25%)	156 (52%)	86:1	300	620/27
Sustacal Liquid (Mead Johnson)	1.0	61 (24%)	23 (21%)	140 (55%)	79:1	625	940/41

*Characteristics: Moderate to low residue
  Protein—intact; semipurified isolates; high molecular weight; derived from casein salts or egg
  Carbohydrate—starches, maltodextrins; glucose oligosaccharides; corn syrup solids
  Fat—contributes greater percentage of calories; corn oil; soy oil; as well as MCT
  Isomolar as well as hyperosmolar
  Palatable

Lactose Free* *(continued)*

Potassium (mg/mEq)	Vol (ml) to meet Vitamin Requirements	Protein Sources	Fat Sources	Carbohydrate Sources
1,320/34	1,887	Calcium and sodium caseinates, and soy protein isolate	Soy oil (80%), MCT oil (20%)	Maltodextrin
960/25	1,560	Egg albumin	Soy oil	Glucose oligosaccharides, sucrose
1,250/32	2,000	Sodium and calcium caseinates	Corn oil	Maltodextrin
1,564/40	1,887	Sodium and calcium caseinates, soy protein isolate	Corn oil	Hydrolyzed corn starch
1,564/40	1,391	Sodium and calcium caseinates, soy protein isolate	Corn oil	Hydrolyzed corn starch, sucrose, soy polysaccharide
1,266/33	1,896	Sodium and calcium caseinates, soy protein isolate	Corn oil	Sucrose, corn syrup solids
888/22	1,710	Egg albumin	Soy oil	Maltodextrin, sucrose
910/23	2,850	Egg albumin	Soy oil	Maltodextrin, sucrose
1,564/40	1,320	Sodium and calcium caseinates, soy protein isolate	Corn oil	Corn syrup, sucrose
1,564/40	1,320	Sodium and calcium caseinates, soy protein isolates	MCT oil (50%) Corn, and soy oil (50%)	Hydrolyzed corn starch, sucrose
1,070/27	1,770	Delactosed lactalbumin	Soybean oil (N/A), MCT (N/A)	Maltodextrin, monosaccharides
2,080/53	1,080	Calcium and sodium caseinates, soy protein isolate	Soy oil	Sucrose, corn syrup

white solids

Monomeric (Elemental)

Formula	Caloric Density (Kcal/ml)	Protein (g) (% Kcal)	Fat (g) (% Kcal)	Carbo-hydrate (g) (% Kcal)	Non-protein Kcal:N	mOsm/kg	Sodium (mg/mEq)
				Nutrients per 1,000 Milliliters			
Vivonex Std (Norwich Eaton)	1.0	20 (8%)	1.5 (1%)	231 (91%)	281:1	550	468/20
Vivonex HN (Norwich Eaton)	1.0	46 (18%)	0.9 (1%)	210 (81%)	125:1	810	529/23
Vivonex TEN (Norwich Eaton)	1.0	38 (15%)	3.0 (2.5%)	206 (82%)	149:1	630	460/20
Vital HN (Ross)	1.0	42 (17%)	11 (9%)	185 (74%)	125:1	460	467/20
Criticare HN (Mead Johnson)	1.06	38 (14%)	3 (3%)	222 (83%)	148:1	650	634/27
Travasorb HN (Travenol)	1.0	45 (18%)	13 (12%)	175 (70%)	126:1	560	920/40
Travasorb STD (Travenol)	1.0	30 (12%)	13 (12%)	190 (76%)	202:1	560	920/40

*Characteristics: Minimal residue, lactose free, assimilated readily with little or no digestion
Protein—predigested (hydrolyzed protein, dipeptides and tripeptides, or crystalline amino acids)
Fat—small amount of essential fatty acids with or without medium chain triglycerides
Hyperosmolar
Poor palatability, designed primarily for tube feeding

Formulations*

Potassium (mg/mEq)	Vol (ml) to meet Vitamin Requirements	Protein Sources	Fat Sources	Carbohydrate Sources
1,172/30	1,800	L-amino acids	Safflower oil (100%)	Glucose oligosaccharides
1,173/30	3,000	L-amino acids	Safflower oil (100%)	Glucose oligosaccharides
782/20	2,000	L-amino acids (33% BCAA)	Safflower oil (100%)	Maltodextrins, modified starch
1,333/34	1,892	Whey, soy and meat protein hydrolysates, free amino acids	Safflower oil (60%) MCT oil (40%)	Hydrolyzed cornstarch, sucrose
1,320/34	1,892	Casein hydrolysates, peptides, amino acids	Safflower oil (100%)	Maltodextrins, cornstarch
1,170/30	2,000	Lactalbumin peptides	Sunflower oil (60%), MCT oil (40%)	Glucose oligosaccharides
1,170/30	2,000	Lactalbumin peptides	Sunflower oil (60%) MCT oil (10%)	Glucose oligosaccharides

Special

		Nutrients per 1,000 Milliliters					
Formula	Caloric Density (Kcal/ml)	Protein (g) (% Kcal)	Fat (g) (% Kcal)	Carbo-hydrate (g) (% Kcal)	Non-protein Kcal:N	mOsm/kg	Sodium (mg/mEq)
Hepatic							
Hepatic Aid II (Kendall McGaw)	1.1	44 (15%)	36 (27.7%)	169 (57.3%)	1:148	560	<345/<15
Travasorb Hepatic (Tra-venol)	1.1	29 (11%)	14 (12%)	209 (77%)	1:218	690	445/19
Renal							
Amin Aid (Kendall McGaw)	2.0	19 (4.0%)	46.1 (21.2%)	366 (75%)	1:830	1,095	<345/<15
Travasorb Renal (Tra-venol)	1.35	23 (7%)	18 (12%)	271 (81%)	1:363	590	%
Stress							
Stresstein (San-doz)	1.2	70 (23%)	28 (20%)	170 (57%)	1:97	910	650/28
Traum-Aid HBC (Kendall McGaw)	1.0	56 (22%)	12 (11%)	166 (67%)	1:102	675	533/23
Traumacal/Fulfil (Mead John-son)	1.5	82 (22%)	68 (40%)	143 (38%)	1:90	550	1,200/52
Pulmocare (Ross)	1.5	63 (17%)	92 (55%)	106 (28%)	1:125	490	1,310/57

*Characteristics: Formulated to meet nutrient requirements for patients with specific medical conditions

Formulas*

Potassium (mg/mEq)	Vol (ml) to meet Vitamin Requirements	Protein Sources	Fat Sources	Carbohydrate Sources
<234/<6	—	Amino acids: high branched chain amino acids (46%), low aromatic amino acids	Partially hydrogenated soy oil	Maltodextrins, sucrose
1,140/29	2,100	Amino acids: high branched chain amino acids (50%), low aromatic amino acids	MCT, sunflower oil	Glucose oligosaccharides
<234/<6	—	Essential amino acids, histidine	Partially hydrogenated soy oil	Maltodextrins, sucrose
0/0	2,100	Essential amino acids, histidine	MCT, sunflower oil	Glucose oligosaccharides, sucrose
1,100/28.2	2,000	Branched chain amino acids (44%), plus essential amino acids	MCT, soy oil	Maltodextrin
1,166/30	3,000	High branched chain amino acids (50%) plus essential and nonessential amino acids	MCT, soy oil	Maltodextrin
1,400/36	2,000	Branched chain amino acid (23%) plus essential and nonessential amino acids	MCT, soy oil	Corn syrup, sucrose
1,902/49	960	Sodium and calcium caseinates	Corn oil	Sucrose, hydrolyzed corn starch

Supplemental Nutrient

Formula	Caloric Density (Kcal/ml)	Nutrients per 1,000 Milliliters				
		Protein (g) (% Kcal)	Fat (g) (% Kcal)	Carbo-hydrate (g) (% Kcal)	Non-protein Kcal:N	mOsm/kg
Carbohydrate						
Polycose (Ross)	2.0 (3.8 Kcal/g)			500 (100%)		850
Modular (Mead Johnson)	2.0 (3.8 Kcal/g)			500 (100%)		725
Sumacal (Sherwood)	2.0 (3.8 Kcal/g)			500 (100%)		—
Fat						
MCT Oil (Mead Johnson)	7.7 (8.3 Kcal/g)		927 (100%)			
Microlipid (Sherwood)	4.5		500 (100%)			60
Protein						
Casec (Mead Johnson)	1.0 (3.7 Kcal/g)	238 (95%)	5 (5%)	0 (0%)		
RDP (Navaco)	1.0 (3.6 Kcal/g)	209 (84%)	11 (10%)	14 (6%)		
Pro Mod (Ross)	1.0 (4.2 Kcal/g)	179 (71%)	21.4 (19%)	24 (10%)		
Propac (Chesebrough-Ponds)	1.0 (4.0 Kcal/g)	192 (77%)	20 (18%)	13 (5%)		

* Characteristics: Specific nutrients to be added
  Not nutritionally complete
  Contents per 1,000 ml unless otherwise specified

Sources*

Sodium (mg/mEq)	Potassium (mg/mEq)	Vol (ml) to meet Vitamin Require-ments	Protein Sources	Fat Sources	Carbohydrate Sources
700/30	60/1.5				Hydrolysis of cornstarch
360/16	20/0.6				Maltodextrin
520/23	—				Maltodextrin
				Fractionated coconut oil	
				Safflower oil	
410/18	27/0.7		Calcium caseinate		
640/28	2,300/58		Whey protein		
460/21	2,300/59		Whey protein		
580/25	1,300/33		Whey protein		

PARENTERAL NUTRITION SOLUTIONS

General Amino Acid Injections

AMINO ACIDS (% of total AA, w/w)	8.5% TRAVASOL	8.5% TRAVASOL WITH LYTES	8.5% AMINOSYN	8.5% FREAMINE III	15% NOVAMINE
Isoleucine	4.78%	4.78%	7.29%	6.94%	5.00%
Leucine	6.19	6.19	9.53	9.06	6.93
Lysine	5.79	5.79	7.34	7.29	7.87
Methionine	5.79	5.79	4.00	5.29	5.00
Phenylalanine	6.19	6.19	4.47	5.65	6.93
Threonine	4.19	4.19	5.41	4.00	5.00
Tryptophan	1.79	1.79	1.76	1.53	1.67
Valine	4.59	4.59	8.00	6.59	6.40
	39.31	39.31	47.80	46.35	44.80
Alanine	20.7	20.7	12.94	7.06	14.47
Arginine	10.35	10.35	10.00	9.53	9.80
Histidine	4.38	4.38	3.06	2.82	5.96
Proline	4.19	4.19	8.82	11.18	5.96
Serine	—	—	4.35	5.88	3.95
Tyrosine	0.4	0.4	0.52	—	0.26
Glycine	20.7	20.7	12.94	14.00	6.93
Cysteine	—	—	—	<0.24	—
Glutamate	—	—	—	—	5.00
Aspartate	—	—	—	—	2.89
Total AA/100 ml	8.5 g	8.5 g	8.5 g	8.5 g	15.0 g
Total N/100 ml	1.42 g	1.42 g	1.34 g	1.3 g	2.37 g

ELECTROLYTES (mEq/L)					
Na	3	73	—	10	—
K	—	60	5.4		—
Cl	34	70	35	<3	—
Acetate	73	141	90	72	151
Mg	—	10	—	—	—
P (mM/L)	—	30	—	10	—
mOsm/L	860	1,160	850	810	1,388
Bottle Volume	500 ml	500 ml	500 ml	500, 1,000 ml	500 ml
Other AA%	5.5, 10	5.5	5, 7, 10	10	—
Manufacturer	Baxter	Baxter	Abbott	McGaw	Baxter

Amino Acid Injections for Renal or Hepatic Diseases

AMINO ACIDS (% of total AA, W/W)	6.5% RENAMIN	5.2% AMINOSYN-RF	5.2% AMINESS	5.4% NEPHRAMINE	8% HEPATAMINE
Isoleucine	7.69%	8.88%	10.14%	10.37%	11.25%
Leucine	9.23	13.96	15.93	16.30	13.75
Lysine	6.92	10.29	11.58	11.85	7.63
Methionine	7.69	13.96	15.93	16.30	1.25
Phenylalanine	7.54	13.96	15.93	16.30	1.25
Threonine	5.85	6.35	7.24	7.41	5.63
Tryptophan	2.46	3.17	3.63	3.70	0.83
Valine	12.62	10.15	11.58	11.58	10.5
	60.00	80.72	91.96	94.08	52.09
Alanine	8.62	—	—	—	9.63
Arginine	9.69	11.54	—	—	7.50
Histidine	6.46	8.25	7.95	4.63	3.00
Proline	5.38	—	—	—	10.00
Serine	4.62	—	—	—	6.25
Tyrosine	0.62	—	—	—	—
Glycine	4.62	—	—	—	11.25
Cysteine	—	—	—	<0.37	<0.25
Total AA/100 ml	6.5 g	5.2 g	5.18 g	5.4 g	8.0 g
Total N/100 ml	1.0 g	0.79 g	0.66 g	0.65 g	1.2 g
ELECTROLYTES (mEq/L)					
Na	3	—	—	5	10
K	—	5.4	—	—	—
Cl	31	—	—	<3	<3
Acetate	60	105	50	44	62
P (mM/L)	—	—	—	—	10
Osm (mOsm/L)	600	475	416	440	785
Bottle Volume	200 and 500 ml	300 ml	400 ml	250 ml	500 ml
Manufacturer	Baxter	Abbott	Baxter	McGaw	McGaw

Amino Acid Injections for Stress or Trauma

AMINO ACIDS (% of total AA, W/W)	6.9% FREEAMINE HBC	7.0% AMINOSYN-HBC	4.0% BRANCHAMINE
Isoleucine	11.01%	11.27%	34.5%
Leucine	19.86	22.51	34.5
Lysine	8.41	3.79	
Methionine	3.62	2.94	
Phenylalanine	4.64	3.26	
Threonine	2.90	3.89	
Tryptophan	1.30	1.26	
Valine	12.75	11.27	31.0
	64.49	60.19	100.0
Alanine	5.80	9.43	
Arginine	8.41	7.24	
Histidine	2.32	2.20	
Proline	9.13	4.48	
Serine	4.78	3.16	
Tyrosine	—	0.47	
Glycine	4.78	9.43	
Cysteine	<0.29	—	
Total AA/100 ml	6.9 g	7.0 g	4.0 g
Total N/100 ml	0.973 g	1.12 g	0.443 g
ELECTROLYTES (mEq/L)			
Na	10	7	
K	—	—	
Cl	<3	<40	
Acetate	57	72	
mOsm/L	620	665	316
Bottle Volume	750 ml	500 & 1,000 ml	500 ml
Manufacturer	McGaw	Abbott	Travenol

Electrolyte Products Used in Parenteral Nutrition

Sodium Chloride	2.5 mEq/ml
Sodium Acetate	2.0 mEq/ml
Sodium Phosphate	Each ml contains 4.0 mEq of Na and 3.0 mM of P
Potassium Chloride	2.0 mEq/ml
Potassium Acetate	2.0 mEq/ml
Potassium Phosphate	Each ml contains 4.4 mEq of K and 3.0 mM of P
Magnesium Sulfate	50%, 8.1 mEq/2 ml
Calcium Gluconate	10%, 4.7 mEq/10 ml

Intravenous Multivitamins

Total Contents per Vial:

	AMA/NAG[†]	
VITAMINS	*ADULT**	*PEDIATRIC[‡]*
A, IU	3,300	2,300
D, IU	200	400
E, IU	10	7
C, mg	100	80
Folic Acid, μg	400	140
B_1, mg	3	1.2
B_2, mg	3.6	1.4
B_6, mg	4	1.0
Niacin, mg	40	17
B_{12}, μg	5	1
Dexpanthenol, mg	15	5
Biotin, μg	60	20
K_1, mg	—	0.2
Dose:	1 vial/day ($\geq$11 years)	1 vial/day (<11 years & $\geq$3 kg) 65% vial/day ($\geq$1 kg & <3 kg) 30% vial/day (<1 kg)

*M.V.I.-12, MVC Plus, MVC 9 + 3, Berocca PN
[†]American Medical Association and Nutrition Advisory Group
[‡]M.V.I. Pediatric

Intravenous Fat Emulsions

	Intralipid	Liposyn II	Nutrilipid	Soyacal
Fat content	10% 20%	10% 20%	10% 20%	10% 20%
Oil source	Soybean oil	Safflower oil & soybean oil	Soybean oil	Soybean oil
Egg phospho-lipids	1.2%	1.2%	1.2%	1.2%
Glycerin	2.25%	2.5%	2.21%	2.21%
Osmolarity (mOsm/L)	260 268	320 340	280 315	280 315
pH	8.0	8.0 8.3	6.0–7.9	6.0–7.9
Particle size	0.5 μm	0.4 μm	0.33 μm	0.33 μm
Caloric value (Kcal/ml)	1.1 2.0	1.1 2.0	1.1 2.0	1.1 2.0
Fatty Acids				
Linoleic acid	50%	65.8%	49–60%	49–60%
Linolenic acid	9%	4.2%	6–9%	6–9%
Oleic acid	26%	17.7%	21–26%	21–26%
Palmitic acid	10%	8.8%	9–13%	9–13%
Stearic acid	3.5%	3.4%	3–5%	3–5%
Container volumes (ml)	50,100 50,100 250,500 250,500	50,100 25,500 200,500 200,500	250,500 250,500	250,500 250,500
Manufacturer	Baxter	Abbott	American McGaw	Alpha Therapeutic

Composition of Intralipid
(per 1,000 ml)

Component	10%	20%
Triglycerides	100 g	200 g
Phospholipid	12 g	12 g
Glycerol	22.5 g	22.5 g
Water	867	766
Polyunsaturated fatty acids (PUFA)	62 g	121 g
Saturated fat	21 g	37 g
P/S ratio	3.0	3.3
Tocopherol		
Total Tocopherol	71 mg (41–111 mg)	148 mg (107–203 mg)
Alpha Tocopheral	6 mg (2–19 mg)	12 mg (6–24 mg)
Gamma Tocopherol	40 mg (15–72 mg)	92 mg (63–130 mg)
Delta Tocopherol	24 mg (11–58 mg)	44 mg (26–67 mg)
Vitamin E Activity*	15 mg (22 I.U.)	31 mg (47 I.U.)
Vitamin E Activity/PUFA (min reg = 0.4)	0.24	0.24
Sterols		
Cholesterol	304 mg (85–409 mg)	304 mg (85–409 mg)
Total plant sterols	370 mg	740 mg
Campesterol	84 mg	168 mg
Stigmasterol	76 mg	152 mg
Sitosterol	210 mg	410 mg
Electrolytes and Trace Minerals		
Mg^{++}	0.011 mEq	0.008 mEq
Ca^{++}	0.027 mEq	0.014 mEq
Na^+	3.4 mEq	3.5 mEq
K^+	0.82 mEq	0.87 mEq
Zn^{++}	0.002 mEq	0.001 mEq
Cu^{++}	0.001 mEq	<0.001 mEq
Cl^-	3.0 mEq	3.1 mEq
Phosphorus (from phospholipids)	15 mmoles	15 mmoles
Kilocalories (Total)	1100 Kcal	2000 Kcal
Triglycerides (9.3 cal/g)	930 Kcal	1860 Kcal
Phospholipid (6.0 cal/g)	72 Kcal	72 Kcal
Glycerol (4.2 cal/g)	94.5 Kcal	94.5 Kcal
Osmolarity	260 mOsm/L emulsion	268 mOsm/L emulsion
Osmolality	300 mOsm/kg H_2O	350 mOsm/kg H_2O

*Vitamin E activity is the same as α-tocopherol equivalent and is based on α:γ:δ- 1.0:0.2:0.01. 1 mg of α-tocopherol = 1 IU (International Unit).

CONVERSION OF MILLIGRAMS TO MILLIEQUIVALENTS

To convert milligrams (mg) to milliequivalents (mEq):

$$\frac{\text{Milligrams}}{\text{Atomic weight}} \times \text{Valence} = \text{Milliequivalents}$$

Mineral Element	Chemical Symbol	Atomic Weight	Valence
Chlorine	Cl	35.4	1
Potassium	K	39	1
Sodium	Na	23	1
Calcium	Ca	40	2
Magnesium	Mg	24.3	2
Sulfur	S	32	
Sulfate	SO_4	96	2

To convert specific weight of sodium to sodium chloride:
Milligrams of sodium $\times$ 2.54 = Milligrams of sodium chloride

To convert specific weight of sodium chloride to sodium:
Milligrams of sodium chloride $\times$ 0.393 = Milligrams of sodium

Sodium mg	Sodium mEq	Sodium Chloride g
500	21.8	1.3
1,000	43.5	2.5
1,500	75.3	3.8
2,000	87.0	5.0

APPROXIMATE CONVERSIONS TO AND FROM METRIC MEASURES

Approximate Conversions To Metric Measures*

When You Know	Multiply By	To Find
Length		
Inches	2.5	Centimeters
Feet	30	Centimeters
Yards	0.9	Meters
Miles	1.6	Kilometers
Area		
Square inches	6.5	Square centimeters
Square feet	9.09	Square meters
Square yards	0.8	Square meters
Square miles	2.6	Square kilometers
Acres	0.4	Hectares
Mass (weight)		
Ounces	28	Grams
Pounds	0.45	Kilograms
Short tons (2,000 lb)	0.9	Tonnes
Volume		
Teaspoons	5	Milliliters
Tablespoons	15	Milliliters
Fluid ounces	30	Milliliters
Cups	0.24	Liters
Pints	0.47	Liters
Quarts	0.95	Liters
Gallons	3.8	Liters
Cubic feet	0.03	Cubic meters
Cubic yards	0.76	Cubic meters
Temperature (exact)		
Fahrenheit temperature	5/9 (after subtracting 32)	Celsius temperature

*From United States Department of Commerce, National Bureau of Standards: Metric Conversion Card (NBS Special Publication 365). Washington, D. C., Government Printing Office, 1972.

Approximate Conversions from Metric Measures*

When You Know	Multiply By	To Find
Length		
Millimeters	0.04	Inches
Centimeters	0.4	Inches
Meters	3.3	Feet
Meters	1.1	Yards
Kilometers	0.6	Miles
Area		
Square centimeters	0.16	Square inches
Square meters	1.2	Square yards
Square kilometers	0.4	Square miles
Hectares (10,000 m^2)	2.5	Acres
Mass (weight)		
Grams	0.035	Ounces
Kilograms	2.2	Pounds
Tonnes (1,000 kg)	1.1	Short tons
Volume		
Milliliters	0.03	Fluid ounces
Liters	2.1	Pints
Liters	1.06	Quarts
Liters	0.26	Gallons
Cubic meters	35	Cubic feet
Cubic meters	1.3	Cubic yards
Temperature (exact)		
Celsius temperature	9/5 (then add 32)	Fahrenheit temperature

* From United States Department of Commerce, National Bureau of Standards: Metric Conversion Card (NBS Special Publication 365). Washington, D. C., Government Printing Office, 1972.

Prefixes for Metric Units

10^6	Mega-	M
10^3	kilo-	k
10^{-1}	deci-	d
10^{-2}	centi-	c
10^{-3}	milli-	m
10^{-6}	micro-	μ
10^{-9}	nano-	n
10^{-12}	pico-	p

MEDICAL ABBREVIATIONS, PREFIXES, AND SUFFIXES

AAA–aortic abdominal aneurysm
ABGs–arterial blood gases
ADL–activities of daily living
AIDS–acquired immune deficiency syndrome
ALL–acute lymphoblastic leukemia
ALS–amyotrophic lateral sclerosis
AML–acute myelocytic leukemia
AODM–adult onset diabetes mellitus
AP–angina pectoris
ARC–aids related complex
ARDS–adult respiratory distress syndrome
ARF–acute renal failure
ASA–aspirin (acetylsalicylic acid)
ASHD–atherosclerotic heart disease
ASO–atherosclerosis obliterans
ATN–acute tubular necrosis
AVM–arteriovenous malformation
BKA–below knee amputation
BMR–basal metabolic rate
BMT–bone marrow transplantation
BPH–benign prostatic hypertrophy
Bx–biopsy
CA–cancer
CAD–coronary artery disease
CAH–chronic active hepatitis
CAH–congenital adrenal hyperplasia
CALD–chronic active liver disease
CAPD–continuous ambulatory peritoneal dialysis
CAT–computerized axial tomography
CBC–complete blood count
CBD–common bile duct
CC–chief complaint

CCK–cholecystokinin
CCU–coronary care unit
CDE–common duct exploration
CHD–coronary heart disease
CHF–congestive heart failure
CHI–closed head injury
CIIP–chronic idiopathic intestinal obstruction
CMV–chronic cytomegalovirus infection
CNS–central nervous system
C/O–complains of
COPD–chronic obstructive pulmonary disease
CPN–central parenteral nutrition
CRF–chronic renal failure
CSF–cerebrospinal fluid
CT–collagenous/connective tissue (disease)
CVA–cerebral vascular accident
CVI–cerebral vascular insufficiency
CVP–central venous pressure
D & C–dilatation and curettage
D/C–discontinue
DIC–disseminated intravascular coagulopathy
DIP–distal interphalangeal (joint)
DJD–degenerative joint disease
DKA–diabetic ketoacidosis
DM–diabetes mellitus
DOA–dead on arrival
DOE–dyspnea on exertion
DU–duodenal ulcer
DVT–deep vein thrombosis
Dx–diagnosis
ECG, EKG–electrocardiogram
ECT–electric convulsive therapy
EEG–electroencephalogram
EENT–eye, ear, nose, and throat
ERCP–endoscopic retrograde cholangiopancreatography
ESR–erythrocyte sedimentation rate
ESRD–end-stage renal disease
FBG–fasting blood glucose
FBS–fasting blood sugar
FFA–free fatty acid
FTT–failure to thrive
FUO–fever of unknown origin
Fx–fracture
GB–gallbladder
GE–gastroenteritis, gastroenterology
GI–gastrointestinal
GSE–gluten sensitive enteropathy
GTT–glucose tolerance test
GU–genitourinary

GYN—gynecology
HA—headache
Hb or Hgb—hemoglobin
HBP—high blood pressure
HCM—hypertrophic cardiomyopathy
HEN—home enteral nutrition
HPI—history of present illness
HPN—home parenteral nutrition
HPT—hyperparathyroidism
HTN—hypertension
Hx—history
ICU—intensive care unit
IDDM—insulin-dependent diabetes mellitus
IDA—iron deficiency anemia
IHD—ischemic heart disease
IHSS—idiopathic hypertrophic subaortic stenosis
IM—intramuscular
IMP—impression
IPJ—interphalangeal joint
IPPB—intermittent positive pressure breathing
IV—intravenous
IVC—inferior vena cava
J—joule
KUB—kidney, ureter, bladder
LBP—low back pain
LFT—liver function tests
LLQ—left lower quadrant
LMD—local medical doctor
LOC—loss of consciousness
LUQ—left upper quadrant
MCA—middle cerebral artery
MCT—medium chain triglyceride
MCTD—mixed convertive tissue disease
MI—myocardial infarction, mitral insufficiency
MOM—milk of magnesia
MS—multiple sclerosis, mitral stenosis
MUGA—multiple-graded acquisition study
NAD—no apparent distress
NG—nasogastric
NIDDM—noninsulin dependent diabetes mellitus
NPN—nonprotein nitrogen
NPO—nothing by mouth
NTS—nontropical sprue
N & V—nausea and vomiting
OBS—organic brain syndrome
OHD—organic heart disease
OR—operating room
ORIF—open reduction (surgical alignment) internal fixation
OT—occupational therapy

Medical Abbreviations, Prefixes, and Suffixes *(continued)*

PA–pulmonary atresia, pernicious anemia
PAME–preanesthesia medical exam
PAN–para-arteritis nodosa
PAT–paroxysmal atrial tachycardia
PBI–protein-bound iodine
PCM–protein calorie malnutrition
PEG–percutaneous endoscopic gastrostomy
PID–pelvic inflammatory disease
PND–paroxysmal nocturnal dyspnea
PNH–paroxysmal nocturnal hemoglobinuria
PPN–peripheral parenteral nutrition
PS–pulmonary stenosis
PSE–portal systemic encephalopathy
Pt–patient
PT–physical therapy, prothrombin time
PTA–prior to admission
PTCA–percutaneous transluminal coronary angiography
PTT–partial thromboplastin time
PVC–premature ventricular contractions
PVD–peripheral vascular disease
PU–peptic ulcer
RE–reticulo-endothial system
REE–resting energy expenditure
RHD–rheumatic heart disease
RIND–reversible ischemic neurologic deficit
RLQ–right lower quadrant
R/O–rule out
ROS–review of systems
RöRx–radiation therapy
RUQ–right upper quadrant
SAH–subarachnoid hemorrhage
SBE–subacute bacterial endocarditis
SBO–small bowel obstruction
SCI–spinal cord injury
SCUF–slow continuous ultra filtration
SIADH–syndrome of inappropriate antidiuretic hormone
SLE–systemic lupus erythematosis
SMAS–superior mesenteric artery syndrome
SOB–shortness of breath
S/P–status postop
STA–superior temporal artery
STSG–split-thickness skin graft
SVC obst—superior vena cava obstruction
Sx–symptoms
T & A–tonsillectomy and adenoidectomy
TCE–transitional cell epithelioma
TE–tracheoesophageal fistula
TG–triglycerides
THA–total hip arthroplasty

THC–transhepatic cholangiogram
TI–tricuspid insufficiency
TIA–transient ischemic attacks
TKA–total knee arthroplasty
TLA–translumbar aortogram
TPN–total parenteral nutrition
TUR–transurethral resection
U/A–urinary analysis
UGI–upper gastrointestinal
URI–upper respiratory infection
UTI–urinary tract infection
V & P–vagotomy and pyloroplasty
VH–vaginal hysterectomy
VIP–vasoactive intestinal peptides
VS–vital signs
WDHA–watery diarrhea, hypokalemia, achlorhydria (pancreatic chlorea)
WNL–within normal limits
ZE–Zollinger-Ellison (syndrome)

Abbreviation	Derivation	Meaning
aa	ana	of each
ac	ante cibum	before meals
ad lib	ad libitum	as needed or desired
alt dieb	alternis diebus	every other day
alt hor	alternis horis	every other hour
alt noc	alternis noctibus	every other night
bid	bis in die	twice a day
c	cum	with
contin	continuetur	let it be continued
dil	dilutus	dilute
div	divide	divide
fl	fluidus	fluid
h	hora	hour
hd	hora decubitus	at bedtime
hs	hora somni	at sleeping time
m et n	mane et nocte	morning and night
nb	nota bene	note well
od	omni die	daily
om	omni mane	every morning
on	omni nocte	every night
part vic	partibus vicibus	in divided doses
pc	post cibum	after food
prn	pro re nata	as required
pulv	pulvis	powder
qd	quaque die	every day
qh	quaque hora	every hour
q2h	quaque secunda hora	every 2 hours
q3h	quaque tertia hora	every 3 hours
qid	quater in die	four times a day
qs	quantum suffisit	as much as is sufficient
Rx	recipe	take
S or sig	signa	give the following directions
s	sine	without
sos	si opus sit	if necessary
ss	semis	one half
stat	statim	at once
tid	ter in die	three times a day

Common Prefixes

Prefix	Meaning
a- or an-	without
cardi-	heart
chol-	bile
col-	colon
cyst-	bladder
enter-	intestine
gastr-	stomach
hepat-	liver
hydr-	water
hyper-	too much
hypo-	too little
myel-	marrow
nephr-	kidney
neur-	nerve
oste-	bone
poly-	many
proct-	anus, rectum
pseud-	false
pulm-	lung
pyel-	pelvis

Common Suffixes

Suffix	Meaning
-algia	pain
-clysis	drenching
-cyte	cell
-ectomy	excision
-emia	presence in blood (usually implies excess)
-genic or -genesis	formation
-gnosis	knowledge
-itis	inflammation
-lytic or -lysis	destruction
-malacia	softening
-opia	vision
-pathy	disease of
-phagia	eating
-phobia	fear of
-pnea	breath
-privia or -penia	poverty of: without
-ptosis	fallen
-sclerosis	hardening
-scopy	inspection
-stenosis	narrowing
-stomy	mouth (new opening)
-tomy	cutting operation
-trophy	nutrition or growth
-uria	urine

INDEX